ANNALS OF THE NEW YORK ACADEMY OF SCIENCES
Volume 940

# NEURO-CARDIOVASCULAR REGULATION

## From Molecules to Man

*Edited by Mark W. Chapleau and François M. Abboud*

*The New York Academy of Sciences*
*New York, New York*
*2001*

**Library of Congress Cataloging-in-Publication Data**

Neuro-cardiovascular regulation: from molecules to man / edited by Mark W. Chapleau and François M. Abboud.
    p.; cm. — (Annals of the New York Academy of Sciences, ISSN 0077-8923 ; v. 940)
Includes bibliographical references and index.
ISBN 1-57331-344-0 (cloth : alk. paper) — ISBN 1-57331-345-9 (paper: alk. paper)
    1. Vasomotor system. 2. Cardiovascular system —Innervation. 3. Baroreflexes. 4. Baroreceptors. 5. Blood pressure—Regulation. I. Chapleau, Mark W. II. Abboud, François M. III. Series.
    [DNLM: 1. Baroreflex—physiology—Congresses. 2. Blood Pressure—physiology—Congresses. 3. Pressoreceptors—physiology—Congresses. WG 102 N4944 2001]

Q11.N5 vol. 940
[QP109]
500 s—dc21
[612.1'8]                                                                                        2001030936

GYAT/PCP

*Printed in the United States of America*
**ISBN 1-57331-344-0** (cloth)
**ISBN 1-57331-345-9** (paper)
**ISSN 0077-8923**

ANNALS OF THE NEW YORK ACADEMY OF SCIENCES

*Volume 940*
*June 2001*

# NEURO-CARDIOVASCULAR REGULATION

## From Molecules to Man

*Editors*
MARK W. CHAPLEAU AND FRANÇOIS M. ABBOUD

*Conference Organizers*
MARK W. CHAPLEAU, FRANÇOIS M. ABBOUD, GERALD F. DIBONA,
ROBERT B. FELDER, A. KIM JOHNSON, ALLYN L. MARK,
AND WILLIAM T. TALMAN

*Advisory Board*
MICHAEL C. ANDRESEN, VERNON S. BISHOP, JEANNE L. SEAGARD,
VIREND K. SOMERS, AND IRVING H. ZUCKER

This volume is the result of a conference entitled **Baroreceptor and Cardiopulmonary Receptor Reflexes** sponsored by the American Physiological Society and held August 23–27, 2000, in Iowa City, Iowa.

## CONTENTS

### Part II. Nucleus Tractus Solitarius: Afferent Processing, Neurotransmision, and Integration

## Part V. Autonomic Mechanisms of Cardiovascular Dysregulation

## Part VI. Reflex Control of Circulation in Humans

**Financial assistance was received from:**

- **ASTRAZENECA**
- **MERCK & CO., INC.**
- **PHARMACIA & UPJOHN**
- **THE AMERICAN PHYSIOLOGICAL SOCIETY**
- **THE NATIONAL HEART, LUNG AND BLOOD INSTITUTE OF THE
  NATIONAL INSTITUTES OF HEALTH**

# NEURO-CARDIOVASCULAR REGULATION

## REGULATION

### From Molecules to Man

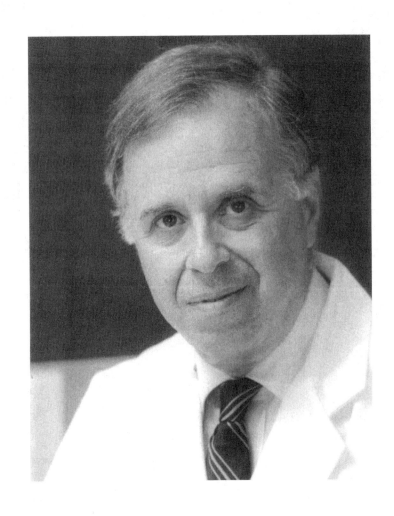

DONALD J. REIS

# In Memoriam: Donald J. Reis

Donald J. Reis could not join us at our scientific feast on the regulation of the arterial baroreflex held in Iowa City in August 2000 because of the devastating illness that robbed him from us on November 1, 2000.

Our admiration for his work, our gratitude for his legacy, and our delight in his friendship are deep feelings that will keep his memory vibrantly alive in our minds. He inspired us with his scientific integrity, challenged us with the novelty of his concepts, and dazzled us with the eloquence of his presentations and the prowess of his double-carousel lectures. He was a paragon in our community of neuro-cardio-vascular physiologists.

An obituary published in *The Physiologist* (**44:** 53–54 [2001]) refers to the diversity of his enormous talent. The richness of his soul was expressed in the music he composed as a young man and in his frequent piano renditions. We could have lost him to the Metropolitan Opera said one of our friends. We are happy we didn't.

For so many of us Don Reis was a critical consultant. He challenged you with his tough questions, always probing to the heart of the problem. With swiftness and intellectual agility he was the essence of the razor-sharp scientist. Yet you could also see in his eyes the gentleness of his spirit, helping you toward the answers and engaging you in formulating exciting new ideas.

For 30 years as an adviser for our program project grant Don was the best. He could focus on the depth of molecular mechanisms and simultaneously envision the beauty of the integrated whole.

Don, we will miss you during our upcoming program project renewal. We will seek guidance from your science and inspiration from our memories of you. We know it will be hard work, but will remember that with you the endeavor was always passion and fun.

—FRANÇOIS ABBOUD

# Neuro-Cardiovascular Regulation: From Molecules to Man

## Introduction

MARK W. CHAPLEAU[a,b,c] AND FRANÇOIS M. ABBOUD[a,b,d]

The [a]Cardiovascular Center, [b]Department of Internal Medicine, and
[d]Department of Physiology and Biophysics,
University of Iowa, Iowa City, Iowa 52242, USA

[c]Veterans Affairs Medical Center, Iowa City, Iowa 52242, USA

The contents of this book reflect the proceedings of a conference entitled "Baroreceptor and Cardiopulmonary Receptor Reflexes," sponsored by the American Physiological Society (APS) and held on August 23–27, 2000 in Iowa City, Iowa. Baroreceptor and cardiopulmonary reflexes are of major importance in the regulation of arterial blood pressure and autonomic and cardiovascular functions.

The history and progress of discovery in an area of science can be appreciated by reviewing the published proceedings of major symposia and conferences. Key symposia in the area of reflex control of the circulation were held in Dayton, Ohio (USA) in 1965 (*Baroreceptors in Hypertension*[1]); in Leeds, UK in 1969 (*Cardiac Receptors*[2]); in Oxford, UK in 1979 (*Baroreceptors and Hypertension*[3]); in Leeds, UK in 1985 (*Cardiogenic Reflexes*[4]); and in Glascow, Scotland in 1993 (*Cardiovascular Reflex Control in Health and Disease*[5]). The Iowa APS Conference brought together major investigators in the field to discuss recent advances and to identify key areas in need of further investigation. We are hopeful that the published proceedings of this conference will provide a valuable resource to present and future investigators and clinicians interested in the broad field of cardiovascular regulation. The book reflects the overall content of the conference, with the majority of invited speakers contributing chapters. The chapter manuscripts were peer-reviewed prior to acceptance for publication.

### THE APS CONFERENCE

The Iowa APS Conference was organized through the efforts of an internal Organizing Committee and external Steering Committee (TABLE 1). The conference was truly an international event: 35% of the 233 registrants came from countries outside the United States and a total of 15 countries were represented. There was strong par-

Address for correspondence: Mark W. Chapleau, Ph.D., Department of Internal Medicine, Division of Cardiovascular Diseases, Room E327-1, GH, 200 Hawkins Drive, Iowa City, Iowa 52242. Voice: 319-356-7760; fax: 319-353-6343.
mark-chapleau@uiowa.edu

**TABLE 1. Members of the organizing committee and steering committee for APS Conference entitled Baroreceptor and Cardiopulmonary Receptor Reflexes**

| Organizing Committee | Steering Committee |
|---|---|
| Mark W. Chapleau, Ph.D.* | Michael C. Andresen, Ph.D.<br>Oregon Health Sciences University<br>Portland, OR |
| François M. Abboud, M.D. | |
| Gerald F. DiBona, M.D.* | Vernon S. Bishop, Ph.D.<br>University of Texas<br>Health Science Center-San Antonio |
| Robert B. Felder, M.D.* | San Antonio, TX |
| Alan Kim Johnson, Ph.D. | Jeanne L. Seagard, Ph.D.<br>Medical College of Wisconsin<br>and VA Medical Center |
| Allyn L. Mark, M.D. | Milwaukee, WI |
| William T. Talman, M.D.* | Virend K. Somers, D.Phil., M.D.<br>Mayo Clinic, Rochester, MN |
| University of Iowa and<br>*Veterans Affairs Medical Center<br>Iowa City, IA | Irving H. Zucker, Ph.D.<br>University of Nebraska Medical Center<br>Omaha, NE |

**TABLE 2. Session moderators for APS conference**

| Session | Moderators |
|---|---|
| Cardiovascular Sensory Afferents-Physiology | François M. Abboud and Thomas E. Pisarri |
| Molecular Mechanisms of Sensory Transduction | Michael J. Welsh and Ellis Cooper |
| Cellular Mechanisms of Vagal Sensory Neuron Function | Diana L. Kunze and Michael C. Andresen |
| NTS: Afferent Processing and Integration | K. Michael Spyer and Julian F.R. Paton |
| NTS: Neurotransmitters and Modulators | Hreday N. Sapru and Patrick J. Mueller |
| Central Baroreflex Mechanisms | Patrice G. Guyenet and Sue A. Aicher |
| Transgenic and Knockout Animal Models and Gene Transfer | Gerald F. DiBona and Edward Johns |
| Regulation of Sympathetic Nerve Activity | Frank J. Gordon and Maria Claudia Irigoyen |
| Baroreflex Control During Exercise | Allyn L. Mark and Lisete Michelini |
| Rhythmic Oscillations in Cardiovascular Control | Alberto Malliani and Gianfranco Parati |
| Integrative Regulation of Arterial Pressure and Circulation | Roger Hainsworth and Mark Drinkhill |
| Autonomic Balance and Baroreflex Sensitivity in Health and Disease | Michael J. Joyner and Richard Hughson |
| Neural Cardiovascular Dysregulation in Heart Failure | Marc D. Thames and Mark E. Dunlap |
| Mechanisms of Orthostatic Hypotension and Intolerance | Alan Kim Johnson and Julia Moffitt |

**TABLE 3. Recipients of Trainee Travel Awards for APS Conference**

| Recipient | Mentor | University |
|---|---|---|
| Madhusudan Natarajan | Shaun Morrison, Ph.D. | Northwestern University |
| Monica Sato | Shaun Morrison, Ph.D. | Northwestern University |
| Carolyn J. Hoang | Meredith Hay, Ph.D. | University of Missouri |
| Peter Larsen | Susan Barman, Ph.D. | Michigan State University |
| Xiao-Hong Xia | Harold Schultz, Ph.D. | University of Nebraska |
| Yong-Chun Zeng | Harold Schultz, Ph.D. | University of Nebraska |

ticipation of young investigators, who represented 29% of the registrants, including 32 graduate students and 36 postdoctoral research fellows. Leaders in the field along with selected young investigators moderated the invited speaker sessions (TABLE 2). There were 114 poster presentations. The abstracts submitted by graduate students and postdoctoral research fellows were judged and Trainee Travel Awards were presented to the winners (TABLE 3). The abstracts related to presentations at the conference were published in *The Physiologist*.[6] Financial support for the conference was provided by the American Physiological Society, the National Heart, Lung and Blood Institute of the National Institutes of Health, AstraZeneca, Merck Inc., and Pharmacia & Upjohn.

## BACKGROUND ON BARORECEPTOR AND CARDIOPULMONARY REFLEXES

The general pathways involved in arterial and cardiopulmonary reflex control of autonomic and cardiovascular functions are illustrated in FIGURES 1 and 2.

**Arterial baroreceptors** are sensory nerve endings that innervate large arteries (carotid sinuses, aortic arch, and origin of the right subclavian artery). Increases or decreases in arterial pressure and vascular stretch alter the frequency of action potential discharge (baroreceptor activity) transmitted along the carotid sinus and aortic depressor nerves to the nucleus tractus solitarii (NTS) in the central nervous system (CNS). The afferent activity is integrated and relayed through a network of central neurons that lead to reflex adjustments that buffer the initial changes in pressure. For example, increased baroreceptor activity during a rise in pressure triggers reflex inhibition of sympathetic activity, parasympathetic activation, and subsequent decreases in vascular resistance and heart rate. Conversely, a decrease in arterial pressure reduces barorecepter afferent discharge and triggers a reflex increase in sympathetic activity, parasympathetic inhibition, and increases in vascular resistance and heart rate. Changes in baroreceptor activity also influence the release of vasopressin and renin that contribute to the reflex adjustment to changes in arterial pressure. *Thus, the baroreceptor reflex provides powerful moment-to-moment negative feedback regulation of arterial pressure that minimizes the fluctuations (lability) in pressure.* In addition to responding to changes in arterial pressure, the baroreflex also provides tonic inhibition of sympathetic activity and vasopressin release and

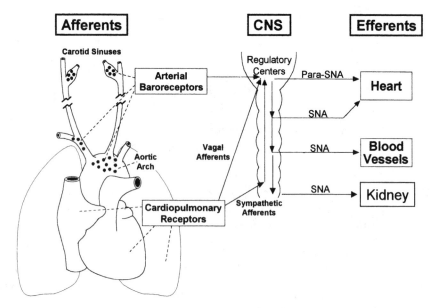

**FIGURE 1.** Afferent, central nervous system (CNS), and efferent pathways involved in baroreceptor and cardiopulmonary reflexes. SNA, sympathetic nerve activity; para-SNA, parasympathetic nerve activity. See text for description.

tonic excitation of parasympathetic activity under resting baseline conditions. These are important regulatory mechanisms in normal and pathological states.

Sensory nerve endings in the heart and lungs are referred to as **cardiopulmonary receptors**. The activity of these receptors is transmitted along **vagal afferent fibers** terminating in NTS and spinal **sympathetic afferent fibers** terminating in the spinal cord. Although there is a variety of cardiopulmonary receptors with varying influences on the circulation, the predominant effect of stimulating cardiopulmonary vagal afferents closely resembles that seen with baroreceptor activation (i.e., bradycardia, vasodilation, and inhibition of vasopressin release). In contrast, activation of sympathetic afferents triggers reflex sympathetic activation, parasympathetic inhibition, vasoconstriction, and tachycardia. Increased activity of sympathetic afferents also mediates the sensation of chest pain (angina) in patients suffering from myocardial ischemia.

Cardiopulmonary receptors also play a major role in the regulation of body fluid balance. For example, mechanosensitive cardiopulmonary vagal afferents are activated by cardiac distension during increases in central blood volume. The subsequent reflex inhibition of both renal sympathetic activity and vasopressin release promote increased sodium and water excretion and a return of central blood volume towards normal levels. Conversely, decreased central blood volume, as occurs during blood loss (hemorrhage), decreases activity of these vagal afferents, leading to sodium and water reabsorption. *Thus, this reflex functions in a negative feedback manner to regulate blood volume.*

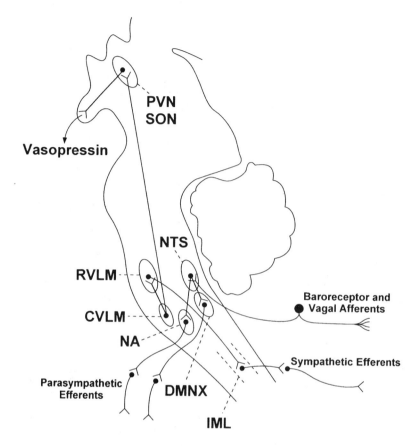

**FIGURE 2.** Key central nervous system nuclei that participate in the central mediation of the baroreceptor and cardiopulmonary reflexes. NTS, nucleus tractus solitarius; CVLM, caudal ventrolateral medulla; RVLM, rostral ventrolateral medulla; IML, intermediolateral column of spinal cord; NA, nucleus ambiguus; DMNX, dorsal motor nucleus of the vagus; PVN, paraventricular nucleus of hypothalamus; and SON, supraoptic nucleus. See text for description.

Cardiopulmonary receptors exhibit **chemosensitivity** as well as **mechanosensitivity**. Subsets of both vagal and sympathetic afferents are responsive to various chemical substances, including prostanoids, bradykinin, protons, reactive oxygen species, serotonin, adenosine, and adenosine triphosphate (ATP). *Some of these factors are responsible for activation of the sensory nerve endings during myocardial ischemia and reperfusion and in other pathological states.*

The **CNS circuitry and integration** responsible for the central mediation of arterial and cardiopulmonary reflexes are complex. Some of the key CNS nuclei are illustrated in FIGURE 2. Neurons in the NTS receive and integrate inputs from the sensory nerves. The NTS subsequently influences the activity of the principal hindbrain nuclei governing efferent parasympathetic and sympathetic drive. There are direct projections from NTS to parasympathetic preganglionic neurons in the nucleus ambiguus (NA) and the dorsal motor nucleus of the vagus (DMNX). Neurons in NTS also project to the caudal ventrolateral medulla (CVLM), which in turn sends inhibitory projections to neurons in the rostral ventrolateral medulla (RVLM). RVLM neurons project to sympathetic preganglionic neurons in the intermediolateral column (IML) of the spinal cord. The inhibitory influence of baroreceptor activity on vasopressin release from the paraventricular nucleus (PVN) and the supraoptic nucleus (SON) also utilizes the NTS-CVLM pathway. Other brainstem regions and higher centers also contribute to the modulation of parasympathetic and sympathetic outflows.

## OVERVIEW OF CONFERENCE PROCEEDINGS

The main objectives of this book are to summarize the most recent advances related to baroreceptor and cardiopulmonary reflexes and to identify important areas for future investigation. The book is divided into six sections, beginning with the sensory afferents and progressing in sequence to CNS pathways and mechanisms, integrative regulation of the circulation, and ending with mechanisms of cardiovascular dysregulation in animal models of disease and in humans.

### Sensory Afferents (Part I)

A major effort is currently under way to identify the mechanisms, at the molecular level, that confer mechanosensivity and chemosensitivity to cells. Several chapters in Part I of this book provide evidence of specific molecules that function as mechanotransducers and/or sensors of chemical stimuli in sensory neurons. Furthermore, it is clear that in addition to direct activation of sensory neurons, chemical factors may modulate the spike-firing frequency of cardiovascular afferents through effects on voltage-gated and ligand-gated ion channels. Other chapters in Part I address the specific mechanisms involved in modulation of afferent activity by chemical factors and the importance of this modulation in pathologic states. The impact of hypertension, atherosclerosis, diabetes mellitus, and myocardial ischemia–reperfusion on baroreceptor and cardiopulmonary receptor afferents is reviewed. In addition to mechanisms of sensory transduction at the peripheral terminals, it is important to understand the molecular basis and physiologic regulation of neurotransmitter release from the central terminals of the afferent fibers. Recent work in this area is presented.

### CNS Mechanisms (Parts II and III)

The major neurotransmitters and ligand receptors mediating neurotransmission in NTS, RVLM, NA, and DMNX are reviewed. Glutamate is the primary neurotransmitter released from the sensory afferent terminals in NTS. The relative roles of NMDA and non-NMDA glutamate receptors in NTS and elsewhere are discussed. Substantial evidence suggests important roles of other transmitters and neuromodulators in NTS including peptides (e.g., substance P, neurotensin, oxytocin, angiotensin) and nitric oxide (NO). Differences in the central processing of myelinated A-fiber vs. nonmyelinated C-fiber afferent baroreceptor inputs to NTS are reviewed. Functional differences among subtypes of neurons within the same central nuclei, including NTS ("adapting" vs. "nonadapting" cells) and RVLM (C1 vs. non-C1 cells), are described. Novel CNS areas important in generation of sympathetic outflow are discussed, including neurons in lateral tegmental field (LTF) that receive barosensitive inputs and project to RVLM and neurons in rostral raphe pallidus (RP) that are relatively unresponsive to baroreceptor input and selectively regulate thermogenesis. In addition, central neural mechanisms responsible for low-frequency and high-frequency variability of heart rate and arterial pressure and sympathovagal balance are described. Lastly, heterogenous receptor distribution to the dendritic tree and to post- vs. pre-synaptic membranes is demonstrated for RVLM and IML neurons using anatomical and histochemical approaches.

## *Integrative Regulation of Circulation (Part IV)*

Chapters in this section focus on integrated cardiovascular regulation. In the first chapter, the integrated baroreflex control of arterial pressure is decomposed into a mechano-neural arc representing the reflex effect of changes in arterial pressure on sympathetic nerve activity, and a neural-mechanical arc representing the effect of changes in sympathetic nerve activity on arterial pressure. Modeling these processes provides new insights into how the reflex provides optimal stability and rapidity of blood pressure control.

Subsequent chapters explore the influence of a variety of environmental and behavioral states on cardiovascular regulatory mechanisms and blood pressure regulation, including effects of acute exercise, chronic exercise training, pregnancy, and changes in dietary salt intake. These states, acting through multiple mechanisms, result in significant changes in baroreceptor and cardiopulmonary reflex control of the circulation.

Hormones exert important effects on neural mechanisms of cardiovascular regulation. For example, it is shown that ovarian hormones acting in RVLM modulate reflex control of sympathetic nerve activity and mimic the changes that occur in pregnancy. Different aspects of central actions of angiotensin on sympathetic tone and baroreflex control of renal sympathetic nerve activity and heart rate are addressed in several chapters. Both local angiotensin acting within the brainstem and circulating angiotensin acting at circumventricular organs lacking a blood–brain barrier influence resting sympathetic nerve activity and modulate baroreflex control of the circulation. Angiotensin exerts a sympathoexcitatory influence in pathological states such as heart failure and in response to a low-salt diet. Increased dietary salt may increase sympathetic nerve activity secondary to increased plasma osmolality and/or failure to suppress angiotensin levels in susceptible, salt-sensitive subjects. The effects of interactions between the sympathetic nervous system and angiotensin, along with blood pressure variability on renal function are reviewed with important consequences for the longer-term regulation of arterial pressure. The final chapter in the section characterizes changes in the rhythmicity of sympathetic nerve activity during normal postnatal development with potential implications for mechanisms of sudden infant death syndrome.

*Mechanisms of Cardiovascular Dysregulation in Animals and Humans*
*(Parts V and VI)*

These sections focus on mechanisms that contribute to autonomic dysfunction and impaired baroreceptor and cardiopulmonary receptor reflexes in animal models (Part V) and humans (Part VI). Novel central mechanisms responsible for excessive sympathetic nerve activity and altered reflex control of the circulation in heart failure are reviewed. Activation of the renin–angiotensin system within the CNS and loss of nitric oxide–mediated sympathoinhibition contribute to sympathoexcitation in animals with heart failure. Chronic exercise training reduces both sympathetic activity and angiotensin. The PVN in hypothalamus and perhaps other forebrain regions appears to play a major role in maintaining the sympathoexcitatory state in heart failure. Possible mechanisms responsible for increased sympathetic activity in human heart failure is also discussed. Evidence is presented that favors a role of activation of a cardiac sympathoexcitatory reflex over impaired baroreflex sensitivity.

Potential mechanisms leading to orthostatic hypotension and intolerance are summarized. Rats subjected to sustained hindlimb unweighting, a model that mimics effects of exposure to microgravity, demonstrate impaired baroreflex-mediated increases in sympathetic nerve activity. The mechanism involves enhanced $GABA_A$-mediated inhibition of RVLM neurons, providing a new potential mechanism that may contribute to orthostatic intolerance in astronauts returning from space. In human studies, altered cerebral blood flow autoregulation is investigated as a possible contributing factor to orthostatic intolerance in patients with postural orthostatic tachycardia syndrome (POTS) or neurally-mediated syncope. A defective norepinephrine transporter has been identified in a subset of patients with orthostatic intolerance. A specific mutation in the gene has been identified, encouraging future studies of possible genetic determinants of orthostatic intolerance.

Methods used for assessment of arterial baroreflex sensitivity in humans as well as chemoreceptor and pulmonary stretch receptor reflexes are reviewed. The impact of various pathologic states, including myocardial infarction, heart failure, diabetes, and sleep apnea, on reflex control of the circulation are discussed.


## FUTURE DIRECTIONS

In recent years we have made striking progress in our understanding of baroreceptor and cardiopulmonary reflexes. The rapid pace of gene discovery and the implementation of molecular and genetic approaches have opened up entirely new areas of investigation. Fundamental discoveries in cell and molecular biology (often using non-mammalian organisms) have led to, and will continue to lead to important advances in the area of cardiovascular regulation. For example, the sequencing of genomes and the use of model systems amenable to genetic studies (e.g. *Drosophila* and *C. elegans*) provide a powerful means of discovering new molecules of fundamental importance. Subsequent identification of mammalian homologues enables study of their functional role in physiological systems.

The ability to genetically manipulate cells and whole organisms now allows us to identify the functions of newly discovered genes and to create novel and more specific animal models of disease. Functional data from physiologic studies can be strengthened considerably through measurement of gene expression at the mRNA and protein levels. The unique susceptibility of mice to genetic manipulation encourages increasing the use of mice in physiological studies. The ability to measure and manipulate gene expression will be particularly advantageous in studies of chronic regulation of the circulation throughout development, with aging and in pathological states.

The molecular and genetic approaches and new technologies described above, combined with traditional hemodynamic and electrophysiological measurements, promise to provide a powerful strategy for important discoveries in numerous areas related to baroreceptor and cardiopulmonary reflexes. For example, the molecular identification of specific mechanosensitive and chemosensitive receptors/channels on sensory nerve terminals has only just begun. The tremendous plasticity and adaptability of the nervous system are widely appreciated. Future studies are needed to determine the potential for phenotypic changes to occur in baroreceptor and cardiopulmonary receptors and the conditions that may evoke these changes in physiological and pathological states. For example, does chronic hypertension or inflammation alter expression of mechanosensitive or chemosensitive ion channels on sensory nerves? Can a mechanosensitive neuron acquire chemosensitivity, and vice versa? Similar questions can be asked related to central and efferent mechanisms of cardiovascular regulation.

The role of neurotransmitters other than glutamate in the central mediation of baroreceptor and cardiopulmonary reflexes remains unclear. Further studies are needed to clarify the role of co-transmitters and neuromodulators at the various CNS synapses. Another promising area for future study relates to the increasing appreciation of distinct subtypes of neurons (e.g., within cardiovascular sensory nerves, within NTS, and within RVLM). The different functional roles of these neuronal subtypes have been difficult to elucidate because of the anatomical proximity to other cells and technical limitations. New techniques can be used to gain insights into the functions of neuronal subtypes. For example, neurons expressing a particular receptor or enzyme can be selectively modified by knockout of the relevant molecule using gene targeting and cell-specific promoters or destroyed by suicide transport of saporin-conjugated antibodies.

Baroreceptor and cardiopulmonary reflexes are altered in pathological states, including chronic hypertension, myocardial ischemia, heart failure, atherosclerosis, diabetes, and various autonomic nervous system disorders. The altered reflexes, reduced resting vagal tone, and excessive sympathetic activity are associated with high morbidity and mortality in these patients. The mechanisms responsible for these changes differ to varying extent among the different diseases and are not well understood. More work is needed to clarify the relative roles of decreased sensitivity of baroreceptors and cardiac vagal afferents, increased sensitivity of cardiac sympathetic afferents, increased chemoreceptor sensitivity, and altered CNS mechanisms in causing autonomic and reflex dysfunction in disease. The effects of pathological states on gene expression in sensory, CNS, and efferent autonomic neurons and its functional consequences remain relatively unexplored and is a promising area for future study. A lot can be learned from transgenic models of disease. Transgenic animals can be created that represent the interaction of more than one pathological process, as so often occurs in patients. The enormous power of this technology coupled with sophisticated measurements of phenotypic expression is just beginning to be realized.

As a result of the Human Genome Project and the increasing knowledge of human genetics and individual gene function, there is tremendous potential for human studies to advance our understanding of neural mechanisms of cardiovascular regulation. Recent studies have suggested that resting baseline sympathetic nerve activity and baroreflex sensitivity are determined in part by heredity. It will be important to define the genetic determinants of autonomic nervous system activity and baroreceptor and cardiopulmonary reflex sensitivity. Studies in patients with profound autonomic and cardiovascular reflex dysfunction may identify gene mutations that provide clues to identifying key molecules important in reflex regulation of the circulation. Genotyping of human subjects will enable linkage analysis of candidate genes to autonomic and cardiovascular reflex phenotypes to be performed.

We believe the future is bright for investigators interested in neural mechanisms of cardiovascular regulation, including the baroreceptor and cardiopulmonary reflexes. Many interesting and critical questions remain to be answered. The complexity of the cardiovascular and nervous systems and their interactions pose difficult challenges to the investigator. Nevertheless, the availability of new experimental approaches and technologies make this an opportune time for discovery and the advancement of knowledge. A multidisciplinary approach including studies at molecular, cellular, and whole-animal/human levels will be required to optimize our progress.

## REFERENCES

1. KEZDI, P., Ed. 1967. Baroreceptors and Hypertension. Pergamon Press. Oxford, UK.
2. HAINSWORTH, R., C. KIDD & R.J. LINDEN, Eds. 1979. Cardiac Receptors. Cambridge University Press. Cambridge, UK.
3. SLEIGHT, P., Ed. 1980. Arterial Baroreceptors and Hypertension. Oxford University Press. Oxford, UK.
4. HAINSWORTH, R., P.N. MCWILLIAM & D.A.S.G. MARY, Ed. 1987. Cardiogenic Reflexes. Oxford University Press. Oxford, UK.
5. HAINSWORTH, R. & A.L. MARK, Eds. 1993. Cardiovascular Reflex Control in Health and Disease. W.B. Saunders. London.
6. 2000. APS Conference: Baroreceptor and Cardiopulmonary Receptor Reflexes. The Physiologist **43(4)**:237–292.

# Mechanisms Determining Sensitivity of Baroreceptor Afferents in Health and Disease

MARK W. CHAPLEAU,[a,b,c] ZHI LI,[d] SILVANA S. MEYRELLES,[e] XIUYING MA,[a,b] AND FRANÇOIS M. ABBOUD[a,b,f]

[a]The Cardiovascular Center, and the Departments of [b]Internal Medicine and [f]Physiology & Biophysics, University of Iowa, Iowa City, Iowa 52242, USA

[c]Veterans Affairs Medical Center, Iowa City, Iowa 52246, USA

[d]Department of Medicine, University of Louisville Health Sciences Center, Louisville, Kentucky 40202, USA

[e]Department of Physiology, Federal University of Espirito Santo, Vitoria, ES, Brazil

ABSTRACT: Baroreceptors sense and signal the central nervous system of changes in arterial pressure through a series of sensory processes. An increase in arterial pressure causes vascular distension and baroreceptor deformation, the magnitude of which depends on the mechanical viscoelastic properties of the vessel wall. Classic methods (e.g., isolated carotid sinus preparation) and new approaches, including studies of isolated baroreceptor neurons in culture, gene transfer using viral vectors, and genetically modified mice have been used to define the cellular and molecular mechanisms that determine baroreceptor sensitivity. Deformation depolarizes the nerve endings by opening a new class of mechanosensitive ion channel. This depolarization triggers action potential discharge through opening of voltage-dependent sodium ($Na^+$) and potassium ($K^+$) channels at the "spike initiating zone" (SIZ) near the sensory terminals. The resulting baroreceptor activity and its sensitivity to changes in pressure are modulated through a variety of mechanisms that influence these sensory processes. Modulation of voltage-dependent $Na^+$ and $K^+$ channels and the $Na^+$ pump at the SIZ by membrane potential, action potential discharge, and chemical autocrine and paracrine factors are important mechanisms contributing to changes in baroreceptor sensitivity during sustained increases in arterial pressure and in pathological states associated with endothelial dysfunction, oxidative stress, and platelet activation.

KEYWORDS: Pressoreceptors; Carotid sinus; Aortic arch; Blood pressure; Sympathetic nerve activity; Parasympathetic nerve activity; Hypertension; Atherosclerosis; Gene transfer; Sodium channels; Potassium channels; Reactive oxygen species; Nitric oxide; Prostacyclin; Platelets; Endothelium

Address for correspondence: Mark W. Chapleau, Ph.D., Department of Internal Medicine, Division of Cardiovascular Diseases, University of Iowa College of Medicine, Room E327-1, GH, 200 Hawkins Drive, Iowa City, IA 52242. Voice: 319-356-7760; fax: 319-353-6343.
    mark-chapleau@uiowa.edu

## INTRODUCTION

Arterial baroreceptors are mechanosensitive nerve endings that innervate adventitia of carotid sinuses and aortic arch.[1,2] Changes in arterial blood pressure are sensed indirectly through the baroreceptors' responsiveness to mechanical deformation during vascular stretch. Changes in the frequency of baroreceptor afferent discharge transmitted to the central nervous system (CNS) trigger reflex adjustments that buffer or oppose the change in pressure; that is, the baroreceptor reflex provides a powerful negative feedback mechanism of blood pressure regulation.

The purpose of this review is to define the mechanisms that determine the sensitivity of baroreceptor afferents in health and disease. First, we summarize the fundamental mechanisms of how changes in arterial pressure lead to changes in frequency of action potential discharge of baroreceptor afferents. Second, we discuss the mechanisms involved in modulation of baroreceptor activity, focusing on the changes that occur in response to sustained increases in arterial pressure and in pathological states associated with altered production of paracrine/autocrine factors (e.g., in atherosclerosis and hypertension).

## HOW DO BARORECEPTORS SENSE CHANGES IN ARTERIAL PRESSURE?

The process by which changes in arterial pressure alter baroreceptor activity occurs through several steps, which are briefly summarized below.

### Vascular Compliance and Viscoelastic Coupling

The vascular compliance defines the extent of blood vessel distension for a given increase in arterial pressure and therefore is a major determinant of the magnitude of deformation and activity of baroreceptors.[2] Decreased vascular compliance contributes to decreased baroreceptor sensitivity in diseases such as atherosclerosis and chronic hypertension and with aging.[3,4] The viscoelastic characteristics of the vessel wall and the coupling elements between the wall and nerve endings also importantly influence baroreceptor deformation and activity.[5] How does deformation generate an electrical signal?

### Baroreceptor Mechanoelectrical Transduction

Elucidation of the mechanism of transducing mechanical deformation into membrane depolarization is of tremendous interest in many areas of biology. Recent efforts have identified molecular components of mechanosensitive ion channels that may be gated directly by membrane tension. Evidence suggests that such channels are present on baroreceptor nerve endings, that the channels are generally permeable to cations, and that sodium and calcium influx through these channels is responsible for depolarization of baroreceptors during increased arterial pressure[6–12] (FIG. 1). Recent work strongly suggests that *degenerin/epithelial $Na^+$ channel (DEG/ENaC) subunits are components of mechanosensitive ion channels in baroreceptors and other mechanosensitive nerves.* This work is reviewed in other chapters in this volume.[12,13]

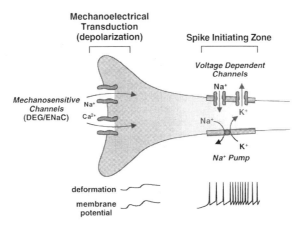

**FIGURE 1.** Schematic depiction of mechanisms of baroreceptor activation during increases in arterial pressure. Mechanoelectrical transduction involves opening of mechanosensitive ion channels on baroreceptor nerve endings that depolarize the terminals in relation to the magnitude of deformation. Evidence suggests that DEG/ENaC subunits are components of the baroreceptor mechanosensitive channel.[11,12] Sufficient depolarization of the "spike initiating zone" (SIZ) evokes action potentials that are transmitted along the afferent fibers at frequencies related to the magnitude of depolarization and the properties and activity of voltage-dependent ion channels and pumps at the SIZ.

## *Encoding of Depolarization into Action Potential Discharge*

Depolarization of mechanosensitive nerve endings is localized to the sensory terminals and rapidly decays with distance from the site of stimulation.[14] The depolarization, often referred to as the *receptor* or *generator potential*, is graded in relation to the magnitude of mechanical stimulation (FIG. 1). In order to inform the CNS of the signal, it is necessary to generate action potentials at a "spike initiating zone" (SIZ) near the nerve terminals[14] (FIG. 1). Action potentials are generated when the depolarization reaches a specific threshold for opening of voltage-dependent sodium ($Na^+$) and potassium ($K^+$) channels. The frequency of action potential discharge increases with further depolarization and is critically dependent on the expression and activity of voltage-dependent ion channels and membrane pumps (e.g., $Na^+/K^+$-ATPase) near the SIZ (FIG. 1). Since these molecules are regulated by membrane potential (depolarization), they represent attractive candidates for modulating baroreceptor sensitivity during sustained changes in arterial pressure (e.g., in acute or chronic hypertension).

## MODULATION OF BARORECEPTOR AFFERENT DISCHARGE

Most of our knowledge of baroreceptor physiology has come from studies in which the frequency of action potential discharge was recorded from baroreceptor afferent fibers during changes in arterial pressure. Baroreceptor activity can be recorded with the circulation intact or from the vascularly isolated carotid sinus or aor-

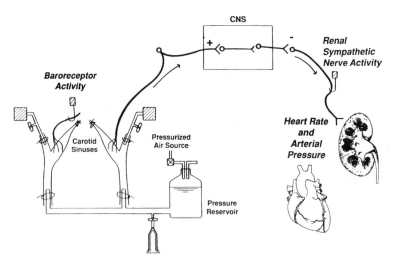

**FIGURE 2.** Illustration of *in situ* isolated carotid sinus preparation (bilateral). Either one or both carotid sinuses are vascularly isolated in anesthetized dogs or rabbits. The carotid sinuses are filled with an oxygenated physiologic buffer solution and attached to a reservoir that enables control of carotid sinus pressure. Baroreceptor activity is recorded from the whole carotid sinus nerve or from single baroreceptor fibers in dissected nerve bundles. Mechanical deformation can be estimated by measuring changes in carotid sinus diameter using sonomicrometer crystals or a videomicrometer (not shown). Corresponding reflex changes in sympathetic nerve activity and systemic arterial pressure can be measured by leaving one or both carotid sinus nerves intact. Aortic depressor nerves and vagi are sectioned to prevent reflex buffering of blood pressure changes.

tic arch, which enables much better control of the pressure stimulus and the composition of fluid bathing the sensory terminals. The isolated carotid sinus preparation *in situ* is illustrated in FIGURE 2.

## *Modulation of Activity during Increased Arterial Pressure*

During a sustained increase in arterial pressure baroreceptor activity increases initially but declines or *adapts* over time as the elevated pressure is maintained.[15–17] Furthermore, after a period of acute hypertension, baroreceptor activity is suppressed (*postexcitatory depression*) and the pressure threshold is increased (*reset*).[3,17–19] Adaptation and resetting occur rapidly within seconds to minutes of the rise in pressure. Baroreceptors, at least those with myelinated afferents, continue to adapt at a slower rate, with baroreceptor activity returning essentially to normal prehypertensive levels despite sustained chronic hypertension.[15] Several mechanisms are thought to contribute to baroreceptor adaptation, resetting, and postexcitatory depression.

### *Viscoelastic Relaxation*

Vascular distension is effectively translated to deformation of the nerve endings as arterial pressure rises; but as the elevated pressure is maintained, the viscoelastic

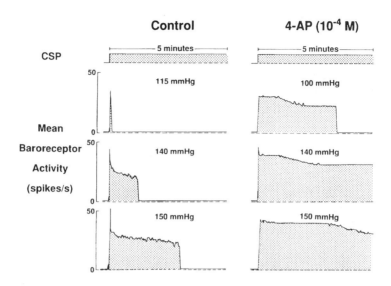

**FIGURE 3.** Effect of $K^+$ channel blocker 4-aminopyridine (4-AP) on baroreceptor adaptation in anesthetized dog. Shown are measurements of activity recorded from a single baroreceptor fiber in response to step increases in isolated carotid sinus pressure to several levels during control (*left*) and in the presence of 4-AP ($10^{-4}$ M) (*right*). 4-AP did not alter the peak nerve activity reached at the beginning of the pressure step but markedly reduced adaptation that occurred as the elevated pressure was maintained. (Reprinted from Chapleau *et al.*[16] by permission.)

relaxation of elements in series with baroreceptors may reduce the tension transmitted to the nerve endings despite an even greater vessel diameter.[5]

## $Na^+$ Pump Activation

Depolarization, increased action potential discharge, and $Na^+$ influx into baroreceptor terminals during increases in arterial pressure activate an electrogenic $Na^+/K^+$ pump at the SIZ that leads to membrane hyperpolarization and postexcitatory depression of baroreceptors upon return of pressure to normal levels. *$Na^+$ pump inhibition with ouabain or low-potassium ($K^+$) solutions prevents or significantly attenuates post-excitatory depression and resetting of pressure threshold after a period of elevated pressure.*[19,20] Interestingly, ouabain does not attenuate baroreceptor adaptation during the period of elevated pressure, suggesting that a different mechanism may cause adaptation.[16]

## $K^+$ Channel Activation

The $K^+$ channel blocker 4-aminopyridine (4-AP), injected into the isolated carotid sinus of dogs, profoundly reduces the magnitude of baroreceptor adaptation observed during step increases in carotid sinus pressure[16] (FIG. 3). 4-AP does not influence the peak nerve activity measured during the initial rise in pressure and does not influence vascular compliance.[16] These results suggest that *activation of 4-AP–sensitive $K^+$ channels on baroreceptor nerve endings is a major contributor to* *baroreceptor adaptation during acute increases in arterial pressure.* 4-AP does not prevent resetting of the baroreceptor pressure threshold after a period of acute hypertension,[21] confirming that adaptation and resetting appear to be mediated through different mechanisms. Baroreceptor subtypes have been described based on characteristics of the pressure–activity relation and the presence or absence of myelinated fibers.[1,2,21,22] Interestingly, 4-AP selectively alters activity of type I myelinated baroreceptor afferents with little or no effect on type II nonmyelinated C-fiber afferents,[22] suggesting differential expression of 4-AP–sensitive $K^+$ channels on type I baroreceptors.

### C-Fiber–Induced Paracrine Inhibition

Neural and mechanical viscoelastic mechanisms can be difficult to distinguish in preparations subjected to changes in arterial pressure. Therefore, we performed studies in which multifiber baroreceptor activity in the rat aortic depressor nerve (ADN) was measured *in vivo* before and after brief periods of antidromic electrical activation of ADN terminals.[23] The ADN was crushed centrally to prevent stimulation-evoked reflex changes in arterial pressure. Brief (5- to 20-s) electrical stimulation of both myelinated A-fiber and nonmyelinated C-fiber afferents, but not selective A-fiber stimulation, caused marked and sustained (>60-s) inhibition of baroreceptor activity.[23] These preliminary results suggest that activation of C-fiber terminals may evoke an additional powerful mechanism of postexcitatory depression, perhaps mediated by chemical factors released from C-fibers acting on neighboring baroreceptor A-fibers. The concept of chemical paracrine-mediated modulation of baroreceptor sensitivity is expanded in the next section.

## Modulation of Baroreceptor Sensitivity by Paracrine/Autocrine Factors

Circulating hormones and locally produced chemical factors have been shown to modulate baroreceptor activity. For example, norepinephrine released from sympathetic nerves innervating carotid sinuses and aortic arch or circulating in blood may decrease baroreceptor activity by reducing vessel diameter due to vasoconstriction or may increase baroreceptor sensitivity through direct actions on the nerve endings.[24,25] Vasoconstrictor substances generally shift the pressure-activity curve, particularly for myelinated baroreceptor fibers, to higher pressures without changing the slope of the curve (gain) or the maximum activity.[24,26] Conversely, vasodilators may shift the function curve to lower pressures.[24,26] Other chemical factors alter the slope of the pressure-activity relation and maximum baroreceptor activity independently of changes in vascular tone. The effects of several paracrine factors, produced by cells near the baroreceptor nerve endings, on the sensitivity of the afferents are summarized below.

### Prostacyclin

The predominant prostanoid produced in large arteries is prostacyclin. Increased blood flow (shear stress) and pulsatile pressure stimulate prostacyclin release from endothelium. Prostacyclin is a vasodilator and a powerful inhibitor of platelet aggregation.[27] *Injection of prostacyclin into the isolated carotid sinus increases baroreceptor sensitivity* without altering the carotid pressure-diameter relation, suggesting a direct action on baroreceptors.[28,29] Inhibitors of prostanoid production such as in-domethacin decrease baroreceptor activity, suggesting a role of endogenous prosta-cyclin in activation of baroreceptors.[28,29] Decreased production of prostacyclin in atherosclerosis and chronic hypertension may contribute to decreased baroreceptor sensitivity in these pathologic states.[29]

## Nitric Oxide

Nitric oxide (NO) is another endothelial factor with potent vasodilator and anti-platelet actions.[27] In contrast to prostacyclin, *NO injected into the isolated carotid sinus decreases baroreceptor sensitivity* independently of its vasodilator action.[30] The neuronal isoform of NO synthase (nNOS or type I NOS) is expressed in a sub-population of vagal afferent nerves[31] (probably C-fibers), raising the possibility that it may function as an autocrine regulator of sensory nerve activity (see section on isolated baroreceptor neurons below).

## Reactive Oxygen Species

Reactive oxygen species (ROS) produced in various pathological conditions in-cluding ischemia/reperfusion, atherosclerosis, diabetes, and aging contribute to dys-function of multiple organ systems. The carotid sinuses are particularly susceptible to development of atherosclerotic lesions. We hypothesized that ROS produced in carotid sinuses may contribute to decreased baroreceptor sensitivity in atherosclero-sis. Rabbits fed a high-cholesterol diet for 7–8 months demonstrate hypercholester-olemia, atherosclerotic lesions in carotid arteries, and decreased baroreceptor activity.[32] *Acute exposure of the carotid sinus to the ROS scavengers superoxide dis-mutase (SOD) and catalase for 10–15 minutes significantly increases baroreceptor activity in atherosclerotic rabbits* but fails to alter activity in normal healthy rab-bits.[32] Catalase alone also increases activity, implicating hydrogen peroxide as a key endogenous factor causing decreased baroreceptor activity in atherosclerotic states.[32] Chemical generation of ROS in the isolated carotid sinus with the reaction of xanthine and xanthine oxidase significantly decreases baroreceptor activity in normal rabbits, confirming that ROS suppress baroreceptor activity.[32]

## Platelet Factors

Carotid sinuses are common sites of platelet aggregation in patients with cardio-vascular disease.[33] We hypothesized that factors released from activated platelets may significantly influence baroreceptor sensitivity with implications for blood pressure regulation. Platelets were isolated from human or rabbit blood, suspended in buffer, activated with thrombin, and injected into the isolated carotid sinus of rabbits[34–38] (FIG. 4).

*Platelet activation in carotid sinuses with carotid sinus pressure maintained con-stant rapidly increases the activity of type II baroreceptors and reflexly abolishes re-nal sympathetic nerve activity, resulting in profound hypotension*[34,35] (FIG. 5). The rapid platelet-induced inhibition of sympathetic activity and hypotension is mediat-ed by platelet-derived serotonin acting on $5\text{-}HT_3$, and to a lesser extent $5\text{-}HT_2$ recep-tors on the type II baroreceptors.[34] Sympathetic activity and systemic arterial pressure gradually recover to normal or above-normal levels within 10–20 minutes of continued exposure to the activated platelets (FIG. 5). The recovery of sympathetic

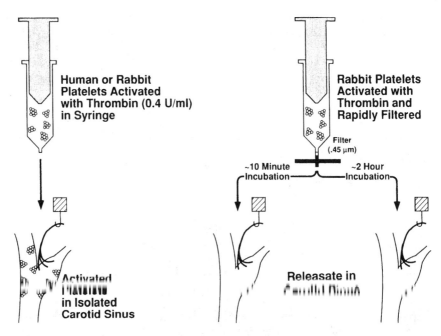

**FIGURE 4.** Schematic illustration of the protocol used to test effects of activated platelets on baroreceptor sensitivity. Platelets were isolated from rabbit or human blood and suspended in physiologic buffer solution. Platelets were activated by thrombin (0.4 units/mL) just before injection of the platelet suspension into the isolated carotid sinus(es) of anesthetized rabbits (*left*). Baroreceptor activity or renal sympathetic nerve activity was measured while holding carotid sinus pressure constant and during ramp increases in pressure before and after addition of the activated platelets. In some experiments, the platelet releasate was filtered through a 0.45-μm Millipore filter, and the releasate was injected into the isolated carotid sinus in the absence of platelets (*right*).

activity and arterial pressure correlates with a delayed impairment of baroreceptor sensitivity to changes in carotid sinus pressure[35–38] (FIG. 6). Impaired baroreceptor sensitivity is also observed after injecting the filtered cell-free "releasate" obtained from the activated platelets into the isolated carotid sinus in the absence of platelets.[38] These results demonstrate that the *delayed platelet-induced inhibition of baroreceptor sensitivity is mediated by a stable diffusible mediator* whose identity is unknown.[38]

## MECHANISMS REVEALED BY STUDY OF ISOLATED BARORECEPTOR NEURONS

The results summarized in the preceding section strongly suggest that certain paracrine factors alter baroreceptor activity by acting directly on the nerve endings. The presence of endothelium and vascular muscle along with other cell types in the vascular wall make it difficult to prove a direct action of a given substance on barore-

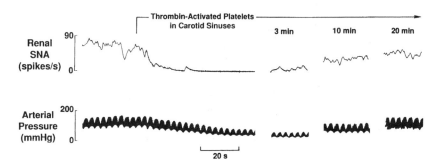

**FIGURE 5.** Rapid sympathoinhibition and hypotension in response to bilateral injection of thrombin-activated platelets into the isolated carotid sinuses of rabbit. Carotid sinus pressure was maintained constant at 80 mmHg. Renal sympathetic nerve activity and systemic arterial pressure gradually returned to control levels within ~20 min despite the continued presence of the platelet suspension in the carotid sinuses. (Reprinted from Mao et al.[34] by permission.)

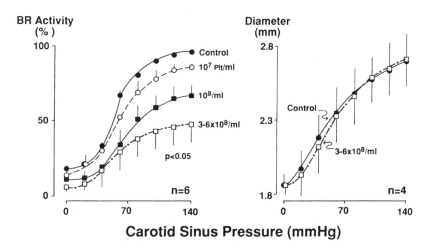

**FIGURE 6.** Sustained platelet activation in carotid sinus decreases baroreceptor sensitivity. Shown are the effects of thrombin-activated human platelets injected into isolated carotid sinuses of rabbits on the baroreceptor pressure-activity relationship (*left*) and the pressure-diameter relationship (*right*). The carotid sinus was exposed to the activated platelets for ~15 min. Activated platelets decreased baroreceptor activity in a concentration-dependent manner without altering the pressure-diameter relationship. Concentrations indicate number of platelets per mL. Thrombin alone did not influence baroreceptor activity (not shown). (Modified from Li et al.[36])

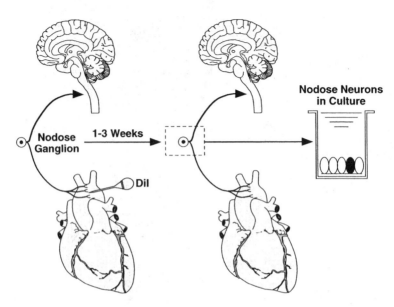

**FIGURE 7.** Schematic illustration of the procedures used to label aortic baroreceptor nerves with the fluorescent dye diI *in vivo*, enabling later identification of the labeled neurons in culture for functional studies. The diI is applied to the aortic arch adventitia in anesthetized rats and mice. The animals are allowed to recover and are maintained for 1–3 weeks to allow sufficient time for transport of the diI along the aortic depressor nerves to the nodose ganglia. At this time, the nodose ganglia are removed and the nodose neurons dissociated and maintained in culture for 1–5 days. The diI-labeled neurons are identified by their fluorescence (*indicated by black neuron*), and functional electrophysiologic or calcium imaging studies are performed.

ceptor endings. Furthermore, the small size and complex architecture of the baroreceptor terminals embedded in the vascular wall prevents direct measurement of membrane potential in the terminals and limits investigation into mechanisms of baroreceptor activation. The inability to measure the mechanically induced depolarization of the terminals has prevented determination of whether a factor modulates baroreceptor sensitivity through an action on mechanosensitive channels or on voltage-dependent channels at the SIZ. These limitations motivated us to develop an *in vitro* preparation of isolated baroreceptor neurons in culture[7–11,39–43] (FIG. 7). Aortic baroreceptor neurons are labeled *in vivo* by application of the fluorescent dye diI to the aortic arch adventitia of rats and mice. One to two weeks later nodose neurons are dissociated from nodose ganglia and maintained in culture. Functional studies are performed on individual fluorescently labeled aortic baroreceptor neurons.

### Cultured Baroreceptor Neuron as a Model of Mechanosensory Transduction

An important consideration is whether molecules expressed at the sensory terminals *in vivo* are also expressed on isolated baroreceptor neurons in culture. *Consid-*

*erable evidence has accumulated suggesting that specific ligand receptors and ion channels present on the nerve endings are also present on the soma of cultured nodose neurons.*[9–11,41–46] Furthermore, spike frequency adaptation of dorsal root ganglion neurons during sustained mechanical stimulation of cutaneous mechanoreceptor endings correlates with the adaptation during sustained depolarization of the same neuron by current injection into the soma.[47] Very importantly, we have shown that *cultured baroreceptor neurons are mechanosensitive,* the hallmark of baroreceptors.[7–11,42,43] In preliminary experiments we have demonstrated that the DEG/ENaC channel blocker amiloride prevents mechanically induced depolarization of mechanosensitive nodose neurons but does not attenuate action potential discharge evoked by depolarizing current injection.[42] In contrast, the voltage-dependent $Na^+$ channel blocker tetrodotoxin suppresses action potential discharge but does not attenuate mechanical stimulation–evoked depolarization.[42] Although there are surely some differences in the amount of expression and the regulation of key sensory molecules in sensory terminals versus isolated neuron somata, we believe that the isolated baroreceptor neuron is a valid and useful model that enables investigation of mechanisms of sensory transduction.

### Voltage-Dependent $K^+$ and $Na^+$ Channels as Targets for Chemical Modulators

We hypothesized that voltage-dependent $K^+$ and $Na^+$ channels are the effector molecules that mediate the prostacyclin-induced increase and the NO-induced decrease in baroreceptor sensitivity.

#### Prostacyclin Analog Carbacyclin

Exposure of isolated baroreceptor neurons to carbacyclin causes depolarization and enhances the action potential discharge evoked by depolarizing current injection[43] (FIG. 8). Carbacyclin does not enhance the depolarization evoked by mechanical stimulation, suggesting a lack of effect on mechanosensitive channels.[43] The mechanism of the *carbacyclin-induced increase in membrane excitability* was investigated with voltage-clamp experiments and *was found to involve inhibition of charybdotoxin-sensitive, calcium-activated $K^+$ current*[39] (FIG. 8).

#### Nitric Oxide

Exposure of isolated baroreceptor neurons to NO donors suppresses action potential discharge evoked by current injection (unpublished observation). Voltage-clamp studies demonstrated that *NO inhibits voltage-dependent $Na^+$ current in baroreceptor neurons through a cyclic GMP–independent, nitrosylation-dependent mechanism*[40,41] (FIG. 9). Interestingly, NO scavengers and the NO synthase inhibitor L-nitroarginine increase baseline $Na^+$ current in isolated baroreceptor neurons, suggesting that *endogenous NO is produced in sensory neurons and that it tonically restrains $Na^+$ channel opening.*[40] A subpopulation of nodose neurons including baroreceptor neurons, contain the neuronal isoform of NO synthase.[31,40]

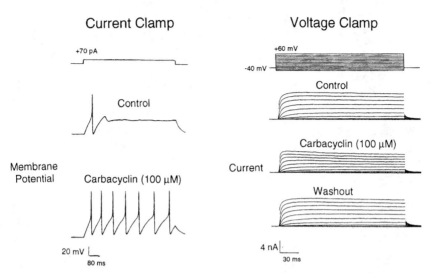

**FIGURE 8.** Recordings from isolated baroreceptor neurons in culture demonstrating increased membrane excitability (current clamp) (*left*) and inhibition of outward $K^+$ current (voltage clamp) (*right*) in the presence of the stable prostacyclin analog carbacyclin. (Modified from Li *et al.*[39] and from *Fundam. Clin. Pharmacol.* 11 [Suppl. 1]: 61s [1997]).

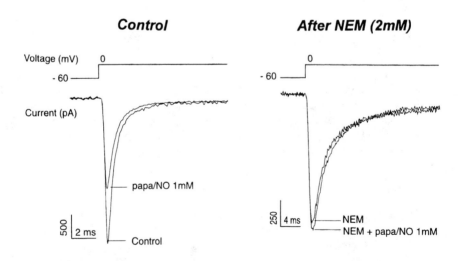

**FIGURE 9.** Inhibition of voltage-dependent $Na^+$ current by the NO donor papa-NONOate (papa/NO). Shown are recordings of inward $Na^+$ current evoked by depolarization before and after addition of the stable NO donor papa-NONOate to the bath solution. Responses to papa-NONOate under control conditions (*left*) and after administration of the sulfhydryl modifier *N*-ethylmaleimide (NEM) (*right*) are illustrated.

## GENETIC DISSECTION OF DETERMINANTS OF BAROREFLEX SENSITIVITY

The current explosion of gene discovery and the development of techniques enabling genetic manipulation of cells and animals open up new opportunities to advance our understanding of baroreceptor function. Viral vectors provide an efficient means of transferring genes into cells and tissues.[48] Strategies are available to either overexpress a gene of interest or to reduce endogenous gene expression using dominant negative or antisense approaches. Creation of transgenic or gene knockout animals allows one to test the role of a specific gene and protein product in chronic regulatory mechanisms *in vivo* and to generate novel animal models of disease.[49] Gene expression can be targeted to specific tissues and turned on or off by using appropriate inducible promoters. Genetic manipulation is often more specific than pharmacological approaches and can preserve normal regulation of an overexpressed molecule, which generally cannot be mimicked by agonist administration.

### *Neural Mechanisms of Cardiovascular Regulation Studied in Mice*

The unique susceptibility of mice to genetic manipulation encourages development of expertise in carrying out physiological studies in mice. We have successfully implemented multiple techniques for assessment of baroreflex and autonomic function in mice[50–58] (TABLE 1). Most relevant to the study of baroreceptor afferents are the measurements of baroreceptor activity in the ADN, renal sympathetic nerve activity, responses to carotid artery occlusion, and the depolarization and action potential discharge evoked by mechanical stimulation of isolated nodose neurons in culture.

Preliminary results suggest that *baroreflex control of renal sympathetic nerve activity is impaired in mice with chronic angiotensin-dependent hypertension (renin/ angiotensinogen transgenics)[56] and in normotensive apolipoprotein E (apoE) knockout mice with atherosclerosis.*[57] ApoE knockout mice (~35–45 weeks of age) also exhibit a reduced pressor response to bilateral carotid artery occlusion during 100% oxygen ventilation, but not during room air ventilation, suggesting a selective impairment of carotid baroreflex control of blood pressure accompanied by an enhanced chemoreceptor reflex activation.[58]

### *Gene Transfer Using Viral Vectors*

We are using two general experimental approaches: gene transfer to carotid sinus (or aortic arch) adventitia *in vivo* and gene transfer to isolated nodose sensory neurons in culture (FIG. 10). One aim of our studies is to restore baroreflex sensitivity in pathological states by altering paracrine influences through gene transfer–induced overexpression of antioxidant enzymes and/or cyclooxygenases in carotid sinus adventitia. A second aim is to identify the molecules that confer mechanosensitivity and modulate membrane excitability of isolated baroreceptor neurons. For example, gene transfer of dominant negative constructs to isolated neurons can be used to inhibit expression of candidate subunits of mechanosensitive channels.

**TABLE 1. Assessment of baroreflex and autonomic function in mice**

| Conscious | Anesthetized | Culture |
| --- | --- | --- |
| Arterial pressure and heart rate variability (spectral analysis) | Baroreceptor activity from aortic depressor nerve (ADN) | Nodose sensory neurons dissociated from nodose ganglia (diI-labeled aortic baroreceptor neurons) |
| Baroreflex control of heart rate (phenylephrine/ nitroprusside) | Renal sympathetic nerve activity | Sympathetic neurons dissociated from aortic/renal and celiac ganglia |
| Chemoreceptor reflex control of respiration (plethysmograph) | Central mediation of baroreflex (responses to ADN stimulation) | Membrane potential (sharp microelectrode-current clamp) |
| | Responsiveness to vagal stimulation (HR responses to electrical stimulation of efferent vagus) | Ionic currents (patch-voltage clamp) |
| | Response to carotid artery occlusion with and without $O_2$ (baro- and chemoreflex) | Intracellular calcium imaging (fura-2) |

*Gene Transfer to Carotid Sinus Adventitia*

Adenoviral vectors containing reporter genes (β-galactosidase or green fluorescent protein) and/or functional genes are applied topically to carotid sinus adventitia in rabbits[59,60] and mice.[61] Transgene expression is evident within one day and is maximal ~4–5 days after virus application. Our results and those of others demonstrate that topical application of adenoviral vectors to adventitia transduces primarily adventitial fibroblasts with no transgene expression in the blood vessel media or in baroreceptor nerves.[59,62,63] Thus, this approach is ideal for selective manipulation of paracrine influences on baroreceptor sensitivity without directly affecting gene expression in vascular muscle or baroreceptors. Neither expression of β-galactosidase nor the virus itself alters baroreceptor function as assessed by measuring baroreceptor activity from the isolated carotid sinus of rabbits[59] and by the pressor response to carotid occlusion in mice.[61] We have demonstrated that *gene transfer of the endothelial isoform of NOS to carotid sinus adventitia of rabbits resets the baroreceptor pressure-activity curve* to higher pressures and increases carotid artery diameter measured 4–5 days after virus application.[60] Gene transfer of superoxide dismutase (SOD) and catalase to carotid sinus adventitia enhances the carotid artery occlusion pressor reflex in apoE knockout mice with atherosclerosis but does not influence the reflex in normal control C57BL/6 mice.[61] These results suggest that *ROS generated close to the nerve endings contribute to baroreflex dysfunction in atherosclerosis and that gene transfer of antioxidant enzymes to carotid sinus can restore reflex sensitivity.*

*Gene Transfer to Isolated Sensory Neurons*

Unlike the carotid sinus nerves *in vivo* discussed above, isolated nodose sensory neurons are easily transduced by adenoviral vectors. Exposure of dissociated rat no-

## Gene Transfer to Carotid Sinus Adventitia in Vivo

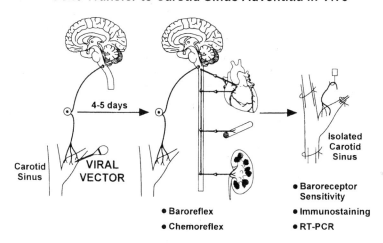

## Gene Transfer to Isolated Baroreceptor Neurons (BRN)

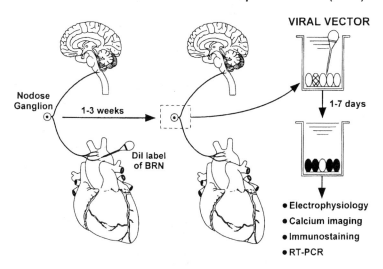

**FIGURE 10.** Schematic illustration of the strategies for gene transfer to carotid sinus adventitia *in vivo*[59–61] and to isolated baroreceptor (nodose) neurons *in vitro*.[64] Gene transfer to carotid sinus transduces adventitial fibroblasts to alter paracrine influences on baroreceptor sensitivity. The same approach can be used for gene transfer to aortic arch adventitia. For *in vitro* gene transfer, aortic baroreceptor neurons (BRN) are labeled with diI applied to aortic arch *in vivo* and identified in culture by fluorescence (*cross-hatching*). Exposure of the culture to viral vector for 1–2 h leads to transgene expression (*black neurons*).

dose neurons to adenoviral vectors containing the reporter gene β-galactosidase ($10^9$ pfu/mL for 30 min) resulted in transgene expression in >80% of neurons.[64] This approach will enable us to test the functional role of specific candidate ion channels and regulatory molecules in mechanoelectrical transduction and modulation of membrane excitability of baroreceptor neurons. For example, one could determine whether overexpression of dominant negative constructs of candidate subunits of DEG/ENaC channels interferes with mechanoelectrical transduction in baroreceptor neurons and whether replacement of missing subunits in neurons from knockout mice can restore or "rescue" mechanosensitivity.

## SUMMARY AND FUTURE DIRECTIONS

Baroreceptor activity is modulated through a variety of mechanisms under physiological conditions and in pathological states. These mechanisms may involve changes in the mechanical properties of the vascular wall of the carotid sinuses and aortic arch, actions on a new class of mechanosensitive ion channel that blunts or enhances the magnitude of depolarization evoked by mechanical stimulation of the endings, and/or by actions on voltage-dependent $Na^+$ and $K^+$ channels at the SIZ that alter the threshold for action potential discharge and the frequency of afferent activity. Modulation of voltage-dependent channels at the SIZ by changes in membrane potential, action potential discharge, and paracrine factors released from nearby cells is an important mechanism contributing to changes in baroreceptor activity during acute hypertension and in pathological states associated with endothelial dysfunction, oxidative stress, and platelet activation.

Promising areas for future investigation include: (1) identification of key molecules involved in mechanoelectrical transduction and modulation of membrane excitability at the molecular level; (2) elucidation of the independent and interacting roles of membrane potential and chemical factors in regulating voltage-dependent $Na^+$ and $K^+$ channels on baroreceptors; and (3) measurement of the expression of ion channels and key regulatory molecules in baroreceptors and delineation of the factors that regulate their expression in normal and pathological states. These future challenges will require a multidisciplinary approach including studies at molecular, cellular, and whole animal levels.

## ACKNOWLEDGMENTS

The authors would like to acknowledge the important contributions of Dr. Xin Su, Dr. Hui Zhen Mao, Dr. Klaus Bielefeldt, Dr. Vladislav Snitsarev, Dr. Wei Sun, Dr. Rubens Fazan, Jr., Greg Davis, and Carol Whiteis to the work summarized in this review. The research was supported by the National Institutes of Health (HL14388), the Department of Veterans Affairs, and the Iowa Affiliate of the American Heart Association. Adenoviral vectors were constructed in the Gene Transfer Vector Core at the University of Iowa. The Vector Core is supported in part by funds from the University of Iowa Carver Trust.

## REFERENCES

1. LANDGREN, S. 1952. On the excitation mechanism of the carotid baroceptors. Acta Physiol. Scand. **26:** 1–34.
2. KIRCHHEIM, H.R. 1976. Systemic arterial baroreceptor reflexes. Physiol. Rev. **56:** 100–176.
3. ANDRESEN, M.C. & M. YANG. 1989. Arterial baroreceptor resetting: contributions of chronic and acute processes. Clin. Exp. Pharmacol. Physiol. (Suppl.) **15:** 19–30.
4. ANGELL-JAMES, J.E. 1974. Arterial baroreceptor activity in rabbits with experimental atherosclerosis. Circ. Res. **34:** 27–39.
5. COLERIDGE, H.M., J.C.G. COLERIDGE, E.R. POORE, *et al.* 1984. Aortic wall properties and baroreceptor behavior at normal arterial pressure and in acute hypertensive resetting in dogs. J. Physiol. (Lond.) **350:** 309–326.
6. HAJDUCZOK, G., M.W. CHAPLEAU, R.J. FERLIC, *et al.* 1994. Gadolinium inhibits mechano-electrical transduction in rabbit carotid baroreceptors: implication of stretch-activated channels. J. Clin. Invest. **94:** 2392–2396.
7. SHARMA, R.V., M.W. CHAPLEAU, G. HAJDUCZOK, *et al.* 1995. Mechanical stimulation increases intracellular calcium concentration in nodose sensory neurons. Neuroscience **66:** 433–441.
8. CUNNINGHAM, J.T., R.E. WACHTEL & F.M. ABBOUD. 1995. Mechanosensitive currents in putative aortic baroreceptor neurons in vitro. J. Neurophysiol. **73:** 2094–2098.
9. KRASKE, S., J.T. CUNNINGHAM, G. HAJDUCZOK, *et al.* 1998. Mechanosensitive ion channels in putative aortic baroreceptor neurons. Am. J. Physiol. **275** (Heart Circ. Physiol. **44**): H1497–H1501.
10. SULLIVAN, M.J., R.V. SHARMA, R.E. WACHTEL, *et al.* 1997. Non-voltage-gated calcium influx through mechanosensitive ion channels in aortic baroreceptor neurons. Circ. Res. **80**(6): 861–867.
11. DRUMMOND, H.A., M.P. PRICE, M.J. WELSH & F.M. ABBOUD. 1998. A molecular component of the arterial baroreceptor mechanotransducer. Neuron **21:** 1435–1441.
12. DRUMMOND, H.A., M.J. WELSH & F.M. ABBOUD. 2001. ENaC subunits are molecular components of the arterial baroreceptor complex. Ann. N.Y. Acad. Sci. This volume.
13. TAVERNARAKIS, N. & M. DRISCOLL. 2001. Degenerins: at the core of the Metazoan mechanotransducer? Ann. N.Y. Acad. Sci. This volume.
14. KATZ, B. 1950. Depolarization of sensory terminals and the initiation of impulses in the muscle spindle. J. Physiol. (Lond.) **111:** 261–282.
15. MCCUBBIN, J.W., J.E. GREEN & I.H. PAGE. 1956. Baroceptor function in chronic renal hypertension. Circ. Res. **4:** 205–210.
16. CHAPLEAU, M.W., J. LU, G. HAJDUCZOK & F.M. ABBOUD. 1993. Mechanism of baroreceptor adaptation in dogs: attenuation of adaptation by the $K^+$ channel blocker 4-aminopyridine. J. Physiol. (Lond.) **462:** 291–306.
17. CHAPLEAU, M.W. & F.M. ABBOUD. 1993. Mechanisms of adaptation and resetting of the baroreceptor reflex. *In* Cardiovascular Reflex Control in Health and Disease. R. Hainsworth & A.L. Mark, Eds.: 165–193. W.B. Saunders. London.
18. KORNER, P.I. 1989. Baroreceptor resetting and other determinants of baroreflex properties in hypertension. Clin. Exp. Pharmacol. Physiol. (Suppl.) **15:** 45–64.
19. HEESCH, C.M., F.M. ABBOUD & M.D. THAMES. 1984. Acute resetting of carotid sinus baroreceptors, II: Possible involvement of electrogenic $Na^+$ pump. Am. J. Physiol. **247:** H833–H839.
20. SAUM, W.R., A.M. BROWN, A.M. & F.H. TULEY. 1976. An electrogenic sodium pump and baroreceptor function in normotensive and spontaneously hypertensive rats. Circ. Res. **39:** 497–505.
21. DRUMMOND, H.A. & J.L. SEAGARD. 1994. Lack of effect of 4-aminopyridine on acute resetting of the type I carotid baroreceptor. Neurosci. Lett. **173:** 45–49.
22. VAN BREDERODE, J.F.M., J.L. SEAGARD, C. DEAN, *et al.* 1990. An experimental and modeling study of the excitability of carotid sinus baroreceptors. Circ. Res. **66:** 1510–1525.
23. DAVIS, G.J., R. FAZAN, JR., F.M. ABBOUD & M.W. CHAPLEAU. 1998. Brief activation of baroreceptor C-fibers causes sustained inhibition of baroreceptor activity: possible

mechanism of baroreceptor resetting following acute hypertension (abstr.). J. Invest. Med. **46**(3): 200A.

24. MUNCH, P.A., P.N. THOREN & A.M. BROWN. 1987. Dual effects of norepinephrine and mechanisms of baroreceptor stimulation. Circ. Res. **61**: 409–419.

25. MUNCH, P.A. & A.M. BROWN. 1987. Sympathetic modulation of rabbit aortic baroreceptors *in vitro*. Am. J. Physiol. **253** (Heart Circ. Physiol. **22**): H1106–H1111.

26. YANG, M. & M.C. ANDRESEN. 1990. Peptidergic modulation of mechanotransduction in rat arterial baroreceptors. Circ. Res. **66**: 804–813.

27. MOMBOULI, J.-V. & P.M. VANHOUTTE. 1999. Endothelial dysfunction: from physiology to therapy. J. Mol. Cell. Cardiol. **31**: 61–74.

28. CHEN, H.I., M.W. CHAPLEAU, T.S. MCDOWELL & F.M. ABBOUD. 1990. Prostaglandins contribute to activation of baroreceptors in rabbits. Possible paracrine influence of endothelium. Circ. Res. **67**(6): 1394–1404.

29. XIE, P., M.W. CHAPLEAU, T.S. MCDOWELL, et al. 1990. Mechanism of decreased baroreceptor activity in chronic hypertensive rabbits. Role of endogenous prostanoids. J. Clin. Invest. **86**: 625–630.

30. MATSUDA, T., J.N. BATES, S.J. LEWIS, et al. 1995. Modulation of baroreceptor activity by nitric oxide and S-nitrosocysteine. Circ. Res. **76**(3): 426–433.

31. RUGGIERO, D.A., E.P. MTUI, K. OTAKE & M. ANWAR. 1996. Central and primary visceral afferents to nucleus tractus solitarii may generate nitric oxide as a membrane-permeant neuronal messenger. J. Comp. Neurol. **364**: 51–67.

32. LI, Z., H. MAO, F.M. ABBOUD & M.W. CHAPLEAU. 1996. Oxygen derived free radicals contribute to baroreceptor dysfunction in atherosclerotic rabbits. Circ. Res. **79**(4): 802–811.

33. ISAKA, Y., K. KIMURA, A. UEHARA, et al. 1989. Platelet aggregability and in vivo platelet deposition in patients with ischemic cardiovascular disease—evaluation by indium-111 platelet scintigraphy. Thromb. Res. **56**: 739–749.

34. MAO, H.Z., Z. LI & M.W. CHAPLEAU. 1996. Platelet activation in carotid sinuses triggers reflex sympathoinhibition and hypotension. Hypertension **27**(Part 2): 584–590.

35. CHAPLEAU, M.W., X. SU & Z. LI. 1995. Platelets aggregating in carotid sinus selectively modulate activity of baroreceptor fiber types (abstr.). FASEB J. **9**(3): A7.

36. LI, Z., F.M. ABBOUD & M.W. CHAPLEAU. 1992. Aggregating human platelets in carotid sinus of rabbits decrease sensitivity of baroreceptors. Circ. Res. **70**(4): 644–650.

37. LI, Z., X. SU & M.W. CHAPLEAU. 1995. Role of cyclooxygenase metabolites in platelet-induced baroreceptor dysfunction. Am. J. Physiol. **269** (Heart Circ. Physiol. **38**): H599–H608.

38. LI, Z. & M.W. CHAPLEAU. 1995. Platelet-induced suppression of baroreceptor activity is mediated by a stable diffusible factor. J. Auton. Nerv. Syst. **51**(1): 59–65.

39. LI, Z., H.C. LEE, K. BIELEFELDT, et al. 1997. The prostacyclin analogue carbacyclin inhibits $Ca^{2+}$-activated $K^+$ current in aortic baroreceptor neurones of rats. J. Physiol. (Lond) **501.2**: 275–287.

40. LI, Z., M.W. CHAPLEAU, J.N. BATES, et al. 1998. Nitric oxide as an autocrine regulator of sodium currents in baroreceptor neurons. Neuron **20**(5): 1039–1049.

41. BIELEFELDT, K., C.A. WHITEIS, M.W. CHAPLEAU & F.M. ABBOUD. 1999. Nitric oxide enhances slow inactivation of voltage-dependent sodium currents in rat nodose neurons. Neurosci. Lett. **271**(3): 159–162.

42. SNITSAREV, V., C.A. WHITEIS, F.M. ABBOUD & M.W. CHAPLEAU. 2001. Distinction between activation of mechanosensitive channels and membrane excitability in isolated nodose sensory neurons (abstr.). FASEB J. **15**(5)Pt. II: A1150.

43. SNITSAREV, V., C.A. WHITEIS, F.M. ABBOUD & M.W. CHAPLEAU. 2001. Effect of prostacyclin analog on mechanosensitive vs. voltage-gated ion channels in nodose neurons (abstr.). Soc. Neurosci Abstr. In press.

44. FOWLER, J.C., W.F. WONDERLIN & D. WEINREICH. 1985. Prostaglandins block a $Ca^{2+}$-dependent slow spike after hyperpolarization independent of effects on $Ca^{2+}$ influx in visceral afferent neurons. Brain Res. **345**: 345–349.

45. CHRISTIAN, E.P., G.E. TAYLOR & D. WEINREICH. 1989. Serotonin increases excitability of rabbit C-fiber neurons by two distinct mechanisms. J. Appl. Physiol. **67**: 584–591.

46. STANSFELD, C.E., S.J. MARSH, J.V. HALLIWELL & D.A. BROWN. 1986. 4-Aminopyridine– and dendrotoxin-induced repetitive firing in rat visceral sensory neurons by blocking a slowly inactivating outward current. Neurosci. Lett. **64:** 299–304.
47. HARPER, A.A. 1991. Similarities between some properties of the soma and sensory receptors of primary afferent neurones. Exp. Physiol. **76:** 369–377.
48. LAFONT, A., C. GUEROT & P. LEMARCHAND. 1996. Prospects for gene therapy in cardiovascular disease. Eur. Heart J. **17:** 1312–1317.
49. SMITHIES, O. 1997. A mouse view of hypertension. Hypertension **30:** 1318–1324.
50. FAZAN, R., JR., R.A. SHAFFER, F.M. ABBOUD & M.W. CHAPLEAU. 1999. Parasympathetic and sympathetic contributions to heart rate and arterial pressure variability in conscious mice (abstr.). FASEB J. **13**(4)Pt I: A453.
51. MA, X.Y., R.A. SHAFFER, F.M. ABBOUD & M.W. CHAPLEAU. 1998. Functional genomics: analysis of afferent, central and efferent components of baroreceptor reflex in mice (abstr.). FASEB J. **12**(4)Pt I: A359.
52. MA, X.Y., F.M. ABBOUD & M.W. CHAPLEAU. 1998. Baroreceptor sensitivity and baroreflex control of renal sympathetic nerve activity in mice (abstr.). J. Invest. Med. **46**(3): 200A.
53. MA, X., F.M. ABBOUD & M.W. CHAPLEAU. 2001. A novel effect of angiotensin on renal sympathetic nerve activity in mice. J. Hypertension **19**(3): 609–618.
54. SUN, W., F.M. ABBOUD & M.W. CHAPLEAU. 2000. Evaluation of baroreflex and chemoreflex by carotid artery occlusion in mice: a method for phenotypic analysis of deletion of candidate sensory molecules (abstr.). Circulation **102**(18): II-700.
55. MA, X., M.W. CHAPLEAU, C.A. WHITEIS, *et al.* 2001. Angiotensin selectively activates a subpopulation of post-ganglionic sympathetic neurons in mice. Circ. Res. **88:** 787–793.
56. MA, X.Y., R.A. SHAFFER, C.D. SIGMUND, *et al.* 1999. Mechanisms of impaired baroreflex control of sympathetic nerve activity in hypertensive renin-angiotensinogen double transgenic mice (abstr.). FASEB J. **13**(5)Pt II: A775.
57. MA, X.Y., F.M. ABBOUD & M.W. CHAPLEAU. 2000. Altered baroreflex control of renal sympathetic nerve activity in normotensive apo-E deficient atherosclerotic mice (abstr.). Physiologist **43**(4): 275.
58. SUN, W., F.M. ABBOUD & M.W. CHAPLEAU. 2001. Altered baro- and chemoreflex sensitivity revealed by carotid artery occlusion reflex in apo-E knockout mice (abstr.). FASEB J. **15**(5)Pt. II: A1146.
59. MEYRELLES, S.S., H.Z. MAO, D.D. HEISTAD & M.W. CHAPLEAU. 1997. Gene transfer to carotid sinus *in vivo*: a novel approach to investigation of baroreceptors. Hypertension **30**(3) [part 2]: 708–713.
60. MEYRELLES, S.S., H.Z. MAO, R.V. SHARMA & M.W. CHAPLEAU. 1998. Baroreceptor resetting and vessel remodeling after gene transfer of nitric oxide synthase to carotid sinus (abstr.). FASEB J. **12**(5)PtII: A687.
61. MEYRELLES, S. & M. CHAPLEAU. 2000. Impaired carotid occlusion reflex in apoE deficient mice and its reversal by gene transfer to carotid sinus (abstr.). J. Hypertens. **18**(Suppl. 4): S202.
62. RIOS, C.D., H. OOBOSHI, D. PIEGORS, *et al.* 1995. Adenovirus-mediated gene transfer to normal and atherosclerotic arteries: a novel approach. Arterioscler. Thromb. Vasc. Biol. **15:** 2241–2245.
63. CHEN, A.F.Y., S.-W. JIANG, T.B. CROTTY, *et al.* 1997. Effects of *in vivo* adventitial expression of recombinant endothelial nitric oxide synthase gene in cerebral arteries. Proc. Natl. Acad. Sci. USA **94:** 12568–12573.
64. MEYRELLES, S.S., R.V. SHARMA, C.A. WHITEIS, *et al.* 1997. Adenovirus-mediated gene transfer to cultured nodose sensory neurons. Mol. Brain Res. **5**(1–2): 33–41.

# Arterial Baroreceptors and Experimental Diabetes

HELIO C. SALGADO,[a] RUBENS FAZAN, JR.,[b] VALÉRIA P. S. FAZAN,[b]
VALDO J. DIAS DA SILVA,[b] AND AMILTON A. BARREIRA[c]

[a]Department of Physiology, School of Medicine of Ribeirão Preto,
University of São Paulo, Ribeirão Preto, SP, Brazil

[b]Department of Biological Science, School of Medicine of Triângulo Mineiro,
Uberaba, MG, Brazil

[c]Department of Neurology, School of Medicine of Ribeirão Preto,
University of São Paulo, Ribeirão Preto, SP, Brazil

ABSTRACT: Alterations of the autonomic reflex control of the cardiovascular
system have been demonstrated in clinical and animal models of insulin-
dependent diabetes mellitus. Established neuroaxonal dystrophy is considered
the neuropathological hallmark of chronic experimental diabetes. However,
the afferent arm of the arterial baroreflex, that is, the carotid sinus nerve and
the aortic depressor nerve, has received much less attention in studies dealing
with this physiopathological model. The attenuation of the pressure response
to bilateral carotid occlusion in conscious rats indicates a derangement of the
baroreflex, probably involving an alteration of the carotid sinus nerve. There
is histological evidence obtained from adult spontaneous insulin-dependent
diabetic rats (strain BB/S) of a carotid sinus nerve with signs of axonal swelling
and intramyelinic edema, suggesting diabetic neuropathy. The study of aortic
baroreceptor activity in anesthetized rats with short- and long-term streptozotocin diabetes by means of cross-spectral analysis of baroreceptor activity
versus arterial pressure revealed a dysfunction in the afferent arm of the
baroreflex even during a short period of diabetes. The morphology of the aortic
depressor nerve of streptozotocin-diabetic rats indicated axonal atrophy by
visual analysis remarkably at the distal segments of the nerves. This finding
was confirmed by morphometric study of the myelinated fibers. In conclusion,
although studies of the arterial baroreceptors related to experimental diabetes
are scanty in the literature, there is electrophysiological and histological evidence demonstrating that the carotid sinus and the aortic depressor nerves are
abnormal in this experimental model.

KEYWORDS: Streptozotocin; Aortic depressor nerve; Carotid sinus nerve;
Baroreflex; Neuroaxonal dystrophy; Diabetic neuropathy; Cross-spectral
analysis

Address for correspondence: Helio C. Salgado, M.D., Ph.D., Department of Physiology,
School of Medicine of Ribeirão Preto, University of São Paulo, 14049-900 Ribeirão Preto, SP,
Brazil. Fax: (55) 16 633 0017.
hcsalgad@fmrp.usp.br

20

Diabetes mellitus, a metabolic disease caused by a deficiency in pancreatic insulin secretion and/or impaired tissue responsiveness to insulin, is commonly associated with a large number of complications. Neuropathy, involving not only the somatic, but also the autonomic nervous system, is often associated with diabetes mellitus with reported frequencies ranging from 5% to 60%.[1–3] Symptoms like orthostatic hypotension, painless myocardial infarction, and decreased exercise tolerance, as well as clinical findings like decreased heart rate variability and impaired cardiac baroreflex, have been considered to be a consequence of the involvement of cardiac innervation by diabetic autonomic neuropathy. Diabetic patients with abnormal cardiovascular reflexes have a higher incidence of mortality than those with normal reflex function.[4]

Animal models of diabetes have been widely used in biomedical studies because they offer promise of new insights into human diabetes. Streptozotocin (STZ)–treated rats are an animal model of insulin-dependent diabetes mellitus (IDDM) commonly used to study cardiovascular alterations caused by diabetes even though their change in cardiovascular function does not fully match the alterations observed under clinical conditions.[5]

## BAROREFLEX AND DIABETES

Dysfunction of baroreflex control of arterial pressure and heart rate has been well described in the literature not only in diabetic patients, but also in experimental models of diabetes. Rats with STZ-induced diabetes present baroreflex dysfunction as early as 5 days after the administration of STZ.[6] It has been well documented that the neuropathy associated with diabetes affects the autonomic nervous system in both of its arms (sympathetic and parasympathetic).[5] Most of the reports showing impairment of baroreflex sensitivity attribute it to the autonomic efferent neuropathy. The afferent arm of the baroreflex, that is, the arterial baroreceptors (carotid and aortic nerves), has received much less attention in diabetes.

## CAROTID SINUS NERVE

Bilateral carotid occlusion (BCO) has been used as a tool to cause overactivity of the peripheral sympathetic drive in either conscious[7–9] or anesthetized[10,11] animals. The cardiovascular effects of BCO consist of an increase in arterial pressure, tachycardia, and an increase in myocardial contractility. BCO in the experimental model of diabetes has been used in dogs and rats, usually to promote ischemia or sympathetic activation to examine some aspects of the disease, such as metabolism of the ischemic brain,[12,13] insulin secretion,[14] or the effect of controlled changes of plasma insulin and glucose concentration on the cardiac response to an increase of the sympathetic drive.[15] The pressure response to BCO in conscious rats presents two components: an initial peak of carotid reflex origin followed by a sustained response probably of ischemic brain origin.[16,17] Recent findings from our laboratory have demonstrated that chronic experimental diabetes elicited by STZ blunted the initial peak of the pressure response to BCO in conscious rats, providing evidence of an impairment of the carotid sinus nerve.[18] Although no studies have been conducted to

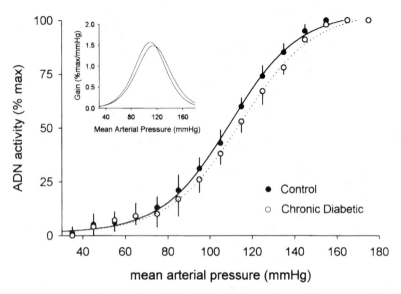

**FIGURE 1.** Plots showing the relationship between mean arterial pressure and aortic depressor nerve activity, expressed as percentage of maximal activity, fitted by logistic-sigmoidal regression. Curves were obtained in control (●) or chronic (12 weeks) STZ-diabetic (○) rats. The inset shows the gain of aortic baroreceptors (first derivate of sigmoidal regression).

determine the effect of diabetes on carotid sinus nerve activity, there is histological evidence from adult spontaneous insulin-dependent diabetic rats (strain BB/S) of a carotid sinus nerve with signs of diabetic neuropathy, that is, axonal swelling and intramyelinic edema.[19]

## AORTIC DEPRESSOR NERVE

Baroreceptor function studied by means of electroneurography in single fibers of an isolated aortic arch/aortic nerve preparation from STZ-diabetic rats[20] and in a multifiber preparation of the aortic nerve of chronic alloxan-diabetic rabbits[21] has been shown to be unaltered. In agreement with previous studies, we found no evidence of any alteration of the aortic depressor nerve (ADN) activity in anesthetized chronic STZ-diabetic rats[22] evaluated by means of pressure/nerve activity curves. We also demonstrated that the ADN of chronic STZ-diabetic rats preserved its ability to rapidly (30 min) reset to hypertensive levels[22] (FIG. 1).

Nevertheless, we also examined[23] the aortic baroreceptor activity in anesthetized rats with short-term (10–20 days) or long-term (12–18 weeks) STZ diabetes by means of spontaneous (respiratory) oscillations of arterial pressure. The arterial pressure variability spectra of pentobarbital-anesthetized rats showed a single peak at the respiratory frequency containing almost all the pressure variability (FIG. 2). Cross-spectral analysis showed a high coherence between arterial pressure and ADN

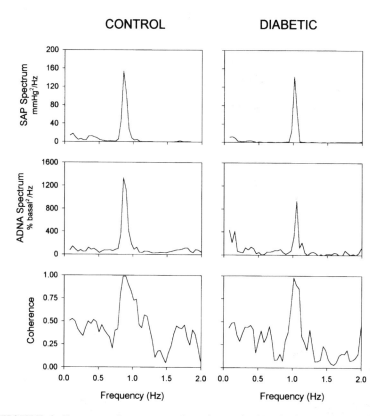

**FIGURE 2.** Representative spectrum from time series beat-by-beat mean arterial pressure (*top*), beat-by-beat integrated ADN activity (*middle*), and coherence between both spectra (*bottom*) from a control (left column) and a long-term (12 weeks) STZ-diabetic rat (right column).

activity at the respiratory frequency with a positive phase, indicating that the respiratory-mediated oscillations in arterial pressure led to ADN activity variability at this frequency. Therefore, we used the magnitude of the transfer function obtained by cross-spectral analysis[24] between beat-by-beat time series of mean arterial pressure and ADN activity as the index of baroreceptor sensitivity (FIG. 3). This new approach has the advantage of permitting the assessment of baroreceptor function under more physiological conditions when compared to the pressure/nerve activity curve studied previously,[22] that is, within a narrow range of arterial pressure variation, contrasting with the wide range (threshold pressure through saturation of the baroreceptors) employed to obtain the pressure/nerve activity curve. The results obtained indicated that both diabetic groups presented a similar remarkable impairment of the baroreceptor sensitivity.[23] Thus, in contrast to previous observations that the aortic baroreceptors were not affected by chronic STZ diabetes,[22] the cross-spectral analysis of baroreceptor activity versus arterial pressure revealed a dysfunction in the afferent arm of the baroreflex, even during a shorter period of diabetes.[22]

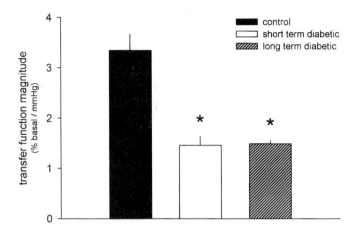

**FIGURE 3.** Bar graph showing the aortic baroreceptor sensitivity assessed by the transfer function magnitude obtained by cross-spectral analysis between mean arterial pressure and ADN activity spectra at the frequency of maximum coherence in control and diabetic groups. *$p < 0.01$ compared to control group.

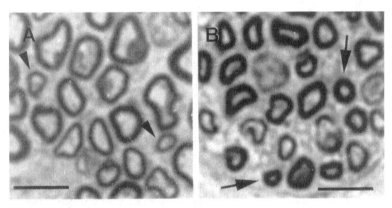

**FIGURE 4.** Endoneural cross-sectional area of the ADN of a control **(A)** and a 15-day diabetic rat **(B)**, under oil immersion lens. Arrows in B indicate fibers with axonal atrophy, compared to normal fibers of approximately the same size shown in A (*arrowheads*). Toluidine blue stained; bar = 5 μm.

We also evaluated in our laboratory the morphology of the ADN myelinated fibers in short-term (15 days) STZ diabetes.[25] Visual morphological analysis of the ADN of STZ-diabetic rats indicated characteristics of axonal atrophy (FIG. 4) in 5 of the 10 nerves studied. As the axon atrophies, the myelin occupies an increasing fraction of the cross-sectional area. The cross-sectional area of the axoplasm is reduced as the myelin collapses into the axonal space, so an abnormally large proportion of the fiber's cross section is occupied by myelin. These characteristics were more marked on the distal (close to the aorta) segments of the nerves and were confirmed by the morphometric study. The axonal atrophy was confirmed by the $G$ ratio (ratio between the axon diameter and whole fiber diameter) histograms, which showed, by the chi-square goodness-of-fit test, a shift to the left for the diabetic nerves ($N = 10$) compared to the normal nerves ($N = 6$). Our findings are in agreement with the reports of axonal changes in myelinated fibers of peripheral nerves from diabetic patients that can be selective to small myelinated fibers[26] and that are predominant distally.[27] Therefore, these data provide morphological support for altered baroreceptor afference in STZ-diabetic rats.

## AORTIC BARORECEPTOR TERMINALS

The aortic baroreceptors (mechanoreceptors) are neural endings present in the ascending aorta, consisting of afferent myelinated (fast conducting) and unmyelinated (slow conducting) nerve fibers. In mammals commonly used as experimental models, the nerve fibers originating from these receptors travel to the central nervous system through the vagus nerve or they can originate as a slender isolated nerve (the ADN or Cyon's nerve) that joins the trunk of the vagus (close to the nodose ganglion) or the superior laryngeal nerve. Cyon and Ludwig,[28] who first described the ADN in rabbits, believed that its fibers were mixed with those of the cardiac plexus, although small branches to the aorta were also described. Köster and Tschermak[29] were the first to document the pathway of the ADN fibers to the aorta and innominate artery with the aid of histological techniques and showed that this nerve ends as small branches, forming a neural plexus on the aortic wall. They also described that most of the fibers were restricted to the adventitia, with some of them reaching the muscular layer (tunica media). In histological preparations of the ADN of rabbits, Sarkar[30] identified myelinated fibers of medium and small caliber and unmyelinated fibers. These findings were confirmed for the ADN of rats by electron microscopy technique.[31]

The terminals of the ADN and the baroreceptors were studied by light[32] and electron microscopy.[33] By light microscopy, Aumonier[32] identified baroreceptor terminals in the adventitia and the muscular layer of the aorta of rabbits, dogs, and cats. These results were in agreement with those of Köster and Tschermak.[29] On the other hand, an ultrastructural study of the baroreceptors of rats[33] showed that, although some receptors are located close to the muscular layer of the aorta, they are located in regions of the adventitia that invaginate into the muscular layer without entering it. Pathologic processes like hypertension and diabetes are known to cause reduction of the distensibility of blood vessels. Dysfunction of the baroreceptors has been found in hypertensive animals and has been ascribed, at least in part, to the morphological alterations of the aortic wall, such as hypertrophy.[34] Very little is known about diabetic dysfunction of the baroreceptors and there are no reports in the literature on the morphological alterations in experimental models of diabetes.

## CONCLUDING REMARKS

Alterations of the autonomic reflex control of the cardiovascular system have been demonstrated in clinical and animal models of insulin-dependent diabetes mellitus (IDDM). The identification of the site (afference, central nervous system, and efference) of impairment of the baroreflex in diabetes has been the objective of a number of studies in the literature. While it is well documented that motor, sensory, and autonomic nerves are affected by the diabetic neuropathy, the afferent arm of the baroreflex, that is, the arterial baroreceptors (carotid and aortic nerves), has received much less attention.

*Carotid sinus nerve:* Recent findings from our laboratory demonstrated an attenuation of the pressure response to bilateral carotid occlusion in conscious chronic STZ-treated rats, providing evidence of an impairment of the carotid sinus nerve.[18] A study on adult spontaneous insulin-dependent diabetic rats (strain BB/S) has reported a carotid sinus nerve with axonal swelling and intramyelinic edema suggestive of diabetic neuropathy.[19]

*Aortic depressor nerve:* In contrast to previous observations that the aortic baroreceptors were not affected by chronic STZ diabetes,[20–22] the cross-spectral analysis of baroreceptor activity versus arterial pressure revealed a dysfunction in the afferent arm of the baroreflex even during a shorter period of diabetes.[23] The morphological analysis of the aortic depressor nerve of STZ-diabetic rats indicated characteristics of axonal atrophy, more marked at the distal segments of the nerves, which were confirmed by the morphometric study. These data provide morphological support of altered baroreceptor afference in STZ-diabetic rats.[25]

## ACKNOWLEDGMENTS

This research has been supported by FAPESP, CAPES CNPq, and FINEP (PRONEX Grant No. 357/96).

## REFERENCES

1. OLEFSKY, J.M. 1985. Diabetes mellitus. *In* Cecil Textbook of Medicine, pp. 1320–1341. Saunders. Philadelphia.
2. NIAKAN, E., Y. HARATI & J.P. COMSTOCK. 1986. Diabetic autonomic neuropathy. Metabolism **35**: 224–234.
3. VINIK, A. & B. MITCHELL. 1988. Clinical aspects of diabetic neuropathies. Diabetes Metab. Rev. **4**: 223–253.
4. EWING, D.J., I.W. CAMPBELL & B.F. CLARKE. 1980. The natural history of diabetic autonomic neuropathy. Q. J. Med. **49**: 95–108.
5. HICKS, K.K. *et al.* 1998. Effects of streptozotocin-induced diabetes on heart rate, blood pressure, and cardiac autonomic nervous control. J. Auton. Nerv. Syst. **69**: 21–30.
6. MAEDA, C.Y. *et al.* 1995. Autonomic dysfunction in short-term experimental diabetes. Hypertension **26**: 1100–1104.
7. DiCARLO, S.E. *et al.* 1989. The role of vasopressin in the pressor response to bilateral carotid occlusion. J. Auton. Nerv. Syst. **27**: 1–10.
8. MACHADO, B.H. *et al.* 1992. Changes in vascular resistance during carotid occlusion in normal and baroreceptor-denervated rats. Hypertension **19**: 149–153.
9. KUMAGAI, K. & I.A. REID. 1994. Losartan inhibits sympathetic and cardiovascular responses to carotid occlusion. Hypertension **23**: 827–831.
10. WANG, H.H. *et al.* 1970. Participation of cardiac and peripheral sympathetics in carotid occlusion response. Am. J. Physiol. **218**: 1548–1554.
11. DAMPNEY, R.A.L., M. KUMADA & D.J. REIS. 1979. Characterization, effect of brainstem and cranial nerve transections, and simulation by electrical stimulation of restricted regions of medulla oblongata in rabbit. Circ. Res. **44**: 48–62.

12. SUGIMORI, H. *et al.* 1996. Mild hyperglycemia and insulin treatment in experimental cerebral ischemia in rats. Brain Res. Bull. **40:** 263–268.
13. LANIER, W.L., R.E. HOFER & W.J. GALLAGHER. 1996. Metabolism of glucose, glycogen, and high-energy phosphates during transient forebrain ischemia in diabetic rats: effect of insulin treatment. Anesthesiology **84:** 917–925.
14. LEE, K.C. & R.E. MILLER. 1985. Bilateral carotid occlusion and the sympathetic regulation of insulin secretion. J. Auton. Nerv. Syst. **14:** 181–190.
15. FITZOVICH, D.E. & D.C. RANDALL. 1990. Modulation of baroreflex by varying insulin and glucose in conscious dogs. Am. J. Physiol. **258:** R624–R633.
16. MAIO, A.A. *et al.* 1981. Cardiovascular responses of conscious rats due to arterial occlusion [abstract]. Braz. J. Med. Biol. Res. **14:** 115.
17. BEDRAN-DE-CASTRO, M.T., E.D. MOREIRA & E.M. KRIEGER. 1986. Reflex and central components of carotid occlusion in conscious rats: effect of lesion of the medial forebrain bundle. Hypertension **8:** 147–151.
18. SALGADO, H.C. *et al.* 2000. Pressure response to bilateral carotid occlusion in conscious chronic diabetic rats: effect of insulin therapy [abstract]. J. Hypertens. **18**(suppl. 4): S138.
19. CLARKE, J.A. *et al.* 1999. The carotid body of the spontaneous insulin-dependent diabetic rat. Braz. J. Med. Biol. Res. **32:** 85–91.
20. REYNOLDS, P.J. *et al.* 1990. Aortic baroreceptor function in long term streptozotocin diabetic rats [abstract]. Soc. Neurosci. Abstr. **16:** 221.
21. MCDOWELL, T.S. *et al.* 1994. Baroreflex dysfunction in diabetes mellitus. II. Site of baroreflex impairment in diabetic rabbits. Am. J. Physiol. **266:** H244–H249.
22. FAZAN, R., JR. *et al.* 1997. Heart rate variability and baroreceptor function in chronic diabetic rats. Hypertension **30:** 632–635.
23. FAZAN, R., JR., V.J.D. SILVA & H.C. SALGADO. 2000. Baroreceptor function in streptozotocin-induced diabetes in rats: a spectral analysis approach [abstract]. J. Hypertens. **18**(suppl. 4): S136.
24. DE BOER, R.W., J.M. KAREMAKER & J. STRACKEE. 1987. Hemodynamic fluctuations and baroreflex sensitivity in humans: a beat-to-beat model. Am. J. Physiol. **253:** H680–H689.
25. FAZAN, V.P.S., H.C. SALGADO & A.A. BARREIRA. 2000. Early stages of experimental diabetes in rats induce morphological alterations of the aortic depressor nerve myelinated fibers [abstract]. Physiologist **43:** 261.
26. BROWN, M.J., J.R. MARTIN & A.K. ASBURY. 1976. Painful diabetic neuropathy: a morphometric study. Arch. Neurol. **33:** 167–171.
27. SAID, G., G. SLAMA & J. SELVA. 1983. Progressive centripetal degeneration of axons in small fiber type diabetic polyneuropathy: a clinical and pathological study. Brain **106:** 791–807.
28. CYON, E. & C. LUDWIG. 1866. Die Reflexe eines der sensiblen Nerven des Herzens auf die motorischen der Blutgefässe. Arb. Physiol. Anst. Leipz. **1:** 128–150.
29. KÖSTER, G. & A.A. TSCHERMAK. 1902. Über Ursprung und Endigung des n. depressor und n. laryngeus superior beim Kaninchen. Arch. Anat. Entwickelungeschicht. **25:** 255–294.
30. SARKAR, B.B. 1922. The depressor nerve of the rabbit. R. Soc. Proc. **93:** 230–235.
31. FAZAN, V.P.S., H.C. SALGADO & A.A. BARREIRA. 1997. A descriptive and quantitative light and electron microscopy study of the aortic depressor nerve in normotensive rats. Hypertension **30:** 693–698.
32. AUMONIER, F.J. 1972. Histological observations on the distribution of baroreceptors in the carotid and aortic regions of the rabbit, cat, and dog. Acta Anat. **82:** 1–16.
33. KRAHUS, J.M. 1979. Structure of rat aortic baroreceptors and their relationship to connective tissue. J. Neurocytol. **8:** 401–414.
34. SAPRU, H.N. & S.C. WANG. 1976. Modification of aortic baroreceptor resetting in the spontaneously hypertensive rat. Am. J. Physiol. **230:** 664–674.

# Degenerins

## At the Core of the Metazoan Mechanotransducer?

NEKTARIOS TAVERNARAKIS AND MONICA DRISCOLL

*Department of Molecular Biology and Biochemistry, Rutgers,*
*The State University of New Jersey, Piscataway, New Jersey 08855, USA*

ABSTRACT: Mechanosensory signaling, believed to be mediated by mechanically gated ion channels, constitutes the basis for the senses of touch and hearing, and contributes fundamentally to the development and homeostasis of all organisms. Despite this profound importance in biology, little is known of the molecular identities or functional requirements of mechanically gated ion channels. Genetic analyses of touch sensation and locomotion in *Caenorhabditis elegans* have implicated a new class of ion channels, the degenerins (DEG) in nematode mechanotransduction. Related fly and vertebrate proteins, the epithelial sodium channel (ENaC) family, have been implicated in several important processes, including transduction of mechanical stimuli, pain sensation, gametogenesis, sodium reabsorption, and blood pressure regulation. Still-to-be-discovered DEG/ENaC proteins may compose the core of the elusive human mechanotransducer.

KEYWORDS: *Caenorhabditis elegans*; Degenerin; ENaC; Ion channel; Mechanosensation; Neurodegeneration; Proprioception

## INTRODUCTION

Cell-volume regulation, gravitaxis, proprioception, touch sensation, and auditory transduction all depend on the conversion of mechanical energy into cellular responses.[1,2] Still, little is known about the molecular properties of ion channels specialized for mechanotransduction. Genetic studies in the nematode *Caenorhabditis elegans* were the first to identify eukaryotic genes that encode subunits of candidate mechanically gated ion channels involved in mediating touch transduction, proprioception, and coordinated locomotion.[3–6] These channel subunits belong to a large family of related proteins in *C. elegans* referred to as degenerins, because unusual gain-of-function mutations in several family members induce swelling or cell degeneration[3,7] (see DEGENERINS AND DEGENERATION below).

*C. elegans* degenerins exhibit approximately 25–30% sequence identity to subunits of the vertebrate amiloride-sensitive epithelial Na$^+$ channels (ENaCs; see Ref. 8), which are required for ion transport across epithelia.[9] Together the *C. elegans* and vertebrate proteins define the degenerin/epithelial sodium channel (DEG/ENaC) superfamily of ion channels.[10,11] DEG/ENaC proteins range from about 550 to 950

Address for correspondence: Nektarios Tavernarakis, Nelson Biological Laboratories A220, 604 Allison Road, Piscataway, NJ 08855. Voice: 732-445-7187; fax: 732-445-4213.
email: tavernarakis@mbcl.rutgers.edu

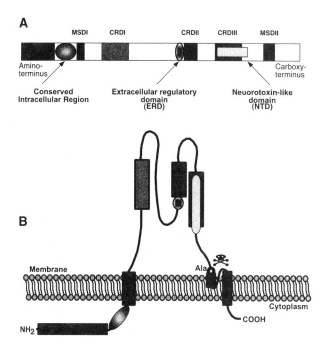

**FIGURE 1.** Schematic representation of DEG/ENaC ion-channel subunit structure and topology. (**A**) General features: *Shaded boxes* indicate defined channel modules. These include the two membrane-spanning domains (MSDs), and the three cysteine-rich domains (CRDs; the first CRD is absent in mammalian channels). The *small oval* depicts the putative extracellular regulatory domain (ERD) identified by García-Añoveros and co-workers in *C. elegans* degenerins.[30] The *box* overlapping with CRDIII denotes the neurotoxin-related domain (NTD; see Ref. 12). The conserved intracellular region is also shown. (**B**) Transmembrane topology: Both terminals are intracellular, with the largest part of the protein situated outside the cell. The *dot* near MSDII represents the amino-acid position (Alanine 713 in MEC-4) affected in dominant, toxic degenerin mutants.

amino acids in length and share several distinguishing blocks of sequence similarity[12] (FIGURE 1A). Subunit topology is invariable: all members of the DEG/ENaC superfamily have two membrane-spanning domains with cysteine-rich domains (CRDs; the most conserved is designated CRDIII) situated between the transmembrane segments.[13,14] N- and C-terminals project into the intracellular cytoplasm, while most of the protein, including the CRDs, is extracellular (FIGURE 1B).

Members of the DEG/ENaC superfamily have been identified from nematodes, snails, flies, and many vertebrates, including humans, and are expressed in tissues as diverse as kidney epithelia, muscle, and neurons. With the sequence analysis of the *C. elegans* genome now complete, it is possible to survey the entire gene family within this organism. At present 25 members of the DEG/ENaC superfamily have

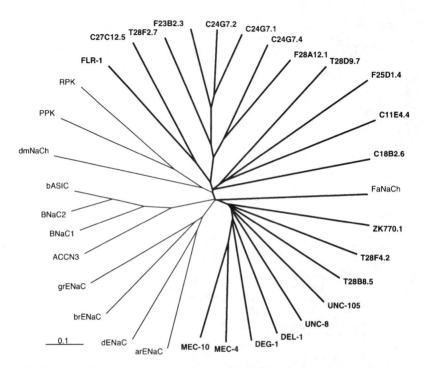

**FIGURE 2.** Phylogenetic relations between DEG/ENaC proteins. The degenerin content of the complete nematode genome is shown in bold. Other DEG/ENaC proteins from a variety of organisms, ranging from snails to humans, are also included. The *scale bar* denotes evolutionary distance equal to 0.1 nucleotide substitutions per site.

been identified in the *C. elegans* genome (FIGURE 2). An experimental challenge is to decipher the biological functions of all these channel subunits and their mammalian counterparts. Here we review analysis of the *C. elegans* family members directly implicated in mechanotransduction and discuss potential roles of their mammalian counterparts in mechanical signaling.

## FEATURES OF THE *C. elegans* MODEL SYSTEM: ADVANTAGES FOR GENETIC AND MOLECULAR STUDIES OF MECHANICAL SIGNALING

*C. elegans* is a small (1-mm) free-living hermaphroditic nematode that completes a life cycle in 2.5 days at 25°C. Mutations can be easily induced and large screens can be performed to isolate mutants having specific phenotypes. The simple body plan and transparent nature of both the egg and the cuticle of this nematode have facilitated an exceptionally detailed developmental characterization of the animal. The complete sequence of cell divisions and the normal pattern of programmed cell deaths that occur as the fertilized egg develops into the 959-celled adult are known.[15]

One considerable advantage of the *C. elegans* system is that it is the first metazoan for which the genome was sequenced to completion.[16] Investigators can take advantage of genome data to perform "reverse genetics," directly knocking out genes. In addition, a novel method of generating mutant phenocopies, called double-stranded RNA-mediated interference (RNAi), enables probable loss-of-function phenotypes to be rapidly evaluated.[17] Another advantage of this system is that construction of transgenic animals is rapid; DNA injected into the hermaphrodite gonad concatamerizes and is packaged into embryos, hundreds of which can be obtained within a few days of the injection.[18]

The anatomical characterization and understanding of neuronal connectivity in *C. elegans* are unparalleled in the metazoan world. Serial section electron microscopy has identified the pattern of synaptic connections made by each of the 302 neurons of the animal (including 5000 chemical synapses, 600 gap junctions, and 2000 neuromuscular junctions), so that the full "wiring diagram" of the animal is known.[19] Although the overall number of neurons is small, 118 different neuronal classes, including many neuronal types present in mammals, can be distinguished. Other animal model systems contain many more neurons of each class (there are about 10,000 more neurons in *Drosophila* with approximately the same repertoire of neuronal types). Overall, the broad range of genetic and molecular techniques applicable in the *C. elegans* model system allow a unique line of investigation into fundamental problems in biology, such as mechanical signaling.

## BEHAVIORS THAT DEPEND UPON MECHANOTRANSDUCTION IN *C. elegans*

Mechanical stimuli regulate many *C. elegans* behaviors, including locomotion, foraging, egg laying, feeding (pharyngeal pumping), and defecation. The mechanosensitive response best characterized at the cellular, genetic, and molecular levels is the movement away from a light touch delivered to the body with an eyelash hair referred to as body touch sensation.[20] Another behavioral paradigm that has been elegantly utilized to study mechanosensory control of locomotion is the response to nose touch, the reversal of direction as a consequence of head-on collision or a light touch on the side of the nose (reviewed in Ref. 21). Other touch-mediated locomotory responses, such as a reaction to harsh touch (a strong prod with a metal wire, best assayed in the absence of gentle touch mechanosensory neurons; see Ref. 22) or to tap (a diffuse stimulus as delivered by a tap on the plate on which worms are reared; Ref. 23), have been less extensively studied at the genetic level.

## CELLULAR REQUIREMENTS FOR BODY TOUCH SENSATION

In the laboratory, *C. elegans* moves through a bacterial lawn on a petri plate with a readily observed sinusoidal motion. When gently touched with an eyelash hair (typically attached to a toothpick) on the posterior, an animal will move forward; when touched on the anterior body, it will move backward (FIGURE 3A). This gentle body touch is sensed by the touch receptor neurons anterior lateral microtubule cell left, right (ALML/R), anterior ventral microtubule cell (AVM), and posterior lateral

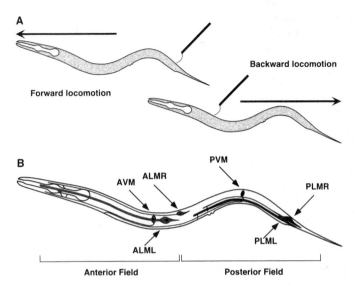

**FIGURE 3.** The nematode touch response. (**A**) The behavior. When animals are stimulated with an eyelash hair attached to a toothpick at the anterior field, they respond by moving backwards. Stimulation at the posterior field results in moving to the opposite direction. (**B**) The neurons: Schematic diagram showing the position of the six touch receptor neurons in the body of the adult nematode. Two fields of touch sensitivity are defined by the arrangement of these neurons along the body axis. The ALMs and AVM mediate the response to touch over the anterior field, whereas PLMs mediate the response to touch over the posterior field. PVM does not mediate touch response by itself.

microtubule cell left, right (PLML/R); FIGURE 3B).[20,24] Posterior ventral microtubule (PVM) is a neuron that is morphologically similar to the touch receptor neurons and expresses genes specific for touch receptor neurons but has been shown to be incapable of mediating normal touch response by itself. The touch receptors are situated so that their processes run longitudinally along the body wall embedded in the hypodermis adjacent to the cuticle. The position of the processes along the body axis correlates with the sensory field of the touch cell. Laser ablation of AVM and the ALMs, which have sensory receptor processes in the anterior half of the body, eliminates anterior touch sensitivity, and laser ablation of the PLMs, which have posterior dendritic processes, eliminates posterior touch sensitivity. In addition to mediating touch avoidance, the touch receptor neurons appear to control the spontaneous rate of locomotion, since animals that lack functional touch cells are lethargic. The mechanical stimuli that drive spontaneous locomotion are unknown, but could include encounters with objects in their environments or body stretch induced by locomotion itself.

Touch receptor neurons have two distinguishing features. First, they are surrounded by a specialized extracellular matrix called the mantle, which appears to attach the cell to the cuticle. Second, they are filled with unusual 15-protofilament microtubules.[20] Genetic studies suggest that both features are critical for the function of these neurons as receptors of body touch (reviewed in Ref. 21).

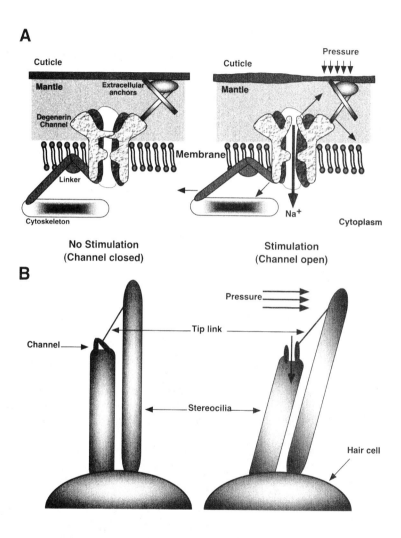

**FIGURE 4.** Models of mechanotransduction: (**A**) A touch transducing complex in *C. elegans* touch receptor neurons. In the absence of mechanical stimulation the channel is closed, and therefore the sensory neuron is idle. Application of a mechanical force to the body of the animal results in distortion of a network of interacting molecules that opens the degenerin channel. Na$^+$ influx depolarizes the neuron initiating the perceptory integration of the stimulus. (**B**) Mechanical gating of the channels in vertebrate hair cells. Mechanosensory channels situated at the stereocilla tips are pulled open by the tip-link when stereocilia are deflected.(Adapted from Pickles and Corey.[40] Reproduced by permission.)

## IDENTIFICATION OF PROTEINS REQUIRED SPECIFICALLY
## FOR BODY TOUCH

Elegant genetic analysis has identified approximately 15 genes that, when mutated, specifically disrupt gentle body touch sensation, and are therefore thought to encode candidate mediators of touch sensitivity (these genes were named *mec* genes, since when they are defective, animals are *mec*hanosensory abnormal[25]). Many of the *mec* genes have now been molecularly identified and most of them encode proteins postulated to make up a touch-transducing complex.[26,27] The core elements of this mechanosensory complex are the channel subunits MEC-4 and MEC-10,[27,28] which can interact genetically and physically.[28–30] Both these proteins are DEG/ENaC family members.[8] Genetic arguments support that at least two MEC-4 and at least two MEC-10 subunits are assembled in the heteromeric touch-transducing channel.[4] The MEC-4 and MEC-10 extracellular domains are postulated to be linked to a touch cell-specific specialized extracellular matrix.[31] Channel intracellular domains are hypothesized to be tied to the cytoskeleton.[32] The tethering of channel subunits to the extracellular matrix and the intracellular cytoskeleton is postulated to confer channel gating tension. In this model, the minute mechanical deflection produced by light touch causes a conformational change in the channel, which is stretched between two attachment points, directly opening a gate for ion flow.[27,28] Below, we discuss a model accommodating the information available on the structure of a nematode mechanotransducing complex (see section on modeling mechanical signaling in *C. elegans* and FIGURE 4).

## DEGENERINS AND PROPRIOCEPTION

Unusual, *semi*dominant gain-of-function mutations in another degenerin gene, *unc-8*, [*unc-8(sd)*] induce transient neuronal swelling[33] and severe uncoordination.[34,35] *unc-8* encodes a degenerin expressed in several motor neuron classes and in some interneurons and nose touch sensory neurons.[6] Interestingly, semidominant *unc-8* alleles alter an amino acid in the region hypothesized to be an extracellular channel-closing domain defined in studies of *deg-1* and *mec-4* degenerins[6,30] (see also FIGURE 1A). The genetics of *unc-8* are further similar to those of *mec-4* and *mec-10*; specific *unc-8* alleles can suppress or enhance *unc-8(sd)* mutations *in trans*, suggesting that UNC-8::UNC-8 interactions occur. Another degenerin family member, *del-1*(for *d*egenerin-*l*ike) is coexpressed in a subset of neurons that express *unc-8* (the VA and VB motor neurons) and is likely to assemble into a channel complex with UNC-8 in these cells.[6]

What function does the UNC-8 degenerin channel serve in motorneurons? *unc-8* null mutants have a subtle locomotion defect.[6] Wild-type animals move through an *E. coli* lawn with a characteristic sinusoidal pattern (this occurs by localized alternating contraction and relaxation of body-wall muscles; see more detailed discussion in Refs. 16 and 22). *unc-8* null mutants inscribe a path in an *E. coli* lawn that is markedly reduced in both wavelength and amplitude, as compared to wild-type. This phenotype indicates that the UNC-8 degenerin channel functions to modulate the locomotory trajectory of the animal.

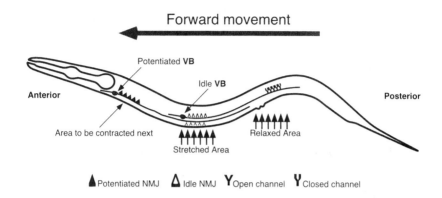

**FIGURE 5.** Model for modulation of locomotion by stretch-responsive channels in motor neurons. Two VB motor neurons in the ventral nerve cord are shown with stretch-sensitive channels postulated to be situated in their undifferentiated processes. The anterior VB signal to muscle is potentiated by the opening of ion channels in its process that experiences stretch due to local body bend. This motor neuron will signal to the anterior muscles to then become fully contracted. At the same time another motor neuron in the middle of the body remains idle because its process does not receive a stretch stimulus. Sequential activation of motor neurons that are distributed along the ventral nerve cord and signal nonoverlapping groups of muscles amplifies and propagates the sinusoidal body wave (NMJ: neuromuscular junction).

How does the UNC-8 motor neuron channel influence locomotion? One highly interesting morphological feature of some motorneurons (in particular, the VA and VB motorneurons that coexpress *unc-8* and *del-1*) is that their processes include extended regions that do not participate in neuromuscular junctions or neuronal synapses (see FIGURE 5). These "undifferentiated" process regions have been hypothesized to be stretch sensitive (discussed in Ref. 36). Given the morphological features of certain motor neurons and the sequence similarity of UNC-8 and DEL-1 to candidate mechanically gated channels, we have proposed that these subunits coassemble into a stretch-sensitive channel that might be localized to the undifferentiated regions of the motor neuron process.[6] When activated by the localized body stretch that occurs during locomotion, this motor neuron channel potentiates signaling at the neuromuscular junction, which is situated at a distance from the site of stretch stimulus (FIGURE 5). The stretch signal enhances motorneuron excitation of muscle, increasing the strength and duration of the pending muscle contraction and directing a full-size body turn. In the absence of the stretch activation, the body wave and locomotion still occur, but with significantly reduced amplitude because the potentiating stretch signal is not transmitted. This model bears similarity to the chain-reflex mechanism of movement pattern generation. However, it does not exclude a central oscillator that would be responsible for the rhythmic locomotion. Instead, we suggest that the output of such an oscillator is further enhanced and modulated by stretch-sensitive motorneurons.

One important corollary of the *unc-8* mutant studies is that the UNC-8 channel does not appear to be essential for motor-neuron function; if this were the case, animals lacking the *unc-8* gene would be severely paralyzed. This observation strengthens the argument that degenerin channels function directly in mechanotransduction rather than merely serving to maintain the osmotic environment so that other channels can function. As is true for the MEC-4 and MEC-10 touch receptor channels, the model of UNC-8 and DEL-1 function that is based on mutant phenotypes, cell morphologies, and molecular properties of degenerins remains to be tested by determining subcellular channel localization, subunit associations and, most importantly, channel gating properties.

## A MODEL FOR MECHANICAL SIGNALING IN *C. elegans*

The molecular features of cloned touch cell and motorneuron structural genes, together with genetic data that suggest interactions between them, constitute the basis of a model for the nematode mechanotransducing complex (FIGURE 4A; see Refs 26 31, 37, 38 for discussion). The central component of this model is the candidate mechanosensitive ion channel, which includes multiple MEC-4 and MEC-10 subunits in the case of touch receptor neurons, and UNC-8 and DEL-1 in the case of motorneurons. These subunits assemble to form a channel pore that is lined by hydrophilic residues in membrane-spanning domain II. Subunits adopt a topology in which the Cys-rich and NTD domains extend into the specialized extracellular matrix outside the touch cell and the amino- and carboxy-termini project into the cytoplasm.

Regulated gating is expected to depend on mechanical forces exerted on the channel. Tension is hypothesized to be delivered by tethering the extracellular channel domains to the specialized extracellular matrix and anchoring intracellular domains to the microtubule cytoskeleton. Outside the cell, channel subunits may contact extracellular matrix components. Inside the cell, channel subunits may interact with the cytoskeleton either directly or via protein links. A touch stimulus could deform the microtubule network, or could perturb the mantle connections to deliver the gating stimulus. In either scenario, $Na^+$ influx would activate the touch receptor to signal the appropriate locomotory response.

Interestingly, the model proposed for mechanotransduction in the touch receptor neurons shares features of the proposed gating mechanism of mechanosensory channels that respond to auditory stimuli in the hair cells of the vertebrate inner ear (FIGURE 4B; see Refs. 39 and 40). Stereocilia situated on the hair-cell apical surface are connected at their distal ends to neighboring stereocilia by filaments called tip links. Directional deflection of the stereocilia relative to each other introduces tension on the tip links, which is thought to open the mechanosensitive hair cell channels directly.

## DEGENERINS AND DEGENERATION

MEC-4, MEC-10, and several related nematode degenerins have a second, unusual property: specific amino-acid substitutions in these proteins result in aberrant channels that induce the swelling and subsequent necrotic death of the cells in which they are expressed.[3,7] This pathological property is the reason that proteins of this subfamily were originally called degenerins.[7]

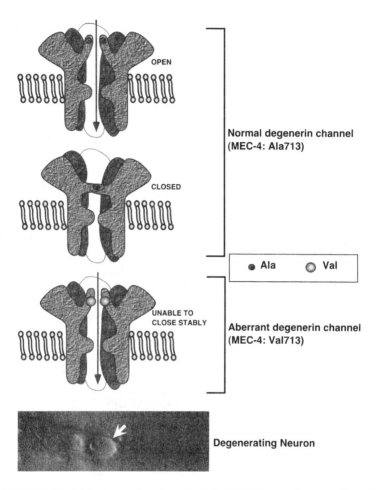

**FIGURE 6.** Model for degenerin-induced toxicity. MEC-4 is used as a paradigm. Gain-of-function mutations in the degenerin gene *mec-4* encode substitutions for a conserved alanine adjacent to MSDII and result in neuronal degeneration. Amino acids with bulkier side chains at this position are thought to lock the channel in an open conformation by causing steric hindrance, resulting in ion influx (ionic selectivity, for the MEC-4-containing channel has not been established yet, but by analogy it is most likely selective for $Na^+$) which triggers the necrotic-like cell death shown at the bottom.

For example, unusual gain-of-function (dominant; *d*) mutations in the *mec-4* gene induce degeneration of the six touch receptor neurons required for the sensation of gentle touch to the body. In contrast, most *mec-4* mutations are recessive loss-of-function mutations that disrupt body touch sensitivity without affecting touch receptor ultrastructure or viability.[41] *mec-4(d)* alleles encode substitutions for a conserved alanine that is positioned extracellularly, adjacent to the pore-lining membrane-spanning domain (see FIGURE 1B). The size of the amino-acid side chain at this position is correlated with toxicity; substitution of a small side-chain amino acid does not induce degeneration, whereas replacement of the Ala with a large side-chain amino acid is toxic.[3] This suggests that steric hindrance plays a role in the degeneration mechanism and supports the following working model for *mec-4(d)*-induced degeneration: MEC-4 channels, like other channels, can assume alternative open and closed conformations. In adopting the closed conformation, the side chain of the amino acid at MEC-4 position 713 is proposed to come into close proximity to another part of the channel. Steric interference conferred by a bulky amino-acid side chain prevents such an approach, causing the channel to close less effectively. Increased cation influx results, initiating neurodegeneration (FIGURE 6). That ion influx is critical, for degeneration is supported by the fact that amino-acid substitutions that disrupt the channel conducting pore can prevent neurodegeneration when present *in cis* to the A713 substitution. In addition, large side-chain substitutions at the analogous position in some neuronally expressed mammalian superfamily members do markedly increase channel conductance.[42,43] Interestingly, the cell death that occurs appears to involve more than the burst of a cell in response to osmotic imbalance.[44] Rather, it appears that the necrotic cell death induced by these channels may activate a death program that is similar in several respects to that associated with the excitotoxic cell death that occurs in higher organisms in response to injury in stroke. Electron microscopy studies of degenerating nematode neurons that express the toxic *mec-4(d)* allele have revealed a series of distinct events that take place during degeneration, involving extensive membrane endocytosis and degradation of cellular components.[44] Thus the toxic degenerin mutations provide the means with which to examine the molecular genetics of injury-induced cell death in a highly manipulable experimental organism.

## FUTURE PROSPECTS: DEGENERINS AND MECHANICAL SIGNALING

DEG/ENaC proteins mediate diverse biological functions and may be gated via several different mechanisms. Beyond this diversity, however, lies a highly conserved subunit structure. This strong conservation across species suggests that DEG/ENaC family members shared a common ancestor early in evolution. The basic subunit structure may have been adapted to fit a range of biological needs by the addition or modification of functional domains. This conjecture remains to be tested by identifying and isolating such structural modules within degenerins.

The detailed model for touch transduction in the *C. elegans* body touch receptor neurons accommodates genetic data and molecular properties of cloned *mec* genes. However, it should be emphasized that, apart from findings that MEC-4 and MEC-10 coimmunoprecipitate *in vitro*, no direct interactions between proteins proposed to be present in the mechanotransducing complex have been demonstrated. Given that genes for candidate interacting genes are in hand, it should now be possible to test hypothesized associations biochemically.

More challenging and most critical, the hypothesis that a degenerin-containing channel is mechanically gated must be addressed. This may be particularly difficult since, at present, it is not straightforward to record directly from tiny *C. elegans* neurons. Expression of the MEC-4/MEC-10 or (UNC-8/DEL-1) channel in heterologous systems such as *Xenopus* oocytes will be complicated by the presence of the many endogenous mechanically gated ion channels (see, for example, Ref. 45) and by the likely possibility that not only the multimeric channel, but essential interacting proteins, will have to be assembled to gate the channel. However, the development of the necessary technology that will allow direct recordings from nematode neurons[46] will facilitate electrophysiological studies on degenerin ion channels while they are kept embedded in their natural surroundings. This approach, combined with the powerful genetics of *C. elegans*, will, it is hoped, allow the complete dissection of a metazoan mechanotransducing complex.

A major question that remains to be addressed is whether the mammalian counterparts of the *C. elegans* degenerins play specialized roles in mechanical signaling in humans. Indeed, some evidence suggests that related molecules are in the right place at the right time. For example, ENaC immunoreactivity has been found in mechanosensory lanceolate nerve endings of the rat mystacial pad[47] in the vibrassae (whisker), and γENaC immunoreactivity is localized to baroreceptor nerve terminals that innervate the aortic arch and carotid sinus, and mediate blood pressure regulation.[48] With the sequence of the human genome due to be released in the near future, additional members of the human ENaC family (which we anticipate could include hundreds of members) should be identified. Some of these may be more closely related to nematode proteins specialized for mechanotransduction than currently identified family members and may be the long-sought human mechanosensors.

NOTE ADDED IN PROOF: While this paper was under review, elegant work by Price and coworkers[49] demonstrated a requirement for the mammalian DEG/ENaC family member BNC1 in normal mechanosensation in the mouse. This finding further supports the involvement of specialized DEG/ENaC ion channels in mechanotransduction in higher organisms.

## REFERENCES

1. FRENCH, A.S. 1992. Mechanotransduction. Annu. Rev. Physiol. **54:** 135–152.
2. SACKIN, H. 1995. Mechanosensitive channels. Annu. Rev. Physiol. **57:** 333–353.
3. DRISCOLL, M. & M. CHALFIE. 1991. The *mec-4* gene is a member of a family of *Caenorhabditis elegans* genes that can mutate to induce neuronal degeneration. Nature **349:** 588–593.
4. HUANG, M. & M. CHALFIE. 1994. Gene interactions affecting mechanosensory transduction in *Caenorhabditis elegans*. Nature **367:** 467–470.
5. LIU, J., B. SCHRANK & R. WATERSTON. 1996. Interaction between a putative mechanosensory membrane channel and a collagen. Science **273:** 361–364.
6. TAVERNARAKIS, N., W. SHREFFLER, S.L.WANG & M. DRISCOLL. 1997. *unc-8*, a member of the DEG/ENaC superfamily, encodes a subunit of a candidate stretch-gated motor neuron channel that modulates locomotion in *C. elegans*. Neuron **18:** 107–119.
7. CHALFIE, M. & E. WOLINSKY. 1990. The identification and suppression of inherited neurodegeneration in *Caenorhabditis elegans*. Nature **345:** 410–416.
8. CHALFIE, M., M. DRISCOLL & M. HUANG. 1993. Degenerin similarities. Nature **361:** 504.
9. HUMMLER, E. & J.D. HORISBERGER. 1999. Genetic disorders of membrane transport. V. The epithelial sodium channel and its implication in human diseases. Am. J. Physiol. **276:** G567–G571.
10. COREY, D.P. & J. GARCÍA-AÑOVEROS. 1996. Mechanosensation and the DEG/ENaC ion channels. Science **273:** 323–324.
11. MANO, I. & M. DRISCOLL. 1999. The DEG/ENaC Channels: a touchy superfamily that watches its salt. Bioessays **21:** 568–578.

12. TAVERNARAKIS, N. & M. DRISCOLL. 2000. *Caenorhabditis elegans* degenerins and vertebrate ENaC ion channels contain an extracellular domain related to venom neurotoxins. J. Neurogenet. **13**: 257–264.
13. RENARD, S., *et al.* 1994. Biochemical analysis of the membrane topology of the amiloride-sensitive Na⁺ channel. J. Biol. Chem. **269**: 12981–12986.
14. LAI, C.C., *et al.* 1996. Sequence and transmembrane topology of MEC-4, an ion channel subunit required for mechanotransduction in *C. elegans*. J. Cell. Biol. **133**: 1071–1081.
15. SULSTON, J.E., E. SCHIERENBERG, J.G. WHITE & J.N. THOMSON. 1983. The embryonic cell lineage of the nematode *Caenorhabditis elegans*. Dev. Biol. **100**: 64–119.
16. CAENORHABDITIS ELEGANS GENOME SEQUENCING CONSORTIUM. 1998. Genome sequence of the nematode caenorhabditis elegans. A platform for investigating biology. Science **282**: 2012–2018.
17. FIRE, A., *et al.* 1998. Potent and specific genetic interference by double-stranded RNA in *Caenorhabditis elegans*. Nature **391**: 806–811.
18. MELLO, C.C., J.M. KRAMER, D. STINCHCOMB & V. AMBROS. 1991. Efficient gene transfer in *C. elegans*: extrachromosomal maintenance and integration of transforming sequences. EMBO J. **10**: 3959–3970.
19. WHITE, J.G., E. SOUTHGATE, J.N. THOMSON & S. BRENNER. 1996. The structure of the nervous system of *Caenorhabditis elegans*. R. Soc. London B: Biol. Sci. **314**: 1–340.
20. CHALFIE, M. & J. SULSTON. 1981. Developmental genetics of the mechanosensory neurons of *Caenorhabditis elegans*. Dev. Biol. **82**: 358–370.
21. DRISCOLL, M. & J. M. KAPLAN. 1996. Mechanotransduction. *In* The Nematode *C. elegans*, II, D.L. Riddle, T. Blumenthal, B.J Meyer, and J.R. Pries, Eds.: 645–677. Cold Spring Harbor Laboratory Press. Cold Spring Harbor, N.Y.
22. WAY, J.C. & M. CHALFIE. 1989. The mec-3 gene of *Caenorhabditis elegans* requires its own product for maintained expression and is expressed in three neuronal cell types. Genes & Dev. **3**: 1823–1833.
23. WICKS, S.R., C. ROEHRIG & C.H. RANKIN. 1996. A dynamic network simulation of the nematode tap withdrawal circuit: predictions concerning synaptic function using behavioral criteria. J. Neurosci. **16**: 4017–4031.
24. CHALFIE, M., *et al.* 1985. The neural circuit for touch sensitivity in *C. elegans*. J. Neurosci. **5**: 956–964.
25. CHALFIE, M. & M. AU. 1989. Genetic control of differentiation of the *Caenorhabditis elegans* touch receptor neurons. Science **243**: 1027–1033.
26. GU, G., G.A. CALDWELL & M. CHALFIE. 1996. Genetic interactions affecting touch sensitivity in *Caenorhabditis elegans*. Proc. Natl. Acad. Sci. USA **93**: 6577–6582.
27. TAVERNARAKIS, N. & M. DRISCOLL. 1997 Molecular modeling of mechanotransduction in the nematode *Caenorhabditis elegans*. Annu. Rev. Physiol. **59**: 659–689.
28. DRISCOLL, M. & N. TAVERNARAKIS. 1996 Molecules that mediate touch transduction in the nematode *Caenorhabditis elegans*. Am. Soc. Grav. Space Biol. Bull. **10**: 33–42.
29. CANESSA, C.M., A.M. MERILLAT & B.C. ROSSIER. 1994. Membrane topology of the epithelial sodium channel in intact cells. Am. J. Physiol. **267**: C1682– C1690.
30. GARCÍA-AÑOVEROS, J., C. MA & M. CHALFIE. 1995. Regulation of *Caenorhabditis elegans* degenerin proteins by a putative extracellular domain. Curr. Biol. **5**: 441–448.
31. DU, H., G. GU, C. WILLIAMS & M. CHALFIE. 1996. Extracellular proteins needed for *C. elegans* mechanosensation. Neuron **16**: 183–194.
32. SAVAGE, C., *et al.* 1989. *mec-7* is a beta tubulin gene required for the production of 15 protofilament microtubules in *Caenorhabditis elegans*. Genes & Dev. **3**: 870–881.
33. SHREFFLER, W., T. MARGARDINO, K. SHEKDAR & E. WOLINSKY. 1995. The *unc-8* and *sup-40* genes regulate ion channel function in *Caenorhabditis elegans* motorneurons. Genetics **139**: 1261–1272.
34. BRENNER, S. 1974. The genetics of *Caenorhabditis elegans*. Genetics **77**: 71–94.
35. PARK, E.-C. & R.H. HORVITZ. 1986. Mutations with dominant effects on the behavior and morphology of the nematode *C. elegans*. Genetics **113**: 821–852.
36. WHITE, J.G, E. SOUTHGATE, J.N. THOMSON & S. BRENNER. 1986. The structure of the nervous system of *Caenorhabditis elegans*. Philos. Trans. R. Soc. London **314**: 1–340.
37. HERMAN, R.K. 1996. Touch sensation in *Caenorhabditis elegans*. BioEssays **18**: 199–206.

38. Huang, M., G. Gu, E.L. Ferguson & M. Chalfie. 1995. A stomatin-like protein is needed for mechanosensation in *C. elegans*. Nature **378:** 292–295.
39. Hudspeth, A.J. 1989. How the ear's works work. Nature. **341:** 397–404.
40. Pickles, J.O. & D.P. Corey. 1992. Mechanoelectrical transduction by hair cells. Trends Neurosci. **15:** 254–259.
41. Hong, K., I. Mano & M. Driscoll. 2000. Structure/function analysis of *C. elegans mec-4*, a component of a $Na^+$ channel required for mechanotransduction. J. Neurosci. **20:** 2575–2588.
42. Waldmann, R., G. Champigny & M. Lazdunski. 1995. Functional degenerin-containing chimeras identify residues essential for amiloride-sensitive $Na^+$ channel function. J. Biol. Chem. **270:** 11735–11737.
43. García-Añoveros, J., J.A. García, J.-D. Liu & D.P. Corey. 1998. The nematode degenerin UNC-105 forms ion channels that are activated by degeneration- or hyper-contraction-causing mutations. Neuron **20:** 1231–1241.
44. Hall, D.H., *et al.* 1997. Neuropathology of degenerative cell death in *C. elegans*. J. Neurosci. **17:** 1033–1045.
45. Lane, J.W., D.W. McBride & O.P. Hamill. 1991. Amiloride block of the mechanosensitive cation channel in *Xenopus* oocytes. J. Physiol. **441:** 347–366.
46. Avery, L., D. Raizen & S. Lockery. 1995. Electrophysiological methods. *In* Methods in Cell Biology. Caenorhabditis Elegans: Modern Biological Analysis of an Organism, Vol. 48, H.F. Epstein and D.C. Shakes, Eds.: 251-269. Academic Press. San Diego.
47. Fricke, B., *et al.* 2000. Epithelial $Na^+$ channels and stomatin are expressed in rat trigeminal mechanosensory neurons. Cell Tissue Res. **299:** 327–334.
48. Drummond, H.A., M.P. Price, M.J. Welsh & F.M. Abboud. 1998. A molecular component of the arterial baroreceptor mechanotransducer. Neuron **21:** 1435–1441.
49. Price, M.P., G.R. Lewin, S.L. McIlwrath, *et al.* 2000. The mammalian sodium channel BNC1 is required for normal touch sensation. Nature **407:** 1007–1011.

# ENaC Subunits Are Molecular Components of the Arterial Baroreceptor Complex

HEATHER A. DRUMMOND, MICHAEL J. WELSH, AND FRANÇOIS M. ABBOUD

*Department of Internal Medicine, College of Medicine, University of Iowa, Iowa City, Iowa 52242, USA*

ABSTRACT: Mechanosensation is essential to the perception of our environment. It is required for hearing, touch, balance, proprioception, and blood pressure homeostasis. Yet little is known about the identity of ion-channel complexes that transduce mechanical stimuli into neuronal responses. Genetic studies in *Caenorhabditis elegans* suggest that members of the DEG/ENaC family may be mechanosensors. Therefore we tested the hypothesis that mammalian epithelial $Na^+$-channel (ENaC) subunits contribute to the mechanosensor in baroreceptor neurons. The data presented here show that ENaC transcripts and proteins are expressed in mechanosensory neurons and at the putative sites of mechanotransduction in baroreceptor sensory-nerve terminals. Additionally, known ENaC inhibitors, amiloride and benzamil, disrupt mechanotransduction in arterial baroreceptor neurons. These data are consistent with the hypothesis that DEG/ENaC proteins are components of mechanosensitive ion-channel complexes.

KEYWORDS: Arterial baroreceptor; Baroreflex; Blood pressure; Mechanosensation; Mechanoreception; Epithelial sodium channel; Ion channel; Degenerin; Merkel-cell–neurite complex; Meissner-like corpuscle; Pacinian-like corpuscle

## INTRODUCTION

The molecular basis of arterial baroreceptor mechanotransduction is poorly understood. However, the recent identification of the *deg*enerin (DEG)/*E*pithelial $Na^+$ *C*hannel (ENaC) family of proteins has provided insight into the identity of mechanosensitive ion-channel complexes. The DEG/ENaC family of proteins is an interesting family of proteins because it is expressed in a broad range of species and may be involved in diverse sensory functions. Members of this family were first identified in the nematode *Caenorhabditis elegans*. Mutations produced animals that developed neuronal degeneration, responded abnormally to light touch, or displayed uncoordinated movement.[1–8] In the fly, members of this family may be required for mechanosensation and proprioception.[9] Another family member functions as a neurotransmitter receptor, *F*MRF-amide $Na^+$ *C*hannel (FaNaCh) in the snail, *helix as-*

Corresponding author: Heather A. Drummond, Ph.D., Department of Internal Medicine, 500 EMRB, University of Iowa, Iowa City, IA 52242. Voice: 319-335-7574.
heather_drummond@uiowa.edu

*persa.*[10] There are two groups of DEG/ENaC proteins found in mammals: acid-gated members and ENaC members. *Brain Na+ Channel 1* (BNC1), *Acid-Sensing Ion Channel* (ASIC), and *Dorsal Root Acid-Sensing Ion Channel* (DRASIC) form acid-gated channels.[11–19] This group of proteins is expressed predominantly in neuronal tissue, and may play a role in acid sensation and mechanosensation. In kidney, colon, and lung epithelia, αENaC, βENaC, and γENaC form a heteromultimeric channel critical in Na+ and water transport.[20–23] Most DEG/ENaC proteins form amiloride-sensitive, non-voltage-gated cation channels.[9,11–19,20,21,23] Because ENaC and pro-ton-gated proteins are related to proteins required for mechanosensation in the nematode, they may also play a role in mechanosensation in mammals.

The arterial baroreceptors are crucial to the short-term control of blood pressure and modulation of sympathetic tone.[24,25] The baroreceptors, located in the aortic arch and carotid sinuses, are activated by pressure-induced vessel-wall stretch.[24,25] The mechanosensitive ion channel may lie in the nerve endings innervating the aortic arch and carotid sinuses. To test the hypothesis that DEG/ENaC proteins are components of the mechanosensitive ion channel in baroreceptor neurons, we asked if (1) DEG/ENaC family members are expressed in baroreceptor neurons, and (2) inhibition of DEG/ENaC channel function alters baroreceptor function.

## EXPRESSION OF ENAC SUBUNITS IN NODOSE NEURONS

We used RT-PCR to determine if mRNA transcripts for αENaC, βENaC, and γENaC are expressed in nodose ganglia. Using lung as a positive control, we found that βENaC and γENaC, but not αENaC, are expressed in nodose ganglia.[26] Since αENaC is required for constitutive activity of the ENaC channel expressed in epithelial tissue, the absence of αENaC expression suggests that the channel formed in nodose tissue behaves differently than the channel in epithelial tissue, that is, the channel in nodose tissue may not be constitutively active.

Since nodose ganglia contain a heterogeneous population of neurons, we used immunofluorescence in retrogradely labeled baroreceptor neurons to determine if they express βENaC and γENaC. Baroreceptor neurons in the nodose ganglia were labeled by the application of Di-I, a lipophilic tracer dye to the aortic arch (FIG. 1A). The dye is incorporated into neuronal membranes, diffuses along the axons, and labels baroreceptor cell bodies in the nodose ganglia. Following labeling the ganglia were removed, the neurons grown in culture, and then immunolabeled for βENaC and γENaC expression. Immunolabeling results indicate that βENaC and γENaC are expressed in Di-I-labeled baroreceptor neurons (FIG. 1B). To determine if γENaC is expressed at the site of mechanotransduction in aortic-arch baroreceptor nerve endings, we used immunolabeling for γENaC in Di-I-labeled nerve endings.[26] Baroreceptor nerve endings in the aortic arch were labeled by injection of Di-I into the nodose ganglia (FIG. 1C). Following this, the arch was removed and immunostained for γENaC and examined using confocal microscopy. We found γENaC expressed in the small Di-I-labeled nerve terminals in the aortic arch (FIG. 1D). We also detected expression of γENaC in baroreceptor nerve endings in the carotid sinus by immunofluorescence. These results demonstrate that message and protein for βENaC and γENaC are expressed in baroreceptor neurons.

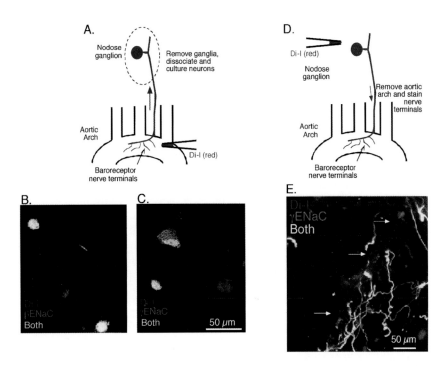

**FIGURE 1.** Immunofluorescence localization of βENaC and γENaC in cultured aortic baroreceptor neurons. (**A**) Labeling of baroreceptor neurons in nodose ganglia. Di-I injected onto aortic arch diffused retrogradely to label the soma of nerves innervating the aortic arch. The nodose ganglia were removed 2 weeks after labeling, dissociated, and maintained in culture for 3 days, then immunolabeled for βENaC or γENaC. (**B** and **C**) Di-I colocalizes with βENaC (in B) and γENaC (in C) immunostaining in cultured baroreceptor neurons. (**D** and **E**) Immunofluorescence localization of γENaC in rat aortic-arch baroreceptor nerve terminals. (D) Di-I labeling of aortic-arch baroreceptor nerve terminals. Di-I injected into the nodose ganglia diffused anterogradely to baroreceptor nerve endings. The arch was removed 2 weeks after injection and immunostained for γENaC. (E) Colocalization of γENaC and Di-I in aortic baroreceptor nerve terminals in a 150-μm-thick section of the aortic arch. Nerves containing γENaC alone appear green, nerves containing Di-I alone appear red, and nerves containing both appear yellow. A bundle of Di-I-labeled nerves (*arrows*) courses from the upper right to lower left-hand corner. The smaller nerve fibers contain γENaC.

## RESPONSES OF BARORECEPTOR NEURONS TO MECHANICAL STIMULATION

To evaluate the role of DEG/ENaC proteins in baroreceptor activation, we assessed the effect of DEG/ENaC inhibitors *in vitro* and *in vivo*.[26] Di-I-labeled aortic baroreceptor neurons were grown in culture for 4–7 days, loaded with Fura-2, a $Ca^{2+}$ indicator dye, then mechanically activated by puffing with small amounts of buffer solution in the presence and absence of amiloride, a known inhibitor of most DEG/ENaC channels. One hundred nM amiloride reversibly attenuated mechanically activated $Ca^{2+}$ transients in these neurons (FIG. 2A). We used the isolated carotid sinus

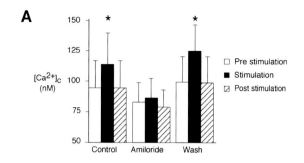

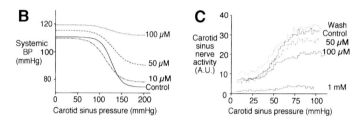

**FIGURE 2.** Effect of amiloride on baroreceptor function *in vitro* and *in vivo*. (**A**) Effect of amiloride on mechanically activated $Ca^{2+}$ transients in cultured baroreceptor neurons. Data are percent increase in $[Ca^{2+}]_c$ in cultured baroreceptor neurons (Di-I positive) before, immediately following, and 30 s after mechanical stimulation with a brief puff with buffer solution. Responses were measured under control conditions, in the presence of 100 nM amiloride, and after amiloride removal (wash). *Asterisk* denotes significant difference from prestimulation ($p < .05$). (**B**) Effect of benzamil, an amiloride analog, on carotid baroreflex control of systemic blood pressure (BP). Reflex changes in blood pressure ($n = 5$) were measured in response to a ramp increase in carotid sinus pressure. The concentration of benzamil in the perfusate is indicated. Benzamil decreased the slope of the response (mmHg systemic BP/mmHg carotid sinus pressure). (**C**) Effect of benzamil on carotid baroreceptor discharge in one animal. Carotid sinus nerve activity (in arbitrary units) was measured in response to a ramp increase in carotid sinus pressure in the presence of intraluminal benzamil. Benzamil reversibly blunts baroreceptor activation.

preparation in the rabbit to determine if benzamil, an amiloride analog, inhibits baroreceptor function. Luminal benzamil produced a reversible and dose-dependent inhibition of baroreceptor activation and reflex control of blood pressure during the increase in carotid sinus pressure (FIG. 2B and 2C). These results suggest that DEG/ENaC proteins may be required for mechanotransduction in baroreceptor neurons.

## ENAC SUBUNITS IN SKIN TOUCH RECEPTORS

To determine whether ENaC proteins are expressed in nonbaroreceptor mechanoreceptors, we evaluated ENaC expression in hairless-skin touch receptors.[27] Hairless skin receives a rich mechanosensory innervation. The cell bodies of these nerves are located in lumbar and cervical dorsal-root ganglia (DRG). Using RT-PCR, we detected expression of βENaC and γENaC, but not αENaC, in cervical and lumbar DRG. Results of immunostaining experiments demonstrated that βENaC and γENaC are expressed in DRG neurons and in the nerve endings that innervate Merkel cell–neurite complexes, Meissner-like corpuscles, and Pacinian-like corpuscles.[27]

## DISCUSSION AND CONCLUSION

Our data demonstrate that βENaC and γENaC are expressed in baroreceptor nerve endings and the nerve fibers innervating Merkel cells, Meissner-like corpuscles, and Pacinian-like corpuscles. The sensors that respond to mechanical stress may be located in the neuronal structures. The location of β and γ subunits in the baroreceptor nerve endings and at the interface of the nerve ending and the Merkel cell, Meissner-like, and Pacinian-like corpuscle lamellar cells places them at a location where mechanotransduction is thought to occur. βENaC and γENaC are also expressed in lanceolate nerve endings in the rat whisker.[28] Exciting recent data from Price et al. provide the first genetic evidence that BNC1, a DEG/ENaC family member, is required for normal mechanosensation in mouse hair follicles.[29]

If βENaC and γENaC are part of a mechanosensitive ion channel in tactile and baroreceptor sensory neurons, then that channel is not the same channel as ENaC in epithelial tissue. In epithelia, αENaC, βENaC, and γENaC form a constitutively active channel that plays an important role in sodium transport. Expression of the αENaC protein is required for this constitutive activity. The lack of expression of αENaC in sensory neurons suggests that αENaC is not part of the mechanosensitive ion channel. Thus βENaC and γENaC probably have different functions in sensory neurons and epithelial tissue. It is not known if some other unidentified DEG/ENaC protein may also contribute to the mechanosensor.

Because mammalian ENaC proteins are related to proteins that are believed to form the pore of the mechanosensitive ion channel in C. elegans touch neurons, we speculate that ENaC proteins may contribute to the pore of mechanosensitive ion channels in mammals. Our results are consistent with this hypothesis and lay the foundation for understanding mechanotransduction in mammalian sensory neurons.

## REFERENCES

1. CHALFIE, M. & E. WOLINSKY. 1990. The identification and suppression of inherited neurodegeneration in Caenorhabditis elegans. Nature 345: 410–416.
2. DRISCOLL, M. & M. CHALFIE. 1991. The mec-4 gene is a member of a family of Caenorhabditis elegans genes that can mutate to induce neuronal degeneration. Nature 349: 588–593.
3. TAVERNARAKIS, N. & M. DRISCOLL. 1997. Molecular modeling of mechanotransduction in the nematode Caenorhabditis elegans. Annu. Rev. Physiol. 59: 659–689.
4. GARCIA-ANOVEROS, J. & D.P. COREY. 1997. The molecules of mechanosensation. Annu. Rev. Neurosci. 20: 567–594.
5. MANO, I. & M. DRISCOLL. 1999. DEG/ENaC channels: a touchy superfamily that watches its salt. Bioessays 21: 568–578.
6. HUANG, M. & M. CHALFIE. 1994. Gene interactions affecting mechanosensory transduction in Caenorhabditis elegans. Nature 367: 467–470.

7. LIU, J., B. SCHRANK & R.H. WATERSTON. 1996. Interaction between a putative mechanosensory membrane channel and a collagen. Science **273:** 361–364.
8. TAVERNARAKIS, N., *et al.* 1997. *Unc-8* a DEG/ENaC family member, encodes a subunit of a candidate mechanically gated channel that modulates *C. elegans* locomotion. Neuron **18:** 107–119.
9. ADAMS, C.M., *et al.* 1998. Ripped pocket and pickpocket, novel Drosophila DEG/ENaC subunits expressed in early development and in mechanosensory neurons. J. Cell Biol. **140:** 143–152.
10. LINGUEGLIA, E., *et al.* 1995. Cloning of the amiloride-sensitive FMRF-amide peptide-gated sodium channel. Nature. **378:** 730–733.
11. PRICE, M.P., P.M. SNYDER & M.J. WELSH. 1996. Cloning and expression of a novel human brain Na$^+$channel. J. Biol. Chem. **271:** 7879–7882.
12. WALDMANN, R., *et al.* 1996. The mammalian degenerin MDEG, an amiloride-sensitive cation channel activated by mutations causing neurodegeneration in Caenorhabditis elegans. J. Biol. Chem. **271:** 10433–10436.
13. GARCIA-ANOVEROS, J., *et al.* 1997. BNaC1 and BNaC2 constitute a new family of human neuronal sodium channels related to degenerins and epithelial sodium channels. Proc. Natl. Acad. Sci. USA **94:**1459–1464.
14. BASSILANA, F., *et al.* 1997. The acid-sensitive ionic channel subunit ASIC and the mammalian degenerin MDEG form a heteromultimeric H$^+$-gated Na$^+$ channel with novel properties. J. Biol. Chem. **272:** 28819–28822.
15. LINGUEGLIA, E. , *et al.* 1997. A modulatory subunit of acid sensing ion channels in brain and dorsal root ganglion cells. J. Biol. Chem. **272:** 29778–29783.
16. WALDMANN, R., *et al.* 1997. Molecular cloning of a non-inactivating proton-gated Na$^+$ channel specific for sensory neurons. J. Biol. Chem. **272:** 20975–20978.
17. WALDMANN, R., *et al.* 1997. A proton-gated cation channel involved in acid sensing. Nature **386:** 173–177.
18. WALDMANN, R. & M. LAZDUNSKI. 1998. H$^+$-Gated cation channels: neuronal acid sensors in the ENaC/DEG family of ion channels. Curr. Opin. Neurobiol. **8:** 418–424.
19. BABINSKI, K., K.T. LE & P. SEGUELA. 1999. Molecular cloning and regional distribution of a human proton receptor subunit with biphasic functional properties. J. Neurochem. **72:** 51–57.
20. CANESSA, C.M., J.D. HORISBERGER & B.C. ROSSIER. 1993. Epithelial sodium channel related to proteins involved in neurodegeneration. Nature **361:** 467–470.
21. CANESSA, C.M., *et al.* 1994. Amiloride sensitive epithelial Na$^+$ channel is made of three homologous subunits. Nature **367:** 463–467.
22. LINGUEGLIA, E., *et al.* 1994. Different homologous subunits of the amiloride-sensitive Na$^+$ channel are differently regulated by aldosterone. J. Biol. Chem. **269:** 13736–13739.
23. MCDONALD, F.M., *et al.* 1995. Cloning and expression of the beta and gamma- subunits of the human epithelial sodium channel. Am. J. Physiol. **268:** C1157–C1163.
24. SHEPERD, J.T. & G. MANCIA. 1986. Reflex control of the human cardiovascular system. Rev. Physiol. Biochem. Pharmacol. **105:** 3–99.
25. KUMADA, M., N. TERUI & T. KUWAKI. 1990. Arterial baroreceptor reflex: its central and peripheral neural mechanisms. Prog. Neurobiol. **35:** 331–361.
26. DRUMMOND, H.A., *et al.* 1998. A molecular component of the arterial baroreceptor mechanotransducer. Neuron **21:** 1435–1441.
27. DRUMMOND, H.A., F.M. ABBOUD & M.J. WELSH. 2000. Localization of β and γ subunits of ENaC in sensory nerve endings in the rat foot pad. Brain Res. **884:** 1–12.
28. FRICKE, B., *et al.* 2000. Epithelial Na$^+$ channels and stomatin are expressed in rat trigeminal mechanosensory neurons. Cell Tissue Res. **299:** 327–334.
29. PRICE, M.P., *et al.* 2000. The mammalian sodium channel BNC1 is required for normal touch sensation. Nature. **407:** 1007–1011.

# The Bezold-Jarisch Reflex

## A Historical Perspective of Cardiopulmonary Reflexes

DOMINGO M. AVIADO AND DOMINGO GUEVARA AVIADO

*Atmospheric Health Sciences, Short Hills, New Jersey 07078, USA*

ABSTRACT: The Bezold-Jarisch reflex is an eponym for a triad of responses (apnea, bradycardia, and hypotension) following intravenous injection of veratrum alkaloids in experimental animals. The observation was first reported in 1867 by von Bezold and Hirt, and confirmed in 1938–1940 by Jarisch. The triad depends on intact vagi and is mediated through cranial nervous medullary centers controlling respiration, heart rate, and vasomotor tone. The respiratory effects are mediated through pulmonary vagal afferents and the bradycardia and vasodepression through cardiac vagal afferents. The veratrum alkaloids activate all known receptors in the carotid–aortic and cardiopulmonary areas. The cardiopulmonary receptors (baroreceptors, cough receptors, and parenchymal stretch receptors) also respond to other chemical substances: nicotine, capsaicin, venom, antihistaminics, halogenated anesthetics, diguanides, and serotonin (5-hydroxytryptamine). Derivatives of last-mentioned amine activate Type 1, 2, or 3 receptors and have potential therapeutic use. Since several types of cardiopulmonary receptors participate in the Bezold-Jarisch reflex, it has been difficult to develop a blockade to one type of receptor for therapeutic use (cough, bronchospasm, pulmonary hypertension, or coronary vasospasm). Axon reflexes influence pulmonary blood vessels, bronchial blood vessels, and bronchial smooth muscles. These intrapulmonary reflexes need further study as to how they relate to the Bezold-Jarisch reflex in health and disease. The cardiopulmonary and carotid–aortic reflexes can serve as defense mechanisms against chemical hazards that are likely to be inhaled in the workplace and in the environment.

KEYWORDS: Autonomic nervous system; Baroreceptors; Bezold-Jarisch reflex; Bronchopulmonary system; Cardiopulmonary control; Carotid–aortic receptors; Chemoreceptors; Nicotine; Respiratory control; Serotonin; Vasovagal syncope, Vagus; Veratrum alkaloids

## I. INTRODUCTION

This article is a historical review of carotid-aortic and cardiopulmonary reflexes. The first international conferences on this subject were sponsored by the Section on Pharmacology (SEPHAR) of the International Union of Physiological Sciences during their First Congress (1961) held in Stockholm,[1] and the Second Congress (1963) held in Prague.[2] SEPHAR, which later became the International Union of Pharmacology, was organized by Carl F. Schmidt from the University of Pennsylvania and

Address for correspondence: Domingo Guevara Aviado, Atmospheric Health Sciences, 225 Hartshorn Drive, Short Hills, New Jersey 07078. Voice/fax: 973-564-9156.
agadma@msn.com

TABLE 1. Cardiopulmonary eponyms

| Eponyms (year) | Location of receptors and afferent innervation (cranial nerve) |
|---|---|
| *Carotid–aortic reflexes*: baroreceptors and chemoreceptors | |
| Cyon-Ludwig's nerve (1866) | Aortic depressor (X) |
| Hering's nerve (1927) | Carotid sinus (IX) |
| Heymans and Heymans reflex (1927–1938) | Carotid body chemoreceptors (IX) |
| *Cardiopulmonary reflexes*: baroreceptors and other receptors | |
| Hering-Breuer reflex (1868) | Pulmonary stretch (X) |
| Kratschmer reflex (1870) | Upper respiratory cough (I, V, IX) |
| Bainbridge reflex (1914–1915) | Right atrium (X) |
| McDowall reflex (1924) | Right atrium (X) |
| Harrison reflex (1932) | Right atrium |
| von Bezold and Hirt reflex (1867) | Vagal receptors (X) |
| Jarisch effect (1938) | Vagal receptors (X) |
| Bezold-Jarisch reflex (1940) | Cardiac and pulmonary (X) |
| Starling's law of the heart (1927) | Heart–lung preparation |

Corneille Heymans from the University of Ghent (Belgium), who trained pharmacologists and physiologists on reflex control of respiration and circulation.[3] It is comforting for basic scientists active during the 1940s to note that clinical researchers are currently interested in cardiopulmonary reflexes. The present conference was organized largely through the efforts of the Cardiovascular Center and Department of Internal Medicine at the University of Iowa and the American Physiological Society.

The senior author of this article, Domingo M. Aviado (DMA), was born in the Philippines and migrated to the United States in 1946 as a transfer medical student from the University of the Philippines to the University of Pennsylvania, where he obtained his medical degree in 1948. Dr. Carl F. Schmidt, then head of the Department of Pharmacology, selected cardiopulmonary reflexes as DMA's first research project,[4] which dictated his interest in the search of new therapeutic agents. DMA later became interested in developing new drugs for the treatment of cardiopulmonary diseases and wrote the first monographs devoted to lung circulation,[5] antitussive agents,[6] sympathomimetic drugs,[7] and propellants to dispense bronchodilators.[8] These monographs, as well as a pharmacology textbook,[9] were written primarily to improve the contents of lectures for medical students. Carl F. Schmidt often reminded his younger associates that their primary function at Penn was teaching and that pharmacologic research should be directed so that students can understand the mechanism of drug action.

As a Penn medical student, DMA was aware that William Bennett Bean, the Professor of Internal Medicine at the University of Iowa, was also born in the Philippines. In 1950 Professor Bean edited a small handbook that was required reading for Penn students: *Sir William Osler: Aphorisms from Bedside Teachings and Writings*.[10]

Sir William Osler was a Professor of Clinical Medicine at Penn from 1884 to 1889 before moving to Johns Hopkins Medical School and Oxford University. The *Aphorisms* were collected by Professor Bean's father, Robert Bennett Bean, who founded the Department of Anatomy at the University of the Philippines. Shortly after Professor William Bennett Bean was born in Manila, his father returned to the United States to become the Professor of Anatomy at the University of Virginia.[11]

Dr. William Bennett Bean was Professor of Internal Medicine at Iowa Medical School and wrote several articles on medical history relating to fingernail growth.[12] During the centennial celebration of Iowa Medical School (founded in 1879), Bean recalled events leading to the formation as the first continually existing coeducational medical school in the United States.[13] There were six physician-founders, including one on Materia Medica, who undoubtedly discussed U.S. pharmacopeia remedies such as *Veratrum* plant alkaloids used in the treatment of hypertension.[14] There was no chair in Physiology, although the respiratory and circulatory reflexes had already been discovered by professors at European medical schools (see TABLE 1).

## II. CARDIOPULMONARY REFLEXES

Cardiopulmonary reflexes belong to the autonomic or involuntary nervous system and consist of the following: (a) sensory receptors in the heart and lungs; (b) the sensory or afferent fibers in the parasympathetic X cranial nerves, including nodose ganglia of vagus; (c) medullary centers regulating visceral function by reciprocal activity on parasympathetic, and sympathetic innervations; (d) preganglionic synapses to thoracic ganglia for sympathetic efferent innervation, and to intravisceral ganglia for parasympathetic efferent innervation; (e) postganglionic fibers from sympathetic thoracic ganglia, anatomically longer than postganglionic fibers from parasympathetic intravisceral ganglia; and (f) neuroeffector junctions for parasympathetic mediated by acetylcholine, and for sympathetic mediated by norepinephrine. The Bezold-Jarisch reflex is interrupted by cervical vagotomy, indicating that the parasympathetic innervation of the cardiopulmonary area is essential in the transmission of the afferent and/or efferent groups of nerve impulses.

### Definition of Bezold-Jarisch Reflex

In 1867, von Bezold and Hirt[15] described in experimental animals the triad of responses (bradycardia, hypotension, and apnea) as a result of intravenous injection of an alkaloidal extract of *Veratrum viride* or *Viscum album*. The response was eliminated by cutting both cervical vagi (X cranial). The 1867 publication was forgotten until, when Jarisch reported the results of veratrum alkaloidal injections in animal experiments, revealing that the responses were reflex in nature and introduced the eponym of *Bezold reflex*.[16,17] Subsequent investigators, mostly pharmacologists and physiologists, referred to the triad of responses as *Bezold-Jarisch reflex* or Bezold-Jarisch effect, the latter, to emphasize that veratrum alkaloids have multiple actions on several groups of reflexes and also directly on the medullary centers.

## Cardiopulmonary Eponyms

After Jarisch confirmed and elaborated on the 1867 report of von Bezold and Hirt, there was considerable effort made to identify the mechanism of action of veratrum alkaloids. Since several cardiopulmonary reflexes had been discovered prior to 1940, it was necessary to compare the veratrum response to each known reflex, most of them with eponyms commemorating the discoverer. TABLE 1 lists two groups of eponyms: carotid–aortic reflexes and cardiopulmonary reflexes. The last entry is *Starling's law of the heart* derived from heart–lung preparation, without any functional connection to the medulla, and refers to the nonvagal or automatic response of ventricular stroke volume to atrial venous return. Cardiac rate is dependent on intact autonomic innervation; an increase in venous return accelerated the heart rate (Bainbridge reflex) and also influenced respiration (Harrison reflex) and blood pressure (McDowall reflex). The right atrial receptors, which are presumed to be responsible for these three reflexes, are diametrically opposed to the triad of responses composing the Bezold-Jarisch reflex.

## A Catalogue of Cardiopulmonary Reflexes

During the 1950s, the growing literature on cardiopulmonary reflexes was reviewed by Heymans and Neil,[18] Dawes and Comroe,[19] and Aviado and Schmidt.[20] These reviews identified the areas for further research, and a more complete catalogue of reflexes was compiled by DMA in a 1965 monograph entitled *The Lung Circulation.*[5] This monograph included a discussion of reflex control of pulmonary circulation, bronchial circulation, and cross influences from bronchopulmonary anastomoses and bronchial muscles. These areas are influenced not only by cardiopulmonary reflexes involving the medullary centers of the brain but also by bronchopulmonary axon reflexes that extend only to autonomic ganglia of the peripheral nerve.

At the present time, the catalogue of reflexes remains essentially unchanged from the 1965 list, and is summarized in TABLE 2. The four types of reflexes refer to the nature of influences on vasoconstrictor, cardioaccelerator and respiratory centers in the medulla: Type 1, perfect inhibition; Type 2, imperfect inhibition; Type 3, perfect stimulation; Type 4, mixed stimulation or inhibition of medullary centers. The type of reflexes depend on the intramedullary connections of the afferent nerves: X cranial or vagus, with distinct branches from heart, lungs, and aortic nerves (Cyon and Ludwig's); IX cranial or glossopharyngeal, limited to carotid sinus nerve (Hering's); I, V, and IX cranial nerves mediating afferent impulses from the upper respiratory tract (Kratschmer reflex); and somatic sensory nerves from extremities responsible for hyperpnea of muscular exercise. Each type of cardiopulmonary and carotid–aortic receptors has been identified by histological examination, recording of nerve impulses and functional separation for chemostimulation (sodium cyanide or hypoxemia), baroreceptor stimulation (elevation of intravascular or intracardiac blood pressure), lung-volume stretch receptor (inflation and deflation), and chemical or physical irritation (upper and lower respiratory tract cough receptors).

The types of respiratory and circulatory reflexes reported in the literature[5] are listed in TABLE 2. The baroreceptor types are activated by distension of the heart chamber or vascular lumen by balloon distension or by innervated organ perfusion

**TABLE 2. Classification of reflexes based on nature of medullary central effects**

| Type | Location of receptors | Afferents in cranial nerves |
|---|---|---|
| Type 1. | Reflexes from baroreceptors producing *perfect inhibition* of vasoconstrictor, cardioaccelerator and respiratory centers | |
| | Carotid sinuses | IX (Hering's nerve) |
| | Aortic arch | X (aortic depressor or Cyon and Ludwig's nerve) |
| | Pulmonary conus | X (pulmonary branch) |
| | Left ventricle | X (cardiac branch) |
| Type 2. | Reflexes from baroreceptors and stretch receptors producing *imperfect inhibition* | |
| Type 2a. | Lacking only respiratory inhibition. | |
| | Right atrium | X (cardiac branch) |
| Type 2b. | Lacking only cardiac inhibition | |
| | Pulmonary veins | X (pulmonary branch) |
| Type 2c. | Cardiac inhibition only | |
| | Left atrium | X (cardiac branch) |
| Type 2d. | Respiratory inhibition only | |
| | Lung parenchyma | X (pulmonary branch: Hering-Breuer inflation reflex) |
| Type 3. | Reflexes from chemoreceptor producing *pure stimulation.* | |
| | Carotid bodies | IX (Heymans and Heymans' reflex) |
| | Aortic bodies | X (aortic depressor or Cyon and Ludwig's nerve) |
| | Glomus pulmonale | X (pulmonary branch) |
| Type 4. | Reflexes from various receptor types producing *stimulation or inhibition.* | |
| | Great veins and right atrium | X (cardiac branch: Bainbridge, McDowall, and Harrison reflexes) |
| | Lung parenchyma | X (pulmonary branch: Hering-Breuer deflation reflex) |
| | Lower respiratory tract | X (pulmonary branch for cough reflex) |
| | Upper respiratory tract | I, V, IX (Kratschmer reflex) |
| | Limbs during muscular exercise | Somatic noncranial (stretch receptors in tendon and joints) |

in experimental animals, usually the anesthetized dog. The responses are uniformly similar to the triad of responses composing the Bezold-Jarisch reflex.

### *Chemical Sensitivity of Cardiopulmonary Receptors*

Veratrum alkaloids activate all receptors listed in TABLE 2. It is for this reason that the Bezold-Jarisch reflex has been referred to as *chemoreflexes,*[19] defined as responses to nonspecific irritation by veratrum alkaloids and other chemical agents.

The term is not applicable to chemoreceptor reflexes (sensitive to cyanide and hypoxia), but to other forms of reflexes, including baroreceptor and stretch reflexes. The reflex elicited by intracoronary injection of veratrum alkaloids is caused by chemical excitation of baroreceptors in the cardiac wall supplied by coronary arteries. Although there are respiratory effects from left ventricular baroreceptors, this is not included in the Bezold-Jarisch reflex evoked when veratrum alkaloids are administered by pulmonary artery injection or by inhalation. The pulmonary venous receptors are activated by inhalation, although the inhalation also influences the Hering-Breuer receptors that may contribute to the apnea component of the Bezold-Jarisch reflex.

The triad of response can be elicited by chemical agents that can be grouped into the following: (a) plant alkaloids, including other veratrum alkaloids identified by Krayer.[17] Veriloid and protoveratrine were used for the treatment of systemic hypertension, but were discarded during the 1960s because of the narrow safety margin between depressor dose and dose that caused medullary effects such as vomiting and gastrointestinal hyperactivity. (b) Nicotine and capsaicin also elicit the triad of responses, but are not used for therapeutics. (c) Venoms from snake, insects (bee, scorpion), and marine animals elicit the Bezold-Jarisch reflex that contributes to their lethality. (d) Tissue constituents, such as potassium chloride, histamine, and serotonin, also elicit the Bezold-Jarisch reflex. Some antihistaminic agents have been reported to cause the reflex that is independent of their therapeutic use as antiallergen. Some derivatives of serotonin have selective actions on Type 1, Type 2, or Type 3 receptors and are being tested for therapy of gastrointestinal diseases. (e) Synthetic organic compounds, such as phenyldiguanide, ethylacetoacetate, thioureas, and halogenated anesthetics, also elicit the Bezold-Jarisch reflex, but these observations have not been applied to the development of selective antagonistic agents.

## III. CARDIOPULMONARY RECEPTORS IN HEALTH AND DISEASE

The interest of physiologists and pharmacologists in the Bezold-Jarisch reflex is based on the premise that the reflex is more than an experimental curiosity for researchers to test chemical agents for treatment of diseases yet to be identified. It is anticipated that scientists now will be encouraged to explore this research so that new preventive and therapeutic agents can be developed. The 1965 review of cardiopulmonary baroreceptors[5] is a starting point for the study of physiology and pathologic physiology of cardiopulmonary receptors. The National Library of Medicine, which started Medline in 1965, introduced *Bezold-Jarisch Reflex* as a Mesh Heading in 1972. Publications of original research articles are readily available from Medline, as is the 1965 monograph. This section summarizes current concepts of the role of reflexes in the pathogenesis of cardiopulmonary diseases.

### *Cardiovascular Regulation*

The most widely accepted theory for function of cardiopulmonary baroreceptors is as follows: regulation of right ventricular and left ventricular outputs to compensate for changes in systemic venous return, with optimum levels of pulmonary circulatory parameters: pulmonary arterial pressure, pulmonary venous pressure, and pulmonary capillary blood flow. The baroreceptors in the systemic vena cava, right atrium, pulmonary conus, pulmonary veins, left atrium, and left ventricle are sensing elements that regulate heart rate, systemic vasomotor tone, and respiration.[5,22]

## Vasovagal Syncope

The syndrome of cardiac slowing with hypotension or vasodepression (vasovagal syncope) has been attributed to activation of the Bezold-Jarisch reflex. The reports that appeared prior to 1965[5] are confirmed in more recent case studies of vasovagal syncope associated with deglutition syncope,[23] shoulder arthroscopy in supine position,[24] and orthostatic intolerance among astronauts.[25] Vasovagal syncope has also been reported in the following cardiac procedures: coronary arteriography,[26] coronary injection of thrombolytic agents,[27] and radio frequency catheter ablation of accessory pathway in patients with Wolff-Parkinson White syndrome.[28] Vasovagal syncope has been attributed to the Bezold-Jarisch reflex in the following situations: sudden death among athletes,[29] syncope in patients with Chagas myocarditis,[30] hemolyses-related syncope,[31] microwave hyperthemia syncope,[32] high-altitude syncope,[33] and fainting after closure of arteriovenous fistula.[34] The last mentioned occurring of vasovagal syncope has been referred to as Branham's sign,[34] for diagnosis of arteriovenous fistula in the extremities. Vasovagal syncope is a common emergency room diagnosis.

## Bronchopulmonary Axon Reflexes

This review of the Bezold-Jarisch reflex that is dependent on intact vagus and participation of medullary centers, requires a consideration of bronchopulmonary axon reflexes that are not mediated through the medulla. After acute denervation of canine lung, the smooth muscle components of the airways, pulmonary blood vessels, and bronchial blood vessels still respond to chemical irritants. Chronic denervation to allow degeneration of preganglionic and postganglionic nerve fibers eliminates the responses, referred to as *bronchopulmonary axon reflexes* (see references cited in *The Lung Circulation*, pp. 171–173, and the Index page, 1345).

In the somatic nervous system, the axon reflex is as follows: dermal pain is accompanied by vasodilation, which is simulated by intradermal application of histamine, or by electrical stimulation of the dorsal (sensory) root of the spinal nerve. Cutaneous injection of histamine transmits nerve impulses through a sensory nerve antidromically to another sensory branch to initiate vasodilation. This form of somatic axon reflex cannot be elicited if the sensory afferent fibers undergo degeneration by severing its connections to dorsal root ganglia.

A pulmonary vascular axon reflex has been postulated to occur in pulmonary embolism. Embolism in one lobe causes pulmonary vasoconstriction in another lobe, provided the sympathetic innervation is intact. Thoracic sympathectomy eliminates postembolism vasoconstriction and reduces the intensity of sulfur-dioxide-induced pulmonary venous spasm. Definitive studies consisting of recording of action potentials in the sympathetic nerves are lacking.

A pulmonary bronchoconstrictor response triggered by bronchial irritation has been postulated as a vagal axon reflex. The vagal ganglia in the lung parenchyma

**TABLE 3.** A unified concept of cardiopulmonary receptors as defense mechanism in response to inhalation of atmospheric pollutants

| Receptor areas | Defense mechanisms |
| --- | --- |
| Upper respiratory tract | Apnea to reduce lower respiratory tract absorption |
| Bronchial mucosa, blood vessels and smooth muscles | Bronchial vasoconstriction and bronchoconstriction to reduce airway absorption and alveolar concentration |
| Lower respiratory tract | Inspiratory gasp followed by expiratory blast (cough reflex) |
| Atria and ventricles | Asystole and bradycardia to reduce systemic blood distribution of absorbed chemical inhalant |
| Cardiopulmonary receptor areas | Depressor reflex to reduce cerebral blood flow |
| Extracardiopulmonary areas | Other mechanisms to promote excretion and metabolism of absorbed chemical |

mediate the bronchospasm through the short ganglionic axon branches to bronchial mucosa and bronchial smooth muscles. Irritation of bronchial mucosa can send antidromic nerve impulses to bronchial smooth muscle, resulting in bronchospasm. This response is part of the defense mechanism discussed in the next and final section.

## IV. CARDIOPULMONARY REFLEXES AS A DEFENSE MECHANISM AGAINST TOXIC CHEMICAL HAZARDS

A more recent hypothesis is being proposed in this article, centered on a unified concept that cardiopulmonary reflexes are defense mechanisms against chemical inhalants. We are suggesting that the cardiopulmonary reflexes serve initially to reduce the degree of inspired pollutant absorbed in the blood, then protect the vital organs from the potential toxicity of absorbed pollutant, and finally facilitate the elimination and deactivation of pollutant. The six defense mechanisms against atmospheric pollutants are summarized in TABLE 3 and listed as receptor areas in the following order.

(1) *Upper Respiratory Tract Receptors:* When irritated by chemical substances or dust particles, these receptors send impulses via olfactory, trigeminal for taste, and pharyngeal nerves (I, V, IX cranials). The end result is apnea or breath-holding, which reduces the amount of inhalant reaching the lower respiratory tract. This is the Kratschmer reflex that is accompanied by bradycardia and vasodepressor response followed by a vasopressor response from systemic vasoconstriction. This sequence of events from irritation of the upper respiratory tract has been confirmed to occur in human subjects. The practice of using spirit of ammonia to arouse a patient who has fainted is explained by chemical irritation of receptors in the upper respiratory tract.

(2) *Bronchial Mucosal Receptors:* Bronchial mucosal blood flow is reduced, based on thermocouple recordings derived in intact, as well as in denervated or excised lungs of experimental animals. Bronchopulmonary axon reflexes responsi-

ble for reduction of bronchial blood flow are difficult to differentiate from a direct effect on bronchial vascular smooth muscle or vasoconstriction. There is also immediate bronchospasm, which can be explained by axon reflexes or local effect on bronchial smooth muscle. Both bronchial vasoconstriction and bronchospasm serve, respectively, to reduce absorption of pollutant in bronchial passages and decrease pollutant concentration in pulmonary alveoli.

(3) *Lower Respiratory Tract Cough Receptors:* Chemical or physical irritation initiates inspiratory gasp, followed by expiratory blast. The act of coughing serves the purpose of immediate expulsion of the inspired pollutant. The components of the cough reflex and evolution of antitussive drugs are reviewed in a monograph published under SEPHAR sponsorship.[6] A search for drugs to selectively block cough receptors without influencing other bronchopulmonary receptors has failed.

(4) *Atria and Ventricles:* The atria and ventricles can be influenced if the chemical inhalant activates the cardiac component of the Bezold-Jarisch reflex (asystole and bradycardia). This chemoreflex response retards systemic distribution of the absorbed chemical pollutant, after escaping constriction of pulmonary veins that are more reactive than the proximal arterioles.

(5) *Cardiopulmonary Receptor Areas:* The baroreceptors in the pulmonary circulation and coronary circulation can respond to chemical irritants. The reflex depressor response caused by systemic vasodilation results in reduction in cerebral blood flow and syncope. Any chemical pollutant absorbed in the blood is less likely to reduce blood flow to the brain, since cerebral blood vessels are less likely to constrict than other vascular beds (splanchnic, renal, and extremities).

(6) *Systemic Circulation and Carotid–Aortic Chemoreceptors:* Carotid–aortic chemoreceptor activation would initiate opposite effects to those originating from cardiopulmonary baroreceptors. Chemoreceptor activation by absorbed chemical inhalant initiates tachycardia and hyperpnea that accelerate respiratory tract elimination. As blood flows through abdominal organs, the pollutant can be excreted through renal and intestinal circulation. Hepatic distribution of blood ultimately can metabolize or inactivate the foreign substance if susceptible to hepatic enzymes.

## Summary of Defense Mechanisms

The preceding six defense mechanisms are not applicable to all inhaled pollutants. The extent of participation depends on the chemical and physical properties of the pollutant. It should be noted that inhaled chemical substances do not introduce new mechanisms in the lungs, heart, systemic circulation, and visceral organs. Like pharmaceutical agents, chemical toxic pollutants do not introduce new mechanisms, but simply activate existing cardiopulmonary reflexes that serve as defense mechanisms. If these defense mechanisms fail, the end result is disease of the heart and lung that are initially reversible, and later, irreversible and fatal. Chemical hazards in the workplace and in the environment have been classified according to the nature of predominant diseases associated with inhalation exposure.[37]

## ACKNOWLEDGMENT

Copies of post-1965 articles were obtained by Mr. Jimmie Staton, George F. Smith Library, University of Medicine & Dentistry of New Jersey, Newark, NJ 07103.

# REFERENCES

1. AVIADO, D.M., Ed. 1963. Pharmacology of the Lung. *In* Proceedings of the First International Pharmacological Meeting, Vol. 9, Part 2: 97–193. Pergamon Press. Oxford.
2. AVIADO, D.M. & F. PALECEK, Eds. 1964. Drugs and respiration. *In* Proceedings of the Second International Pharmacological Meeting, Vol. 11: 1–141. Pergamon Press. Oxford.
3. AVIADO, D.M. 1992. Nicotinic receptors in healthy and ischemic heart with special reference to the Bezold-Jarisch reflex. Arch. Int. Pharmacodyn. **319:** 7–23
4. AVIADO, D.M., R. G. PONTIUS & C. F. SCHMIDT. 1949. J. Pharmacol. Exp. Ther. **97:** 420–431.
5. AVIADO, D.M. 1965. The Lung Circulation. Vol. 1, Physiology and Pharmacology: 1–590; Vol. 2, Pathological Physiology and Therapy of Diseases: 591–1405. Pergamon Press. Oxford.
6. AVIADO, D.M. & H. SALEM, Eds. 1969. Antitussive Agents. Section 27 of International Encyclopedia of Pharmacology and Therapeutics, Vols. 1, 2, and 3: 1–834. Pergamon Press. Oxford.
7. AVIADO, D.M. 1970. Sympathomimetic Drugs: 1–615. Charles C Thomas. Springfield, IL.
8. AVIADO, D.M., S. ZAKHARI & T. WATANABE. 1977. Nonfluorinated Propellants and Solvents for Aerosols: 1–106. CRC Press. Cleveland, OH.
9. AVIADO, D.M. 1972. Pharmacologic Principles of Medical Practice, 8th ed.: 1–1345. Williams & Wilkins. Baltimore, MD.
10. BEAN, W. B., Ed. 1950. Sir William Osler: Aphorisms from His Bedside Teachings and Writings: 1–159. Schuman. New York.
11. BEAN, R.B. 1965. Obituary. Science. **101:** 345–348.
12. BEAN, W.B. 1974. Nail growth: 30 years of observation. Arch. Intern. Med. **134:** 497–502.
13. BEAN, W.B. 1970. The University of Iowa College of Medicine: 100 years ago. J. Iowa Med. Soc. **60:** 237–240.
14. OSOL, A., *et al.*, Eds. 1955. The Dispensatory of the United States of America. Veratrum Viride, 25th ed.: 1486–1488.Lippincott. Philadelphia, Pa.
15. BEZOLD, A. VON & L. HIRT. 1867. Uber die physiologischen Wirkungen des essigsauren Veratrine. Unters. Physiol. Lab. Wurzburg. **1:** 73–122.
16. JARISCH, A. & C. HENZE. 1937. Uber Blutdrucksenkung durch chemische Erregung depressorischer Nerven. Naunyn-Schmiedeberg's Arch. Exp. Pathol. Pharmak. **187:** 706–730.
17. JARISCH, A. 1940. Vom Herzen ausgehende Kreislaufreflexe. Arch. Kreislaufforsch. **7:** 260–274.
18. HEYMANS, C. & E. NEIL. 1958. Reflexogenic Areas of the Cardiovascular System: 1–271. Little, Brown. Boston.
19. DAWES, G.S. & J.H. COMROE, JR. 1954. Chemoreflexes from the heart and lungs. Physiol. Rev. **34:** 167–201.
20. AVIADO, D.M. & C.F. SCHMIDT. 1955. Reflexes from stretch receptors in blood vessels, heart and lungs. Physiol. Rev. **35:** 247–300.
21. KRAYER, O. & G.H. ACHESON. 1946. Pharmacology of veratrum alkaloids. Physiol. Rev. **26:** 383-446.
22. SOMERS, V.K. & F.M. ABBOUD. 1996. Neurocardiogenic syncope. Adv. Intern. Med. **41:** 399–435.
23. MARSHALL, T.M., H.F. MIZGALA & J.A. YEUNG-LAI-WAH. 1993. Successful treatment of deglutition syncope with oral beta-adrenergic blockade. J. Clin. Pharmacol. **34:** 460–465.
24. KAHN, R.L. & M.J. HARGETT. 1999. Beta-adrenergic blockers and vasovagal episodes during shoulder surgery in the sitting position under interscalene block. Anesth. Analg. **88:** 378–381.
25. SMITH, R.M.L. 1994. Mechanisms of vasovagal syncope: relevance to postflight orthostatic intolerance. J. Clin. Pharmacol. **34:** 460–465.
26. MARK, A.L. 1983. The Bezold-Jarisch reflex revisited: clinical implications of inhibitory reflexes originating in the heart. J. Am. Coll. Cardiol. **1:** 90–102.

27. VARRIALE, P., A. INGUAGGIATO & W. DAVID. 1992. Bradyarrhythmias incident to thrombolysis for acute inferior wall infarction. A caveat. Chest. **101:** 732–735.
28. TSAI, C.F., *et al.* 1999. Bezold-Jarisch reflex during radiofrequency ablation of the pulmonary vein tissues in patients with paroxysmal focal atrial fibrillation. J. Cardiovasc. Electrophysiol. **10:** 27–35.
29. ROSSI, L. 1995. Structural and non-structural disease underlying high-risk cardiac arrhythmias relevant to sports medicine. J. Sports Med. Phys. Fitness **35:** 79–86.
30. TORRES, A., *et al.* 1996. Heart rate responses to intravenous serotonin in rats with acute chagasic myocarditis. Braz. J. Med. Biol. Res. **29:** 817–822.
31. LIGTENBERG, G. 1999. Regulation of blood pressure in chronic renal failure: determinants of hypertension and dialysis-related hypotension. Neth. J. Med. **55:** 13–18.
32. SCOTT, R.S. & J.D. DEL ROWE. 1986. A transient hypotensive episode (Bezold-Jarisch effect) occurring in a patient treated with microwave hyperthermia. Am. J. Clin. Oncol. **9:** 170–172.
33. WESTENDROP, R.G., *et al.* 1997. Hypoxic syncope. Aviat. Space Environ. Med. **68:** 410–414.
34. WATTANASIRICHAIGOON, S. & F.B. POMPASELLI, JR. 1997. Branham's sign is an exaggerated Bezold-Jarisch reflex of arteriovenous fistula. [Lett.] J. Vasc. Surg. **26:** 171–172.
35. AVIADO, D.M. 1975. Regulation of bronchomotor tone during anesthesia. Anesthesiology **42:** 68–80.
36. NIDEN, A.H. & D.M. AVIADO. 1952. Effects of pulmonary embolism on the pulmonary circulation with special reference to arteriovenous shunts in the lung. Circ. Res. **4:** 67–73.
37. AVIADO, D.M. & E.I. CUYEGKENG. 1996. Occupational and environmental chemical hazards: a disease classification for students of medicine and allied professions. J. Clean Technol. Environ. Toxicol. Occup. Med. **5:** 297–324.

# Cardiac Vagal Chemosensory Afferents
## Function in Pathophysiological States

HAROLD D. SCHULTZ

*Department of Physiology and Biophysics, University of Nebraska
College of Medicine, Omaha, Nebraska 68198-4575*

ABSTRACT: Stimulation of cardiac vagal afferent endings evokes reflex hypotension and bradycardia, also known as a Bezold-Jarisch effect. The physiological importance of this reflex pathway remains uncertain today, but it is increasingly apparent that cardiac vagal afferents can play an important role in modulating cardiovascular control in pathophysiological states, particularly myocardial ischemia. The afferent endings that compose this vagal input are functionally diverse. Ventricular endings exist that are stimulated by wall motion. However, cardiac chemosensitive endings, stimulated by a variety of metabolically active substances known to be produced by the stressed myocardium (e.g., bradykinin, prostaglandins, reactive oxygen species), play a major role in mediating reflex adjustments during myocardial ischemia. Data are presented highlighting the importance of arachidonic acid metabolites and oxygen radicals in activating cardiac vagal endings during myocardial ischemia and reperfusion, and their role in modulating cardiac afferent sensitivity in the disease states of heart failure and insulin-dependent diabetes.

KEYWORDS: Bezold-Jarisch reflex; Ventricular receptors; Oxygen radicals; Prostaglandins; Antioxidants; Myocardial ischemia; Heart failure; Diabetes

## INTRODUCTION

The heart possesses a sensory innervation of mechanically and chemically sensitive endings that send signals to the central nervous system via vagal and sympathetic afferent pathways. Stimulation of cardiac vagal afferent endings evokes reflex hypotension and bradycardia (sympathoinhibitory) also known as a Bezold-Jarisch effect.[1] By contrast, stimulation of cardiac sympathetic afferent endings evokes reflex hypertension (sympathoexcitatory effect), as well as the perception of cardiac pain.[2] The possible clinical implications of these receptors with regard to autonomic control of the cardiovascular system have been a subject of debate for many years. The complexity of these sensory networks consisting of multiple sensory modalities, divergent afferent pathways, and opposing central influences on autonomic outflow makes it difficult to predict their functional significance in any situation. As a result, we speak more confidently about "functional effects" from studies in which afferent

Address for correspondence: Harold D. Schultz, Ph.D., Department of Physiology and Biophysics, 984575 University of Nebraska Medical Center, Omaha, NE 68198-4575. Voice: 402-559-7167; fax: 402-559-4438.
hschultz@unmc.edu

pathways and stimuli are carefully isolated and controlled. As yet, we can only infer their contribution to function in the intact state.

In the present review, attention is focused only on those receptors whose afferent fibers traverse the vagi and whose sensory endings respond to chemical mediators. These cardiac vagal afferent endings mediate the Bezold-Jarisch reflex (a.k.a. coronary chemoreflex) characterized by bradycardia, hypotension, and active cholinergic coronary vasodilatation.[1] These endings, found predominately but not exclusively in ventricular muscle, are activated by exposure to irritant chemicals such as capsaicin and phenyl diguanide, and most do not readily respond to changes in cardiac pressures or volume.[3] They are also stimulated by a variety of metabolically active substances known to be produced by the stressed myocardium (e.g., bradykinin, prostaglandins, adenosine, $H^+$), and thus are thought to serve a protective function to reduce energy demands on myocardial tissue during stress.[1–4]

This review focuses on our study of the function of these endings during pathophysiological states of myocardial ischemia and reperfusion, heart failure, and diabetes mellitus.

## MYOCARDIAL ISCHEMIA AND REPERFUSION

Studies during the last two decades have suggested that myocardial ischemia represents a potent stimulus capable of exciting cardiac vagal sensory endings. Occlusion of the circumflex coronary artery in dogs results in a decrease in arterial pressure and renal sympathetic nerve activity and inhibition of the baroreflex.[5] In addition, clinical studies[6] have shown that reperfusion of the ischemic myocardium by thrombolysis in patients with acute myocardial infarction is associated with bradycardia and hypotension. It was assumed that these cardiodepressor effects during reperfusion are also the result of stimulation of sympathoinhibitory reflexes mediated by these vagal afferents from the left ventricle.

Previous studies have suggested that during myocardial ischemia, prostaglandins (PGs) serve as a major stimulus to ventricular chemosensitive endings with sympathoinhibitory vagal afferent fibers.[5] However, another important metabolic event that occurs in ischemia, and especially in reperfusion, is reactive oxygen species activation.[7] In studies in rats, we investigated the contribution of reactive oxygen species and arachidonic acid metabolism to activation of cardiac chemosensitive vagal endings during acute myocardial ischemia and reperfusion.[8]

We recorded single-fiber activity from fine slips of the left cervical vagus in anesthetized Sprague-Dawley rats. Afferent fibers identified as chemosensitive exhibited an irregular pattern of discharge at rest, failed to responded to small changes in cardiac pressure, showed no evidence of cardiac or respiratory modulation, and were classified as C-fibers. The results of this study demonstrate that regional ischemia produced by occlusion of the left anterior descending coronary artery (LAD) in rats causes rapid activation of chemosensitive vagal endings located only within the ischemic area (FIGS. 1 and 2). The same correlation was found by Coleridge and coworkers, who recorded impulses from afferent vagal endings in the left ventricle in dogs after the occlusion of the left anterior descending or left circumflex artery.[9]

We examined whether afferent responses to coronary occlusion were mediated by PGs, since the ischemic myocardium releases PGs, which are known to stimulate

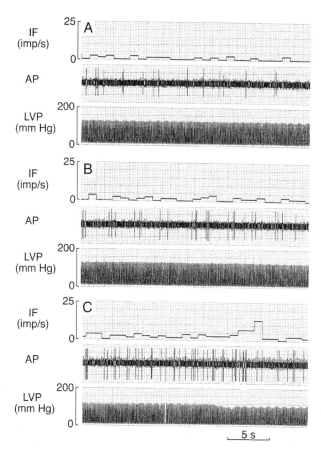

**FIGURE 1.** Effect of LAD occlusion and reperfusion on the activity of a $H_2O_2$-sensitive vagal afferent fiber with its ending within the ischemic zone. (**A**) Final minute of the control period. (**B**) Two minutes after occlusion of LAD. (**C**) One minute after reperfusion (IF: impulse frequency; AP: action potentials; LVP: left ventricular pressure). (Reproduced from Ustinova and Schultz,[8] with permission from the American Heart Association.)

these nerve endings in dogs and to evoke a cardiogenic depressor reflex mediated by these afferents.[5] We found, in rats, that inhibition of cyclooxygenase with indomethacin abolished activation of chemosensitive endings within the ischemic zone at the onset of LAD occlusion (FIG. 2).

Sustained recordings of single afferent fibers during 30 minutes of coronary occlusion and 10 minutes of reperfusion allowed us to observe a second wave of activation that developed at the end of the ischemic period and, even more prominently, at the beginning of reperfusion. This activation was not abolished with indomethacin, and thus was mediated by factors other than cyclooxygenase products. Only chemosensitive fibers that were found to be responsive to chemically induced formation of free radicals (by application of $H_2O_2$ to the heart) increased their activity at

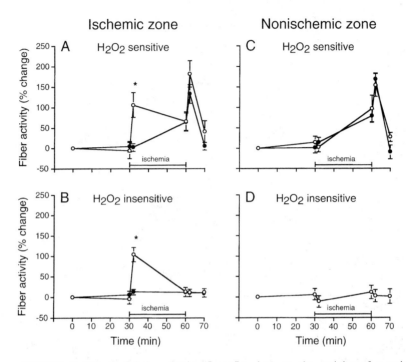

**FIGURE 2.** Effect of indomethacin (5 mg/kg, i.v.) on the activity of ventricular chemosensitive endings during 30 minutes of LAD occlusion and 10 minutes of reperfusion. Afferent fibers were grouped according to the location of the sensory field with respect to the ischemic zone and its responsiveness to epicardial application of $H_2O_2$. Afferent responses in the indomethacin-treated groups (*closed circles*) are compared to those of the untreated groups (*open circles*). Indomethacin abolished afferent responses to ischemia only at the onset of LAD occlusion, from both $H_2O_2$-sensitive and $H_2O_2$-insensitive endings, located only within the ischemic zone. * $p < .05$ compared to untreated (control) group. (Reproduced from Ustinova and Schultz,[8] with permission from the American Heart Association.)

the end of the ischemic period and during reperfusion (FIG. 3). Thus, it is quite likely that this activation was mediated by reactive oxygen species.

We found that activation of cardiac vagal afferent endings in late ischemia and at reperfusion could be abolished by the antioxidants deferoxamine and dimethylthiourea (FIG. 3). Deferoxamine is known to prevent the formation of hydroxyl radicals, and dimethylthiourea is a specific scavenger of hydroxyl radicals. In an accompanying study on rats, we found that both deferoxamine and dimethylthiourea abolished activation of cardiac chemosensitive vagal afferents in response to application of xanthine/xanthine oxidase and $H_2O_2$ to the heart.[10] Thus, there is supportive evidence that deferoxamine prevented activation of chemosensitive afferent endings in the heart during prolonged ischemia and at reperfusion by limitation of reactive oxygen species formation.

Antioxidants had no effect on the activation of the endings at the beginning of coronary occlusion, which suggests that reactive oxygen species do not contribute to

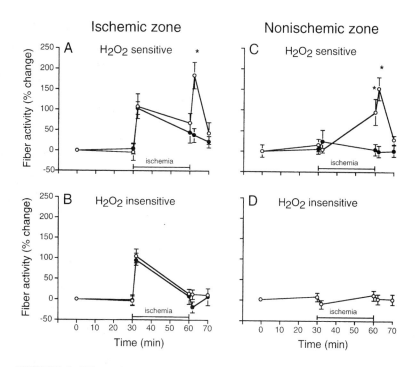

**FIGURE 3.** Effect of deferoxamine (20 mg/kg, i.v.) on the activity of ventricular chemosensitive endings during 30 minutes of LAD occlusion and 10 minutes of reperfusion. Afferent fibers were grouped as in FIGURE 2. Afferent responses in the deferoxamine-treated groups (*closed circles*) are compared to those of the untreated groups (*open circles*). Deferoxamine abolished afferent responses to ischemia only after prolonged LAD occlusion, only from $H_2O_2$ sensitive endings, located both inside and outside the ischemic zone. $*p < .05$ compared to untreated (control) group. (Reproduced from Ustinova and Schultz,[8] with permission from the American Heart Association.)

excitation of cardiac chemosensitive endings in early ischemia. Several studies have shown that enhanced formation of free radicals does not begin immediately after the onset of ischemia. In the rat heart, an increase in hydroxyl radical production begins about 10 minutes after occlusion of the LAD, and the activity of antioxidant enzymes decreases 20–30 minutes thereafter.[11] Nevertheless, 10–15 minutes of coronary occlusion in rats is sufficient to lead to a burst of free radical production during subsequent reperfusion.

An interesting observation from our study was that all of the $H_2O_2$-sensitive endings found in the left ventricle were stimulated by prolonged ischemia and by reperfusion regardless of their location in relation to the ischemic zone (FIG. 3). Because these afferent responses were abolished by deferoxamine, these results would suggest that oxygen free radical formation is enhanced throughout the left ventricle in response to coronary occlusion and reperfusion. In support of this notion, other studies have shown that occlusion of the LAD in the rat decreases the activity of antioxidant enzymes and increases free radical formation in both ischemic and nonischemic areas of the heart.[11,12]

Our results, using electroneurographic recordings in rats, corroborate the notion that the stimulation of chemosensitive vagal afferents in response to production and release of PGs or other cyclooxygenase products from the ischemic tissue initiate these reflex changes at the onset of myocardial ischemia.[5] Our results further suggest that during more prolonged periods of ischemia, and during reperfusion, these reflex responses are more likely to be mediated by these afferents in response to reactive oxygen species production.

The mechanisms responsible for enhancement of free radical formation in the nonischemic myocardium during acute ischemia are not yet well understood. In addition to partial inactivation of endogenous enzymatic antioxidant systems, myocardial ischemia produces an excessive release of catecholamines, which are known to increase energy demand of the tissue and to activate lipases and phospholipases, that is, metabolic changes that facilitate free radical peroxidation in the myocardium.[13,14] Autooxidation of norepinephrine also results in free radical formation.[14] In our study, one could speculate that these metabolic changes enhanced free radical production in the nonischemic areas of the myocardium during the 30-min period of ischemia. By contrast, in the ischemic zone, the lack of oxygen may limit activation of free radical production during ischemia, and a more marked increase in free radical production would occur at the beginning of reperfusion. This hypothesis could explain why the activity of $H_2O_2$-sensitive endings in the nonischemic zone of the left ventricle gradually increased over the course of 30 minutes of ischemia, while activation of $H_2O_2$-sensitive endings within the ischemic zone occurred more prominently at the onset of reperfusion.

The functional significance of the effects of myocardial ischemia and reperfusion on cardiac chemosensitive vagal afferents remains unresolved. Needleman speculated that the increased parasympathetic tone and decreased sympathetic tone reflexly evoked by these afferents in response to PGs is beneficial to the ischemic myocardium.[15] Thus, the bradycardia, decreased contractility, and peripheral vasodilatation would decrease the work of the heart and reduce oxygen demand of the compromised myocardium. Furthermore, the cholinergic-mediated increase in coronary blood flow would increase oxygen delivery. The functional implications of these reflex changes at the onset of reperfusion of the ischemic myocardium is less clear, but certainly the increased parasympathetic drive could help to stabilize the excitability of the myocardium and impede potentially dangerous arrhythmias, which are known to occur with myocardial reperfusion.[16] Thus, despite the pronounced detrimental effects of free radicals on the function and excitability of cardiac myocytes, the stimulatory effect of these reactive oxygen species on chemosensitive vagal reflexes during reperfusion could be of some benefit.

## HEART FAILURE

It is generally assumed that cardiac reflexes are attenuated in congestive heart failure (HF). Studies carried out in anesthetized dogs with congestive heart failure confirm that, in general, cardiovascular mechanoreflexes, including arterial, atrial, and ventricular mechanoreflexes, are significantly blunted in this state.[17] Although

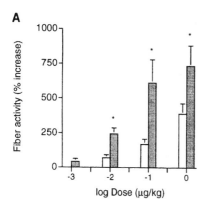

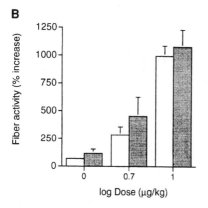

**FIGURE 4.** Afferent response of cardiac vagal chemosensitive endings from sham-operated (*open bars*) and heart failure (HF) dogs (*shaded bars*) in response to left atrial injection of graded doses of (**A**) bradykinin and (**B**) capsaicin. *$p < .05$ sham-operated vs. HF. (Reproduced from Schultz *et al.*,[16] with permission from the American Physiological Society.)

the mechanisms responsible for mechanoreflex abnormalities in heart failure are not completely understood, it is clear that mechanoreceptor endings themselves exhibit a depressed sensitivity to change in pressure. However, unlike the mechanoreflexes, evidence suggests that the cardiac vagal chemoreflex is potentiated in dogs with pacing-induced heart failure.[18] Because the Bezold-Jarisch reflex is so potent under normal conditions, it is of interest to determine whether this reflex behaves differently in states in which the myocardium is either chronically dilated or hypertrophied.

We examined the discharge characteristics and chemical sensitivity of chemosensitive endings in the left ventricle in dogs after chronic ventricular pacing as a model of low-output HF.[19] We found that there was no difference in the rate or pattern of resting discharge of cardiac vagal fibers between HF and sham-operated dogs. However, the afferent response to bradykinin (BK) was significantly enhanced in HF dogs (FIG. 4). The $B_2$ receptor antagonist HOE-140 inhibited this effect. This enhanced sensitization of the cardiac vagal chemosensitive afferents appeared to be receptor specific, because there was no enhancement of the afferent response to capsaicin.

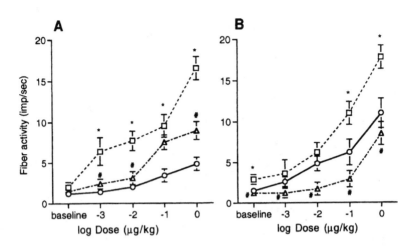

**FIGURE 5.** Effect of captopril (2 mg/kg, i.v.) and then indomethacin (5 mg/kg, i.v.) on afferent responses to BK in (**A**) sham-operated and (**B**) HF dogs. *Open circles*: Control; *open squares*: captopril; *triangles*: indomethacin. *$p < .05$ compared with control responses. #$p < .05$ compared with response after captopril. (Reproduced from Schultz et al.,[16] with permission from the American Physiological Society.)

Increased levels of PGs may mediate sensitization of the cardiac chemosensitive endings to BK in HF because the enhancement was reversed by indomethacin (FIG. 5). In addition, indomethacin more effectively inhibited resting discharge from the afferents in the HF state than in the sham-operated state (FIG. 5). PG production is known to be elevated in cardiac tissue during HF. Furthermore, evidence indicates that PGs potentiate both afferent and reflex responses evoked by stimulation of cardiac vagal endings with BK.[20]

In this study, we also found that captopril enhanced afferent sensitivity of chemosensitive endings to exogenous BK in both the sham-operated and HF animals to a similar degree (FIG. 5). These results suggest that angiotensin-converting enzyme (ACE) activity significantly reduces the ability of BK to stimulate cardiac vagal endings in both the normal and HF state, presumably by metabolic inactivation of the peptide. Cardiac ACE activity is known to be elevated in experimental HF, and thus one would anticipate that ACE activity should inhibit afferent responses to BK more effectively in the HF state. Our observation that ACE inhibition by captopril markedly enhanced basal discharge from cardiac afferents only in the HF state (FIG. 5) is consistent with this notion. However, our results also indicate that cardiac chemosensitive afferents in the failing heart are sensitized to exogenous BK. Such an effect would be paradoxical in the face of elevated ACE activity.

One possible explanation of the paradoxical result is that enhanced PG synthesis and ACE activity in cardiac tissue during HF exert opposing influences on cardiac vagal afferent responsiveness to BK. A high level of ACE activity in failing cardiac tissue may counter the ability of endogenous BK and PGs to enhance spontaneous discharge at rest. On the other hand, elevations in BK (as with exogenous administration) would tip the balance toward enhancing afferent sensitivity due to the synergistic effects between BK and PGs.[20]

Undoubtedly, many yet unexplored factors also may contribute to altered cardiac vagal chemosensory function in heart failure in addition to BK, PGs, and ACE activity. The role of free radicals and other metabolic changes in HF is of obvious concern that awaits future exploration. Of these, one important factor that must be taken into consideration is the influence of ventricular distension on cardiac chemoreflex responses. In a recent study, Wang and coworkers have found that acute volume expansion enhances cardiac sympathetic afferent reflex responses to epicardial application of BK.[21] The mechanism of this interaction between wall stress and chemosensory function in heart is not yet clear, but may be related to increased $O_2$ demand in response to the heightened work load.

The importance of our findings calls into question the established etiology of the sympthoexcitation of HF. The sympathoexcitation that parallels the severity of HF is generally thought to be due to the blunted arterial and cardiopulmonary mechanoreflex inhibition of sympathetic outflow. We must now reevaluate the net effect on sympathetic outflow with respect to the relative reduction of mechanoreceptor sensitivity versus the increase in sensitivity of chemosensitive endings. In this regard, it is important to note recent studies demonstrating that the cardiac sympathetic afferent chemoreflex is enhanced in the HF condition.[22] Unlike the vagal afferent reflex, the cardiac sympathetic afferent reflex provides a positive stimulus to sympathetic outflow, and thus, could play an important role in tipping the balance of control of sympathetic outflow toward higher levels.

Our studies also may shed light on a contributory mechanism to the beneficial effect of ACE inhibitors in HF by our observation that captopril elevates resting discharge from cardiac vagal afferent endings in the HF state. It is possible that the increased central input from these cardiac afferents contributes to the decrease in sympathetic outflow that is known to occur after ACE inhibition. This enhanced sympathoinhibitory reflex may help to improve cardiac performance by reducing the sympathoexcitation of HF.

## DIABETES MELLITUS

Silent myocardial ischemia and cardiac arrhythmias are frequent and major complications of diabetes mellitus that place the patient at risk of sudden cardiac death. Autonomic neuropathy is thought to play an important role in the pathogenesis of these complications. Cardiac parasympathetic and sympathetic fibers are affected, leading to a decrease in heart-rate variability and impaired baroreflex function.[23] This impairment in autonomic control, in concert with other disease processes occurring in the diabetic heart, can contribute to life-threatening arrhythmias. Diabetic patients also have a blunted perception of cardiac pain.[24] As a result, myocardial ischemia or infarction may be associated with only mild symptoms that go unrecognized. These observations suggest an impairment of cardiac afferent as well as efferent autonomic function, which may compound the risk for cardiac death in diabetic patients.

It is reasonable to suggest that the function of cardiac chemosensory endings is depressed consistent with generalized peripheral autonomic neuropathy characteris-

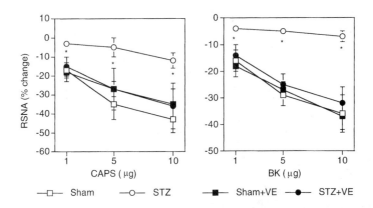

**FIGURE 6.** Effect of VE treatment on the reflex inhibition of RSNA in response to epicardial application of CAPS and BK in sham-operated and STZ-induced diabetic rats with cardiac sympathetic denervation (cardiac vagal afferent reflex). *$p < .05$ compared to sham-operated. (Reproduced from Ustinova et al.,[23] with permission from the American Physiological Society.)

tic of chronic diabetes. Nevertheless, direct evidence has been lacking to document whether the sensory innervation of the heart is altered in diabetes. One of the primary factors known to contribute to cardiomyopathy and peripheral neuropathy in diabetes is oxidative stress.[25] Since we have previously shown that cardiac afferent endings are known to be sensitive to oxygen-reactive species,[10] it is possible that the elevated presence of free radicals in cardiac tissue during diabetes may lead to alterations in cardiac afferent function.

We investigated the effects of diabetes mellitus and antioxidant treatment on the sensory and reflex function of cardiac vagal chemosensory nerves in rats.[26] Diabetes was induced by streptozotocin (STZ, 85 mg/kg, i.p.). Subgroups of sham-operated and STZ-treated rats were chronically treated with an antioxidant, vitamin E (60 mg/kg *per os*, daily, starting 2 days before STZ). Animals were studied 6–8 weeks after STZ injection. We measured renal sympathetic nerve activity (RSNA) and cardiac vagal and sympathetic afferent activities in response to stimulation of chemosensitive sensory nerves in the heart by epicardial application of capsaicin (CAPS) and bradykinin (BK). Sinoaortic denervation and cardiac sympathetic denervation were performed in order to confine reflex responses to activation of cardiac vagal afferent endings.

Epicardial application of either CAPS or BK (1–10.0 µg) evoked a vagal-afferent-mediated reflex depression of RSNA and mean arterial pressure in sham-operated rats, which was significantly blunted in STZ rats (FIG. 6). Chronic vitamin E treatment effectively prevented these cardiac chemoreflex defects in STZ rats without altering resting blood glucose or hemodynamics (FIG. 6). STZ rats with insulin replacement did not exhibit impaired cardiac chemoreflexes. In afferent studies, CAPS and BK (0.1 g–10.0 µg) increased cardiac vagal afferent nerve activity in a dose-dependent manner in sham-operated rats, which was significantly blunted in STZ-treated rats (FIG. 7). Vitamin E prevented the impairment of afferent discharge

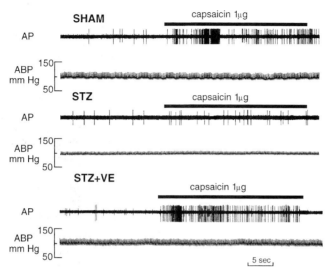

**FIGURE 7.** Recordings of impulse activity from vagal afferent fibers arising from the left ventricle in (**A**) a sham-operated rat, (**B**) a STZ-treated rat, and (**C**) a STZ + VE-treated rat in response to epicardial capsaicin (1 μg in 10 μL). *Bars* indicate the duration of capsaicin application. AP: action potential. (Reproduced from Ustinova *et al.*,[23] with permission from the American Physiological Society.)

to chemical stimulation in STZ rats. The antioxidant efficacy of Vitamin E was assessed by measuring plasma lipid peroxides. The plasma level of lipid peroxides in STZ rats was significantly greater than in sham-operated rats. Chronic treatment with vitamin E prevented this accumulation of lipid peroxides in diabetic animals.

These results indicate that the Bezold-Jarisch reflex is markedly depressed in STZ-induced diabetic rats. The results also indicate that this functional impairment in the diabetic state can be prevented by chronic treatment with vitamin E. From these results we believe that oxidative stress is the major underlying mechanism causing impairment of the chemosensitive and reflex properties of cardiac sensory nerve endings in diabetes.

Oxidative stress is thought to be a major contributor to cardiovascular disease in diabetes mellitus.[25] Morphological studies also have shown that chronic treatment with vitamin E largely prevents the degeneration of autonomic nerve fibers in the hearts of diabetic rats.[27] Hyperglycemia-driven metabolic changes in diabetes increase generation of free radicals though several mechanisms, including glucose autoxidation, protein glycation, increased substrate flux through the polyol pathway, and depression of natural antioxidant systems.[25] One or more of these potential mechanisms is likely to be involved in the impairment of cardiac afferent function in the diabetic rats.

We also found that in sham-operated rats, vagotomy increased resting RSNA; whereas in diabetic rats, vagotomy did not.[26] These results correlate with our observation that resting RSNA appeared to be elevated in the diabetic state.[26] Furthermore, chronic vitamin E treatment prevented this impairment of vagal restraint of sympathetic outflow in diabetic rats. These data suggest that oxidative stress in diabetes impairs vagal influences that limit tonic sympathetic activity. This observation may have important implications for the study of heart-rate variability and the pathogenesis and treatment of arrhythmias in diabetic patients.

One aspect of our afferent and reflex results that is discrepant is the correlation between resting RSNA and resting cardiac chemosensitive afferent activity in sham and diabetic rats. Resting impulse activity from cardiac vagal chemosensitive afferent fibers did not differ between sham and diabetic rats, whereas resting RSNA was elevated and vagal restraint of resting sympathetic outflow was blunted in diabetic animals.[26] The functional significance of this paradox has not yet been resolved, but several possible explanations can be considered. An impairment in central integration of the cardiac vagal chemoreflex may also occur in the diabetic state, causing a reduction in tonic restraint of sympathetic outflow in the face of normal resting afferent activity. In addition, other vagal reflexes may play a comparatively larger role in the tonic control of sympathetic outflow and also may be impaired in the diabetic state. It is known that the neural component of the volume reflex is blunted in STZ diabetic rats.[28] It is possible that cardiopulmonary mechanoreceptors are similarly blunted in the diabetes and that a reduction in afferent input from this vagal reflex pathway can account for the alterations in resting renal sympathetic outflow observed in diabetic rats.

Impairment of the cardiac vagal chemoreflex in diabetic animals may be the result of oxidative injury at any of the many levels of the neural reflex arc: afferent, central, efferent. Because cardiac chemosensitive afferents are stimulated acutely by oxygen reactive species,[10] chronic exposure to free radicals may desensitize or injure the afferent endings and diminish reflexes that arise from their activation. We tested this possibility by directly recording action potentials from cardiac vagal chemosensitive afferents in response to stimulation by CAPS, BK, and veratridine. Our data demonstrate that the responses of cardiac vagal fibers to CAPS and BK were depressed in diabetic rats (FIG. 7). Chronic treatment with vitamin E completely abolished the detrimental effect of diabetes on the chemosensory properties of the cardiac afferent nerves. This defect of the sensory properties of the cardiac afferent nerve endings appears to be mediated by oxidative stress and provides a primary explanation for the depressed cardiac chemoreflexes in our diabetic animals.

We found that the response of cardiac vagal chemosensitive endings to veratridine, unlike CAPS or BK, was not attenuated in diabetic rats.[26] This observation may provide some insight into the mechanism of the oxidative impairment of the afferent endings. Most chemical mediators of chemosensitive endings, including CAPS and BK, evoke depolarization of the afferent neuron by binding to membrane receptors or ligand-gated ion channels in the nerve terminal leading to depolarization. Unlike CAPS and BK, veratridine bypasses the receptor-mediated complex and evokes action potentials by direct activation of the voltage-gated $Na^+$ channel at the level of the spike-initiating zone. As we have shown, the impairment of cardiac vagal afferent discharge in diabetic rats did not extend to the general ability of the afferent fibers to propagate action potentials, since responses to veratridine were normal. Thus the impairment in cardiac afferent responses to CAPS and BK in the diabetic rats appears to involve a dysfunction in the chemical transduction process prior to spike initiation.

It should be noted that the impairment in cardiac vagal afferent responses after chronic exposure to elevated free radical production (diabetes) is opposite to that which occurs in response to acute exposure (acute ischemia), which activates these endings.[8,10] It is possible that this chronic desensitization occurs via downregulation of the receptor-mediated complexes activated by free radicals. This notion is consistent with our recent demonstration that acute exposure to the antioxidant, superoxide dismutase, after 6 weeks of diabetes rapidly restores (within hours) cardiac chemoreflex function in diabetic rats, implying a reversible regulatory mechanism.[29] These results also implicate the superoxide anion as the primary oxidant involved in this desensitization process.

In summary, our studies indicate that the Bezold-Jarisch effect is markedly depressed in diabetic rats, and correspondingly chronic antioxidant treatment can effectively prevent this impairment. Our results show that cardiac chemosensory nerves are desensitized in diabetes as a result of a dysfunction in the chemical transduction process in the sensory terminal. The efficacy of vitamin E and superoxide dismutase in preventing this afferent dysfunction is consistent with a mechanism mediated by superoxide anion. Impairment in cardiac chemosensory function may play an important role in exacerbating diabetic cardiac complications, such as silent ischemia and arrhythmias. In addition, these results provide evidence that chronic antioxidant therapy can be effective in reducing the risk of these complications in diabetic patients. Given the uncertainties in extrapolation of our results from diabetic rats to the human condition, further studies are needed to assess their clinical implications.

## CONCLUSIONS

The sensory and reflex properties of cardiac chemosensitive endings with afferent vagal projections are markedly influenced by conditions associated with changes in the metabolic state of the myocardium. These endings are activated during acute myocardial ischemia and reperfusion as a result of increased myocardial tissue production of ischemic mediators. Of these, cyclooxygenase products and enhanced oxygen-radical formation appear to play an important role. In the setting of HF, these endings exhibit an enhanced responsiveness to bradykinin that appears to involve cyclooxygenase products as well. This enhancement in afferent responsiveness in HF, however, may be offset to a certain degree by an increase in cardiac angiotensin-converting enzyme activity to reduce endogenous bradykinin effects on basal activity. Another important factor that may contribute to enhanced cardiac chemosensitivity in HF is volume overloading of the heart, leading to increased wall stress and increased $O_2$ demand. In the setting of diabetes mellitus, cardiac vagal afferent function is impaired as a result of desensitization of the afferent endings via chronic exposure to oxidative stress. Superoxide anions appear to play an important role in this desensitization process. The functional implications of these changes remain to be fully understood. Although it is logical to suggest that these sensory endings intend to serve a protective reflex to prevent overexertion of cardiac muscle, we cannot discount the possibility that changes in activity of these endings in disease states as we have described may have important detrimental consequences on autonomic control of cardiac performance.

## ACKNOWLEDGMENT

This work was supported in part by Grant HL-52190 from the National Heart, Lung, and Blood Institute, and in part by grants-in-aid from the American Heart Association.

## REFERENCES

1. HAINSWORTH, R. 1991. Reflexes from the heart. Physiol. Rev. **71:** 617–658.
2. MALLIANI, A. 1990. Cardiocardiac excitatory reflexes during myocardial ischemia. Basic Res. Cardiol. **85**(Suppl.1): 243–252.
3. COLERIDGE, H.M., J.C.G. COLERIDGE & C. KIDD. 1964. Cardiac receptors in the dog with particular reference to two types of afferent ending in the ventricular wall. J. Physiol. **174:** 323–339.
4. COLERIDGE, H.M. & CG COLERIDGE. 1980. Cardiovascular afferents involved in regulation of peripheral vessels. Ann. Rev. Physiol. **42:** 413–427.
5. ZUCKER, I.H., M.J. PANZENBECK, J.F. HACKLEY & K. HAIDERZAD. 1989. Baroreflex inhibition during coronary occlusion is mediated by prostaglandins. Am. J. Physiol. (Regulatory, Integrative, and Comp. Physiol.) **257:** R216–R223.
6. WEI, J.Y., J.E. MARKIS, M. MALAGOLD & E. BRAUNWALD. 1983. Cardiovascular reflexes stimulated by reperfusion of ischemic myocardium in acute myocardial infarction. Circulation **67:** 796–801.
7. BOLLI, R. 1991. Oxygen-derived free radicals and myocardial reperfusion injury: an overview. Cardiovasc. Drugs Ther. **5**(Suppl. 2): 249–268.
8. USTINOVA, E.E. & H.D. SCHULTZ. 1994. Activation of cardiac vagal afferents by ischemia and reperfusion: prostaglandins versus oxygen-derived free radicals. Circulation Res. **74:** 904–911.
9. COLERIDGE, J.C., H.M. COLERIDGE, T.E. PISSARI & H.D. SCHULTZ. 1990. Stimulation of cardiac vagal chemosensitive C-fibers by coronary occlusion in dogs. [Abstr.] FASEB J. **4**(1): A707.
10. USTINOVA, E.E. & H.D. SCHULTZ. 1994. Activation of cardiac vagal afferents by oxygen-derived free radicals in rats. Circ. Res. **74:** 895–903.
11. GUTKIN, D.V. & I.A. PETROVICH. 1982. Activity of antioxidative enzymes of the myocardium during ischemia. Bull. Exp. Biol. Med. **93:** 3–35.
12. MEERSON, F.Z. 1982. The role of lipid peroxidation in pathogenesis of ischemic damage and the antioxidant protection of the heart. Basic Res. Cardiol. **77:** 465–485.
13. SCHOMIG, A. 1988. Adrenergic mechanisms in myocardial infarction: cardiac and systemic catecholamines release. J. Cardiovasc. Pharmacol.**12** (Suppl. 1): S1–S7.
14. RUMP, A.F. & W. KLAUS. 1994. Evidence for norepinephrine cardiotoxicity mediated by superoxide anion radicals in isolated rabbit hearts. Naunyn-Schmiedebergs Arch. Pharmacol. **349:** 295–300.
15. NEEDLEMAN, P. 1976. The synthesis and function of prostaglandins in the heart. Fed. Proc. **35:** 2376–2381.
16. BERNIER, M., D.J. HEARSE & A.S. MANNING. 1986. Reperfusion induced arrhythmias and oxygen free radicals. Studies with anti-free radical interventions and a free radical generating system in the isolated perfused rat heart. Circulation Res. **58:** 331–340.
17. ZUCKER, I.H., W. WANG, M. BRANDLE & H.D. SCHULTZ. 1996. Baroreflex and cardiac reflex control of the circulation in pacing-induced heart failure. *In* Pathophysiology of Tachycardia-Induced Heart Failure. F.G. Spinale, Ed.: 193–226. Futura. Armonk, N.Y.

18. Zucker, I.H., W. Wang, M. Brandle, *et al.* 1995. Neural regulation of sympathetic nerve activity in heart failure. Prog. Cardiovasc. Dis. **37:** 397–414.
19. SCHULTZ, H.D., W. WANG, E.E. USTINOVA & I.H. ZUCKER. 1997. Enhanced responsiveness of cardiac vagal chemosensitive endings to bradykinin in heart failure. Am. J. Physiol. (Regulatory, Integrative, and Comp. Physiol.) **273:** R637–R645.
20. STASZEWSKA-BARCZAK, J. 1983. Prostanoids and cardiac reflexes of sympathetic and vagal origin. Am. J. Cardiol. **52:** 36A–45A.
21. WANG, W., H.D. SCHULTZ & M. RONG. 2001. Volume expansion potentiates cardiac sympathetic afferent reflex in dogs. Am. J. Physiol. Heart Circ. Physiol. **280:** H576–H581.
22. WANG, W., H.D. SCHULTZ & M. RONG. 1999. Cardiac sympathetic afferent sensitivity is enhanced in heart failure. Am J. Physiol. Heart Circ. Physiol. **277:** H812–H817.
23. MCDOWELL, T.S., M.W. CHAPLEAU, G. HADJUCZOK & F.M. ABBOUD. 1994. Baroreflex dysfunction in diabetes mellitus. I. Selective impairment of parasympathetic control of heart rate. Am. J. Physiol. Heart Circ. Physiol. **35:** H235–H243.
24. AIRAKSINEN, K.E. & M.J. KOISTINEN. 1992. Association between silent coronary artery disease, diabetes, and autonomic neuropathy. Fact of fallacy? Diabetes Care **15:** 288–292.
25. BAYNES, J.W. 1991. Perspectives in diabetes: role of oxidative stress in development of complications in diabetes. Diabetes **40:** 405–412.
26. USTINOVA, E.E., C.J. BARRETT, S.-Y. SUN & H.D. SCHULTZ. 2000. Oxidative stress impairs cardiac chemoreflexes in diabetic rats. Am. J. Physiol. Heart Circ. Physiol. **279:** H2176–H2187.
27. EWING, D.J. 1996. Diabetic autonomic neuropathy and the heart. Diabetes Res. Clin. Pract. **30**(Suppl. 1): 31–36.
28. PATEL, K.P. 1997. Volume reflex in diabetes. Cardiovascular Res. **34:** 81–90.
29. BARRETT, C.J. & H.D. SCHULTZ. 1999. Superoxide anion mediates impaired cardiac vagal reflex function in streptozotocin-induced diabetic rats. [Abstr.] Circulation (Suppl.) **100**(18): 1–130.

# Cardiac Sympathetic Afferent Activation Provoked by Myocardial Ischemia and Reperfusion

## Mechanisms and Reflexes

JOHN C. LONGHURST, STEPHANIE C. TJEN-A-LOOI, AND LIANG-WU FU

*Department of Medicine, University of California, Irvine, Irvine, California 92697, USA*

ABSTRACT: Cardiac sympathetic afferents are known to reflexly activate the cardiovascular system, leading to increases in blood pressure, heart rate, and myocardial contractile function. During myocardial ischemia, these sensory nerves also transmit the sensation of pain (angina pectoris) and cause tachyarrhythmias. The authors' laboratory has been interested in defining the mechanisms of activation of this neural system during ischemia and reperfusion. During these periods, reactive oxygen species, particularly hydroxyl radicals, are produced from the breakdown of purine metabolites and lead to stimulation of sympathetic (and vagal) ventricular chemosensitive nerve endings. For example, stimulation with hydrogen peroxide leads to a small reflex increase in blood pressure from the predominant sympathetic afferent activation that is reduced by simultaneous activation of cardiac vagal afferents (known to exert predominantly depressor reflexes). Central integration of these two opposing reflexes likely occurs at several regions of the brain stem, including the nucleus tractus solitarii, where neural occlusion occurs during simultaneous cardiac sympathetic and vagal-afferent stimulation. Activation of platelets also appears to play a role during myocardial ischemia, leading to local release of serotonin (5HT), which, through a $5HT_3$ mechanism, stimulates sympathetic afferents. Finally, regional changes in pH from lactic acid (but not hypercapnia), stimulate ventricular afferents and may activate kallikrein to increase bradykinin (BK), which, in turn, breaks down arachidonic acid to form prostaglandins. Prostaglandins sensitize cardiac sympathetic afferents to BK. Thus, stimulation of cardiac sympathetic afferents during ischemia and reperfusion and the resulting reflex events form a multifactorial process resulting from activation of a number of chemical pathways in the myocardium.

KEYWORDS: NTS; ROS, Serotonin, Platelets; Bradykinin; Proton

Author for correspondence: John C. Longhurst, Department of Medicine, Medical Sciences 1, C240, University of California at Irvine, Irvine, CA 92697. Voice: 949-824-5602; fax: 949-824-2200.

jcl@uci.edu

## INTRODUCTION

Cardiac–cardiovascular reflexes are important in both physiological and pathophysiological conditions. In this regard, stimulation of cardiac vagal sensory neurons leads to vasodepressor reflex events, while stimulation of cardiac sympathetic or spinal neurons leads to vasopressor responses. These reflexes become manifested in a number of clinical conditions when the reflexes are either stimulated or blunted by the pathophysiologic process. For instance, during left-ventricular outflow obstruction, there is particularly strong stimulation of cardiac vagal afferents, leading to reflex cardioinhibition and occasionally syncope and collapse.[1,2] During or after cardiopulmonary bypass, sympathetic cardiac afferents are stimulated and remarkable hypertensive emergencies can occur.[3–6] Conversely, in patients with congestive heart failure, the activity of cardiac afferents, particularly the atrial afferents, appears to be blunted, and normal reflex processes that could promote a diuresis, and thereby reverse the volume overload, are not brought into action in an appropriate fashion.[2,7,8] Myocardial ischemia is still another condition when both vagal and sympathetic cardiac-afferent systems are activated.[9–11] During this process, depending upon the location and extent of ischemia, there can either be vasodepressor reflex responses, which include decreases in blood pressure, heart rate, as well as bradyarrhythmias, nausea, and vomiting,[11,12] or be excitatory responses, which include tachyarrhythmias, hypertension, and, of course, the warning sign of angina pectoris.[13,14] The former responses appear to be mainly a function of vagal afferents, while the latter appear to be caused by activation of sympathetic afferents. Thus, relatively important warning signs and symptoms as well as potentially deleterious or even lethal reflex responses from activation of cardiac afferents during ischemia can occur. Despite these recognized autonomic responses, the sensory signaling mechanisms leading to their activation are poorly understood. For many years our laboratory has been exploring the mechanisms underlying stimulation of abdominal visceral afferents, particularly those afferents that ascend through sympathetic pathways and the spinal cord.[15,16] This review describes some of our more recent and ongoing attempts to define those mechanisms, particularly the chemical mechanisms, that are important in activating cardiac afferents during myocardial ischemia. We recognized at the outset that studying the heart was particularly difficult, since ischemia can lead to infarction or perhaps myocardial stunning, and this might, by itself, alter the afferent nerve discharge properties from the heart. Therefore, we limited our studies to relatively brief ischemia of 5–10 min that would not be associated with infarction or stunning and that could be used on at least two successive occasions in a protocol design that incorporated specific inhibitors and receptor antagonists. This experimental design gave us the opportunity to study the independent and interactive actions of a number of chemical mediators that potentially could be important in stimulating cardiac sensory nerve endings during and after ischemia. We were guided, in part, by our previous studies of abdominal sympathetic afferents in which we had observed afferents that discharged not only during ischemia but also during reperfusion, either as a prolonged monophasic discharge or as a secondary wave of increased activity during reperfusion.[17]

We began our studies by looking at those mediators that might be produced and therefore would be available to activate cardiac sensory nerve endings during ischemia *and* reperfusion. Thus, in addition to studying conventional mediators like bradykinin, some of our first studies were designed to investigate the possibility that reactive oxygen species (ROS) could play an important noninjurious role in stimulating cardiac sympathetic afferents.

## STUDIES OF CARDIAC SYMPATHETIC
## AFFERENT MECHANISMS

### Protons

Myocardial ischemia results in local tissue acidosis because of the retention of acid metabolites in the ischemic region. Previous studies have demonstrated that in the ischemic working heart, the concentration of lactic acid rises and the intracellular pH falls rapidly as the acid products of glycolysis and metabolism of abnormal fatty acid accumulate.[18]

Protons play a prominent role in activation of visceral afferents including pulmonary vagal afferents and abdominal sympathetic afferent nerve endings.[19,20] Protons also can evoke a somatic-cardiovascular reflex through activation of somatic afferents. In this regard, Rotto et al.[21] demonstrated that lactic acid reflexly increases heart rate and arterial pressure through stimulation of group III and IV afferent nerve endings in muscle.[21] In a rat skin-saphenous nerve preparation, Steen et al.[22] observed that protons, derived from either lactic acid or $CO_2$, selectively stimulate polymodal cutaneous C-fiber afferents rather than $A\delta$-fibers. During our studies of abdominal visceral afferents we observed, however, that ischemically sensitive abdominal sympathetic $A\delta$- and C-fiber afferents responded to administration of lactic acid but not to hypercapnia, despite the smaller changes in local tissue pH caused by lactic acid compared to hypercapnia.[19] Likewise, it has been observed that hypercapnia does not activate cardiac vagal chemoreceptors.[23] Exogenous lactic acid also stimulates pulmonary unmyelinated fibers[20] and cardiac sympathetic afferents including both myelinated and unmyelinated fibers.[24,25] Therefore, protons produced during myocardial ischemia are thought to play a role in activation and/or sensitization of ischemically sensitive cardiac sympathetic afferents.

To evaluate the importance of protons as a stimulus of cardiac afferents, we investigated the effect of ischemia-induced alterations of epicardial pH on the activity of cardiac afferents in the absence and the presence of an isotonic neutral phosphate buffer. Three major sources of protons during myocardial ischemia include accumulation of lactic acid, generation of $CO_2$, and abnormal fatty acid metabolism.[18,19] Therefore, we also examined the responses of these afferents to hypercapnia, acidic phosphate buffer, lactic acid, or sodium lactate.[26] Epicardial pH was measured continuously with a pH-sensitive needle electrode (0.9 mm o.d.), because cardiac sympathetic afferent nerve endings generally are located near the epicardial surface.[27] We found that epicardial pH decreased progressively during brief (5-min) ischemia, topical application of acidic phosphate buffer, lactic acid, or exposure to hypercapnic gas mixtures. We also observed that lactic acid, but not sodium lactate, stimulated cardiac sympathetic afferents to a greater extent than the acidic phosphate buffer solution (FIG. 1). Conversely, inhalation of a high $CO_2$ gas concentration failed to activate these afferents, despite similar or greater pH changes in the epicardial region. Compared to ischemically sensitive afferents (100%), only 19% of ischemically in-

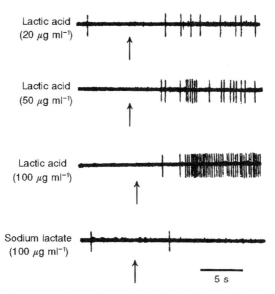

**FIGURE 1.** Representative tracings of an ischemically sensitive cardiac sympathetic afferent (CV = 0.46 m/s) innervating the anterior wall of left ventricle. Topical application (-) of lactic acid (20, 50, and 100 µg/mL), but not sodium lactate (100 µg/mL), to the receptive field of the afferent on left ventricle, stimulated this cardiac afferent in a dose-dependent manner. The epicardial pH values were 7.18, 7.03, 6.83, and 7.34, respectively. (From Pan *et al.*, 1999.[26] Reproduced by permission.)

sensitive afferents responded to epicardial application of lactic acid. Moreover, the neutral phosphate buffer, which prevented tissue acidosis in the epicardial layer of the ischemic region, attenuated the response of these afferents to brief myocardial ischemia (FIGS. 2 and 3). Thus, we believe that endogenous protons, derived from lactic acid, but not from hypercapnia, contribute to activation or sensitization of cardiac sympathetic afferents during myocardial ischemia. Protons could directly stimulate cardiac sympathetic afferent nerve endings, and/or they could cause the production of other mediators such as bradykinin (BK), since an acidic environment favors the activation of kallikrein,[19] the enzyme responsible for production of BK. Future studies will be required to define the specific mechanism by which protons lead to activation of cardiac afferents during ischemia.

### *Bradykinin and Prostaglandins*

Myocardial ischemia produces various metabolites that potentially can stimulate or sensitize cardiac sympathetic afferents. Among many others, BK has been considered to be one of the chemical mediators that plays a role in the activation of cardiac afferents during ischemia.[28] Baker *et al.*[27] originally suggested that BK may be a chemical mediator of cardiac pain. Experimental evidence has shown that the concentration of BK increases in the coronary sinus within 2 to 5 min after occlusion of the left descending coronary artery.[29] In addition, cardiovascular reflexes associated

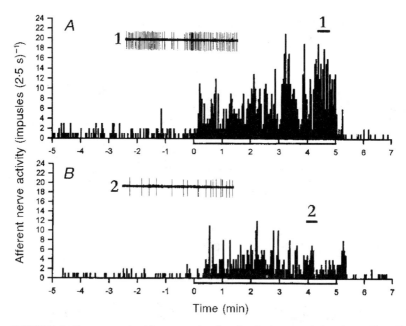

**FIGURE 2.** Representative histogram showing the discharge activity of a cardiac afferent during myocardial ischemia in the absence (**A**) and the presence (**B**) of isotonic neutral
phosphate buffer. *Numbers 1, 2, and the short line* in (A) and (B) indicate period of representative neurograms. This C-fiber (CV= 0.64 m/s) afferent nerve ending was located in the
anterior of ventricle. Impulse activity of this afferent was attenuated during ischemia after
treatment with isotonic neutral phosphate buffer. (From Pan *et al.*, 1999.[26] Reproduced by
permission.)

with myocardial ischemia have been shown to be mediated by BK. In this regard,
Staszewska-Woolley and Woolley[30] demonstrated that the reflex response, induced
by application of BK to the epicardium, can be abolished or attenuated by a kinin $B_2$
receptor antagonist. In a related study, we have shown that prostaglandins (PGs) are
capable of sensitizing abdominal visceral afferents to enhance the afferent activity
during BK and abdominal ischemia.[31] In addition, PGs, whose production is enhanced by BK,[32] have been shown to enhance the role of BK in activation of cardiac–cardiovascular reflexes. Thus, our recent studies have focused on the role of
endogenous BK and the specific BK receptor subtype involved in the activation of
spinal cardiac afferents during myocardial ischemia. We tested the hypothesis that
BK produced during ischemia activates cardiac afferents through stimulation of kinin $B_2$ receptors. We also examined the associated hypothesis that the effect of BK
on the ischemically sensitive cardiac afferents was dependent upon the presence of
PGs.

Our work focused on single-unit activity of cardiac afferents in cats isolated from
the sympathetic chain at $T_2–T_6$. Cardiac afferents, innervating the left ventricle and
sensitive to ischemia upon occlusion of a branch of the coronary artery for 5 min,
were selected to test for the role of BK and PGs. Ischemic-sensitive cardiac-afferent

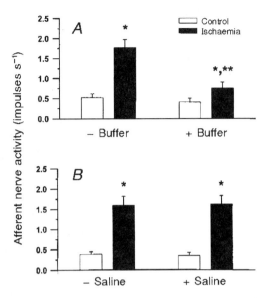

**FIGURE 3.** The response of cardiac afferents to repeated 5 min of ischemia before and after treatment with isotonic neutral phosphate buffer (**A**, $n = 16$) or saline (**B**, $n = 14$). *Columns* and *error bars* are means ± S.E.M. * < .05 compared with respective preischemia control. **$P < .05$ compared with the initial afferent response to ischemia. These data demonstrate that isotonic neutral phosphate buffer attenuates the response of cardiac afferents to ischemia. (From Pan *et al.*, 1999.[26] Reproduced by permission.)

endings have been identified on the anterior and posterior left ventricle near the coronary vessels (FIG. 5A).[28] Our data have shown that exogenous BK, but not the specific kinin $B_1$ receptor agonist, des-Arg[9]-BK, increases the firing rate of cardiac sympathetic afferents. Two structurally dissimilar kinin $B_2$ receptor antagonists, $HOE_{140}$ and NPC-17731, decreased the activity of cardiac fibers during ischemia (FIG. 4). In addition, we demonstrated that, prior to blockade of kinin $B_2$ receptors, inhibition of cyclooxygenase products with indomethacin, decreased activity of ischemically sensitive cardiac afferents during BK stimulation (FIG. 5B). However, we observed a further reduction in responses of cardiac sympathetic afferents to ischemia of subsequent blockade with a kinin $B_2$ receptor antagonist (FIG. 6). Thus, BK activates ischemically sensitive cardiac afferents through the kinin $B_2$ receptor, which is partly dependent and partly independent of cyclooxygenase products.[28] In contrast to the abdominal afferents, cardiac afferents[31] are less dependent upon the action of cyclooxygenase products.

### *Adenosine*

Adenosine is the product of adenosine-5'-triphosphate (ATP). In the presence of normal aerobic metabolism, adenosine-5'-diphosphate (ADP) is converted to ATP. In the absence of normal oxidative phosphorylation (i.e., ischemia) ADP is converted to adenosine-5'-monophosphate (AMP), which in turn is broken down to adenosine and ultimately to inosine, hypoxanthine and xanthine.[33] Previous studies of cardiac-cardiovascular reflexes as well as direct recordings of cardiac afferents' activities suggested that adenosine may be a stimulant of cardiac sympathetic afferents.[34,35] In this regard, previous study has demonstrated that the concentration of adenosine is increased in the ischemic region during brief myocardial ischemia.[36] Clinical evidence also has documented that intracoronary or intravenous adenosine causes anginal-like pain in humans, likely through activation of adenosine $A_1$ receptors,[37–39] whereas aminophylline, a nonselective adenosine receptors antagonist, attenuates the severity of chest pain induced by adenosine.[37,39] Experimental data indicate that intracoronary injection of adenosine or $N^6$-cyclopentyladenosine (CPA), an adenosine $A_1$ receptors agonist, reflexly increases the renal efferent activity.[34] Moreover, Huang et al.[40] observed that adenosine stimulates cardiac sympathetic afferents through activation of $A_1$ and $A_2$ receptors in dogs. Others reported that in cats adenosine activates cardiac sympathetic afferent fibers.[41] These observations have led to the conclusion that adenosine is capable of stimulating cardiac sympathetic afferents through activation of adenosine $A_1$ receptors.

In contrast to these studies, we found that even very high concentrations of adenosine and CPA, an adenosine $A_1$ agonist, failed to stimulate ischemically sensitive cardiac afferent nerve endings in cats.[42] Moreover, blockade of adenosine receptors with aminophylline did not attenuate the response of these C-fiber nerve endings during ischemia (FIG. 7). Consistent with our data, Gnecchi-Ruscone et al.[41] demonstrated that aminophylline does not alter the response of cardiac sympathetic afferents to myocardial ischemia, although they observed that exogenous adenosine stimulates these afferents in cats. Dibner-Dunlap et al.[34] reported that intracoronary injection of adenosine or CPA decreases heart rate and arterial pressure in the presence of vagotomy and sinoaortic denervation, although adenosine or CPA increases renal efferent nerve activity. Other investigators have observed that application of adenosine to epicardium does not evoke reflex responses, including renal efferent nerve activity.[43] Finally, Wilson et al.[44] have reported that intracoronary injection of adenosine fails to elicit cardiac pain in any of their patients. Thus, the effect of adenosine on cardiac sympathetic afferents has led to mixed results. It is possible that the differences in the experimental species and subgroups of afferent fibers lead to the differential results of influence of adenosine on cardiac-afferent nerve endings. One firm conclusion that can be made, however, based on the data from our group and Malliani's group, is that adenosine does not appear to be an important contributor to activation of cardiac sympathetic afferents during myocardial ischemia in cats.

### Reactive Oxygen Species

ROS can stimulate visceral afferent endings during ischemia.[45] Our laboratory previously demonstrated that ROS, produced during abdominal ischemia, stimulate

---

**FIGURE 4.** Histograms display the discharge frequency of an ischemically sensitive cardiac afferent during myocardial ischemia. (**A**) and (**B**) shows the afferent activity before and after the application of $HOE_{140}$, kinin $B_2$ receptor antagonist, respectively. Neurograms 1 to 4 display the activity of the afferent at times indicated in the histograms. (From Tjen-A-Looi et al. 1998.[28] Reproduced by permission.)

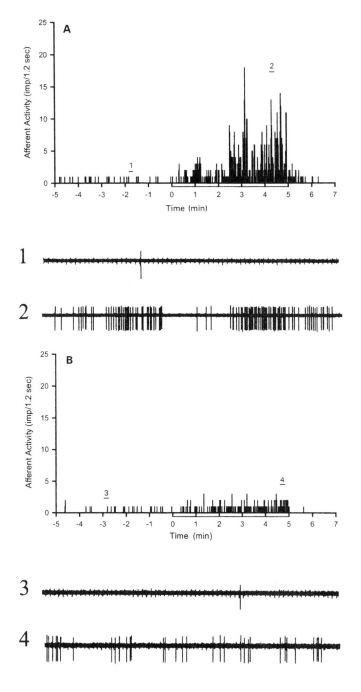

**FIGURE 4.** *See previous page for caption.*

abdominal afferents to reflexly activate the cardiovascular system.[45] Although there is evidence that ROS can stimulate cardiac vagal afferents,[46,47] it was not known whether ROS can stimulate cardiac sympathetic afferents during myocardial ischemia and reperfusion. We first needed to determine, however, if ROS were produced during brief ischemia and/or reperfusion. Using a method of trapping hydroxyl radicals ($\cdot$OH), which involved infusion of phenylalanine and measurement of the end products of various isoforms of tyrosine,[48,49] we found that the ortho- and metatryrosines were produced as early as one minute during ischemia, as well as during reperfusion.[50]

Our second study tested the hypothesis that ROS, like hydrogen peroxide ($H_2O_2$), superoxide radical ($O_2^{\cdot-}$) and hydroxyl radicals ($\cdot$OH), activate cardiac sympathetic afferents during myocardial ischemia. Single-unit afferent activity was measured before and during ischemia and reperfusion while nonspecific scavenger dimethylthiourea (DMTU) was administered. DMTU significantly reduced the increased activity of the afferents stimulated by ischemia and reperfusion. In the presence of iron, $O_2^{\cdot-}$ and $H_2O_2$ form $\cdot$OH by the Haber-Weiss reaction.[51] Therefore, deferoxamine, which chelates iron and thereby inhibits the Haber-Weiss reaction,[52,53] was used to inhibit $\cdot$OH formation to facilitate a better understanding of the chemical mechanism of activation of cardiac sympathetic afferents. Like DMTU, deferoxamine inhibited the increased discharge activity of the afferents during myocardial ischemia and during reperfusion. On the other hand, iron-loaded deferoxamine did not decrease the firing rate of these afferents. Our data thus suggest that $\cdot$OH contribute to activation of cardiac sympathetic afferents during ischemia and reperfusion.[54]

We recently have performed preliminary studies to identify the sources of ROS, such as purine metabolites and polymorphonuclear leukocytes (PMN). During ischemia, purine metabolites, including hypoxanthine and xanthine, accumulate as ATP is broken down.[33] We therefore tested the hypothesis that xanthine oxidase, which converts hypoxanthine to xanthine, is an important source of ROS during myocardial ischemia. Our preliminary results show that oxypurinol, a xanthine oxidase inhibitor, decreases cardiac afferent activity during ischemia,[55] suggesting therefore that purine breakdown constitutes an important source of ROS that plays a role in activating ischemically and reperfusion-sensitive cardiac afferents. We also have begun to test the hypothesis that PMNs are another source of ROS, with regard to activation of cardiac sympathetic afferents during ischemia and reperfusion. In this regard, infusion of antibody against cat PMN appears to attenuate the firing rate of the afferents during myocardial ischemia. However, this antibody reduces platelets following administration of the antibody in addition to PMNs, albeit to a much smaller degree.[56] Thus, purine metabolites, and possibly PMNs, may contribute to production of ROS during myocardial ischemia.

### Platelets

Activation of platelets occurs during myocardial ischemia. In this regard, experimental studies have shown that coronary artery occlusion is associated with platelet activation,[57] and clinical investigations have demonstrated that platelets in patients with spontaneous angina, unstable angina, or myocardial infarction also are activated.[58-60] Four well-defined stages of activation of platelets are recognized: (1) adhesion, (2) shape changes, (3) contraction and release of granule contents, and (4)

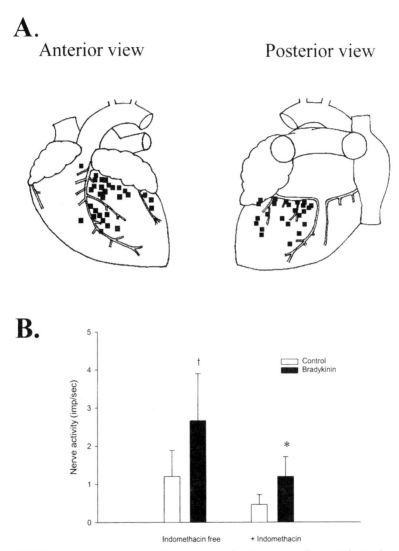

**FIGURE 5.** Ischemically sensitive cardiac afferent nerve endings are located on the epicardial surface of the heart (**A**). *n* Indicates the receptive fields of the afferents (*n* = 54). *Bar histogram* (**B**) demonstrates the effect of indomethacin on the discharge activity of ischemically sensitive sympathetic cardiac afferents. BK increases afferent responses from the spontaneous baseline (control) level of afferent activity, < .05. * Blockade by indomethacin significantly reduced responses of six afferents to BK, *P* < .05. (From Tjen-A-Looi *et al.* 1998.[28] Reproduced by permission.)

aggregation.[61] Although circulating freely in the blood under conditions of normal homeostasis, platelets interact with cell matrix components including collagen, fibronectins, laminin, and von Willebrand factor (vWF), as well as with thrombin, ad-

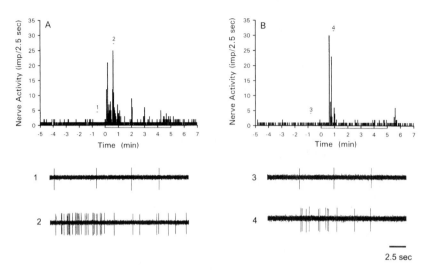

**FIGURE 6.** Representative tracings illustrate the responses of an ischemically sensitive cardiac afferent to ischemia before (**A**) and after (**B**) the application of NPC-17731, kinin $B_2$ receptor antagonist, in indomethacin-pretreated animal. *Numbers in the histograms* correspond with the neurograms 1 to 4. (From Tjen-A-Looi *et al.*, 1998.[28] Reproduced by permission)

enosine-5'-diphosphate (ADP) and epinephrine when vascular injury occurs during rupture of an atherosclerotic plaque, which frequently leads to myocardial ischemia and infarction.[61] These interactions stimulate specific platelet receptors and activate the glycoprotein IIb/IIIa (IIb$_3$) integrin on plasma membranes of platelets, leading subsequently to platelet activation.[61,62]

Platelets contain at least three distinct types of storage granules: dense granules, $\alpha$-granules, and lysosomal vesicles. Dense granules contain mostly small molecules and ions including adenosine-5'-triphosphate (ATP) and ADP, 5-hydroxytryptamine (5-HT, i.e. serotonin), histamine, calcium, inorganic diphosphate, and inorganic phosphate.[61,63] The $\alpha$-granules and lysosomal vesicles primarily contain macromolecular substances including proteins, glycoproteins, proteoglycans, and a number of different acid hydrolytic enzymes.[64] The content of these granules are released when platelets are activated by agonists or by various natural and artificial surfaces. Of the platelet mediators, two major classes of chemical substances: arachidonic acid metabolites, for example, prostaglandins, and biogenic amines, including 5-HT and histamine, may have a role in activation of sensory nerve endings.[65] As noted earlier, prostaglandins are capable of stimulating or sensitizing both cardiac sympathetic and vagal afferents to the action of other observed mediators.[28,47,66] In addition, we previously documented that endogenous serotonin and histamine stimulate ischemically sensitive abdominal visceral afferents.[67,68] These studies led us to hypothesize that ischemia-induced activation of platelets likely contributes to excitation of cardiac sympathetic afferents.

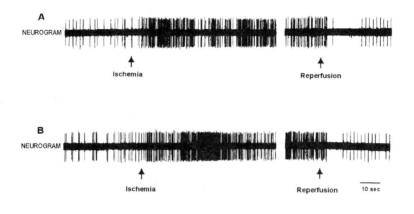

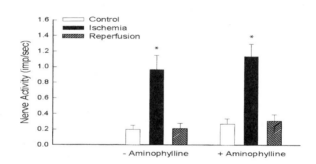

**FIGURE 7.** *Top panel* (neurograms) shows response of one cardiac C-fiber (CV= 0.46 m/s) afferent to 5 min of myocardial ischemia and reperfusion in the absence (**A**) and presence (**B**) of aminophylline (5 mg/kg i.v.). This afferent innervated the posterior wall of left ventricle. *Bottom panel* displays the averaged discharge activity of 10 cardiac C-fiber afferents during 5 min of myocardial ischemia and 2 min after reperfusion before and after treatment with aminophylline (5 mg/kg i.v.). *Columns* and *error bars* represent means ± S.E.M. *$P < .05$ compared with preischemia control. These data indicate that aminophylline does not alter the response of cardiac afferents to ischemia and reperfusion in cats. (From Pan and Longhurst, 1995.[42] Reproduced by pemission.)

To test the hypothesis, we conducted a preliminary study in which we recorded the responses of ischemically sensitive cardiac sympathetic afferents to activated platelets. Platelets in platelet-rich plasma (PRP) were activated by either collagen or thrombin, both functioning as strong agonists that activate platelets. We observed that left atrial injection of a solution of activated platelets (i.e., PRP + collagen or PRP + thrombin) stimulated these afferents.[69] Conversely, PRP containing nonactivated platelets and platelet-poor plasma (PPP) + collagen or thrombin did not change the activity of any of these afferents. Subsequently, we observed that the response of these cardiac afferents to PRP + thrombin was abolished by tropisetron, a specific 5-HT$_3$ receptor antagonist.[70] In a similar vein, Blunk et al.[71] have reported that intra-dermal injection of human platelets induces a distinct sensation of pain in humans. In addition, application of platelets activated by ADP to the receptive field of cuta-neous afferents in rats enhances the discharge activity of the C-fiber afferents.[72] Fi-nally, intravenous injection of platelet-rich solutions is capable of inducing a burning pain and protracted hyperalgesia in human subjects.[73] Taken together, our prelimi-nary studies suggest that activated platelets are capable of stimulating ischemically sensitive cardiac sympathetic afferents through a 5-HT$_3$ receptor mechanism. The contribution of activated platelets to excitation of cardiac sympathetic afferents dur-ing ischemia is under active investigation.

### Serotonin

Serotonin, one of the mediators released from the dense granules of platelets, may be a major chemical stimulus of cardiac sympathetic afferents. In this regard, exper-imental evidence has shown that the plasma concentration of 5-HT is elevated mark-edly (18- to 27-fold) at the site of coronary arterial stenosis and in coronary sinus blood during thrombosis-induced occlusion of coronary arteries.[74,75] The effects of 5-HT in tissue potentially may be mediated by a large family of receptors, which have been divided into at least seven subtypes.[76] Based on the pharmacological data, four major subtypes of 5-HT receptors, designated as 5-HT$_1$, 5-HT$_2$, 5-HT$_3$, and 5-HT$_4$, have been shown to exist in the nervous system.[76] Direct activation of 5-HT$_{1A}$ receptors on the primary afferents produces hyperalgesia.[77] Stimulation of 5-HT$_2$ re-ceptors potentiates pain produced by inflammatory mediators, and increases nocice-ption at the spinal level through stimulation of primary somatic C-fiber afferents.[78] Grundy et al.[79] observed that exogenous 5-HT stimulates vagal gastric mucosal chemosensitive afferents through a 5-HT$_3$ receptor mechanism. 5-HT$_3$ receptors also are thought to mediate an excitatory action on somatic sensory nociceptive neu-rons.[80] Furthermore, data from our laboratory have demonstrated that endogenous 5-HT stimulates ischemically sensitive abdominal visceral afferents through a 5-HT$_3$ mechanism, but not through activation of 5-HT$_1$ or 5-HT$_2$ receptors.[68] Previous studies also have documented that stimulation of 5-HT$_4$ receptors depolarizes the cervical vagus nerve.[81] Additional evidence suggests that 5-HT could contribute to activation of cardiac afferents during ischemia, since exogenous 5-HT stimulates cardiac sympathetic A$\delta$-fiber afferents in cats.[82]

We recently performed a pilot study testing the hypothesis that 5-HT activates cardiac sympathetic afferents during ischemia through stimulation of 5-HT$_3$ recep-tors.[83] Responses of single-unit cardiac sympathetic afferents to ischemia, 5-HT, and specific 5-HT receptor agonists were recorded. Initially, we found that, com-pared to bradykinin, which broadly stimulates a number of different types of cardiac sympathetic afferents,[27,84] 5-HT appears to selectively stimulate ischemically sen-sitive afferents but not ischemically insensitive afferents. Subsequently we observed that phenylbiguanide or 2-methyl-5-HT, a specific 5-HT$_3$ receptor agonist, activates most (83%) ischemically sensitive cardiac afferents studied. Conversely, α-methyl-5-HT, a 5-HT$_2$ receptor agonist, stimulates a minority (33%) of the afferents tested, and specific 5-HT$_1$ and 5-HT$_4$ receptors agonists do not alter the activity of any car-diac afferents. Importantly, tropisetron, a 5-HT$_3$ receptor antagonist, appears to at-

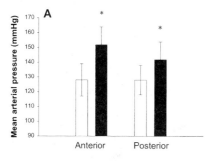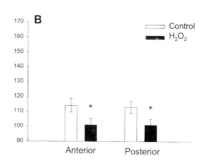

**FIGURE 8.** Changes in mean arterial pressure following topical application of $H_2O_2$ on the anterior and posterior surfaces of the left ventricle (**A**) in bilateral cervical vagotomized and (**B**) in bilateral $T_1$–$T_4$ sympathetic ganglionectomized cats. *Significantly different from control, $P < .05$. (From Huang *et al.*, 1995.[54] Reproduced by permission.)

tenuate the activity of cardiac afferents during brief myocardial ischemia.[83] Taken together, these preliminary studies suggest that serotonin released by activated platelets may constitute an important stimulus of cardiac afferents during myocardial ischemic syndromes. The contribution of 5-HT to activation of cardiac sympathetic afferents during ischemia is under active exploration.

## SYMPATHETIC AND VAGAL AFFERENT REFLEXES FROM THE HEART

Our previous studies of abdominal visceral afferents indicate that ROS induce cardiovascular reflex responses through stimulation of sympathetic or spinal-afferent nerve endings.[85,86] As we have previouslysuggested, during myocardial ischemia there is an increase in the production of ROS such as ·OH, among others, from the breakdown of purines.[87] It was not known, however, if ROS generated during myocardial ischemia were capable of activating sympathetic or vagal afferents to evoke pressor or depressor reflexes. Our studies tested the possibility that $H_2O_2$-induced hydroxyl-radical production reflexly stimulate or inhibit the cardiovascular system when sympathetic or vagal afferents, respectively, are activated. In these studies we applied $H_2O_2$ topically on the anterior or posterior myocardial surface before and after bilateral cervical vagotomy and after $T_1$–$T_4$ ganglionectomy. When both sets of cardiac afferent systems were intact, we observed a small pressor response when $H_2O_2$ was applied to the heart. Conversely, application of $H_2O_2$ on the epicardium in bilaterally vagotomized cats led to significant pressor responses, including increases in mean arterial pressure, heart rate, aortic flow, total peripheral resistance, and left ventricular dP/dt at 40 mmHg developed pressure. These pressor reflexes were abolished by bilateral sympathetic ganglionectomy. On the other hand, application of $H_2O_2$ on the epicardium caused depressor responses in sympathectomized animals (FIG. 8). The depressor responses were eliminated after bilateral cervical vagotomy. The significance of ROS was evaluated with the nonspecific scavenger DMTU.[88] DMTU abolished the $H_2O_2$-induced cardiovascular depressor

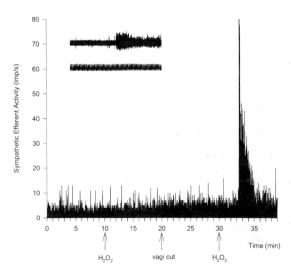

**FIGURE 9.** Histogram in impulses per second (imp/s) represents the activity of cardiac sympathetic efferent fibers before and after vagotomy following application of $H_2O_2$ on the surface of the ventricle. *Inset* displays the neurogram (*top*) and arterial blood pressure (*bottom*) responses to $H_2O_2$ after vagotomy. (From Tjen-A-Looi *et al.*, 1997.[86] Reproduced by permission.)

responses in sympathectomized animals and pressor reflexes in vagotomized ones. Thus, $H_2O_2$ causes both excitatory and inhibitory cardiovascular reflexes that are mediated by sympathetic and vagal afferent pathways, respectively.[85]

The preceding study demonstrated that pressor responses, consequent to stimulation of cardiac afferents by ROS, are augmented by vagotomy and abolished by sympathectomy. Stimulation of cardiac sympathetic afferents excited neurons in the nucleus tractus solitarii (NTS). This excitation was decreased by simultaneous activation of cardiac vagal afferents. This observation has led to our suggestion that there is an occlusive (inhibitory) interaction between sympathetic and parasympathetic afferents in the NTS.[86] We recorded sympathetic efferent activity at the $T_1-T_2$ level before and after application of $H_2O_2$ on the myocardial surface with and without vagotomy, and found that sympathetic outflow was increased after vagotomy with application of $H_2O_2$ on the surface of the myocardium (FIG. 9). This observation reinforced the possibility of an occlusive interaction in the CNS that influences sympathetic outflow. To determine where in the CNS the inhibitory interaction might occur, we noted that previous studies (Bennett *et al.*[89]) demonstrated that vagal afferents from the heart activate neurons in the NTS. We therefore tested the hypothesis that simultaneous stimulation of cardiac sympathetic and vagal afferents, which occurs during application of $H_2O_2$ to the epicardium, leads to an occlusive interaction in interneurons in the NTS. Extracellular recording of neuronal activities in the NTS showed that excitatory responses evoked by stimulation of cardiac sympathetic afferents were decreased (occluded) during simultaneous activation of cardiac vagal afferents in approximately half of the neurons studied (FIG. 10). Thus,

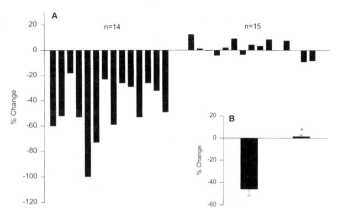

**FIGURE 10.** (**A**) Individual percent changes evoked in activity of 29 NTS neurons . Fourteen afferents demonstrated inhibition of cardiac sympathetic evoked activity during simultaneous stimulation of cardiac vagal pathways. (**B**) represents grouped mean data of neurons taken from (A), demonstrating inhibitory (occlusive) interaction compared to those afferents that demonstrated no effect. About half of the neurons have occlusive interaction, which is judged with more than 18% (2 times standard deviation) change from baseline response. (From Tjen-A-Looi et al., 1997.[86] Reroduced by permission.)

cardiac vagal afferent stimulation decreases the evoked activity of NTS neurons, which receive convergent excitatory input from cardiac sympathetic afferents. We also have found a few units in the NTS that display additive or facilitative interaction upon simultaneous stimulation of both cardiac afferent systems. We concluded, however, that there is an occlusive interaction between cardiac sympathetic and parasympathetic afferents in the NTS.[86]

## CONCLUSIONS AND FUTURE RECOMMENDATIONS

Our studies of mechanisms of activation of cardiac sympathetic afferents are, with a few exceptions, mostly congruent with our previous studies of abdominal visceral afferents. We have shown that protons, BK, prostaglandins, and ROS, particularly ·OH, play important roles in activating cardiac sympathetic afferents during ischemia and reperfusion. At first glance, the sources of ROS appear to be from purine metabolism and possibly from neutrophils. However, these preliminary observations, particularly those concerning the role of PMNs, require confirmation. Although prostaglandins appear to be critical to the afferent responses to BK in the abdominal region, we have observed that kinins are capable of operating more independently in stimulating cardiac afferents. Thus, while prostaglandins clearly are capable of sensitizing cardiac sympathetic afferents, they are not critically required in activation of all such afferents by BK.

The observation that the source of protons is critical to their capability of activating cardiac afferents is an interesting one. At the present time, we have no explanation for this result. However, abdominal visceral afferents also appear to respond differently to proton donors such as lactic acid and hypercapnia.[19] We have provided new data suggesting not only that serotonin is important, but that the principal source for serotonin is platelets. This is a tentative observation that needs to be confirmed. However, if the role of platelets is documented, then we can begin to understand some of the basic underpinnings of not only angina pectoris but also of some very deleterious reflex responses during cardiac ischemic syndromes that clearly have been shown to depend upon platelet activation and aggregation.

Our recent studies also have begun to explore the central neural interactions between the opposing reflex responses that originate from the simultaneous activation of cardiac vagal and sympathetic afferents. To date we have shown that the NTS is one area where a neural occlusive response occurs. Presumably other sites in the CNS are present where interactions between these two important sensory systems also exist. This remains an additional area for future investigation.

One may wonder why two opposing reflexes from the heart exist, one that increases blood pressure and one that reduces it. The answer to this teleologic question is uncertain. However, this situation may provide a mechanism for fine-tuning of the composite reflex response to limit an exaggerated response that might occur if either the sympathetic or vagal nerve response predominated.

Although, many mediators studied have been predicted to play a part in stimulating cardiac afferents during ischemia, we have not been able to confirm a role for all of the possible candidates. For instance, it has been suggested that adenosine is an important mediator in reflex studies from other laboratories.[34,35] In our hands, however, adenosine, even in very large concentrations, does not appear to be capable of activating cardiac sympathetic afferents, either when administered exogenously or during ischemia. Different findings between our studies and those of others remain a puzzle that may depend upon species differences, afferent pathway studied, or in the type of protocol performed. These possibilities have been mentioned by others.[90] We would like to emphasize, however, that ours is the only study in which the influence of mediator on ischemically sensitive cardiac afferent activity has been evaluated directly.

In addition to the mediators studied already, we suspect that there are still other chemical and probably mechanical events that are important in activating cardiac afferents during ischemia. Some of these events will occur in isolation, while others may be part of a complex interactive process involving two or more mediators or events adding together or even influencing the action of other mediators to cause the final cardiac-afferent response. Thus, there remain many areas for fruitful study for the future. However, because of the difficulty in isolating and recording single cardiac-afferent nerves, particularly thin-fiber units, and most particularly those endings that originate in the heart and that specifically are active during ischemia and/or reperfusion, we suspect that further advances in this field will be slowly forthcoming and guided by only a few laboratories with significant experience in this area.

## ACKNOWLEDGMENT

This work is supported, in part, by National Heart, Lung, and Blood Institute Grants HL-51428 and HL-36527 and by American Heart Association, Western

States Affiliates, Beginning Grant-in-Aid #9960007Y. The authors thank Sherry Ong for secretarial assistance.

## REFERENCES

1. MARK, A.L., F.M. ABBOUD & P.G. SCHMID. 1973. Cardiovascular responses to left ventricular outflow obstruction and activation of ventricular baroreceptors in dogs. J. Clin. Invest. **52:** 1147–1153.
2. ABBOUD, F.M., M.D. THAMES & A.L. MARK. 1981. Role of cardiac afferent nerves in regulation of circulation during coronary occlusion and heart failure. *In* Disturbances in Neurological Control of the Circulation, F.M. Abboud, H.A. Fozzard, and J.P. Gilmore, Eds.: 65–86. American Physiological Society. Bethesda, Md.
3. ESTAFANOUS, F.G., R.C. TARAZI, J.F. VILIJOEN & E.I. TAWILMY. 1973. Systemic hypertension following myocardial revascularization [Abstr.]. Am. Heart J. **85:** 732–738.
4. FOUAD, F.M., F.G. ESTAFANOUS & R.C. TATAZI. 1978. Hemodyanamics of postmyocardial revascularization and hypertension [Abstr.]. Am. J. Cardiol. **41:** 564–569.
5. FOUAD, F.M., F.G. ESTAFANOUS, E.L. GRAVO, *et al.* 1979. Possible role of cardioaortic reflexes in postcoronary bypass hypertension. Am. J. Cardiol. **44:** 866–872.
6. TARAZI, R.C., G.F. ESTAFANOUS & F.M. FOUAD. 1978. Unilateral stellate block in the treatment of hypertension after coronary bypass surgery. Am. J. Cardiol. **42:** 1013–1018.
7. ZUCKER, I.H., A.M. EARLE & J.P. GILMORE. 1979. Changes in sensitivity of left atrial receptors following reversal of heart failure. Am. J. Physiol. **237:** H555–H559.
8. THAMES, M.D. & P.G. SCHMID. 1979. Cardiopulmonary receptors with vagal afferents tonically inhibit ADH release in the dog. Am. J. Physiol. **237:** H299–H304.
9. BOSNJAK, Z.J., E.J. ZUPERKU & R.L. COON. 1979. Acute coronary artery occlusion and cardiac sympathetic afferent nerve activity. Proc. Soc. Exp. Biol. Med. **161:** 142–148.
10. MALLIANI, A., P.J. SCHWARTZ & A. ZANCHETTI. 1969. A sympathetic reflex elicited by experimental coronary occlusion. Am. J. Physiol. **217:** 703–709.
11. CONSTANTIN, L. 1963. Extra cardiac factors contributing to hypotension during coronary occlusion. Am. J. Cardiol. **11:** 205–217.
12. CHADDA, K.D., E. LICHSTEIN, P.K. GUPTA & R. CHOY. 1975. Bradycardia-hypotension syndrome in acute myocardial infarction. Am. J. Med. **59:** 158–164.
13. KENT, K.M., E.R. SMITH & D.R. REDWOOD. 1972. The deleterious electrophysiologic effects produced by increasing heart rate during experimental coronary occlusion. Clin. Res. **20:** 379.
14. FIGUERAS, J. & J. CINCA. 1981. Acute arterial hypertension during spontaneous angina in patients with fixed coronary stenosis and exertional angina: an associated rather than a triggering phenomenon. Circulation **64:** 60–68.
15. LONGHURST, J.C. 1991. Reflex effects from abdominal visceral afferents. *In* Reflex Control of the Circulation, I.H. Zucker and J.P.Gillmore, Eds.: 551–577. Telford Press. Caldwell, N.J.
16. LONGHURST, J.C. 1995. Chemosensitive abdominal visceral afferents. *In* Proceedings: Visceral Pain Symposium, G.F. Gebhart, Ed.: 99–132. IASP Press. Seattle, Wash.
17. GREGORY, S.L., H.-L. PAN & J.C. LONGHURST. 1993. Activation of ischemia- and reperfusion-sensitive abdominal visceral C fiber afferents—Role of hydrogen peroxide and hydroxyl radicals. Circ. Res. **72:** 1266–1275.
18. POOLE-WILSON, P.A. 1978. Measurement of myocardial intracellular pH in pathological states. J. Mol. Cell. Cardiol. **10**(6): 511–526.
19. STAHL, G.L. & J.C. LONGHURST. 1992. Ischemically sensitive visceral afferents: importance of $H^+$ derived from lactic acid and hypercapnia. Am. J. Physiol. **262:** H748–H753.

20. HONG, J.L., K. KWONG & L.Y. LEE. 1997. Stimulation of pulmonary C fibers by lactic acid in rats: concentrations of $H^+$ and lactate ions. J. Physiol. (Lond.) **500:** 319–329.
21. ROTTO, D.M., C.L. STEBBINS & M.P. KAUFMAN. 1989. Reflex cardiovascular and ventilatory responses to increasing $H^+$ activity in cat hindlimb muscle. J. Appl. Physiol. **67:** 256–263.
22. STEEN, K.H., A.E. STEEN & P.W. REEH. 1995. A dominant role of acid pH in inflammatory excitation and sensitization of nociceptors in rat skin, *in vivo*. J. Neurosci. **15:** 3982–3989.
23. MARK, A.L., F.M. ABBOUD, D.D. HEISTAD, *et al.* 1974. Evidence against the presence of ventricular chemoreceptors activated by hypoxia and hypercapnia. Am. J. Physiol. **227:** 273–279.
24. UCHIDA, Y. & S. MURAO. 1975. Acid-induced excitation of afferent cardiac sympathetic nerve fibers. Am. J. Physiol. **228:** 27–33.
25. PAL, P., J. KOLEY, S. BHATTACHARYYA, *et al.* 1989. Cardiac nociceptors and ischemia: role of sympathetic afferents in cat. Jpn. J. Physiol. **39:** 131–144.
26. PAN, H.-L., J.C. LONGHURST, J.C. EISENACH & S.-R. CHEN. 1999. Role of protons in activation of cardiac sympathetic C-fiber afferents during ischemia in cats. J. Physiol. (Lond.) **518.3:** 857–866.
27. BAKER, D.G., H.M. COLERIDGE, J.C.G. COLERIDGE & T. NERDRUM. 1980. Search for a cardiac nociceptor: stimulation by bradykinin of sympathetic afferent nerve endings in the heart of the cat. J. Physiol. (Lond.) **306:** 519–536.
28. TJEN-A-LOOI, S., H.-L. PAN & J.C. LONGHURST. 1998. Endogenous bradykinin activates ischaemically sensitive cardiac visceral afferents through kinin $B_2$ receptors in cats. J. Physiol. (Lond.) **510:** 633–641.
29. KIMURA, E., K. HASHIMOTO, S. FURUKAWA & H. HAYAKAWA. 1973. Changes in bradykinin level in coronary sinus blood after the experimental occulsion of a coronary artery. Am. Heart J. **85:** 635–647.
30. STASZEWSKA-WOOLLEY, J. & G. WOOLLEY. 1989. Participation of the kallikrein-kinin-receptor system in reflexes arising from neural afferents in the dog epicardium. J. Physiol. (Lond.) **419:** 33–44.
31. PAN, H.-L., G.L. STAHL, S.V. RENDIG, *et al.* 1994. Endogenous BK stimulates ischemically sensitive abdominal visceral C fiber afferents through kinin $B_2$ receptors in cats. Am. J. Physiol. **267:** H2398–H2406.
32. RANG, H.P., S.J. BEVAN & A. DRAY. 1991. Chemical activation of nociceptive peripheral neurons. Br. Med. Bull. **47**(3): 534–548.
33. JENNINGS, R.B., K.A. REIMER, M.L. HILL & S.E. MAYER. 1981. Total ischemia in dog heart in vitro. 1. Comparison of high energy phosphate production, utilization, an depletion, and of adenine nucleotide catabolism in total ischemia in vitro vs. severe ischemia *in vivo*. Circulation **49:** 892–900.
34. DIBNER-DUNLAP, M.E., T. KINUGAWA & M.D. THAMES. 1993. Activation of cardiac sympathetic afferents: effects of exogenous adenosine and adenosine analogues. Am. J. Physiol. **265:** H395–H400.
35. COX, D.A., J.A. VITA, C.B. TREASURE, *et al.* 1989. Reflex increase in blood pressure during intra-coronary administration of adenosine in man. J. Clin. Invest. **84:** 592–596.
36. DELYANI, J.A. & G.L. VAN WYLEN. 1994. Endocardial and epicardial interstitial purines and lactate during graded ischemia. Am. J. Physiol. **226:** H1019–H1026.
37. SYLVEN, C., B. BEEMANN, B. JONZON & R. BRANDT. 1986. Angina pectoris-like pain provoked by intravenous adenosine. Br. Med. J. **293:** 227–230.
38. CREA, F., G. PUPITA, A. GALASSI, *et al.* 1990. Role of adenosine in pathogenesis of angina pain. Circulation **81**(1): 164–182.

39. CREA, F., A. GASPARDONE, J.C. KASKI, *et al.* 1992. Relation between stimulation site of cardiac afferent nerves by adenosine and distribution of cardiac pain: results of a study in patients with stable angina. J. Am. Coll. Cardiol. **20:** 1498–1502.
40. HUANG, M.H., C. SYLVEN, M. HORACKOVA & J.A. ARMOUR. 1995. Ventricular sensory neurons in canine dorsal root ganglia: effects of adenosine and substance P. Am. J. Physiol. **269**(2, Pt. 2): R318–R324.
41. GNECCHI-RUSCONE, T., N. MONTANO, M. CONTINI, *et al.* 1995. Adenosine activates cardiac sympathetic afferent fibers and potentiates the excitation induced by coronary occlusion. J. Auton. Nerv. Syst. **53:** 175–184.
42. PAN, H.-L. & J.C. LONGHURST. 1995. Lack of a role of adenosine in activation of ischemically sensitive cardiac sympathetic afferents in cats. Am. J. Physiol. **269:** H106–H113.
43. PAGANI, M., R. PIZZINELLI, R. FURLAN, *et al.* 1985. Analysis of the pressor sympathetic reflex produced by intracoronary injections of bradykinin in conscious dogs. Circ. Res. **56:** 175–183.
44. WILSON, R.F., K. WYCHE, B.V. CHRISTENSEN, *et al.* 1990. Effects of adenosine on human coronary arterial circulation. Circulation **82:** 1595–1606.
45. STAHL, G.L., H.-L. PAN & J.C. LONGHURST. 1993. Activation of ischemia and reperfusion-sensitive abdominal visceral C fiber afferents: role of hydrogen peroxide and hydroxyl radicals. Circ. Res. **72:** 1266–1275.
46. USTINOVA, E. & H.D. SCHULTZ. 1994. Activation of cardiac vagal afferents by oxygen-derived free radicals in rats. Circ. Res. **74:** 895–903.
47. STINOVA, E.E. & H.D. SCHULTZ. 1994. Activation of cardiac vagal afferents in ischemia and reperfusion: prostaglandins vs. oxygen free radicals. Circ. Res. **74:** 904–911.
48. MASKOS, Z., J.D. RUSH & W.H. KOPPENOL. 1992. The hydroxylation of phenyalanine and tyrosine: a comparison with salicylate and tryptophan. Arch. Biochem. Biophys. **296:** 521–529.
49. SUN, J.-Z., H. KAUR, B. HALLIWELL, *et al.* 1993. Use of aromatic hydroxylation of phenylalanine to measure production of hydroxyl radicals after myocardial ischemia *in vivo*: direct evidence for a pathogenetic role of the hydroxyl radical in myocardial stunning. Circ. Res. **73:** 534–549.
50. O'NEILL, C.A., L.-W. FU, B. HALLIWELL & J.C. LONGHURST. 1996. Hydroxyl radical production during myocardial ischemia and reperfusion in cats. Am. J. Physiol. **271:** H660–H667.
51. GRISHAM, M.B. & D.N. GRANGER. 1988. Neutrophil-mediated mucosal injury: role of reactive oxygen metabolites. Dig. Dis. Sci. **33:** 6S–15S.
52. HALLIWELL, B. & J.M.C. GUTTERIDGE. 1990. Role of free radicals and catalytic metal ions in human disease. An overview. Methods Enzymol. **186:** 1–85.
53. HALLIWELL, B. 1989. Protection against tissue damage in vivo by desferrioxamine. What is its mechanism of action? Free Radic. Biol. Med. **7:** 645–651.
54. HUANG, H.-S., H.-L. PAN, G.L. STAHL & J.C. LONGHURST. 1995. Ischemia- and reperfusion-sensitive cardiac sympathetic afferents: influence of $H_2O_2$ and hydroxyl radicals. Am. J. Physiol. **269:** H888–H901.
55. TJEN-A-LOOI, S. & J.C. LONGHURST. 1998. Role of xanthine oxidase (XO) in activation of cardiac afferents during myocardial ischemia. FASEB J. **12:** A689.
56. LONGHURST, J.C. & S. TJEN-A-LOOI. 1998. Both neutrophils (PMNs) and xanthine oxidase (XO) contribute to activation of cardiac sympathetic afferents in cats. J. Auton. Nerv. Sys. **8:** 283.
57. FLORES, N.A., N.V. GOULIELMOS, M.J. SEGHATCHIAN & D.J. SHERIDAN. 1994. Myocardial ischemia induces platelet activation with adverse electrophysiological and arrhythmogenic effects. Cardiovasc. Res. **28**(11): 1662–1671.

58. FLORES, N.A. & D.J. SHERIDAN. 1994. The pathophysiological role of platelets during myocardial ischemia. Cardiovasc. Res. **28:** 295–302.
59. GRANDE, P. 1990. Unstable angina pectoris: platelet behavior and prognosis in progressive angina and intermediate coronary syndrome. Circulation **81**(Suppl. I): 116–119.
60. FITZGERALD, D.J. 1991. Platelet activation in the pathogenesis of unstable angina: importance in determining the response to plasminogen activators. Am. J. Cardiol. **68:** 51B–57B.
61. STORMORKEN, H. 1986. Platelets in hemostasis and thrombosis. *In* Platelet Responses and Metabolism, Vol. 1, H. Holmsen, Ed.: 3–32. CRC. Boca Raton, Fla.
62. TOPOL, E.J., T.V. BYZOVA & E.F. PLOW. 1999. Platelet GP IIb-IIIa blockers. Lancet **353:** 227–231.
63. MEYERS, K.M., H. HOLSMEN & C.L. SEACHORD. 1982. Comparative study of platelet dense granule constituents. Am. J. Physiol. **243:** R454–R461.
64. RAO, G.H.R. 1993. Physiology of blood platelet activation. Indian J. Physiol. Pharmacol. **37:** 263–275.
65. HOLMSEN, H. 1985. Platelet metabolism and activation. Semin. Hematol. **22:** 219–240.
66. NERDRUM, T., D.G. BAKER, H.M. COLERIDGE & J.C.G. COLERIDGE. 1986. Interaction of bradykinin and prostaglandin $E_1$ on cardiac pressor reflex and sympathetic afferents. Am. J. Physiol. **250:** R815–R822.
67. FU, L.-W., H.-L. PAN & J.C. LONGHURST. 1997. Endogenous histamine stimulates ischemically sensitive abdominal visceral afferents through $H_1$ receptors. Am. J. Physiol. **273:** H2726–H2737.
68. FU, L.-W. & J.C. LONGHURST. 1998. Role of $5\text{-}HT_3$ receptors in activation of abdominal sympathetic C-fibre afferents during ischemia in cats. J. Physiol. **509:** 729–740.
69. FU, L.-W. & J.C. LONGHURST. 1999. Activated platelets stimulate ischemically sensitive cardiac afferents. Circulation **100**(Suppl. 1): I-132.
70. FU, L.-W. & J.C. LONGHURST. 2000. Activated platelets stimulate cardiac afferents through a 5-HT receptor mechanism. FASEB J. **14:** A377.
71. BLUNK, J., G. OSIANDER, M. NISCHIK & M. SCHMELZ. 1999. Pain and inflammatory hyperalgesia induced by intradermal injections of human platelets and leukocytes. Eur. J. Pain. **3:** 247–259.
72. RINGKAMP, M., M. SCHMELZ, M. KRESS, *et al.* 1994. Activated human platelets in plasma excite nociceptors in rat skin, in vitro. Neurosci. Lett. **170:** 103–106.
73. SCHMELZ, M., G. OSIANDER, J. BLUNK, *et al.* 1997. Intracutaneous injections of platelets cause acute pain and protracted hyperalgesia. Neurosci. Lett. **226**(3): 171–174.
74. ASHTON, J.H. 1986. Serotonin as a mediator of cyclic flow variation in stenosed canine coronoary arteries. Circulation **73:** 572–578.
75. BENEDICT, C.R., B. MATHEW, K.A. REX, *et al.* 1986. Correlation of plasma serotonin changes with platelet aggregation in an in vivo dog model of spontaneous occlusive coronary thrombus formation. Circ. Res. **58:** 58–67.
76. HOYER, D., D.E. CLARKE, J.R. FOZARD, *et al.* 1994. International union of pharmacology classification of receptors for 5-hydroxytryptamine (serotonin). Pharmacol. Rev. **46**(2): 157–203.
77. TAIWO, Y.O. & J.D. LEVINE. 1992. Serotonin is a directly-acting hyperalgesic agent in the rat. Neuroscience **48**(2): 485–490.
78. PEROUTKA, S.J. 1994. 5-Hydroxytryptamine receptors. J. Neurochem. **60:** 408–416.
79. GRUNDY, D., L.A. BLACKSHAE & K. HILLSLEY. 1994. Role of 5-hydroxytryptamine in gastrointestinal chemosensitivity. Dig. Dis. Sci. **39**(Suppl.): 44S–47S.
80. RICHARDSON, B.P., G. ENGEL, P. DONATSCH & P.A. STADLER. 1985. Identification of serotonin M-receptor subtypes and their specific blockade by a new class of drugs. Nature **316:** 126–131.

81. RHODES, K.F., J. COLEMAN & N. LATTIMER. 1992. A component of 5-HT-evoked depolarization of the rat isolated vagus nerve is mediated by a putative 5-HT$_4$ receptor. Naunyn-Schemiedeberg's Arch. Pharmacol. **346:** 496–503.
82. NISHI, K., M. SAKANASHI & F. TAKENAKA. 1977. Activation of afferent cardiac sympathetic nerve fibers of the cat by pain producing substances and by noxious heat. Pflügers Arch. **372:** 53–61.
83. FU, L.-W. & J.C. LONGHURST. 1998. Activation of ischemically sensitive cardiac afferents by serotonin through 5-HT$_3$ receptors. Soc. Neurosci. Abstr. **24:** 1622.
84. MALLIANI, A. 1982. Cardiovascular sympathetic afferent fibers. Rev. Physiol. Biochem. Pharmacol. **94:** 11–74.
85. HUANG, H.-S., G.L. STAHL & J.C. LONGHURST. 1995. Cardiac-cardiovascular reflexes induced by hydrogen peroxide in cats. Am. J. Physiol. **268:** H2114–H2124.
86. TJEN-A-LOOI, S., A. BONHAM & J. LONGHURST. 1997. Interactions between sympathetic and vagal cardiac afferents in nucleus tractus solitarii. Am. J. Physiol. **272:** H2843–H2851.
87. SIMPSON, P.J. & B.R. LUCCHESI. 1987. Free radicals and myocardial ischemia and reperfusion injury. J. Lab. Clin. Med. **110:** 13–30.
88. JACKSON, J.H., C.W. WHITE, N.B. PARKER, *et al.* 1985. Dimethylthiourea consumption reflects H$_2$O$_2$ concentrations and severity of acute lung injury. J. Appl. Physiol. **59:** 1995–1998.
89. BENNETT, J.A., C.S. GOODCHILD, C. KIDD & P.N. MCWILLIAM. 1985. Neurons in the brain stem of the cat excited by vagal afferent fibres from the heart and lungs. J. Physiol. (Lond.) **369:** 1–15.
90. MALLIANI, A., F. LOMBARDI & M. PAGANI. 1986. Sensory innervation of the heart. Prog. Brain Res. **67:** 39–48.

# Toward an Understanding of the Molecules that Sense Myocardial Ischemia

CHRISTOPHER J. BENSON[a] AND STEPHANI P. SUTHERLAND[b]

[a]Department of Medicine, University of Iowa College of Medicine, Iowa City, Iowa 52242

[b]The Vollum Institute, Oregon Health Sciences University, Portland, Oregon 97201

ABSTRACT: Cardiac afferent neurons are activated in the setting of myocardial ischemia and mediate the sensation of angina. However, the precise stimuli and receptive molecules responsible are not completely understood. To further investigate the molecular components involved, cardiac afferents were isolated in dissociated culture and patch-clamp experiments were performed on these cells. It was found that acidic pH evoked large inward currents in almost all cardiac sympathetic afferents. By comparison, the responses to other potential chemical mediators were inconsistent and much smaller. The biophysical properties of the acid-evoked currents in cardiac afferents match the acid-sensing ion channel 3 (ASIC3).

KEYWORDS: ENaC/Deg ion channel; Myocardial ischemia protons; Cardiac afferents

## INTRODUCTION

Cardiac afferents are sensory neurons that continuously respond and relay information about the chemical and mechanical milieu of the heart. However, humans appear to be conscious of this flow of information only during the special circumstance of myocardial ischemia, when the heart is receiving inadequate oxygen and blood flow. The sensation experienced is pain, termed angina pectoris by clinicians, and is most commonly caused by coronary artery disease. Thomas Lewis in the 1930s first proposed that pain associated with myocardial ischemia was due to the activation of cardiac afferents by chemical compounds that are released by the metabolically stressed myocardial tissue.[1] Over the past 30 years, through the recording of cardiac afferents in whole-animal models, significant inroads have been made into the understanding of these potential chemical mediators of angina.[2] Several of these substances have been shown to activate cardiac afferents, with bradykinin[3–5] and adenosine[5–8] receiving the most attention. Other chemicals have also been proposed (see Ref. 2 for review). Nevertheless, the precise stimuli and molecular mechanisms underlying cardiac-afferent activation remain largely unknown. This review focuses

Address for correspondence: Christopher J. Benson, Department of Medicine, University of Iowa College of Medicine, 371 EMRB, Iowa City, IA 52242. Voice: 319-353-5941; fax: 319-353-5942.

chris-benson@uiowa.edu

on our work to identify the specific chemicals and receptors involved in sensing myocardial ischemia and mediating the sensation of angina.[9,10]

Lactic acid, or more specifically protons, is a likely candidate to mediate sensation in the setting of myocardial ischemia. In isolated ischemic hearts, pH is lowered
both intra-[11] and extracellularly[12,13] in myocardial tissue, as well as in the venous
return of blood from the hearts of patients with active coronary artery disease.[14] In
a rat skin preparation, acid plays a dominant role in activating afferents compared to
other potential chemical mediators of inflammation.[15] In the case of skeletal muscle,
human subjects report increasing pain in perfect time with the decreasing pH of their
ischemic forearm.[16] Although there have been relatively few studies examining the
role of protons activating cardiac afferents, Uchida and Murao[17] first showed that
acidic pH stimulated cardiac sympathetic nerve fibers in a dog. More recently, Pan
*et al*.[13] have shown that lactic acid activates cardiac afferents, and also that the addition of a strong pH buffer in the pericardial space inhibits firing of ischemically
sensitive cardiac afferents in response to coronary artery occlusion.

Our first goal was to explore the response of cardiac afferents to various potential
chemical mediators of myocardial ischemic sensation. To better define the molecules
involved in this process, we developed a new method to isolate cardiac afferents. Using a fluorescent tracer dye, we labeled cardiac sensory neurons *in vivo* so that they
could later be identified in primary dissociated culture. This allowed for whole-cell
patch-clamp recording of cardiac afferents and their response to various chemicals.
Our most important initial finding was that relatively modest changes in pH (pH 7.4
to 7.0) evoked large inward depolarizing currents in almost all cardiac sympathetic
afferents.[9] The extremely large amplitude and consistency of these acid-evoked currents imply a critical role in sensing myocardial ischemia. Our second goal was to determine the molecular identity of the pH sensor in cardiac afferents.[10] We found that
ASIC3 appears to be the primary proton sensor in cardiac afferent neurons.

## ISOLATION OF CARDIAC AFFERENTS
## IN PRIMARY CULTURE

Because of the difficulty in teasing apart the molecular components of the cardiac-afferent system in a whole-animal model, we chose to isolate a particular component of the system, using whole-cell electrophysiology of dissociated cardiac
afferents in culture. The problem with the study of sensory neurons in primary culture, however, is that the neuron's original site of innervation and its sensory modal-
ity are unknown. We took advantage of a unique method to solve this problem by
fluorescently labeling afferents *in vivo* so that they can later be identified in dissociated primary culture.[18] For our purposes, we injected a lipid soluble dye (diIC18,
Molecular Probes) into the pericardial space of a rat. The dye diffuses into adjacent
cell membranes, including nerve terminals, and some of the stained membrane is en-
docytosed and transported back to the neuron's cell body. With this technique, afferents innervating both the epicardium (i.e., the outermost layer of cells of the
myocardium) and the pericardium are stained and labeled. The anatomy of the sensory innervation of these two structures is as follows. The cell bodies of the cardiac
afferents (which innervate the myocardium) reside in two distinct sets of sensory
ganglia: those that follow the sympathetic tracts are found in the upper thoracic dor-

sal root ganglia (DRG, $C_8$–$T_3$), and those that follow the vagal tracts are located in the nodose ganglia. The afferents of the parietal pericardium, separate from that of the heart, follow the phrenic nerve tracts to the cervical DRG (C3–C5).[19] Thus, by collecting the upper thoracic DRG and the nodose ganglia, dissociating the ganglia into individual cells in culture, and identifying those cells that are labeled, we isolated pure populations of sensory neurons that innervate the heart.

## CHEMICAL ACTIVATION OF CARDIAC AFFERENTS

Having isolated cardiac afferents in primary dissociated culture, we then recorded from these individual cells with the whole-cell patch-clamp technique. We studied three populations of cells: (1) labeled afferents in the DRG, that is, cardiac sympathetic afferents; (2) labeled afferents in the nodose ganglia, that is, vagal afferents; (3) and randomly chosen unlabeled DRG neurons of similar diameter. We first applied a variety of chemicals that have been implicated as potential mediators of angina to these cells and recorded their responses.

The most important finding of this experiment was that acidic pH evoked large inward currents in almost all cardiac sympathetic afferents (FIG. 1). By comparison, the response to other potential chemical mediators was inconsistent, and the activated currents were far smaller than those evoked by acid. Furthermore, when compared to unlabeled DRG and cardiac vagal afferents, a higher percentage of cardiac sympathetic afferents responded to acid, and the resulting current amplitude was significantly larger.

Another consistent and large response was evoked by ATP in cardiac vagal afferents. The current was slow activating and only partially desensitized (data not shown), suggesting homomeric $P2X_2$ and heteromeric $P2X_{2/3}$ channels as previously described in nodose neurons.[20–22] In contrast, ATP-evoked currents in DRG neurons were substantially smaller and consisted primarily of a fast-activating and -desensitizing current (see FIG. 1A), indicative of the $P2X_3$ receptor subtype.[21–23] Cardiac afferents sometimes responded to the other chemicals in FIGURE 1; however, they did so inconsistently, and the amplitude of the evoked currents in the responders were much smaller than those seen with either pH or ATP. Of the chemicals tested: protons, ATP, 5HT, and capsaicin activate ion channels that are presumed to serve as sensory transducers in sensory neurons (the ASICs,[24] P2X receptors,[20,23] 5HT3 receptor,[25] and vanilloid receptors,[26,27] respectively). No current was evoked by acetycholine, but small currents were occasionally seen in response to bradykinin or adenosine. Presumably, these currents arose from modulation of a channel by an intracellular signaling process; the importance of this may be understated by our methods. Nonetheless, the consistently large pH-evoked responses in cardiac sympathetic afferents indicate that a distinct pH-sensitive molecule is highly expressed in these cells and may be important in sensing myocardial ischemia.

## PROPERTIES OF ACID-EVOKED CURRENTS IN CARDIAC AFFERENTS

In an effort to understand the molecular identity of the cardiac pH sensor, it was necessary to further characterize the biophysical and pharmacological properties of

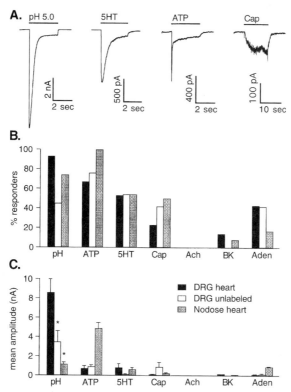

**FIGURE 1.** Cardiac afferents respond to a variety of chemical activators. (**A**) Representative currents evoked by extracellular application of various chemicals to cardiac sensory neurons from the DRG. Note the different *scale bars* and *application times*. (**B**) The percentage of cardiac DRG, cardiac nodose, and unlabeled DRG neurons that responded to various chemicals: [pH, 5.0; adenosine 5′-triphosphate (ATP), 30 µM; serotonin (5HT), 30 µM; capsaicin (Cap), 1 µM; acetylcholine (ACh), 200 µM; bradykinin (BK), 500 nM; or adenosine (Aden), 200 µM]. Each *bar* represents at least 12 cells. (**C**) Mean amplitudes of the evoked currents of the responding neurons. Error bars = SEM. *$P < .01$ vs. pH-evoked current in DRG heart. (From Benson *et al.*[9] Reproduced by permission.)

these acid-evoked currents. The primary acid-evoked currents in cardiac afferents are qualitatively similar to those previously described in unlabeled rat DRG neurons. Consistent with the findings of Bevan and Yeats,[28] we found that pH less than 7 activated a transient (rapidly activating and desensitizing) current, which was followed by a sustained current only when the pH dropped further, to pH 6 and below (FIG. 2). The $EC_{50}$ (pH 6.6) was less acidic than previously reported by other investigators for acid-evoked currents in rat DRG neurons,[29] suggesting that cardiac afferents are particularly sensitive to acidic changes. The transient current was $Na^+$-selective, and the sustained current was nonselective in some neurons (see FIG. 6A), consistent with previous studies.[28-30] Finally, the transient current was inhibited by the potassium-sparing diuretic amiloride (data not shown). Given these defined charac-

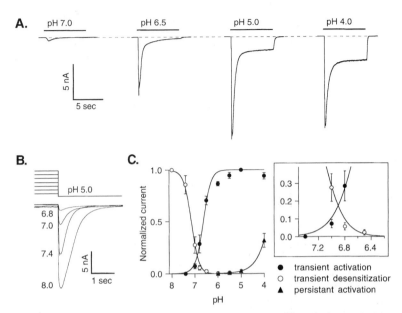

**FIGURE 2.** Activation and desensitization properties of acid-evoked currents in cardiac DRG neurons. (**A**) Typical currents evoked by applying various pH to a cardiac DRG neuron. Note the transient, fast-activating and -desensitizing current that is evoked by relatively low proton concentrations. At higher proton concentrations a nondesensitizing, sustained current is evoked. Resting pH = 8.0 at −70 mV. (**B**) Superimposed currents evoked by pH 5.0 from varying resting pH. (**C**) Dose-response data for acid-evoked transient (*closed circles,* n = 6) and sustained (*triangles,* n = 6) currents. The *open circles* are data obtained using the desensitization protocol in (**B**) (n = 7). The transient responses are normalized to the peak current obtained from application of pH 5.0. The sustained responses are normalized to the saturation level of the curve fit. Half-activation values were pH 6.6 (transient) and pH 3.7 (sustained); half-desensitization was pH 7.2. The *boxed inset* magnifies the region where the transient activation and desensitization curves overlap. Points represent means ±SEM. (From Benson *et al.*[9] Reproduced by permission.)

teristics, and the recent cloning of several pH-sensitive candidate molecules, we set out to determine the molecular identity of the cardiac pH sensor.

## POTENTIAL MOLECULES THAT SENSE PH CHANGES

There exist two classes of molecules that are proposed to sense changes in extracellular pH in sensory neurons: (1) acid-sensing ion channels (ASICs), which are members of the epithelial Na$^+$/degenerin family of ion channels, and (2) vanilloid receptors. Vanilloid receptors are activated by capsaicin (the compound in pepper that tastes "hot"), noxious heat, and protons.[31] Therefore, it is thought that vanilloid receptors, in addition to sensing heat, may mediate sensory responses to acidity caused by inflammation and ischemia. Cardiac afferents detect cardiac ischemia, yet only a small fraction exhibit capsaicin-activated current, and those that do respond have small currents compared to capsaicin-activated currents in unlabeled DRG neurons (FIG. 1). This suggests that vanilloid receptors play a lesser role in cardiac sensation than in sensation from other organs. Furthermore, the distinct kinetics, $Na^+$ selectivity, and amiloride sensitivity of the currents distinguish the proton-sensing channels in cardiac afferents as ASICs.

Two recent studies[32,33] reported diminished proton-activated currents in DRG neurons from mice lacking the vanilloid receptor (VR1). However, both groups studied relatively small-diameter neurons (mean = 23 µm, and <22 µm, respectively), whereas the diameter of cardiac-afferent neurons is typically between 25 and 35 µm. Furthermore, these studies focused on the sustained pH-evoked currents (Davis *et al.*[33] reported that the transient pH currents were intact in the VR1-deficient mice). In a later section, we further the case that the transient, rather than the sustained, component of the current is most likely responsible for pH sensing in the setting of myocardial ischemia. On the whole, our results argue that ASICs are more important than vanilloid receptors for sensing myocardial ischemia.

## THE SPECIFIC ASIC RESPONSIBLE FOR THE PH-EVOKED CURRENT IN CARDIAC AFFERENTS

The ASICs are members of a larger superfamily of ion channels and other membrane proteins that appear to have widely diverse functions. This includes the amiloride-sensitive epithelial $Na^+$ channel, which controls $Na^+$ reabsorption by the kidneys, lungs, and other organs,[34] and the degenerins, which in nematodes causes neuronal cell death when they are constitutively active and are also involved in mechanotransduction.[35] Interestingly, Price *et al.*[36] have recently shown a touch deficit in mice lacking one of the ASIC members, BNC1 (a.k.a. ASIC2). Although in the next section we will make the case that one particular ASIC is poised to act as a pH sensor, it is intriguing to speculate on a potential mechanosensory role for these proteins in cardiac afferents. Coincidentally, there is precedent for dual sensory integration by a single molecule: the vanilloid receptor, VR1, has been shown to mediate multiple stimuli—heat and protons.[31,32]

Currently, ASICs consist of five members in rat: ASIC1a;[37,38] and its splice variant ASIC1b;[39] ASIC2a;[38,40,41] and its splice variant ASIC2b;[42] and ASIC3[43] (nomenclature as in Ref. 24). The proteins are small (~500 aa), with a predicted membrane topology of a large extracellular loop connecting two transmembrane domains, with the amino and carboxyl termini inside the cell. The functional channels may be formed by homomultimeric and/or heteromultimeric combinations of the ASIC subunits.[24] Like the other members of the extended ion-channel family, each ASIC is blocked by amiloride, albeit by relatively high concentrations. The mRNAs for all subtypes except ASIC2a[42] are expressed in rat sensory neurons, and the ASIC3 and ASIC1b mRNAs in the rat are expressed exclusively in sensory neurons.[39,43] Although Lazdunski's group recently reported a tarantula toxin that specifically blocks ASIC1a,[44] there is no readily available pharmacological agent that distinguishes the different ASICs. We therefore studied detailed biophysical characteristics to identify the ASIC(s) responsible for the acid-evoked currents in native cardiac afferents.

**TABLE 1. ASIC3 matches the native cardiac afferent current in all parameters measured, while the other ASIC subtypes do not**

| Functional Property | Cardiac | ASIC3 | ASIC1a | ASIC1b |
|---|---|---|---|---|
| $pH_{0.5}$ activation | 6.6 | 6.7 | 5.7 | $5.9^{39}$ |
| $pH_{0.5}$ desensitization | 7.2 | 7.1 | 7.3 | |
| $\tau$ Act. (ms, at pH 6) | $3.7 \pm 1.3$ | $3.2 \pm 0.96$ | $13.7 \pm 3.5^{a}$ | |
| $\tau$ Densens. (s, at pH 6) | $0.35 \pm 0.04$ | $0.32 \pm 0.07$ | $3.5 \pm 0.39^{a}$ | $1.7 \pm 0.27^{a}$ |
| $\tau$ Recovery (s, at pH 7.4) | 0.61 | 0.58 | 13 | 5.9 |
| % Block by 10 mM $Ca^{2+}$ | $44 \pm 7.3$ | $34 \pm 9.2$ | $82 \pm 4.9^{a}$ | $83 \pm 2.5^{a}$ |
| $I_{30Ca}/I_{10Ca}$ | $3.1 \pm 0.77$ | $2.5 \pm 0.42$ | $0.99 \pm 0.16^{a}$ | |
| $P_{Na}/P_{K}$ | 6.8 | 4.5 | 5.5 | $2.6^{39}$ |
| $IC_{50}$ amiloride ($\mu$M) | 37 | $63^{43}$ | $10^{37}$ | $21^{39}$ |

[a]Denote means that differ from the cardiac afferent with greater than 99% certainty (two-tailed $t$-test, $n = 3-6$). Values without standard errors are derived from curve fits ($n = 3-12$). All measurements were by us unless referenced. $I_{30Ca}/I_{10Ca}$ is the ratio of peak amplitudes when $Ca^{2+}$, at either 30 mM or 10 mM, is the only permeant ion. Activation rates were measured in outside-out patches; all others were made in whole cell. (Modified from Sutherland *et al.*[10] Reproduced by permission.)

## ASIC3 MATCHES THE PH-EVOKED CURRENT IN CARDIAC AFFERENTS

Of the five known ASIC proteins, two were ruled out based on the previously published data: ASIC2a is not present in rat sensory ganglia, and ASIC2b does not form a functional channel as a homomultimer.[42] Thus, we studied the properties of ASIC 1a, 1b, or 3 expressed in COS-7 cells to determine if they might emulate the native currents seen in cardiac afferents.

First, and perhaps most importantly, the pH sensitivity of ASIC3 precisely matches that of the cardiac-afferent channel (FIG. 3). ASIC1a and 1b were less sensitive to protons (TABLE 1). Because the critical pH range that occurs with myocardial ischemia is pH 7.1 to 6.7,[12] we further explored the sensitivity of the various channels in this range (FIG. 4). Clearly, ASIC3 functions best as a pH sensor in this critical range. Another property that readily distinguishes the channels is their recovery from desensitization. FIGURE 5 shows that the native channel and ASIC3 recover more rapidly than the other channels (see figure legend for experimental protocol). Also apparent from FIGURE 5 is that the kinetics of activation and desensitization of ASIC3 match that of cardiac-afferent neurons.

Another important observation from *in vivo* studies is that protons derived from lactic acid excite pulmonary,[45] gastrointestinal,[46] and cardiac afferents[13] more than other acids applied at the same pH. Interestingly, the McCleskey laboratory has recently presented data suggesting that lactate anion potentiates the acid-evoked currents in cardiac-afferent neurons and in heterologously expressed ASIC3.[47]

TABLE 1 summarizes the various measured properties of the native cardiac afferent and the cloned channels. All channel types share two traits: selection of $Na^{+}$ over

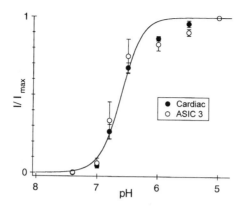

**FIGURE 3.** The pH sensitivity of cardiac afferents matches that of ASIC3. Average (±SEM) fractional current vs. pH for cardiac afferents (*filled circles*, $n$ = 14) and COS7 cells expressing ASIC3 (*open circles*, $n$ = 11), normalized to pH 5. *Solid line* is the fit of the Hill equation for cardiac afferents. (Modified from Sutherland *et al.*[10] Reproduced by permission.)

$K^+$, and weak block by amiloride. However, the following six properties of the native channel are shared only by ASIC3: high proton sensitivity, rapid rates of activation, desensitization, recovery, weak $Ca^{2+}$ block, and low but detectable $Ca^{2+}$ permeability. Because all these functional features match in near-perfect detail, we conclude that ASIC3 is likely the predominant molecule that makes up the native acid-gated channel in cardiac-afferent neurons. Although it probably is not relevant to myocardial ischemia, many cardiac afferents exhibit a nonselective sustained current at very acidic pH that is not mimicked by ASIC3 homomers.

## AN UNIDENTIFIED VARIABLE SUSTAINED CURRENT

As previously stated, the predominant pH-evoked current in cardiac afferents is an extremely large transient current that is evoked by modest pH changes (in the range that occurs in the setting of myocardial ischemia). This current is consistent with ASIC3. However, at extreme acidic pH (half-activation pH = 3.7), a smaller (average $I_{sust}/I_{trans}$ = 0.14 ± 0.04 at pH 5, $n$ = 13) and variable sustained current is elicited. FIGURE 6 demonstrates that the sustained current is small compared to the transient current, and its ion selectivity varies among cells. In agreement with work previously published,[43,48] ASIC3 alone yields sustained currents that are $Na^+$ selective (FIG. 6C). In contrast, we found that coexpression of ASIC3 and ASIC2b yields a sustained current that does not distinguish between monovalent cations (FIG. 6B), as previously reported.[42] Although we did not study all of the properties of the heteromeric channel, the kinetics and $Na^+$ selectivity of the transient current are qualitatively similar to the ASIC3 homomeric channel. Because ASIC2b alone does not form a functional channel, these results suggest that heteromeric channels formed of ASIC3 and 2b subtypes generate a nonselective sustained current at very low pH, and that ASIC2b forms heteromers with ASIC3 in some, but not all, cardiac affer-

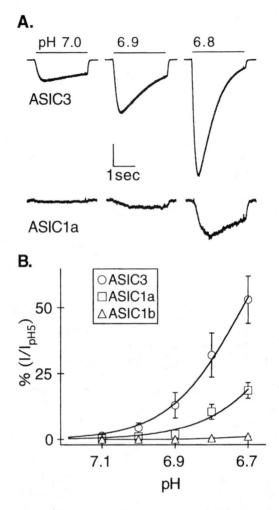

**FIGURE 4.** ASIC3 is extremely sensitive to protons in the range incurred by myocardial ischemia. (**A**) Representative currents from COS7 cells expressing ASIC3 or ASIC1a in
response to pH 7.0, 6.9, and 6.8. *Vertical scale bar* represents 10% of the current evoked by
pH 5.0 (ASIC3 = 2 nA; ASIC1a = 46 pA). (**B**) Average currents of the indicated subunits
normalized to the value at pH 5. *Solid lines* are fits of the Hill equation. (From Sutherland
*et al.*[10] Reproduced by permission.)

ents. ASICs probably do not account for all sustained pH-evoked current in cardiac
afferents. Although we have shown them to be present at low levels in cardiac afferents, vanilloid receptors generate sustained, nonselective currents at such extreme
pH. Furthermore, extreme acidic pH might modulate other ion channels to contribute
small nonselective currents. Regardless, the extreme acidic pH necessary to evoke

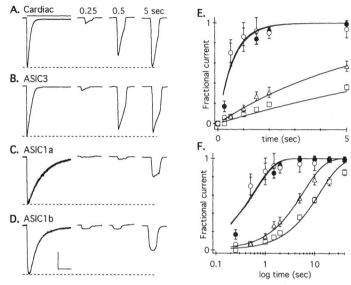

**FIGURE 5.** Only ASIC3 mimics recovery kinetics of cardiac afferents. Current was completely desensitized by a prolonged pulse to pH 6.0 (*bar*), and then the cell was returned to pH 7.4. Recovery from desensitization was tested by a brief pH pulse applied at the indicated times; only one data point was collected after each desensitizing pulse. Currents in (**A**) a cardiac afferent and (**B**) ASIC3 recovered rapidly; currents in (**C**) ASIC1a and (**D**) 1b recovered slowly. *Horizontal scales*: 2 s for desensitizing currents (*left*), 1 s for test currents. *Vertical scales*: (A) 1 nA, (B) 1.25 nA, (C) 0.45 nA, and (D) 0.5 nA. Recovery of average ±SEM) currents, normalized to initial amplitude, for (**E**) the first 5 s (linear) and (**F**) 40 s (*log scale*) is given. *Solid lines* are fits of single exponentials. Cardiac afferents (●, $\tau = 0.61$ s, $n = 4$ for each data point), ASIC3 (○, $\tau = 0.58$ s, $n = 5$), ASIC1a (□, $\tau = 12.99$ s, $n = 4$), ASIC1b △, $\tau = 5.88$ s, $n = 3$). (From Sutherland *et al*.[10] Reproduced by permission.)

sustained currents in cardiac afferents calls into question the physiological relevance of such responses.

Bevan and Geppetti[49] have proposed that a prolonged sensation, such as pain associated with ischemia, must be a consequence of the sustained acid-evoked current in DRG neurons. However, the sustained current is not activated until pH is lowered to 6.0 or lower. In the case of myocardial ischemia, extracellular pH probably rarely if ever reaches this range. Cobbe and Poole-Wilson[12] have shown in an isolated rabbit heart that it takes a full 60 min of total heart ischemia to produce pH drops below 6.0. On the other hand, pH is lowered to 7.0 (the pH that activates the transient current) after 5 min of ischemia. Perhaps coincidentally, there usually is a 5-min time delay from the onset of ischemic signs (ST segment depression on an electrocardiogram) to the onset of reported angina in patients with coronary artery disease.[50] Clinical attempts to measure pH changes in the cardiac veins of patients with active myocardial ischemia have shown even less extreme drops in pH.[14] Most convincingly, Pan *et al*.[13] demonstrated that epicardial tissue pH changes from pH 7.35 to 7.0 stimulate cardiac afferents in cats to fire a sustained train of action potentials.

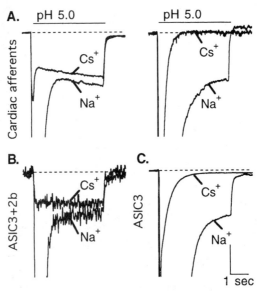

**FIGURE 6.** Variable expression of a sustained, nonselective current in cardiac afferents suggests variable expression of ASIC2b. Peak currents are off scale to emphasize the smaller sustained component. (**A**) Currents, evoked by steps to pH 5, from two cardiac afferents that display sustained components differing in selectivity. (*Left*) the sustained component is nonselective (passes $Cs^+$ and $Na^+$ equally). (*Right*) the sustained component is $Na^+$-selective. (**B**) Coexpression of ASIC3 and 2b yields a nonselective sustained component. (**C**) The ASIC3 homomer yields a $Na^+$-selective sustained component. *Vertical scales*: (A, *left*) 600 pA, (A, *right*) 150 pA, (B) 35 pA, (C) 500 pA . (From Sutherland *et al.*[10] Reproduced by permission.)

It seems clear that persistent activation of a population of sensory neurons occurs when extracellular pH drops from 7.4 to 7.0, a change that would not be expected to activate sustained current through vanilloid receptors or ASICs, but clearly activates a transient current via ASIC3. The molecular basis of this is not yet understood, but our data suggest one explanation. FIGURE 2C reveals a window of overlap of the activation and desensitization curves of the transient acid-evoked current. The channels are activated in this range (pH 7.2–6.5), but incompletely desensitized, and could create a sustained current and depolarization.

## CONCLUSION

For the past 30 years, there has been a vast amount of research focused on the determinants of cardiac sensation. The bulk of this work has been done in whole-animal experimental models, and while much has been learned, results have often been contradictory.[2] By identifying and isolating cardiac afferents in culture, we have developed a novel approach to identify the molecules responsible for the sensation of myocardial ischemia. Having found that lowered pH is a likely mediator of myocardial ischemic sensation, we then defined the primary molecular sensor underlying this response as being the acid sensing ion channel—ASIC3. Although our research has focused on acid as a mediator of cardiac ischemia, other chemical mediators and sensors cannot be ignored. Most likely, activation of cardiac afferents in the setting of myocardial ischemia represents a complex interplay between multiple mediators and molecular sensors.

The practical implications of this work are substantial. Approximately 6 million people in the United States alone suffer from chronic angina. Understanding the molecules that transduce this sensation might lead to new therapies for this common debilitating illness. In addition, the clinical implications of these findings extend beyond relief of pain. A broad range of cardiovascular disease processes, including myocardial ischemia,[51] congestive heart failure,[52] and arrhythmias[53] are precipitated or worsened by perturbations in the autonomic nervous system. Much of the current pharmacological therapies are directed toward blocking the *compensatory*, but often deleterious, neurohormonal reflexes that are activated in these diseases. In skeletal muscle[54] and abdominal viscera,[55] ischemia induces acidic conditions, which activates afferent fibers, which in turn cause potent excitation of the sympathetic efferent system. The same acid-evoked reflex loop may exist in the heart and contribute to the detrimental effect of sympathetic activation in myocardial ischemic conditions. Specific blockade of acid-evoked activation of cardiac afferents, via the pH sensor ASIC3, presents a potential new therapeutic strategy in the treatment of ischemic heart disease.

## ACKNOWLEDGMENTS

This work was supported by the following NIH grants: RO1DAO7415, Cardiovascular Signaling SP Training Grant T32-HL07817, and Neuronal Signal Transduction Training Grant NS07381.

## REFERENCES

1. LEWIS, T. 1932. Pain in muscular ischemia: its relation to anginal pain. Arch. Int. Med. **49:** 713–727.
2. MELLER, S.T. & G.F. GEBHART. 1992. A critical review of the afferent pathways and the potential chemical mediators involved in cardiac pain. Neuroscience **48:** 501–524.
3. BAKER, D.G., H.M. COLERIDGE, J.C. COLERIDGE, *et al.* 1980. Search for a cardiac nociceptor: stimulation by bradykinin of sympathetic afferent nerve endings in the heart of the cat. J. Physiol. (Lond.) **306:** 519–536.
4. EUCHNER-WAMSER, I., S.T. MELLER & G.F. GEBHART. 1994. A model of cardiac nociception in chronically instrumented rats: behavioral and electrophysiological effects of pericardial administration of algogenic substances. Pain **58:** 117–128.
5. PAN, H.L. & J.C. LONGHURST. 1995. Lack of a role of adenosine in activation of ischemically sensitive cardiac sympathetic afferents. Am. J. Physiol. **269:** H106–H113.
6. THAMES, M.D., T. KINUGAWA & M.E. DIBNER-DUNLAP. 1993. Reflex sympathoexcitation by cardiac sympathetic afferents during myocardial ischemia. Role of adenosine. Circulation **87:** 1698–1704.
7. GNECCHI-RUSCONE, T., N. MONTANO, M. CONTINI, *et al.* 1995. Adenosine activates cardiac sympathetic afferent fibers and potentiates the excitation induced by coronary occlusion. J. Auton. Nerv. Syst. **53:** 175–184.

8. HUANG, M.H., M. HORACKOVA, R.M. NEGOESCU, et al. 1996. Polysensory response characteristics of dorsal root ganglion neurones that may serve sensory functions during myocardial ischaemia. Cardiovasc. Res. **32:** 503–515.

9. BENSON, C.J., S.P. ECKERT & E.W. MCCLESKEY. 1999. Acid-evoked currents in cardiac sensory neurons: a possible mediator of myocardial ischemic sensation. Circ. Res. **84:** 921–928.

10. SUTHERLAND, S.P., C.J. BENSON, J.P. ADELMAN, et al. 2001. Acid-sensing ion channel 3 matches the acid-gated current in cardiac ischemia-sensing neurons. Proc. Natl. Acad. Sci. USA **98:** 711–716.

11. JACOBUS, W.E., G.J.I. TAYLOR, D.P. HOLLIS, et al. 1977. Phosphorus nuclear magnetic resonance of perfused working rat hearts. Nature **265:** 756–758.

12. COBBE, S.M. & P.A. POOLE-WILSON. 1980. The time of onset and severity of acidosis in myocardial ischaemia. J. Mol. Cell Cardiol. **12:** 745–760.

13. PAN, H.L., J.C. LONGHURST, J.C. EISENACH, et al. 1999. Role of protons in activation of cardiac sympathetic C-fibre afferents during ischaemia in cats. J. Physiol. (Lond.) **518:** 857–866.

14. COBBE, S.M. & P.A. POOLE-WILSON. 1982. Continuous coronary sinus and arterial pH monitoring during pacing-induced ischaemia in coronary artery disease. Br. Heart J. **47:** 369–374.

15. STEEN, K.H., A.E. STEEN & P.W. REEH. 1995. A dominant role of acid pH in inflammatory excitation and sensitization of nociceptors in rat skin, in vitro. J. Neurosci. **15:** 3982–3989.

16. ISSBERNER, U., P.W. REEH & K.H. STEEN. 1996. Pain due to tissue acidosis: a mechanism for inflammatory and ischemic myalgia? Neurosci. Lett. **208:** 191–194.

17. UCHIDA, Y. & S. MURAO. 1975. Acid-induced excitation of afferent cardiac sympathetic nerve fibers. Am. J. Physiol. **228:** 27–33.

18. ECKERT, S.P., A. TADDESE & E.W. MCCLESKEY. 1997. Isolation and culture of rat sensory neurons having distinct sensory modalities. J. Neurosci. Methods **77:** 183–190.

19. MCNEILL, D.L. & H.W. BURDEN. 1986. Convergence of sensory processes from the heart and left ulnar nerve onto a single afferent perikaryon: a neuroanatomical study in the rat employing fluorescent tracers. Anat. Rec. **214:** 441–444, 396–447.

20. LEWIS, C., S. NEIDHART, C. HOLY, et al. 1995. Coexpression of P2X2 and P2X3 receptor subunits can account for ATP-gated currents in sensory neurons. Nature **377:** 432–435.

21. COCKAYNE, D.A., S.G. HAMILTON, Q.M. ZHU, et al. 2000. Urinary bladder hyporeflexia and reduced pain-related behaviour in P2X3-deficient mice. Nature **407:** 1011–1015.

22. SOUSLOVA, V., P. CESARE, Y. DING, et al. 2000. Warm-coding deficits and aberrant inflammatory pain in mice lacking P2X3 receptors. Nature **407:** 1015–1017.

23. CHEN, C.C., A.N. AKOPIAN, L. SIVILOTTI, et al. 1995. A P2X purinoceptor expressed by a subset of sensory neurons. Nature **377:** 428–431.

24. WALDMANN, R. & M. LAZDUNSKI. 1998. H+-gated cation channels: neuronal acid sensors in the ENaC/DEG family of ion channels. Curr. Opin. Neurobiol. **8:** 418–424.

25. MARICQ, A.V., A.S. PETERSON, A.J. BRAKE, et al. 1991. Primary structure and functional expression of the 5HT$_3$ receptor, a serotonin-gated ion channel. Science **254:** 432–437.

26. CATERINA, M.J., M.A. SCHUMACHER, M. TOMINAGA, et al. 1997. The capsaicin receptor: a heat-activated ion channel in the pain pathway. Nature **389:** 816–824.

27. CATERINA, M.J., T.A. ROSEN, M. TOMINAGA, et al. 1999. A capsaicin-receptor homologue with a high threshold for noxious heat. Nature **398:** 436–441.

28. BEVAN, S. & J. YEATS. 1991. Protons activate a cation conductance in a sub-population of rat dorsal root ganglion neurones. J. Physiol. (Lond.) **433:** 145–161.

29. KRISHTAL, O.A. & V.I. PIDOPLICHKO. 1980. A receptor for protons in the nerve cell membrane. Neuroscience **5:** 2325–2327.

30. KONNERTH, A., H.D. LUX & M. MORAD. 1987. Proton-induced transformation of calcium channel in chick dorsal root ganglion cells. J. Physiol. (Lond.) **386:** 603–633.

31. TOMINAGA, M., M.J. CATERINA, A.B. MALMBERG, et al. 1998. The cloned capsaicin receptor integrates multiple pain-producing stimuli. Neuron **21:** 531–543.

32. CATERINA, M.J., A. LEFFLER, A.B. MALMBERG, *et al*. 2000. Impaired nociception and pain sensation in mice lacking the capsaicin receptor. Science **288**: 306–313.
33. DAVIS, J.B., J. GRAY, M.J. GUNTHORPE, *et al*. 2000. Vanilloid receptor-1 is essential for inflammatory thermal hyperalgesia. Nature **405**: 183–187.
34. GARTY, H. & L.G. PALMER. 1997. Epithelial sodium channels: function, structure, and regulation. Physiol. Rev. **77**: 359–396.
35. TAVERNARAKIS, N. & M. DRISCOLL. 1997. Molecular modeling of mechanotransduction in the nematode *Caenorhabditis elegans*. Annu. Rev. Physiol. **59**: 659–689.
36. PRICE, M.P., G.R. LEWIN, S.L. MCILWRATH, *et al*. 2000. The mammalian sodium channel BNC1 is required for normal touch sensation. Nature **407**: 1007–1011.
37. WALDMANN, R., G. CHAMPIGNY, F. BASSILANA, *et al*. 1997. A proton-gated cation channel involved in acid-sensing. Nature **386**: 173–177.
38. GARCIA-ANOVEROS, J., B. DERFLER, J. NEVILLE-GOLDEN, *et al*. 1997. BNaC1 and BNaC2 constitute a new family of human neuronal sodium channels related to degenerins and epithelial sodium channels. Proc. Natl. Acad. Sci. USA **94**: 1459–1464.
39. CHEN, C.C., S. ENGLAND, A.N. AKOPIAN, *et al*. 1998. A sensory neuron-specific, proton-gated ion channel. Proc. Natl. Acad. Sci. USA **95**: 10240–10245.
40. PRICE, M.P., P.M. SNYDER & M.J. WELSH. 1996. Cloning and expression of a novel human brain $Na^+$ channel. J. Biol. Chem. **271**: 7879–7882.
41. WALDMANN, R., G. CHAMPIGNY, N. VOILLEY, *et al*. 1996. The mammalian degenerin MDEG, an amiloride-sensitive cation channel activated by mutations causing neurodegeneration in *Caenorhabditis elegans*. J. Biol. Chem. **271**: 10433–10436.
42. LINGUEGLIA, E., J.R. DE WEILLE, F. BASSILANA, *et al*. 1997. A modulatory subunit of acid sensing ion channels in brain and dorsal root ganglion cells. J. Biol. Chem. **272**: 29778–29783.
43. WALDMANN, R., F. BASSILANA, J. DE WEILLE, *et al*. 1997. Molecular cloning of a noninactivating proton-gated $Na^+$ channel specific for sensory neurons. J. Biol. Chem. **272**: 20975–20978.
44. ESCOUBAS, P., J.R. DE WEILLE, A. LECOQ, *et al*. 2000. Isolation of a tarantula toxin specific for a class of proton-gated $Na^+$ channels. J. Biol. Chem. **275**: 25116–25121.
45. HONG, J.L., K. KWONG & L.Y. LEE. 1997. Stimulation of pulmonary C fibres by lactic acid in rats: contributions of $H^+$ and lactate ions. J. Physiol. (Lond.) **500**: 319–329.
46. STAHL, G.L. & J.C. LONGHURST. 1992. Ischemically sensitive visceral afferents: importance of $H^+$ derived from lactic acid and hypercapnia. Am. J. Physiol. **262**: H748–H753.
47. SUTHERLAND, S.P., D. IMMKE. L.S. STONE, *et al*. 2000. ASIC3 matches the acid-gated current in cardiac ischemia-sensing neurons. Presented at the 30th Annual Meeting of the Society for Neuroscience. New Orleans, La.
48. BABINSKI, K., K.T. LE & P. SEGUELA. 1999. Molecular cloning and regional distribution of a human proton receptor subunit with biphasic functional properties. J. Neurochem. **72**: 51–57.
49. BEVAN, S. & P. GEPPETTI. 1994. Protons: small stimulants of capsaicin-sensitive sensory nerves. Trends Neurosci. **17**: 509–512.
50. LEVY, R.D., L.M. SHAPIRO, C. WRIGHT, *et al*. 1986. Haemodynamic response to myocardial ischaemia during unrestricted activity, exercise testing, and atrial pacing assessed by ambulatory pulmonary artery pressure monitoring. Br. Heart J. **56**: 12–18.
51. THAMER, V., A. DEUSSEN, J.D. SCHIPKE, *et al*. 1990. Pain and myocardial ischemia: the role of sympathetic activation. Basic Res. Cardiol. **85**: 253–266.
52. FRANCIS, G.S., S.R. GOLDSMITH, T.B. LEVINE, *et al*. 1984. The neurohumoral axis in congestive heart failure. Ann. Intern. Med. **101**: 370–377.
53. MITRANI, R.D. & D.P. ZIPES. 1994. Clinical neurocardiology: arrhythmias. *In* Neurocardiology, J.A. Armour & J.L. Ardell, Eds.: 365–395. Oxford University Press. New York.
54. VICTOR, R.G., L.A. BERTOCCI, S.L. PRYOR, *et al*. 1988. Sympathetic nerve discharge is coupled to muscle cell pH during exercise in humans. J. Clin. Invest. **82**: 1301–1305.
55. RENDIG, S.V., P.S. CHAHAL & J.C. LONGHURST. 1997. Cardiovascular reflex responses to ischemia during occlusion of celiac and/or superior mesenteric arteries. Am. J. Physiol. **272**: H791–H796.

# Nicotinic Acetylcholine Receptors on Vagal Afferent Neurons

ELLIS COOPER

*Department of Physiology, McGill University, Montreal, Quebec, Canada H3G 1Y6*

ABSTRACT: Nicotinic acetylcholine receptors (nAChRs) play an important role in various processes involved in regulating systemic blood pressure. These receptors are expressed at excitatory cholinergic synapses between sympathetic preganglionic neurons and postganglionic sympathetic neurons and link the integrative activities of the CNS with peripheral effector mechanisms of the sympathetic nervous system. Nicotinic AChRs are also expressed on a subset of vagal afferent neurons, including those involved in baroreceptor reflexes. This review discusses the developmental expression of nAChRs on vagal afferent neurons and two factors that influence the differentiation of these neurons: ganglionic satellite cells and neurotrophins. In addition, this review discusses two important properties of neuronal nAChRs: inward rectification and calcium permeability. At the molecular level, intracellular polyamines, acting as gating particles, effectively block the receptor pore in a voltage-dependent manner, producing inward rectification. Moreover, a critical structural determinant underlies both the block by intracellular polyamines and calcium permeability. Finally, this review discusses the modulation and block of neuronal nAChRs by extracellular polyamines and the possible implications for neurodegenerative diseases.

KEYWORDS: Nicotinic acetylcholine receptors; Sympathetic neurons; Nodose neurons; Polyamines; Calcium permeability; Inward rectification; Neurotrophins; Ganglionic satellite cells

## INTRODUCTION

A major determinant of systemic blood pressure is the activity of sympathetic nerves. Sympathetic nerves, by releasing norepinephrine, stimulate smooth muscle contraction in blood vessels, thereby increasing peripheral resistance. The clinical significance of this mechanism is clear: most hypertensives have increased sympathetic nerve activity, as measured by circulating norephinephrine concentrations and by direct microneurography.[1,2] Various central and peripheral factors, such as cardiopulmonary reflexes, exercise, and emotions, particularly those involving stress, combine to influence the activity of sympathetic nerves. To a large extent, the integration of these central and peripheral factors is a function of neurons located in the rostral ventrolateral (RVL) part of the medulla, the major vasomotor area in the brain. These RVL neurons integrate inputs directly or indirectly from all levels of the

Address for correspondence: Ellis Cooper, Ph.D., Department of Physiology, McGill University, McIntyre Medical Science Building, 3655 Promenade Sir William Osler, Montreal, Quebec, Canada H3G 1Y6. Voice: 514-398-4334; fax: 514-398-7452.
Ecooper@med.mcgill.ca

CNS, including those from the hypothalamus, the amygdala, and the nucleus tractus solitarius (NTS); in addition, RVL neurons directly excite sympathetic preganglionic neurons in the intermediate lateral part of the spinal cord.[3] In turn, preganglionic neurons relay activity from RVL neurons to sympathetic neurons located in peripheral paravertebral and prevertebral ganglia through excitatory cholinergic nicotinic synapses. These excitatory nicotinic synapses link the integrative activities of the CNS with peripheral effector mechanisms of the sympathetic nervous system. Moreover, RVL neurons are tonically active and are directly responsible for much of the tonic activity in sympathetic nerves.[3]

Feedback information about systemic blood pressure is conveyed to the brain stem by baroreceptor afferents. Baroreceptors, located in the walls of the aortic arch, the carotid sinus, the atria, and the ventricles, furnish the CNS with moment-to-moment information about the pressure in the arterial system. Inputs from baroreceptors, terminating in the NTS, are among the most potent inhibitors of sympathetic activity.[4] Baroreceptors respond rapidly to changes in arterial pressure, thereby providing a valuable first line of defense against abnormal pressures. In this way, the baroreceptor reflex normally maintains arterial blood pressure within narrow limits; for patients with chronic hypertension, however, functional adaptations occur, changing the sensitivity or the gain of the reflex.[4]

To understand baroreflex function, one must understand the cellular and molecular mechanisms that govern action potential activity in baroreceptor afferent and sympathetic efferent neurons. Specifically, one would like to know more about the mechanisms that regulate the expression, targeting, and clustering of neurotransmitter-gated and voltage-gated ion channels; in general, these mechanisms operate during development and dictate how neurons integrate different synaptic inputs, fire action potentials at various frequencies, and release the appropriate amount of neurotransmitter. A growing number of studies indicate that perturbations in these mechanisms have serious consequences for neuronal function and underlie various diseases.[5] To gain insight into these mechanisms, we have been studying ion channel expression in developing rat nodose and sympathetic neurons. Here, I review some of this work, concentrating on the expression of nicotinic acetylcholine receptors (nAChRs) on nodose neurons.

## DIFFERENTIATION OF DEVELOPING NODOSE NEURONS

Precursors to nodose neurons, migrating cranial placodal cells, undergo their last cell division by embryonic day 15 and start differentiating into sensory neurons.[6] At birth, neurons in nodose ganglia have a distinct sensory neuron phenotype: their unipolar cell bodies lack conventional dendrites and are in close contact with ganglionic nonneuronal satellite cells.[7] Emerging from the cell body is a single axonal process that bifurcates within a few hundred microns of the soma into a central branch and a peripheral branch. During the first few postnatal weeks, the spherical somas, which lack synapses, continue to enlarge and become completely engulfed by satellite cells while the peripheral and central connections mature.

We are interested in the factors that influence the expression of voltage-gated channels on peripheral neurons. Neonatal nodose neurons are electrically excitable and generate rapid, overshooting action potentials. These neurons have various voltage-gated currents: two types of voltage-gated $Na^+$ currents—a rapidly activating, TTX-sensitive current and a slowly activating, TTX-insensitive current;[8,9] at least two types of voltage-gated $Ca^{2+}$ currents;[10,11] and several types of $K^+$ currents.[12–14] We are interested in the expression of both voltage-gated $Na^+$ and voltage-gated $K^+$ channels on neonatal nodose neurons because these channels play an important role in initiating action potentials and modulating their firing frequencies. In general, TTX-sensitive $Na^+$ currents on peripheral neurons are difficult to characterize with conventional whole-cell patch-clamp techniques, in part, because the currents activate so rapidly. Recently, we developed an amplifier with a unique method to compensate for series resistance to overcome this technical limitation; this amplifier has sufficient bandwidth and stability to allow us to voltage-clamp $Na^+$ currents accurately.[15] We are now using this amplifier to measure $Na^+$ currents on both peripheral and central neurons.

Neonatal nodose neurons express at least three distinct voltage-gated $K^+$ channels: a rapidly inactivating channel, a slowly inactivating channel, and a noninactivating channel.[13] Briefly, the rapidly inactivating and slowly inactivating channels have similar single channel conductance and overlapping sensitivities to 4-AP and TEA, but they differ in their voltage-dependence for activation and inactivation and in their kinetics. The expression and properties of these voltage-gated $K^+$ channels change little over the first 3–4 weeks of neonatal development. In an attempt to identify the genes that underlie these $K^+$ channels, mRNA levels for voltage-gated $K^+$ channel genes were measured in neonatal nodose neurons using RNase protection assays. The results demonstrated that nodose neurons express at least seven different voltage-gated $K^+$ channel genes.[16] Like the voltage-gated $K^+$ channels, the expression of these genes changes little over the first 3–4 weeks of neonatal development. Currently, we are determining which genes are responsible for the voltage-gated $K^+$ channels on these neurons.

*Developmental Plasticity.* Neonatal nodose neurons are not completely committed to a sensory neuron phenotype at birth and express several properties untypical for sensory neurons if their *in vivo* environment is perturbed. Two important factors that influence the differentiation of these neurons are ganglionic satellite cells and neurotrophins. For example, when neonatal nodose neurons develop in culture with their ganglionic satellite cells and the neurotrophin BDNF, we find that they continue to express properties typical of nodose neurons in vivo, including a unipolar morphology and sensitivity to capsaicin. However, if these same neurons develop in culture without their ganglionic satellite cells and with NGF, they extend dendrites and develop functional cholinergic nicotinic synapses among one another—characteristics more typical of autonomic neurons than of sensory neurons.[7,17] We have also shown that neurotrophins affect the expression of 5-$HT_3R$ on nodose neurons.[18] From these studies, we conclude that the surrounding ganglionic satellite cells exert an important developmental influence(s) on the developing nodose neurons. Moreover, we find that this influence operates over a brief developmental window, lasting about 2 weeks, before the neurons become fully committed to a sensory phenotype: if neonatal nodose neurons develop with satellite cells for about 2 weeks, either *in vivo* or in culture, removing the satellite cells and adding NGF has little effect on their subsequent differentiation.[19] Our studies on cellular and molecular mechanisms that influence the early postnatal differentiation of nodose neurons are ongoing.

## EXPRESSION OF NICOTINIC ACETYLCHOLINE RECEPTORS
## ON NODOSE NEURONS

To learn more about these developmental influences, we have focused on the expression and appearance of nAChRs. Using whole-cell patch-clamp techniques, we found that about 40% of neonatal nodose neurons have functional nAChRs: among these ACh-sensitive neurons, there was a large variation in ACh-evoked current densities.[20] Neither the proportion of ACh-sensitive neurons nor the distribution of ACh-evoked current densities changed over the first few weeks of postnatal development. Moreover, when these neonatal neurons developed in culture together with their nonneuronal satellite cells for 2–3 weeks, these neurons retained their sensitivity to ACh: we observed no change in the proportion of ACh-sensitive neurons over time in culture, nor in the distribution of ACh-evoked current densities among neurons. Moreover, the addition of neurotrophins to these cultures had no effect on the appearance of functional AChRs on these neurons.[20] However, when these neonatal neurons developed in culture without nonneuronal cells, the addition of NGF caused a significant increase both in the proportion of ACh-sensitive neurons and in the density of functional nAChRs on individual neurons. Our results suggest that NGF upregulates the appearance of functional nAChRs on developing nodose neurons, but only if the nonneuronal cell influence is removed.[20]

To characterize these receptors further, we used RNase protection assays and found that nodose neurons express at least six nAChR transcripts: $\alpha 3$, $\alpha 5$, $\alpha 7$, $\beta 2$, $\beta 3$, and $\beta 4$. Of these, mRNA for $\beta 2$ is the most abundant, whereas levels of $\alpha 5$ and $\beta 3$ are at the limit of detection. In contrast, in sympathetic neurons, $\alpha 3$, $\alpha 7$, and $\beta 4$ are the most abundant transcripts and $\beta 3$ is below detection.[21] Recently, it has been shown that mice with targeted mutations in the $\alpha 7$ gene have an impaired baroreceptor reflex; it is not clear whether this impaired function results from an absence in $\alpha 7$ protein in nodose neurons, in sympathetic neurons, or in other neurons that are involved in the reflex.[22]

*Physiological Role.* Almost 50 years ago, J. Diamond established that baroreceptor afferents have functional nAChRs located on or near the baroreceptor terminals in the periphery.[23] Nicotinic AChRs have no direct role in mechanosensory transduction mechanisms, nor is it likely that they become activated by circulating ACh because cholinesterase in the blood breaks down ACh too rapidly. Currently, the physiological role for nAChRs on sensory terminals in the periphery remains unclear. Vagal afferent neurons also have nAChRs located at presynaptic nerve terminals in the CNS; presumably, these receptors act to modulate transmitter release, as has been shown for nAChRs elsewhere in the CNS.[24] Neuronal nAChRs have several properties that make them ideally suited to modulate transmitter release when located at presynaptic nerve terminals: (1) they have high relative permeability to calcium; (2) they have large single channel conductances, which (coupled with the high input impedance of a nerve terminal) means that only a few receptors need to be activated to trigger an action potential; (3) they allow ions to flow into the cell at negative membrane potentials, but do not permit ions to leave at positive membrane potentials; this mechanism, referred to as inward rectification, prevents nAChRs from short-circuiting the action potential and compromising transmitter release. For nAChRs located in the postsynaptic membrane, like those at synapses between preganglionic nerve terminals and sympathetic neurons, the rectification and high relative calcium permeability act to modulate the effectiveness of these synapses.

## VOLTAGE-DEPENDENT BLOCK OF NEURONAL NICOTINIC ACETYLCHOLINE RECEPTORS BY INTRACELLULAR POLYAMINES

We investigated the underlying mechanisms for both the strong inward rectification and the high relative calcium permeability. Previous work has shown that strong inward rectification is not a property of receptors: nAChRs measured in cell-free patches showed little or no rectification, suggesting that the rectification results from a block of the receptor channel by intracellular molecules.[25,26] One intracellular molecule known to block ion channels is $Mg^{2+}$; however, we found that $Mg^{2+}$ had little effect on the rectification of nAChRs. Other intracellular molecules known to block ion channels are polyamines, ubiquitous positively charged molecules that block inwardly rectifying $K^+$ channels and $Ca^{2+}$-permeable AMPA and kainate glutamate receptors.[27,28] Polyamine concentrations are highly regulated and exist in the mM range inside cells. Most polyamines are bound to negatively charged structures, such as chromatin, whereas about 5% (roughly 50–100 μM) are free in the cytoplasm. We used cell-free outside-out patches to demonstrate that polyamines, acting as gating particles, effectively blocked the receptor pore. We found that the block was voltage-dependent and occurred with a relatively high affinity ($K_d$ of 3 to 4 μM at 0 mV), similar to values needed to block other ion channels.[29] This block by polyamines accounts for the macroscopic rectification of ACh-evoked currents (see FIGURE 1).

In addition to the implications for nAChR function, our results indicate that a common mechanism exists for producing strong inward rectification of cation permeable ion channels. Inward rectifying $K^+$ channels, calcium-permeable glutamate receptors, and neuronal nAChRs are all blocked by intracellular polyamines in a voltage-dependent manner. However, given that the structure of the pore for inwardly rectifying $K^+$ channels and $Ca^{2+}$-permeable glutamate receptors is markedly different from the structure of the pore in nAChRs, this raises the following question: what are the structural determinants for this polyamine interaction with nAChRs?

*Structural Determinants of Polyamine Block.* Strong evidence indicates that the second hydrophobic domain of nAChRs, M2, forms the pore.[30,31] The M2 domain contains three rings of negatively charged residues, one at the extracellular end and two at the intracellular end, the intermediate ring (closest to the pore) and the cytoplasmic ring. These negatively charged residues have an important influence on conduction of cations through the pore. Since positively charged polyamines interact with negatively charged structures in the cell, we reasoned that the negatively charged rings at the intracellular region of the receptor could form a polyamine binding site on the receptor; because this site is near the narrowest part of the pore,[30,31] polyamines binding to this site would block the flow of ions through the pore, resulting in rectification.

To test this, we mutated the negatively charged residues in both the cytoplasmic and the intermediate ring. We found that substituting two or three negatively charged residues with neutral residues at the cytoplasmic ring had no effect on the block by

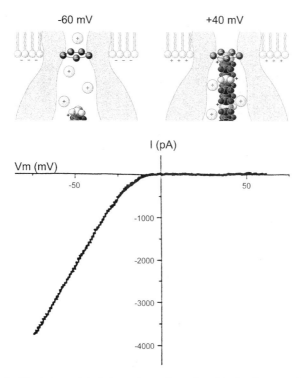

**FIGURE 1. (Top)** A model of the voltage-dependent block of neuronal nAChRs by intracellular polyamines. When the receptors are activated at negative (−60 mV) membrane potentials, inward cations flow through the receptor, producing ACh-evoked inward currents. However, at positive (+40 mV) membrane potentials, intracellular polyamines are attracted to the intermediate ring of the receptor under the influence of the membrane electrical field and are held there through an electrostatic interaction with the negatively charged Glu residues that make up the intermediate ring. This polyamine-nAChR interaction blocks the flow of outward cations through the receptor, a process called inward rectification. **(Bottom)** The graph shows the ACh-evoked current-voltage relationship for neuronal nAChRs on rat sympathetic neurons measured with whole-cell voltage-clamp techniques.

polyamines; even replacing all five negative charges, one from each subunit of the pentamer, did not prevent the receptors from rectifying, although we did observe a significant relief of block at very positive potentials.[32] These results indicate that the negatively charged amino acids at the cytoplasmic ring do not play a large role in the block by intracellular polyamines, except perhaps to help stabilize the polyamine molecule near the inner mouth of the channel. On the other hand, we found that substituting as few as two negatively charged residues with neutral residues at the intermediate ring completely abolished inward rectification.[32] These results indicate that the intermediate ring, located near the narrowest portion of the pore, forms the site where intracellular polyamines interact with the receptor. This interaction produces strong inward rectification.

In addition to the effects on inward rectification, we found that decreasing the charge at the intermediate ring also decreases the relative calcium permeability through the receptor.[32] This indicates that the same structural determinant affects two important functional properties of neuronal nAChRs: inward rectification and calcium permeability. Moreover, our results suggest that polyamines may alter calcium permeability by screening the negative charges at the intermediate ring; this could serve as an important mechanism for modulating receptor function, particularly in the postsynaptic membrane.

*Extracellular Block by Polyamines.* Furthermore, we found that polyamines are potent noncompetitive antagonists for neuronal nAChRs when acting from outside the cell. From dose-inhibition experiments, we determined that spermine blocked neuronal nAChRs with an $IC_{50}$ of roughly 50 μM.[29,32] This blocking action by low extracellular polyamine concentrations has implications for the function of nAChRs during neuronal degenerative disease; when cells die, they can release polyamines into the extracellular milieu. Our results demonstrating that polyamines act as potent noncompetitive antagonists also suggest that polyamine-related molecules might serve as effective open-channel blockers for these receptors.

One hundred years ago, W. E. Dixon showed that injecting spermine into animals altered their heart rate and decreased their blood pressure.[33] From our work on polyamines and nAChR function, we conclude that many of Dixon's observations can be explained by postulating that the injected spermine blocked nAChR function, which resulted in a decrease in the activity of sympathetic nerves. This finding reinforces the importance of nAChR function in regulating systemic blood pressure.

## ACKNOWLEDGMENTS

I thank several current and former colleagues for fruitful discussions about different aspects of this work. In addition, I thank D. Wheeler and L. Cooper for comments on the manuscript. This work was supported by the MRC of Canada and the Canadian Heart and Stroke Foundation.

## REFERENCES

1. TUCK, M.L. 1992. Obesity, the sympathetic nervous system, and essential hypertension. Hypertension **19:** 167–177.
2. DI BONA, G.F. & U.C. KOPP. 1997. Neural control of renal function. Physiol. Rev. **17:** 75–197.
3. SUN, M.K. 1995. Central neural organization and control of sympathetic nervous system in mammals. Prog. Neurobiol. **47:** 157–233.
4. GUYTON, A.C. 1991. Blood pressure control—special role of the kidneys and body fluids. Science **252:** 1813–1816.
5. LEHMANN-HORN, F. & K. JURKAT-ROTT. 1999. Voltage-gated ion channels and hereditary disease. Physiol. Rev. **19:** 1317–1372.
6. ALTAMAN, J. & S.A. BAYER. 1982. Development of the cranial nerve ganglia and related nuclei in the rat. Adv. Anat. Embryol. Cell Biol. **74.**
7. COOPER, E. 1984. Synapse formation among developing sensory neurons from rat nodose ganglia grown in tissue culture. J. Physiol. **351:** 263–274.
8. BACCAGLINI, P.I. & E. COOPER. 1982. Electrophysiological studies on new-born rat nodose neurones in cell culture. J. Physiol. **324:** 429–439.

9. IKEDA, S.R., G.G. SCHOFIELD & F.F. WEIGHT. 1986. $Na^+$ and $Ca^{2+}$ currents of acutely isolated adult rat nodose ganglion cells. J. Neurophysiol. **55:** 527–539.
10. BESSOU, J.J. & A. FELTZ. 1984. Depolarization elicits two distinct calcium currents in vertebrate sensory neurones. Eur. J. Physiol. **403:** 360–368.
11. MENDELOWITZ, D. & D.L. KUNZE. 1992. Characterization of calcium currents in aortic baroreceptor neurons. J. Neurophysiol. **68:** 509–517.
12. COOPER, E. & A. SHRIER. 1989. Inactivation of A currents and A channels on rat nodose neurons in culture. J. Gen. Physiol. **94:** 881–910.
13. MCFARLANE, S. & E. COOPER. 1991. Kinetics and voltage-dependence of A-type currents on rat sensory neurons in culture. J. Neurophysiol. **66:** 1380–1391.
14. JAFRI, M.S., K.A. MOORE, G.E. TAYLOR & D. WEINREICH. 1997. Histamine H1 receptor activation blocks two classes of potassium current, IK(rest) and IAHP, to excite ferret vagal afferents. J. Physiol. **503:** 533–546.
15. SHERMAN, A., A. SHRIER & E. COOPER. 1999. Series resistance compensation for whole-cell patch clamp studies using a membrane state estimator. Biophys. J. **77:** 2590–2601.
16. FRASER, A.B. 1998. Expression of voltage-gated potassium channel genes by neonatal rat peripheral neurons. Ph.D. thesis, McGill University, Montreal, Quebec.
17. DE KONINCK, P., S. CARBONETTO & E. COOPER. 1993. NGF induces neonatal rat sensory neurons to extend dendrites in culture after removal of satellite cells. J. Neurosci. **13:** 577–585.
18. ROSENBERG, M., B. PIE & E. COOPER. 1997. Developing neonatal rat sympathetic and sensory neurons differ in their regulation of 5-HT$_3$ receptor expression. J. Neurosci. **17:** 6629–6638.
19. COOPER, E. & M. LAU. 1986. Factors affecting the expression of acetylcholine receptors on rat sensory neurons in culture. J. Physiol. **377:** 409–420.
20. MANDELZYS, A. & E. COOPER. 1992. Effects of ganglionic satellite cells and NGF on the expression of nicotinic acetylcholine currents by rat sensory neurons. J. Neurophysiol. **67:** 1213–1221.
21. MANDELZYS, A., B. PIE, E.S. DENERIS & E. COOPER. 1994. The developmental increase in ACh current densities on rat sympathetic neurons correlates with changes in nicotinic ACh receptor $\alpha$-subunit gene expression and occurs independent of innervation. J. Neurosci. **14:** 2357–2364.
22. FRANCESCHINI, D., A. ORR-URTREGER, W. YU et al. 2000. Altered baroreflex responses in alpha-7 deficient mice. Behav. Brain Res. **113:** 3–10.
23. DIAMOND, J. 1955. Observations on the excitation by acetylcholine and by pressure of sensory receptors in the cat's carotid sinus. J. Physiol. **130:** 513–532.
24. MACDERMOTT, A.B., L. ROLE & S. SIEGELBAUM. 1999. Presynaptic ionotropic receptors and control of transmitter release. Annu. Rev. Neurosci. **22:** 443–485.
25. IFUNE, C.K. & J.H. STEINBACH. 1993. Modulation of acetylcholine-elicited currents in clonal rat phaeochromocytoma (PC12) cells by internal polyphosphates. J. Physiol. **463:** 431–447.
26. SANDS, S.B. & M.E. BARISH. 1992. Neuronal nicotinic acetylcholine receptors in phaeochromocytoma (PC12) cells: dual mechanism of rectification. J. Physiol. **447:** 467–487.
27. NICHOLS, G.G. & A.N. LOPATIN. 1997. Inward rectifier potassium channels. Annu. Rev. Physiol. **59:** 171–191.
28. BOWIE, D. & M.L. MAYER. 1995. Inward rectification of both AMPA and kainate subtype glutamate receptors generated by polyamine-mediated ion channel block. Neuron **15:** 453–462.
29. HAGHAGHI, A.P. & E. COOPER. 1998. Neuronal nicotinic acetylcholine receptors are blocked by intracellular spermine in a voltage-dependent manner. J. Neurosci. **18:** 4050–4062.
30. KARLIN, A. & M.H. AKABAS. 1995. Toward a structural basis for the function of nicotinic acetylcholine receptors and their cousins. Neuron **15:** 1231–1244.
31. CORRINGER, P.J., N. NOVERE & J.P. CHANGEUX. 2000. Nicotinic receptors at the amino acid level. Annu. Rev. Pharmacol. Toxicol. **40:** 431–458.

32. HAGHAGHI, A.P. & E. COOPER. 2000. A molecular link between inward rectification and calcium permeability of neuronal nicotinic acetylcholine α3β4 and α4β2 receptors. J. Neurosci. **20:** 529–541.
33. DIXON, W.E. 1900. A note on the physiological action of Poehl's spermine. J. Physiol. **25:** 356–363.

# Cellular Mechanisms Regulating Synaptic Vesicle Exocytosis and Endocytosis in Aortic Baroreceptor Neurons

MEREDITH HAY, CAROLINE J. HOANG, AND JAYA PAMIDIMUKKALA

*Dalton Cardiovascular Research Center, Department of Veterinary Biomedical Sciences, University of Missouri, Columbia, Missouri 65251, USA*

ABSTRACT: The purpose of this chapter is to review some of the recent progress in the understanding of the cellular and biophysical mechanisms that are involved in the regulation of arterial baroreceptor neurotransmssion. Synaptic depression or fatigue following repeated neuronal stimulation has been shown at central baroreceptor synapses *in vivo* and *in vitro*. As most of the central neurons have a limited number of vesicles, vesicle retrieval or endocytosis following exocytosis is thought to play a major role in preserving synaptic transmission. We have hypothesized that central baroreceptor terminals may inhibit their own synaptic transmission via feedback activation of presynaptic metabotropic glutamate receptors (mGluRs). We have analyzed the effects of mGluR autoreceptors (group III mGluRs) on voltage-gated calcium channels using standard patch-clamp techniques and on the process of exocytosis and endocytosis in aortic baroreceptor neurons using the quantitative imaging dye FM1-43 and FM2-10. Usng the whole-cell patch-clamp technique, we have found that activation of group III mGluRs with L-AP4 inhibits peak calcium channel current. Furthermore, activation of group III mGluRs with L-AP4 markedly decreases stimulation-induced exocytosis in aortic baroreceptor neurons, as measured with FM1-43, and inhibits synapsin I phosphorylation. These results suggest that activation of group III mGluRs may inhibit synaptic transmission by (1) inhibiting calcium influx, (2) decreasing synaptic vesicle exocytosis, and (3) modulating the mechanisms governing synaptic vesicle recovery and endocytosis. These effects of mGluRs on baroreceptor synaptic vesicles may contribute to the baroreceptor/nucleus tractus solitarius synaptic depression observed *in vivo*.

KEYWORDS: Nodose ganglia; Synaptic transmission; mGluRs; Synapsin

## INTRODUCTION

The purpose of this chapter is to review some of the recent progress in the understanding of the cellular and biophysical mechanisms that are involved in the regulation of arterial baroreceptor neurotransmssion. The emphasis is on the nature of the ion channels required for the activation of baroreceptor neurons and some of the cel-

Address for correspondence: Meredith Hay, Ph.D., Dalton Cardiovascular Research Center, Research Park, University of Missouri, Columbia, MO 65251. Voice: 573-882-0044; fax: 573-884-4232.

haym@missouri.edu

lular mechanisms that have recently been identified as being important in the modulation of central arterial baroreceptor neurotransmssion. The last decade has brought outstanding progress in our understanding of the biophysical mechanisms regulating baroreceptor neurons and potentially new insights into the role of these mechanisms in the physiological and pathophysiological regulation of the cardiovascular system.

Information concerning the level of blood pressure originates from both arterial and cardiac baroreceptors. The arterial baroreceptors provide the high-gain rapid-reflex responses to changes in arterial pressure and are considered to be the predominant mechanism for moment-to-moment regulation of arterial pressure. Peripherally, baroreceptor terminals within the carotid sinus and the aortic arch innervate the adventitia layers of the vessel wall. Deformation of the vessel wall due to alterations in blood pressure are sensed by mechanosensitive ion channels within the terminal fields of the aortic and carotid sinus baroreceptors,[1] Activation of these ion channels is transduced into a depolarization event that triggers the induction of action potentials within the baroreceptor afferents. This activity is then propagated centrally to the neurons of the nucleus of the solitary tract (NTS) and represent the events that initiate the activation the arterial baroreceptor reflex.[2]

Activity and time-dependent integration of baroreceptor information at the level of the NTS is a crucial step in the normal regulation of cardiovascular reflex function. Alteration of synaptic transmission between the baroreceptor afferents and NTS neurons is thought to contribute to inappropriate reflex control of sympathetic outflow. In many central nervous system synapses, it has been suggested that the maintenance of synaptic transmission over a wide range of frequency stimulations requires that nerve terminals maintain pools of synaptic vesicles in reserve that can be recruited to active zones during periods of intense activity.[3,4] Thus, the mechanisms governing synaptic turnover at the baroreceptor terminals may serve as a common site for the regulation of baroreflex function.

## CELLULAR MECHANISMS AND BARORECEPTOR AFFERENT REGULATION

High levels of activation of baroreceptor afferents, as are found during hypertension, have been reported to decrease this reflex response to increases in pressure and to shift the baroreflex response curve to the right, towards the prevailing pressure.[5,6] This hypertension-evoked "resetting" of the reflex allows the reflex to function, but now at a higher arterial pressure. Mechanisms responsible for this resetting are not clear and have been suggested to include peripheral changes in baroreceptor sensitivity as well as possible changes in the activity of central neurons involved in the normal regulation of sympathetic outflow.

Cellular studies on the responses of NTS neurons to high-frequency afferent stimulation have demonstrated that the postsynaptic responsiveness of NTS cells to afferent stimulation is frequency dependent, with a marked decrease in NTS excitatory postsynaptic responses at stimulation frequencies greater than 5 Hz.[7–9] It is reasonable to suggest that activity-dependent decreases in evoked NTS responses could possibly result in a decreased reflex response to baroreceptor input and ultimately a rightward resetting in the reflex. To date, the mechanisms underlying this activity-dependent decrease in NTS responsiveness are unknown. One potential mechanism that may be important in the modulation of baroreceptor afferent synaptic efficacy is an alteration in transmitter release from the presynaptic terminal. This is likely to involve the activation and inactivation of regulatory proteins involved in the exocytosis of synaptic vesicles in afferent nerve terminals. These regulatory proteins include; (1) voltage-gated calcium channels, (2) synaptic vesicle fusion proteins, and (3) proteins involved in maintaining the reserve pool of synaptic vesicles. Thus, the mechanisms governing the recruitment of vesicles to the active zone and the regulation synaptic vesicle turnover at the baroreceptor terminals may serve as a common site for the regulation of baroreflex function. In the case of the baroreceptor/NTS synapses, activation of presynaptic autoreceptors during periods of high activity could be hypothesized to inhibit the exocytosis regulatory processes, thus decreasing synaptic efficacy. This could then result in decreased NTS postsynaptic activation, ultimately allowing an increase in sympathetic outflow.

## BARORECEPTOR NEUROTRANSMISSION

Neurotransmitter candidates for baroreceptor neurons include l-glutamate (l-glu),[10,11] acetylcholine,[12] serotonin,[13,14] SubP,[15,16] and NPY.[17] Some of these transmitters, in particular l-glutamate and NPY, are thought not only to act postsynaptically on NTS neurons, but to act presynaptically to alter transmitter release. Glutamate has been hypothesized to act on multiple receptor subtypes, each of which may play a specific role in baroreceptor signal transduction. In general, L-glu receptors fall into two primary classes. The first class is the ligand-gated ionotropic receptor. There are three general subtypes of ionotropic glutamate receptors, [N-methyl D-Aspartate] (NMDA), kainate, and [2-amino-3-hydroxy-5-methylisoxazole-4-propionic acid] (AMPA), which, when activated, open a nonselective cation channel.[18] These receptors are generally thought to be involved in fast neurotransmission.[19] The second class of L-glu receptor, which is found both pre- and postsynaptically, is the metabotropic glutamate receptor (mGluR). The activation of these receptors activates a G protein–dependent second messenger system such as inositol triphosphate or the adenylate cyclase system to affect neuronal activation.[20–22]

Molecular studies have revealed that mGluRs are a heterogeneous class of G protein–coupled receptors; at least eight different subtypes have so far been characterized.[23] These receptors have been divided into three major groups based on sequence homology, pharmacology, and coupling to signal transduction pathways in expression systems (FIG. 1). Group I are coupled to inositol triphosphate production and are highly sensitive to quisqualate and selectively activated by DHPG; group II are coupled to the inhibition of cAMP formation and are selectively activated by DCG-IV; and group III are also coupled to the inhibition of cAMP but are selectively activated by L-AP4.[23,24] Immunohistochemical studies have identified mGluR1, mGluR2/3, mGluR5, and mGluR7 expressed in autonomic regulatory regions of the medulla.[25] In a number of different neuronal models, it is the mGluR(s) that have been suggested to function as autoreceptors involved in the regulation of neurotransmitter release.[24]

Metabotropic glutamate receptors are thought to modulate synaptic transmission between the nodose ganglia and the NTS neurons and have been shown to be impor-

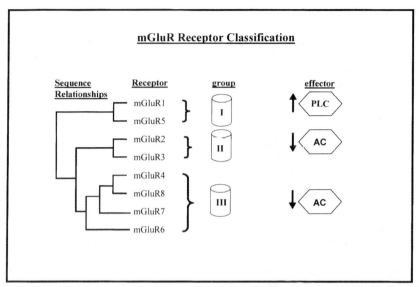

**FIGURE 1.** The three major groups of metabotropic glutamate receptors (mGluRs) and their relationships based on sequence homology, pharmacology, and signal transduction pathways.

tant for arterial baroreflex modulation.[26-28] However, the specific mGluRs involved in the presynaptic nodose ganglia neurons have only recently been resolved. Studies using RT-PCR techniques on both nodose ganglia and NTS tissue have revealed a differential expression pattern of mGluRs in these two tissues. RT-PCR experiments using primers for mGluRs subtypes 1–8 have been performed in both NTS and nodose ganglia.[29] In these studies, nodose ganglia were found to express only mGluRs 4, 6, 7, and 8 but not mGluRs 1, 2, 3, or 5. In contrast, the NTS was found to express all eight subtypes. Thus, visceral afferents of the nodose ganglia express primarily group III mGluRs 4, 6, 7, and 8, all of which have been shown by others to be involved in presynaptic modulation of synaptic transmission. It has been suggested that these receptors may play important roles in the modulation of synaptic transmission between baroreceptor afferents and the NTS.

## PRESYNAPTIC MECHANISMS: METABOTROPIC GLUTAMATE RECEPTORS

As mentioned above, activation of presynaptic autoreceptors such as mGluR receptors have been hypothesized to modulate the processes of vesicle exocytosis and thus regulate the efficacy of neurotransmission. If high activity–induced decreases in baroreceptor afferent synaptic strength involve inhibition of baroreceptor synaptic vesicle exocytosis and turnover, then mechanisms governing synaptic turnover at the baroreceptor terminals may serve as a common site for the regulation of baroreflex function. Neurotransmitters released by baroreceptor neurons, such as l-glu, are hypothesized to feed back onto the presynaptic membrane and modulate their own re-

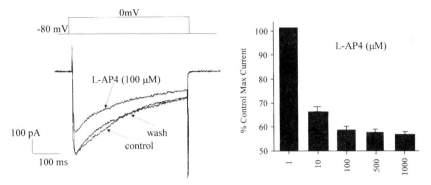

**FIGURE 2.** Inhibitory effects of L-AP4 on aortic baroreceptor calcium currents. (**A**) Calcium currents evoked by 0-mV step depolarizations from a −80-mV holding potential before, during, and following exposure to 100 μM L-AP4. (**B**) Averaged response (mean ± SEM) of evoked peak calcium current to varying concentrations of L-AP4 ($n = 3$, 1.0 μm; $n = 9$, 10.0 μm, $n = 4$, 100 μm; $n = 4$, 1000 μm).

lease. This modulation of vesicle release could potentially be the result of a combination of events including (1) direct mGluR inhibition of $Ca^{2+}$ influx through voltage-gated channels, (2) mGluR modulation of synaptic vesicle exocytosis, or (3) mGluR modulation of synaptic vesicle turnover and recovery.

The influx of $Ca^{2+}$ through voltage-dependent channels into nerve terminals is known to be required for the exocytosis of synaptic vesicles.[30,31] The influx of $Ca^{2+}$ is also known to initiate additional cellular events associated with vesicle release including protein phosphorylation/dephosphorylation and cytoskeletal disassembly.[32] The phosphorylation of synapsin I, for example, is required for the maintenance of neurotransmitter release.[33] However, multiple mechanisms have been suggested to regulate the phosphorylation of synapsins including $Ca^{2+}$-calmodulin–dependent protein kinase II and increases in adenylate cyclase.[34,35] Thus, presynaptic regulation of transmitter release can be achieved by multiple mechanisms including the regulation of $Ca^{2+}$ channel conductance and the regulation of the activity of kinases and phosphatases involved in the phosphorylation of synaptic proteins like the synapsins. FIGURE 2 illustrates the effects of mGluR activation on voltage-gated $Ca^{2+}$ currents in aortic baroreceptor neurons. Studies from our laboratory have shown that activation of mGluR(s) with the group III selective agonist L-AP4 (100 μM) significantly decreases $Ca^{2+}$ current influx.[36] Previous studies have shown that this action is mostly via inhibition of the N-type $Ca^{2+}$ channels.[37] This inhibition of voltage-gated calcium channels would be anticipated to alter calcium-dependent exocytosis as well as calcium dependent phosphorylation of synaptic proteins involved in the regulation of vesicle exocytosis and recycling.

## SYNAPSINS

Synaptic vesicles are thought to be stored within the synapse in (1) a readily releasable pool that is docked with the plasma membrane and (2) a reserve pool that may be associated with the actin cytoskeleton.[30,34,38] Synapsins are a subgroup of phosphoproteins found in virtually all neuronal terminals and account for nearly 6% of total vesicular protein.[39] It is known that the phosphorylation state of the synapsins are increased following membrane depolarization and influx of $Ca^{2+}$. Biochemical experiments indicate that synapsin I binds to both synaptic vesicles and cytoskeletal proteins and is hypothesized to serve as a vesicle tether in its nonphosphorylated form.[33,40] Thus, the dephosphorylated form of synapsin I is thought to provide an inhibitory constraint for vesicle exocytosis, and this constraint is relieved upon phosphorylation. It is hypothesized that upon depolarization-induced $Ca^{2+}$ entry, activation of CaM kinase II phosphorylates the C-terminal domain of synapsin I, resulting in the dissociation of the vesicles from the cytoskeleton and the transformation of these vesicles from the reserve pool to the readily releasable pool of synaptic vesicles.[38]

Since mGluR agonists inhibit visceral sensory neuronal voltage-gated $Ca^{2+}$ channels and calcium influx is important for synapsin I phosphorylation, we also hypothesized that activation of mGluRs may modulate synapsin I phosphorylation in visceral afferent neurons of the nodose ganglia.[36] FIGURE 3 illustrates the effects of mGluR activation on resting and depolarization-induced increases in synapsin I phosphorylation in nodose ganglia neurons. While activation of mGluRs has no effect on resting synapsin I phosphorylation, mGluRs do inhibit depolarization-induced increases in synapsin I phosphorylation. This attenuation of synapsin I phosphorylation is consistent with the hypothesis that activation of mGluR receptors may inhibit synaptic transmission via multiple mechanism including modulation of the phosphorylation state of some synaptic proteins. If synapsin I phosphorylation is important for maintaining synaptic fidelity, then mGluR inhibition of synapsin I phosphorylation in visceral afferents may contribute to the frequency-dependent depression of baroreceptor/NTS neurotransmission.

## SYNAPTIC VESICLE EXOCYTOSIS AND RECYCLING

While a number of studies have used the postsynaptic responses of NTS neurons to postulate about presynaptic mechanisms involved in the regulation of neurotransmission between baroreceptor afferents and NTS neurons,[7,28,41] to date, there have been few studies of the cellular mechanisms involved in synaptic vesicle exocytosis and endocytosis in baroreceptor terminals. Unfortunately, measurements of synaptic vesicle endocytosis and exocytosis from baroreceptor neurons are currently technically not possible *in vivo*. The study of the process of exocytosis and endocytosis in other cell types has been most directly approached by measuring changes in membrane capacitance that are associated with the turnover of synaptic vesicles. These studies have been restricted to relatively large neuroendocrine cells and retinal bipolar cells due to the inaccessibility of most small neuronal synaptic terminals to these types of measurements. However, an optical technique, developed by Betz and colleagues,[42] allows for a functional assay of synaptic vesicle exocytosis and recycling by quantitative fluorescence imaging of styryl dyes such as FM1-43 (N-(3-(triethyl ammonium) propyl)-4-(4-dibutyrlaminostyryl pyridinium, dibromide). This method allows us to study synaptic vesicle recycling at previously inaccessible nerve terminal compartments and to distinguish between exocytosis and endocytosis.[12,24,34] FM dyes are amphipathic molecules that can insert reversibly into the surface of lipid

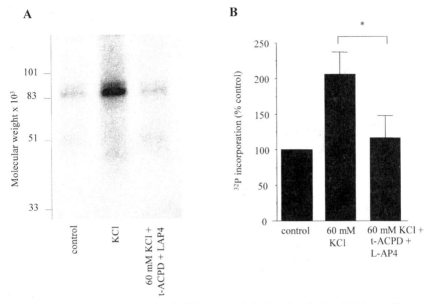

**FIGURE 3.** mGluR activation inhibits synapsin I phosphorylation. **(A)** Autoradiogram from a 10-day exposure at −70 °C of the effects of 1.0 mM ACPD + 1.0 mM L-AP4 on high-K+–induced phosphorylation of synapsin I. **(B)** Quantification of radioactive phosphate incorporation into synapsin I. Values represent mean + standard error percentage change from control phosphorylation ($n = 5$). * = $p < 0.05$.

membranes. They emit little fluorescence in aqueous medium but fluoresce intensely upon membrane binding. When incubated with neuronal preparations, the dyes insert into the outer leaflet of the plasma membrane and are internalized during vesicle retrieval after stimulation of exocytosis. The dye remaining on membranes that have not been internalized can be washed away quickly, leaving labeled synaptic vesicles inside the nerve terminal. The uptake of the dye reflects endocytosis. The loss of fluorescence from these labeled regions upon subsequent stimulation is a measure of vesicle exocytosis, as movement of the dye from the synaptic vesicle membrane into the extracellular solution mimics release of transmitters. The kinetics of endocytosis measured using simultaneous whole-cell capacitance and styryl dyes reveal a brief delay between exocytosis and endocytosis.[42] At most fast synapses exocytosis precedes endocytosis. Exocytosis ceases as soon as the stimulation is stopped, but endocytosis has been shown to continue for up to 2 min following stimulation.[35] This sustained endocytosis can be used to evaluate group III mGluR and $Ca^{2+}$–mediated modulation of endocytosis in aortic baroreceptor neurons. Our laboratory has used FM1-43 and FM2-10 to monitor vesicle exocytosis and endocytosis, and recycling in aortic baroreceptor neurons and unlabeled nodose neurons. We have described the time course of exocytosis during both electrically evoked action potential stimuli and high potassium depolarization. In addition, we have investigated the modulation of aortic baroreceptor exocytosis by selective calcium channel toxins and the metabotropic glutamate receptor agonist L-AP4.[43] FIGURE 4 illustrates the staining and

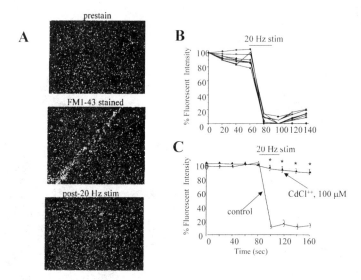

**FIGURE 4.** FM1-43 staining and destaining induced by stimulation with an extracellular bipolar electrode. **(A)** Fluorescent image of baroreceptor terminal stained with FM1-43 by 30 s of 20-Hz stimulation with a bipolar electrode. Additional stimulation in the absence of dye results in a loss of FM1-43 staining. **(B)** The time course of exocytosis for eight regions in one field during a 30-s, 20-Hz stimulation with a bipolar electrode. **(C)** Average FM1-43 destaining in the absence and presence of 100 μM CdCl$_2$. $n = 8$, * = $p < 0.01$.

destaining of an aortic baroreceptor terminal. In the presence of 2.0 μM FM1-43 without stimulation, no dye is visible in the terminal (top panel). After a 20-Hz stimulation with a bipolar electrode for 1 min in the presence of 2.0 μM FM1-43, followed by a 5-min FM1-43 free wash, fluorescent boutons appeared along the terminal (middle panel). Additional stimulation at 20 Hz for 30 s resulted in the release of FM1-43 from the boutons and a decrease in fluorescent intensity (bottom panel). This sequence can be repeated multiple times with nearly identical results (FIG. 4B). Further, inhibition of voltage-gated calcium channels via application of 100 μM CdCl$_2$ inhibits the stimulus-evoked destaining.

Previous studies have shown that the N-type calcium channels are the predominant voltage-gated calcium channel in baroreceptor neurons.[44] To determine the role of this channel in vesicle exocytosis, we examined exocytosis during blockade of the N-type calcium channel with omega-conotoxin GVIA. As seen in FIGURE 5A, application of ω-CgTx had no significant effect on the initial rate or extent of vesicle exocytosis recorded in the first 60 seconds of destaining. However, ω-CgTx did significantly inhibit the slow phase of destaining that occurred following 120 seconds of depolarization (control = 85 ± 9% decreases in fluorescence, ω-CgTx = 56 ± 5% decrease in fluorescence, $p < 0.05$). Results from these studies suggested that a ω-CgTx–insensitive calcium channel may be responsible for initial exocytosis and the w-CgTx–sensitive channel may play a more prominent role during prolonged depolarization. Alternatively, the residual ω-CgTx–insensitive calcium current may be enough to release the docked vesicle pool, and the N-type channels may be essential

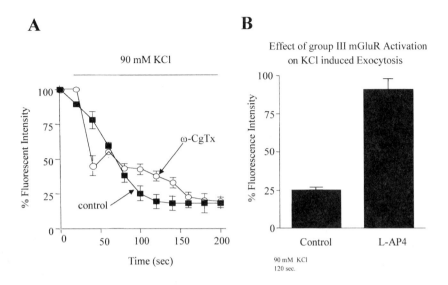

**FIGURE 5.** (A) Averaged effects of 2.0 μM ω-CgTX on the time course of 90 mM KCl induced exocytosis, $n = 9$, * = $p < 0.5$. (B) Averaged effects of 200 μM L-AP4 on exocytosis induced by 90 mM KCl measured at 120 s following the beginning of the depolarization.

for refilling of the readily releasable synaptic vesicle pool. We also examined the effects of group III mGluR activation on synaptic vesicle exocytosis (FIG. 5B). In the control condition, 90 mM KCl for 120 s resulted in exocytosis as measured by a 75% reduction in fluorescent intensity. The addition of L-AP4 markedly inhibited the depolarization-induced exocytosis. These studies were the first to show that activation of group III mGluRs inhibits direct measurements of synaptic vesicle exocytosis in baroreceptor neurons.

Maintenance of synaptic transmission over a wide range of frequency stimulations requires that nerve terminals maintain pools of synaptic vesicles in reserve that can be recruited to active zones during periods of intense activity. Hence, mechanisms governing synaptic turnover at the baroreceptor terminals may serve as a common site for the regulation of baroreflex function. Studies from our laboratory show that the process of endocytosis in aortic baroreceptor neurons can also be studied using FM1-43 and FM2-10. In these studies the FM dye and drugs are added after cessation of electrically evoked action potential stimuli, thereby ensuring that the effects observed were due exclusively to modulation of endocytosis. Endocytosis in baroreceptor neurons exhibits frequency-dependent depression. FIGURE 6 illustrates the decrease in relative endocytosis with increased number of evoked action potentials. Prolonged stimulation decreases the absolute levels of endocytosis. The relationship between endocytosis and the frequency and duration of stimulation of baroreceptor neurons in this study supports observations made *in vivo* that show decreased synaptic fidelity with increased afferent activity.

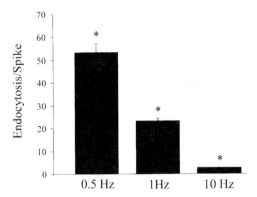

**FIGURE 6.** Endocytosis exhibits frequency-dependent depression. Averaged effects of increasing number of action potentials on endocytosis in baroreceptor neurons. * = $p < 0.5$.

## CONCLUSION

These studies are the first to begin to address the cellular and subcellular mechanisms that may underlie regulation of baroreceptor synaptic transmission. As with most complex systems, the regulation of baroreceptor afferent neurotransmission occurs at multiple levels. Synaptic vesicle exocytosis and recycling is known to be activity dependent and can be modulated by ligand receptors, such as mGluR receptors, possibly acting to affect the phosphorylation state of synaptic vesicle–associated proteins. Therefore, frequency-limited synaptic transmission in baroreceptor afferents may be due to mGluR inhibition of synaptic vesicle exocytosis and endocytosis, and this may involve the modulation of activity-dependent phosphorylation/dephosphorylation of vesicle-associated proteins.

Understanding of the mechanisms regulating synaptic efficacy between baroreceptor afferents and NTS neurons will not only require the gathering of new information regarding the cellular systems involved in the regulation of synaptic vesicle exocytosis and recycling, but will also require that this information be translated back into the whole animal system. In order to understand how these cellular mechanisms may affect cardiovascular homeostasis, a concerted effort must be made to test the validity of cellular hypotheses in an intact system.

FIGURE 7 is a schematic representation of the working hypotheses we have tested and are continuing to test. The metabotropic glutamate receptors (mGluRs) are located on the presynaptic terminal and on the postsynaptic NTS neuron. The baroreceptor presynaptic terminal is hypothesized to release l-glutamate (glu), which acts postsynaptically to excite NTS neurons and presynaptically to inhibit neurotransmitter release by (1) inhibiting voltage-gated $Ca^{2+}$ channels and (2) inhibiting vesicle exocytosis and endocytosis via modulation of the phosphorylation state of synaptic vesicle release–associated proteins such as the synapsins. The sites of neurotransmission regulation currently focused on are: (1) the evaluation of aortic baroreceptor vesicle *exocytosis* during activation of metabotropic glutamate receptors; (2) the evaluation of aortic baroreceptor vesicle *endocytosis* during activation

# Presynaptic Mechanisms Governing Synaptic Transmission at the Central Baroreceptor Terminal

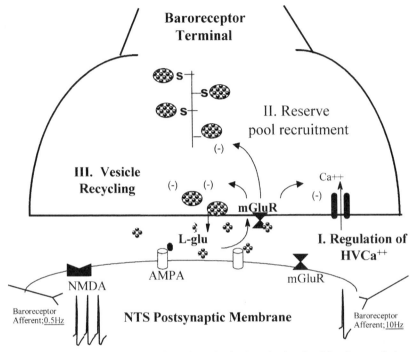

**FIGURE 7.** Cellular mechanisms hypothesized to be involved in the regulation of baroreceptor neurotransmission. Principal sites include (I) regulation of voltage-gated calcium channels, (II) reserve pool recruitment, and (III) vesicle recycling.

of metabotropic glutamate receptors; (3) the evaluation of signal transduction and second messenger systems involved in the mGluR regulation of transmission in aortic baroreceptor neurons; (4) the evaluation of phosphorylation of synapsin I and synapsin II in visceral afferent neurons during activation of mGluR receptors; and (5) the determination the role of mGluR receptor activation on frequency-limited activation of afferent-evoked NTS neuronal activity.

## REFERENCES

1. KRASKE, S., J.T. CUNNINGHAM, G. HAJDUCZOK, *et al.* 1998. Mechanosensitive ion channels in putative aortic baroreceptor neurons. Am. J. Physiol. **275**(44): H1497–H1501.
2. SELLER, H. 1992. Central baroreceptor reflex pathways. *In* Baroreceptor Reflexes: Integrative Functions and Clinical Aspects. P.B. Persson & H.R. Kirchheim, Eds.: 45–74. Springer-Verlag. New York.
3. DE CAMILLI, P. 1995. Keeping synapses up to speed (letter). Nature **375**: 450–451.

4. SOLLNER, T. & J.E. ROTHMAN. 1994. Neurotransmission: harnessing fusion machinery at the synapse. Trends Neurosci. **17:** 344–347.
5. HAYWARD, L.F., M. HAY & R.B. FELDER. 1993. Acute resetting of the carotid sinus baroreflex by aortic depressor nerve stimulation. Am. J. Physiol. **264:** H1215–H1222.
6. TAN, W., M.J. PANZENBECK, M A. HAJDU & I.H. ZUCKER. 1989. A central mechanism of acute baroreflex resetting in the conscious dog. Circ. Res. **65:** 63–70.
7. ANDRESEN, M.C. & M. YANG. 1995. Dynamics of sensory afferent synaptic transmission in aortic baroreceptor regions on nucleus tractus solitarius. J. Neurophysiol. **74**(4): 1518–1528.
8. MIFFLIN, S.W. & R.B. FELDER. 1988. An intracellular study of time-dependent cardiovascular afferent interactions in nucleus tractus solitarius. J. Neurophysiol. **59:** 1798–1813.
9. MILES, R. 1986. Frequency dependence of synaptic transmission in nucleus of the solitary tract. J. Neurophysiol. **55:** 1076–1090.
10. DIETRICH, W.D., O.H. LOWRY & A.D. LOEWY. 1982. The distribution of glutamate, GABA, and aspartate in the nucleus tractus solitarius of the cat. Brain Res. **237:** 254–260.
11. PERRONE, M.H. 1981. Biochemical evidence that L-glutamate is a neurotransmitter of primary vagal afferent nerve fibers. Brain Res. **230:** 283–293.
12. CRISCIONE, L., D.J. REIS & W.T. TALMAN. 1983. Cholinergic mechanisms in the nucleus tractus solitarii and cardiovascular regulation in the rat. Eur. J. Pharmacol. **88:** 47–55.
13. HIGASHI, H. & S. NISHI. 1992. 5-hydroxytryptamine receptors of visceral primary afferent neurons in rabbit nodose ganglia. J. Physiol. **323:** 543–567.
14. LAGUZZI, R., D.J. REIS & W.T. TALMAN. 1984. Modulation of cardiovascular and electrocortical activity through serotonergic mechanisms in the nucleus tractus solitarius of the rat. Br. Res. **304:** 321–328.
15. KUBO, T. & M. KIHARA. 1990. Modulation of the aortic baroreceptor reflex by neuropeptide Y, neurotension and vasopressin microinjected into the nucleus tract solitarii of the rat. Naunyn-Schmiedebergs Arch. Pharmacol. **342:** 182–188.
16. MACLEAN, D.B., F. WHEELER & L. HAYES. 1990. Basal and stimulated release of substance P from dissociated cultures of vagal sensory neurons. Brain Res. **519:** 308–314.
17. WILEY, J.W., R.A. GROSS, Y. LU & R.L. MACDONALD. 1990. Neuropeptide Y reduces calcium current and inhibits acetylcholine release in nodose neurons via a pertussis toxin–sensitive mechanism. J. Neurophysiol. **77:** 1499–1507.
18. MACDONALD, J.F. & L.M. NOWAK. 1990. Mechanisms of blockade of excitatory amino acid receptor channels. Trends Pharmacol. Sci. **11:** 167–172.
19. MAYER, M.L. & R.J. MILLER. 1990. Excitatory amino acid receptors, second messengers and regulation of intracellular Ca2+ in mammalian neurons. Trends Pharmacol. Sci. **11:** 254–260.
20. HOUAMED, K.M., J.L. KUIJPER, T.L. GILBER, *et al.* 1991. Cloning, expression, and gene structure of a G protein–coupled glutamate receptor from rat brain. Science **252:** 1318–1321.
21. SHOEPP, D., J. BOCKAERT & F. SLADECZEK. 1990. Pharmacological and functional characteristics of metabotropic excitatory amino acid receptors. Trends Pharmacol. Sci. **11:** 508–515.
22. SUGIYAMA, H., I. ITO & C. HIRONO. 1987. A new type of glutamate receptor linked to inositol phospholipid metabolism. Nature **325:** 531–533.
23. PIN, J.P. & R. DUVOISIN. 1995. The metabotropic glutamate receptors: structure and functions. Neuropharmacology **34**(1): 1–26.
24. CONN, P.J. & J.P. PIN. 1997. Pharmacology and functions of metabotropic glutamate receptors. Annu. Rev. Pharmacol. Toxicol. **37:** 205–237.
25. HAY, M., K. LINDSLEY, H. MCKINZIE, *et al.* 1999. Heterogeneity of metabotropic glutamate receptors in cardiovascular regulatory regions of the medulla. J. Comp . Neurol. **403:** 486–501.

26. GLAUM, R.R. & R.J. MILLER. 1992. Metabotropic glutamate receptors mediate excitatory transmission in the nucleus of the solitary tract. J.Neurosci. **12:** 2251–2258.
27. FOLEY, C.M., J.A MOFFITT, M. HAY & E.M. HASSER.1998. Glutamate in the nucleus tractus solitarius activates both ionotropic and metabotropic glutamate receptors. Am. J. Physiol. **275:** R1858–R1866.
28. LIU, Z., C.Y. CHEN & A.C. BONHAM. 1998. Metabotropic glutamate receptors depress vagal and aortic baroreceptor signal transmission in the NTS. Am. J. Physiol. **275:** H1682–1694.
29. HOANG, C.J. & M. HAY. Expression of metabotropic glutamate receptors in the nodose ganglia and the nucleus of the solitary tract. Am. J. Physiol. In press.
30. HUANG, E. & E. NEHER. 1996. Calcium dependent exocytosis from the somata of dorsal root ganglion neurons. Neuron **17:** 135–145.
31. REUTER, H. 1995. Measurements of exocytosis from single presynaptic nerve terminals reveal heterogeneous inhibition by Ca2+-channel blockers. Neuron **14:** 773–779.
32. COFFEY, E.T., T.S. SIHRA, D.G. NICHOLLS & J.M. POCOCK. 1994. Phosphorylation of synapsin I and MARCKS in nerve terminals is mediated by Ca2+ entry via an Aga-GI sensitive Ca2+ channel which is coupled to glutamate exocytosis. FEBS Lett. **353:** 264–268.
33. GREENGARD, P., F. VALTORTA, A.J. CZERNIK & F. BENFENATI. 1993. Synaptic vesicle phosphoproteins and regulation of synaptic function. Science **259:** 780–785.
34. GREENGARD, P., F. BENFENATI & F. VALTORTA. 1994. Synapsin I, an actin-binding protein regulating synaptic vesicle traffic in the nerve terminal. Adv. Second Messenger Phosphoprotein Res. **29:** 31–45.
35. ROTHMAN, J.E. 1994. Intrcellular membrane fusion. *In* Molecular and Cellular Mechanisms of Neurotransmitter Release. L. Stjarne, P. Greengard, S. Grillner, *et al.*, Eds.: 81–96. Raven Press. New York.
36. HAY, M., C.J. HOANG, E.M. HASSER & E.M. PRICE. 2000. Activation of metabotropic glutamate receptors inhibits synapsin I phosphorylation in visceral sensory neurons. J. Membr. Biol. **178:** 195–204.
37. HAY, M. & D.L. KUNZE. 1994. Glutamate metabotropic receptor inhibition of voltage-gated calcium currents in visceral sensory neurons. J. Neurophysiol. **72** (No.1): 421–430.
38. PIERIBONE, V.A., O. SHUPLIAKOV, L. BRODIN, *et al.* 1995. Distinct pools of synaptic vesicles in neurotransmitter release (letter). Nature **375:** 493–497.
39. BAJJALIEH, S.M. & R.H. SCHELLER. 1994. Synaptic vesicle proteins and exocytosis. *In* Molecular and Cellular Mechanisms of Neurotransmitter Release. L. Stjarne, P. Greengard, S. Grillner, *et al.*, Eds.: 59–79. Raven Press. New York.
40. CECCALDI, P.E., F. GROHOVAZ, F. BENFENATI, *et al.* 1995. Dephosphorylated synapsin I anchors synaptic vesicles to actin cytoskeleton: an analysis by videomicroscopy. J.Cell Biol. **128:** 905–912.
41. SCHEUER, D.A., J. ZHANG, G.M. TONEY & S.W. MIFFLIN. 1996. Temporal processing of aortic nerve evoked activity in the nucleus of the solitary tract. J. Neurophysiol. **76**(6): 3750–3757.
42. BETZ, W.J., F. MAO & G.S. BEWICK. 1992. Activity-dependent fluorescent staining and destaining of living vertebrate motor nerve terminals. J. Neurosci. **12:** 363–375.
43. HAY, M. & E.M. HASSER. 1998. Measurement of synaptic vesicle exocytosis in aortic baroreceptor neurons. Am. J. Physiol. **275:** H710–H716.
44. MENDELOWITZ, D. & D.L. KUNZE. 1992. Characterization of calcium currents in aortic baroreceptors. J. Neurophysiol. **68:** 509–517.

# Cellular Mechanisms of Baroreceptor Integration at the Nucleus Tractus Solitarius

MICHAEL C. ANDRESEN, MARK W. DOYLE, YOUNG-HO JIN, AND TIMOTHY W. BAILEY

*Department of Physiology and Pharmacology, Oregon Health Sciences University, Portland, Oregon 97201-3098, USA*

ABSTRACT: The autonomic nervous system makes important contributions to the homeostatic regulation of the heart and blood vessels through arterial baroreflexes, and yet our understanding of the central nervous system mechanisms is limited. The sensory synapse of baroreceptors in the nucleus tractus solitarius (NTS) is unique because its participation is obligatory in the baroreflex. Here we describe experiments targeting this synapse to provide greater understanding of the cellular mechanisms at the earliest stages of the baroreflex. Our approach utilizes electrophysiology, pharmacology, and anatomical tracers to identify and evaluate key elements of the sensory information processing in NTS.

KEYWORDS: Baroreceptor; Baroreflex; Glutamate; Visceral sensory; Nucleus of the solitary tract; Synaptic processing

## INTRODUCTION

The autonomic nervous system provides rapid adjustments of the heart and blood vessels as part of the homeostatic regulation of the cardiovascular system and basic integrated life support.[1] One of the most important classes of cardiovascular autonomic reflexes is the arterial baroreflex.[2] Over the past 100 years, despite an improved general understanding of baroreflex control, detailed information concerning the central nervous system (CNS) nuclei and the mechanisms that they utilize to constitute these baroreflexes remains, for the most part, only available as a rough outline.[3]

Considerable research identifies the nucleus of the tractus solitarius (NTS) as the site of the first baroreceptor contacts with CNS neurons.[4–6] Thus, the second-order neurons of the baroreceptor reflex lie generally within the dorsal medial portions of the caudal NTS and constitute the beginning of these reflex pathways within the CNS (FIG. 1). Arterial baroreceptors and other cardiovascular afferents converge onto NTS along with other visceral sensory afferents including prominent representations from the respiratory and gastrointestinal systems (broken line box, FIG. 1).[3] These baroreceptor synapses are obligatory and represent a common point in the reflex pathway through which blood pressure information flows before diverging to a

Address for correspondence: Dr. Michael C. Andresen, Department of Physiology and Pharmacology, Oregon Health Sciences University, Portland, Oregon 97201-3098. Voice: 503-494-5831; fax: 503-494-4352.

andresen@OHSU.edu

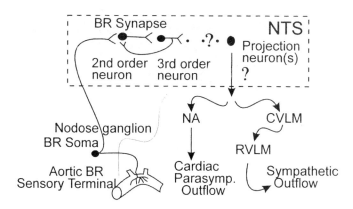

**FIGURE 1.** Basic outline of the baroreceptor reflex. Arterial baroreceptor (BR) sensory neurons including those in the aortic arch travel to the nodose ganglion and project central processes to second-order neurons within NTS (*broken line and shading*). Interneurons (third- order neurons) exist within NTS, although some neurons within NTS act as projection neurons to important autonomic targets including the caudal ventrolateral medulla (CVLM), the rostral ventrolateral medulla, vagal dorsal motor nucleus (DMN), and nucleus ambiguus (NA). The cardiovascular autonomic targets are chiefly the heart and blood vessels via both parasympathetic (e.g., NA) and sympathetic efferent (RVLM) outflow pathways. ? indicates that the precise nature of these pathways are uncertain—especially with regard to the number or existence of intervening neurons between for example second-order neurons in NTS and brainstem autonomic neurons.

variety of central nuclei. Beyond this point, sensory information is broadcast to other regions within the brain stem and beyond to supramedullary regions more broadly involved in integrative control of a variety of regulatory control systems and behaviors.[1,7] Such projections beyond NTS contribute to a broad range of other regulatory mechanisms.

## NTS AND THE BAROREFLEX PATHWAY

Visceral afferents distribute synapses across NTS neurons to some extent viscerotopically.[7] Cardiovascular afferents impinge on dorsomedial NTS, whereas respiratory afferent endings are found ventrally and ventrolaterally. There is clear overlap. NTS receives and sends processes to many other CNS areas as reciprocal connections although few of these are characterized beyond anatomical tracing (see ref. 3). The overall basic brainstem circuit of the baroreflex (FIG. 1) includes NTS, the caudal ventrolateral medulla (CVLM), the rostral ventrolateral medulla, vagal dorsal motor nucleus (DMN), and nucleus ambiguus (NA). To better understand the key steps in this pathway that contribute to the baroreflex, more detailed information is essential about the mechanisms by which baroreceptors communicate with NTS neurons, how NTS processes this sensory information, and how that processing is modulated.

The obligatory nature of the sensory synapse on NTS neurons makes this initial synaptic transmission process particularly important in the overall autonomic regulation scheme (FIG. 1). Clearly, this common step has the potential to affect all subsequent information processing beyond this point in the reflexes. Although the open and closed loop performance of the overall baroreflex has been the subject of intensive investigation, even the most basic mechanisms underlying CNS information processing in autonomic networks are poorly understood.[8]

## NTS INTEGRATION

Even from our present knowledge base, NTS is clearly not simply a relay nucleus. NTS integrates convergent information and is itself the site of substantial modulation. Sensory signal processing may well impact importantly the characteristics of the overall performance of the baroreflex, even at this first stage of the reflex pathway. Few details are firmly established on the number, types, or the nature of the interconnections of neurons within NTS. Only cursory cellular information exists on the nature of the baroreceptor synaptic contacts within NTS, for example. The evidence does suggest that within NTS, baroreceptor input to the CNS is critically conditioned, and this processing profoundly shapes baroreflex performance (see refs. 9 and 10). Clearly, NTS is essential to baroreflex integrity.[11] Lesion or pharmacological blockade of medial portions of NTS eliminates baroreflex responses.[12]

## ELEMENTS OF SYNAPTIC PROCESSING

Our recent studies have tried to identify what are likely to be key elements in these cellular processing mechanisms for sensory signals. In simplest form, these can be divided broadly into pre- and postsynaptic mechanisms at each of the first and subsequent synapses. Clearly, the neurotransmitters delivered by sensory terminals act at ligand-specific receptors located both presynaptically and postsynaptically (FIG. 2). Such receptors are in turn coupled to a number of cellular effector systems in the respective neurons which transduce these neurotransmitter signals via enzymatic cascades and ion channels.[13–16] This neurotransmitter receptor/ intracellular transduction cascade contributes to both the presynaptic and postsynaptic modulation of processing afferents signals. Such elements within the NTS network are in turn also likely to be the targets of descending control by other brain regions via neurotransmitters, possibly even at this critical early stage of the reflex (e.g., refs. 17 and 18).

Recording from single NTS neurons *in vivo* has revealed unique information related to circuitry and sensory afferent mechanisms that affect the discharge and performance properties of the neurons involved in the baroreceptor reflex (e.g., refs. 9 and 19). Heterogeneity across NTS neurons and their synaptic responses is a hallmark finding of such studies. Generally, intracellular recordings offer the most direct approach to issues related to cellular mechanisms of CNS neuron function. As a practical matter, intracellular recording is most successful in isolated brain preparations where experimental control is more stable (reduced movement, close access to the cells of interest, etc.). The daunting complexity of the anatomical inputs to NTS, coupled with the difficulty experimentally accessing these neurons in the intact sit-

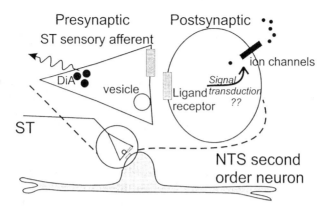

**FIGURE 2.** Outline of key elements in cellular processing mechanisms for sensory signals at NTS. Solitary tract (ST) axons terminate in presynaptic endings. Such endings contain transmitter vesicles that are released during afferent activation. This presynaptic element contains receptors for neuron transmitters (*gray box*). The presynaptic terminal can be dye labeled with tracer (*filled circles*), and in slices the dye is excited to emit fluorescent light (*wavy arrow*) for neuron identification. Postsynaptically, neurotransmitter ligand receptors are coupled to signal transduction cascades, and these in turn affect activity of ion channels (*filled rectangle*) and other targets. Similar transduction occurs presynaptically.

uation, motivated us to approach sensory synaptic transmission in medial portions of NTS to better understand the cellular and subcellular processes.

## PRIMARY SENSORY NEUROTRANSMITTER: GLUTAMATE

The predominant excitatory neurotransmitter in the CNS generally, and in NTS in particular, is glutamate (Glu). Glu is the primary cell-to-cell chemical transmission mode and activates a large family of receptors coupled either to ion channels (ionotropic)[20] or to second messenger systems (metabotropic).[21] Inotropic receptors are divided into *N*-methyl-D-aspartate (NMDA) and two non-NMDA classes, AMPA and kainate. Some details about subcellular localization of specific receptors are beginning to emerge[22] although how this relates to function is as yet unclear. Block of Glu receptors by injection of broad-spectrum Glu antagonists into NTS eliminates baroreflex responses.[3,23] Microinjection of Glu or its agonist analogues into NTS evokes baroreflex like hemodynamic and autonomic responses. Selective Glu antagonists injected into NTS attenuate the baroreflex, and thus both inotropic receptor subtypes contribute to NTS function related to cardiovascular control.

## NMDA AND NON-NMDA RECEPTORS

Over the past five years, a consensus view may have emerged that non-NMDA receptors play a major role in mediating baroreceptor and vagal sensory synaptic transmission.[24–30] Most studies indicate that postsynaptic NMDA receptors contribute as well. Previous work on isolated NTS neurons found generally small NMDA currents (< 15 pA).[3] In a minority (18%) of isolated NTS cells, however, NMDA evoked substantial currents. In addition to postsynaptic NTS sites of NMDA receptors, a recent report provides surprising electron microscopic evidence that NMDA receptors are present presynaptically on visceral sensory endings in NTS.[22] A presynaptic function of NMDA receptors remains unclear at this time but it presents another layer of subcellular complexity that requires explanation.

## SENSORY SYNAPTIC TRANSMISSION

One experimental strategy can be based on the fact that the sensory neuron inflow pathway, the solitary tract (ST), is well established and can be exploited experimentally within brain slices of the medulla. If the brain stem is cut horizontally, lengthy sections of the solitary tract remained synaptically coupled to second-order neurons. This facilitates the electrophysiological dissection of synaptic responses because a small concentric bipolar electrode can be placed some distance from the recorded neurons (FIG. 3). This allows selective electrical activation of ST axons in part by minimizing the possible recruitment of local interneurons and fibers of passage. Such stimuli, however, activate both directly, sensory afferent fibers impinging on NTS neurons as well as other synaptic responses indirectly through more complex pathways that are activated via the ST (FIG. 3). Drugs can be applied to the bath for controlled pharmacological dissection. An important additional approach for our studies is an anatomical one. Lipophilic tracers, carbocyanine dyes including DiA[6] placed on the peripheral nerve trunk of the aortic depressor nerve, are transported centrally.[6] Fluorescence from this dye can be used to identify second-order NTS

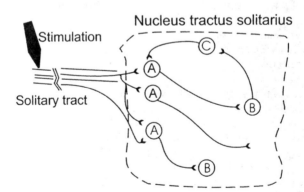

FIGURE 3. Schematic depicting direct and hypothetical indirect synaptic connections activated by solitary tract (ST) stimulation. In horizontal brainstem slices, the stimulation electrode (*left*) is placed on the ST several millimeters distant (*represented as broken line*) from the recorded neurons. **A** represents second-order neurons directly linked to sensory synapses and receiving all ST synapses. **B** represents third-order neurons that are activated by **A**. **C** represents fourth-order neurons—in this case, interneurons. Note that some **A** neurons can receive inputs from both the ST and from interneurons and that these different synapses will both be activated in sequence following ST stimulation.

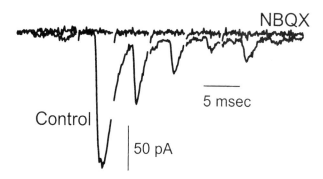

**FIGURE 4.** Representative example of excitatory postsynaptic current (EPSC) responses recorded in an mNTS neuron to a burst of five stimuli at 200 Hz to the solitary tract (ST) recorded under zero bath $Mg^{2+}$. Inward currents are down. Response latency was less than 2 ms. Note the depression of the EPSC to the second and later ST shocks. Application of the non-NMDA receptor selective antagonist NBQX completely blocked the EPSCs.

neurons (FIG. 2) within the living brain slices which receive baroreceptor synaptic contacts.

Activation of the ST evokes short-latency synaptic responses which appear to activate primarily non-NMDA receptors (FIG. 4).[31] Many other patterns of synaptic responses are found in NTS, reflecting the complexity of interconnected neurons retained even within a relatively thin (250 μm) slice of the medulla (see ref. 32). The responses arrive at a variety of latencies and our initial studies have focused on first sorting out monosynaptic from polysynaptic responses and second on characterizing the pharmacological nature of these synaptic connections and receptors upon which they depend.[31]

In a sample of mNTS neurons activated by ST stimulation, latencies ranged from about 1 ms to nearly 8 ms (FIG. 5). The variation of those synaptic latencies within neurons expressed as the standard deviation of the latency or synaptic jitter was better at discriminating second-order from third-order neurons. Such neurons were independently identified by their pharmacological profile or anatomically by dye-tracer labeling. Some of synaptic responses were clearly polysynaptic by pharmacological criteria—being blocked by both the non-NMDA selective antagonist NBQX and by the GABAa receptor antagonist bicuculline.[31–33] Still other neurons within this data set were clearly monosynaptic—based on the presence of fluorescently labeled baroreceptor sensory terminals arising from the aortic depressor nerve clustered on their somas and observed at the time of recording.[31] Thus, unlike sensory transmission in the spinal dorsal horn where NMDA receptors contribute substantially to sensory synaptic responses,[34,35] fast NTS sensory transmission relies primarily on non-NMDA receptors.[29,30]

In the relationship between jitter and synaptic latency, the responses with jitter of less than 100 μs appear to arise from the monosynaptic sensory afferent synapses. All aortic baroreceptor-labeled neurons are within this group.[31] None of these low-jitter neurons are pharmacologically disynaptic or GABAergic. A linear regression

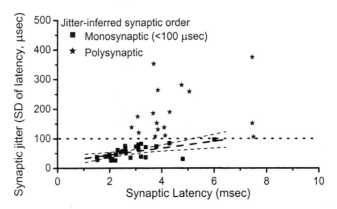

**FIGURE 5.** Representative sample of the latency and jitter values for 44 synaptic responses in mNTS neurons. Jitter is the standard deviation of the synaptic latency and is a measure of the reproducibility of the synaptic latency. *A horizontal dotted line* has been placed at a jitter equal to 100 μs, which we believe is likely close to the division between monosynaptic (*below the line*) and polysynaptic (*above the line*). Pharmacological and anatomic data generally support such a division, but it is likely to be uncertain close to this division. Synaptic responses with jitters less than 100 μs (*filled squares, n = 27*) were subjected to a least squares linear regression. The fit relation for Y = A + B * X resulted in A = 20.7 ± 10.2 and B = 11.8 ± 3.4, R = 0.57, and p = 0.0018. *Short dashed lines* are 95% confidence limits for the fit. Synaptic responses with jitter greater than 100 μs (*filled stars*) had latencies that overlapped individual latency values in the inferred monosynaptic group.

analysis of this group of data suggest that as latency increases within this low-jitter group, there is a small but significant rise in jitter (FIG. 5). Note in this same data set, however, that many other synaptic responses lie very close to this somewhat arbitrary division. Thus, moderate latency responses of about 100 μs jitter could be monosynaptically connected to the ST. At about 3 ms in absolute latency, the relationship displays a number of highly variant data with much higher jitter (stars, FIG. 5). The fact that this change occurs at roughly double the minimum latency value observed is interesting to note because such synaptic events may represent disynaptic ST evoked responses, and many of these are glutamatergic. The baroreceptor-labeled neurons are similar to unlabeled neurons. Such data are consistent with the conclusion that the basic processes of sensory synaptic transmission may not be fundamentally different between baroreceptor and other sensory modalities entering NTS. Clearly, our studies are limited to medial portions of caudal NTS, but it will be interesting to learn whether ST inputs to other regions within NTS conform to such relations.

## FUTURE DIRECTIONS

Such strategies allow identification of synaptic responses due to activation of sensory afferents and baroreceptor-linked second-order neurons. This approach opens several new avenues of interest in sensory processing in NTS and particularly in understanding the mechanisms of baroreceptor integration. One key puzzle is whether myelinated and unmyelinated pathways process baroreceptor sensory information differently and how that impacts reflex performance. A potential experimental strategy is to exploit the well-known differences in the afferent neurons.

Much of our understanding of sensory neurons comes from work in spinal sensory ganglia. Small, dark-staining neurons of dorsal root ganglion are believed to be linked to C-type axons and have distinct morphological, biochemical, and electrophysiological differences from large, light-staining dorsal root ganglion neurons linked to A-type axons.[36] Whether such differences exist in cranial visceral sensory neurons, as well as their meaning, remains unclear. A range of myelinated and unmyelinated afferents innervates virtually all regions and organs of the viscera. The cardiovascular system hosts prominent populations of afferents from all cardiac chambers and major arteries and veins; most have C-type axons.[37] Despite some differences between somatic and cranial visceral sensory neurons, their overall similarities are striking.

Our work has focused on better understanding the mechanisms responsible for transmission of baroreceptor information across the first sensory synapse within NTS. Although this involves many components, clearly the mechanisms controlling presynaptic release of neurotransmitter as well as the postsynaptic receptors are paramount (FIG. 3). At many synapses, more than one transmitter substance may be released either from the same or different vesicles during transmission. There certainly are hints that such is the case in mNTS. Many of these substances have been implicated in both pre- and postsynaptic effects along with the primary transmitter. Experiments need to be designed to determine whether co-transmitters are released during baroreceptor activation and how these participate in synaptic transmission. Targets of such co-transmitters likely reside both on presynaptic or postsynaptic elements (FIG. 3). A key contribution of visualized slice work in NTS will be to exploit optical approaches to the study of these neurons and provide better definition of presynaptic modulation of sensory transmission in NTS. The slice offers the cellular resolution that is quite difficult to establish by other means. Exploitation of key differences in the molecular composition of the presynaptic endings of sensory afferents may provide the entry to better understanding the mechanistic basis of baroreceptor information processing within NTS and its impact on CNS autonomic control.

## ACKNOWLEDGMENTS

This work was made possible by grants from the National Institutes of Health (HL-41119 and HL-56460) and the National Center of the American Heart Association.

## REFERENCES

1. SPYER, K.M. 1990. The central nervous organization of reflex circulatory control. *In* Central Regulation of Autonomic Functions. A.D. Loewy & K.M. Spyer, Eds.: 168–188. Oxford University Press. New York.
2. COLERIDGE, H.M. & J.C.G. COLERIDGE. 1980. Cardiovascular afferents involved in regulation of peripheral vessels. Annu. Rev. Physiol. **42:** 413–427.

3. ANDRESEN, M.C. & D.L. KUNZE. 1994. Nucleus tractus solitarius: gateway to neural circulatory control. Annu. Rev. Physiol. **56:** 93–116.
4. CIRIELLO, J., S.L. HOCHSTENBACH & S. RODER. 1994. Central projections of baroreceptor and chemoreceptor afferent fibers in the rat. *In* Nucleus of the Solitary Tract. R.A. Barraco, Ed.: 35–50. CRC Press. Boca Raton, FL.
5. CZACHURSKI, J., K. LACKNER, D. OCKERT & H. SELLER. 1982. Localization of neurones with baroreceptor input in the medial solitary nucleus by means of intracellular application of horseradish peroxidase in the cat. Neurosci. Lett. **28:** 133–137.
6. MENDELOWITZ, D., M. YANG, M.C. ANDRESEN & D.L. KUNZE. 1992. Localization and retention *in vitro* of fluorescently labeled aortic baroreceptor terminals on neurons from the nucleus tractus solitarius. Brain Res. **581:** 339–343.
7. LOEWY, A.D. 1990. Central autonomic pathways. *In* Central regulation of autonomic functions. A.D. Loewy & K.M. Spyer, Eds.: 88–103. Oxford. New York.
8. KUMADA, M., N. TERUI & T. KUWAKI. 1990. Arterial baroreceptor reflex: its central and peripheral neural mechanisms. Prog. Neurobiol. **35:** 331–361.
9. LIU, Z., C.Y. CHEN & A.C. BONHAM. 2000. Frequency limits on aortic baroreceptor input to nucleus tractus solitarii. Am. J. Physiol. Heart Circ. Physiol. **278:** H577–H585.
10. SELLER, H. & M. ILLERT. 1969. The localization of the first synapse in the carotid sinus baroreceptor reflex pathway and its alteration of the afferent input. Pflügers Arch. **306:** 1–19.
11. REIS, D.J. 1984. The brain and hypertension: reflections on 35 years of inquiry into the neurobiology of the circulation. Circulation **70:** 31–45.
12. SCHREIHOFER, A.M., E.M. STRICKER & A.F. SVED. 1994. Chronic nucleus tractus solitarius lesions do not prevent hypovolemia-induced vasopressin secretion in rats. Am. J. Physiol. Regul. Integr. Comp. Physiol. **267:** R965–R973.
13. TRUSSELL, L.O. 1999. Synaptic mechanisms for coding timing in auditory neurons. Annu. Rev. Physiol. **61:** 477–496.
14. WU, L.G. & P. SAGGAU. 1997. Presynaptic inhibition of elicited neurotransmitter release. Trends Neurosci. **20:** 204–212.
15. MATTHEWS, G. 1996. Neurotransmitter release. Annu. Rev. Neurosci. **19:** 219–233.
16. GARTHWAITE, J. & C.L. BOULTON. 1995. Nitric oxide signaling in the central nervous system. Annu. Rev. Physiol. **57:** 683–706.
17. MIFFLIN, S.W., K.M. SPYER & D.J. WITHINGTON-WRAY. 1988. Baroreceptor inputs to the nucleus tractus solitarius in the cat: postsynaptic actions and the influence of respiration. J. Physiol. (Lond.) **399:** 349–367.
18. MIFFLIN, S.W., K.M. SPYER & D.J. WITHINGTON-WRAY. 1988. Baroreceptor inputs to the nucleus tractus solitarius in the cat: modulation by the hypothalamus J. Physiol. (Lond.) **399:** 369–387.
19. FELDER, R.B. & S.W. MIFFLIN. 1994. Baroreceptor and chemoreceptor afferent processing in the solitary tract nucleus. *In* Nucleus of the Solitary Tract. R.A. Barraco, Ed.: 169–186. CRC Press. Boca Raton, FL.
20. BARNARD, E.A. 1997. Ionotropic glutamate receptors: new types and new concepts. Trends Pharmacol. Sci. **18:** 141–148.
21. NICHOLLS, D.G. 1992. A retrograde step forward. Nature **360:** 106–107.
22. AICHER, S.A., S. SHARMA & V.M. PICKEL. 1999. *N*-Methyl-D-aspartate receptors are present in vagal afferents and their dendritic targets in the nucleus tractus solitarius. Neuroscience **91:** 119–132.
23. OHTA, H. & W.T. TALMAN. 1994. Both NMDA and non-NMDA receptors in the NTS participate in the baroreceptor reflex in rats. Am. J. Physiol. Regul. Integr. Comp. Physiol. **267:** R1065–R1070.
24. SMITH, B.N., P. DOU, W.D. BARBER & F.E. DUDEK. 1998. Vagally evoked synaptic currents in the immature rat nucleus tractus solitarii in an intact *in vitro* preparation. J. Physiol. **512:** 149–162.
25. AYLWIN, M.L., J.M. HOROWITZ & A.C. BONHAM. 1997. NMDA receptors contribute to primary visceral afferent transmission in the nucleus of the solitary tract. J. Neurophysiol. **77:** 2539–2548.

26. AYLWIN, M.L., J.M. HOROWITZ & A.C. BONHAM. 1998. Non-NMDA and NMDA receptors in the synaptic pathway between area postrema and nucleus tractus solitarius. Am. J. Physiol. Heart Circ. Physiol. **44:** H1236–H1246.
27. CHEN, C.Y. & A.C. BONHAM. 1998. Non-NMDA and NMDA receptors transmit area postrema input to aortic baroreceptor neurons in NTS. Am. J. Physiol. Heart Circ. Physiol. **275:** H1695–H1706.
28. ZHANG, J. & S.W. MIFFLIN. 1997. Influences of excitatory amino acid receptor agonists on nucleus of the solitary tract neurons receiving aortic depressor nerve inputs. J. Pharmacol. Exp. Ther. **282:** 639–647.
29. ZHANG, J. & S.W. MIFFLIN. 1998. Differential roles for NMDA and non-NMDA receptor subtypes in baroreceptor afferent integration in the nucleus of the solitary tract of the rat. J. Physiol. **511:** 733–745.
30. SEAGARD, J.L., C. DEAN & F.A. HOPP. 1999. Role of glutamate receptors in transmission of vagal cardiac input to neurones in the nucleus tractus solitarii in dogs. J. Physiol. **520:** 243–253.
31. DOYLE, M.W. & M.C. ANDRESEN. 2001. Synaptic reliability of monosynaptic transmission in brain stem neurons *in vitro*. J. Neurophysiol. **85:** 2213–2223.
32. ANDRESEN, M.C. & D. MENDELOWITZ. 1996. Sensory afferent neurotransmission in caudal nucleus tractus solitarius—common denominators. Chem. Sens. **21:** 387–395.
33. ANDRESEN, M.C. & M. YANG. 1995. Dynamics of sensory afferent synaptic transmission in aortic baroreceptor regions of nucleus tractus solitarius. J. Neurophysiol. **74:** 1518–1528.
34. CERNE, R. & M. RANDIC. 1992. Modulation of AMPA and NMDA responses in rat spinal dorsal horn neurons by *trans*-1-aminocyclopentane-1,3-dicarboxylic acid. Neurosci. Lett. **144:** 180–184.
35. SANDKUHLER, J., J.G. CHEN, G. CHENG & M. RANDIC. 1997. Low-frequency stimulation of afferent Adelta-fibers induces long-term depression at primary afferent synapses with substantia gelatinosa neurons in the rat. J. Neurosci. **17:** 6483–6491.
36. LAWSON, S.N. 1992. Morphological and biochemical cell types of sensory neurons. *In* Sensory Neurons: Diversity, Development, and Plasticity. S.A. Scott, Ed.: 27–59. Oxford University Press. New York.
37. THOREN, P.N. 1979. Role of cardiac vagal c-fibers in cardiovascular control. Rev. Physiol. Biochem. Pharmacol. **86:** 1–94.

# Properties of NTS Neurons Receiving Input from Barosensitive Receptors

J. L. SEAGARD, C. DEAN, AND F.A. HOPP

*Department of Anesthesiology, Medical College of Wisconsin, and the Zablocki VA Medical Center, Milwaukee, Wisconsin 53295, USA*

ABSTRACT: Afferent input from barosensitive receptors, including carotid baroreceptors and cardiac mechanoreceptors, has been found to produce different types of discharge patterns in neurons in the nucleus tractus solitarius (NTS). The discharge patterns of the neurons may be dependent on many factors, including input from the different barosensitive receptor subtypes, the contribution of different ionotropic glutamate receptors [NMDA (N-methyl-D-aspartate) versus nonNMDA receptors] in transmission of the input, effects of different neuropeptide neurotransmitters/neuromodulators on afferent transmission, or the order of the neuron within the barosensitive reflex arc. It is not clear if the roles of the glutamate receptor subtypes are the same for neurons activated by the different barosensitive inputs. In addition, the amount of afferent input from the barosensitive receptors, due to increases or decreases in stimulating pressures, may result in altering the roles of the ionotropic glutamate receptor subtypes. While most evidence suggests that nonNMDA receptors play the greatest role in the transmission of afferent activity to second-order NTS neurons, it is possible that increases in afferent input may lead to an enhanced role for NMDA receptors in the transmission of the barosensitive input, since increased depolarization of the NTS neurons may lead to removal of a $Mg^{2+}$ block of the NMDA channel. Transmission of baroreceptor input at third- and higher-order neurons has been found to involve both nonNMDA and NMDA receptors, suggesting a possible functional role for the distribution of these receptor types. The roles of these different factors in the initiation of NTS neuronal discharge will be discussed.

KEYWORDS: Baroreceptors; Glutamate receptors; NMDA; Medulla

## INTRODUCTION

While the discharge patterns of barosensitive receptors, including arterial baroreceptors and cardiac mechanoreceptors, have been well characterized, the patterns of activity evoked by these inputs in neurons in the NTS has been less well described, particularly in response to pressure-evoked afferent input. Activation of baroreceptors or cardiac ventricular mechanoreceptors through pressure-induced stretching of their receptive fields produces similar reflex depressor and bradycardic responses.[1–3] The similar patterns of reflex responses suggest that at least a portion

Address for correspondence: Jeanne L. Seagard, Ph.D., Research Service 151, VA Medical Center, 5000 W. National Ave., Milwaukee, WI 53295. Voice: 414-384-2000, ext. 41589; fax: 414-645-6550.

jseagard@mcw.edu

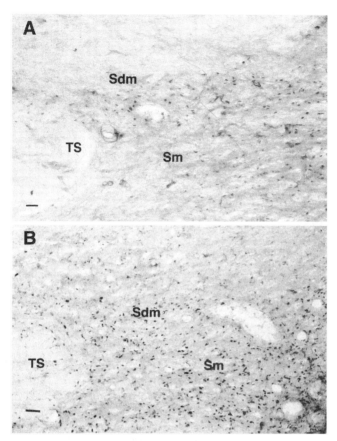

**FIGURE 1.** Digital photomicrographs illustrating Fos distribution in the nucleus tractus solitarius of the dog at the level of the obex, in response to (**A**) stimulation of the ipsilateral carotid sinus baroreceptors and (**B**) stimulation of cardiac mechanoreceptors. Stimulation of the cardiac mechanoreceptors induced a greater degree of Fos expression in the medial subnucleus, relative to stimulation of the carotid baroreceptors. *Bar:* 100 μm. Sm, medial subnucleus; Sdm, dorsomedial subnucleus; TS, tractus solitarius.

of the reflex pathways are similar. Anatomical tracing studies have shown that the sites of first termination of baroreceptor[4,5] and vagal cardiac[6] afferent fibers in the central nervous system have been located in the NTS. Functional neuronal recording studies in which afferent activity was evoked by electrical stimulation of baroreceptor[7–9] or cardiac vagal fibers[7,8,10,11] or by chemical or mechanical activation of baroreceptors[7,9] or cardiac receptors[10–12] have shown activation of neurons within similar subnuclei of the NTS. Studies from this laboratory used *c-fos* expression, an intermediate early gene expressed in the nucleus of neurons excited by synaptic input, to anatomically map and compare the distribution of NTS neurons activated by baroreceptors[13,14] and cardiac mechanoreceptors. Similar to earlier studies, these studies have also shown that afferent input from baroreceptors is directed to subnuclei of the NTS, but there are some small differences in the patterns of innervation between baroreceptors and cardiac mechanoreceptors. Preliminary data for input from activation of cardiac mechanoreceptors indicates that there is a larger degree of innervation of the medial subnucleus in the intermediate and caudal NTS by these cardiac receptors versus baroreceptors (FIG. 1). Using this information to provide location, we have recorded NTS neuronal activity to characterize the responses of NTS neurons produced by pressure-induced activation of carotid sinus baroreceptors and left ventricular cardiac mechanoreceptors and the roles of glutamate receptor subtypes in the transmission of this afferent input. To activate carotid baroreceptors, slow ramp pressure increases in carotid sinus pressure (CSP) in a vascularly isolated carotid sinus were made to ipsilaterally pressure activate the baroreceptors. To activate cardiac mechanoreceptors, slow increases in arterial pressure were made by infusion of phenylephrine (5-10 mL of 1 mg%) in a ganglionically blocked dog (hexamethonium, 20–40 mg). Only the afferent pathway under investigation in each animal was left intact, with all other afferent inputs eliminated by section of the aortic depressor nerves and either the carotid sinus or vagal nerves. Neuronal activity was recorded using a multibarrel pipette, with one recording barrel containing a carbon fiber filament. The remaining three barrels were filled with vehicle (artificial CSF) and the glutamate (GLU) receptor antagonists NBQX [(1,2,3,4-Tetrahydro-6-nitro-2,3-dioxo-benzo(f)quinoxaline-7-sulfonamide disodium), a non-NMDA receptor antagonist; 100 μM] and AP5 [((±)-2-amino-5-phosphonovaleric acid), an NMDA receptor antagonist; 5 mM], which were picoejected onto the recorded neuron in order to determine the role of the respective glutamate receptor subtypes in the transmission of the barosensitive activity.

## CAROTID BARORECEPTOR-MODULATED NTS NEURONS

Previous studies have identified two subtypes of carotid sinus baroreceptors, based on discharge patterns produced in response to slow ramp increases in CSP.[15] Type I baroreceptors are characterized by a sudden onset and higher rate of discharge, while type II baroreceptors have a slower rate of firing, gradually increasing from a spontaneous rate of discharge to a saturation firing rate at higher levels of CSP (FIG. 2). It is not known if afferent input from these two subtypes of baroreceptors induce similar or different firing patterns in neurons in the NTS or if input from these subtypes converge upon the same second-order neurons in the NTS.

Most of the available data regarding baroreceptor-modulated NTS neuronal firing patterns indicates that there are few cells with pulse-synchronous discharges,[7,9,16] which is unexpected given the pulse-synchronous discharge of the baroreceptors themselves. Averaging methods over longer periods (minutes) have shown that some neurons do have a discharge that correlates with the R wave, suggesting some synchronicity with heart rate.[17] One study[16] has found different patterns of extracellular discharge in central baroreceptor-modulated neurons, with some neurons that were silent at resting blood pressure (BP) and fired only sparsely at a specific pressure level during pressure increases or decreases, while other neurons showed an on-going level of discharge that increased with increases in BP. In a study that recorded intracellular activity of neurons that responded to both carotid sinus nerve stimulation and inflation of a balloon in the carotid sinus, the neuronal responses were also var-

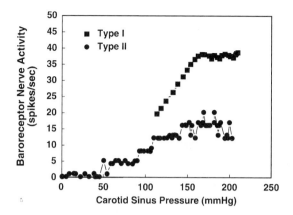

**FIGURE 2.** Examples of discharge curves for a type I and type II baroreceptor. The type I curve shows the greater rate of discharge and sensitivity characteristic of these receptors. The type II curve reflects the spontaneous discharge below pressure threshold and wider operating range of the slower, less sensitive type II baroreceptors.

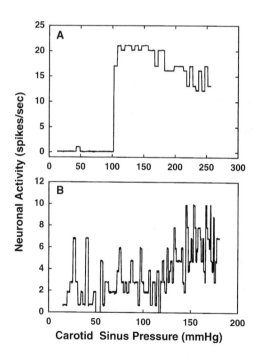

**FIGURE 3.** Examples of discharge patterns of baroreceptor-sensitive NTS neurons produced in response to ramp increases in carotid sinus pressure. Two general patterns of discharge were obtained: **Panel A:** sudden-onset neurons that adapted despite further increases in carotid sinus pressure; **Panel B:** slow-onset neurons that did not adapt to increases in carotid sinus pressure.

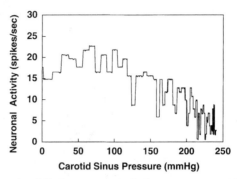

**FIGURE 4.** Example of discharge pattern of a baroreceptor-sensitive NTS neuron that had a decrease in discharge in response to ramp increases in carotid sinus pressure. This type of response was seen in a small number of baroreceptor-modulated NTS neurons.

ied.[7] Neurons displayed excitatory postsynaptic potentials (EPSPs), EPSP plus inhibitory postsynaptic potentials (IPSPs), or IPSPs to both electrical carotid sinus nerve stimulation or carotid sinus distention via intrasinus balloon inflation. Thus, both intracellular and extracellular recording studies have found that there are multiple firing patterns for baroreceptor-modulated neurons in the NTS. The patterns of discharge from these earlier studies have some similarities to responses obtained from baroreceptor-modulated NTS neurons studied in the dog in this laboratory using ramp pressure increases in an isolated carotid sinus to pressure-activate carotid baroreceptors.[18] Neurons that increased activity in response to baroreceptor input displayed either a rapid-onset pattern, in which neurons turned on with a burst of activity at a given pressure threshold and then adapted (FIG. 3A) (12 of 33), or a slow-onset, nonadapting pattern in which neuronal activity increased with increasing CSP (FIG. 3B) (21 of 33). The nonadapting neurons demonstrated a pressure-related increase in discharge up to saturation firing rates similar to those previously reported; however, the rate of discharge of the rapid-onset, adapting neurons was much greater than that reported for the sudden-onset NTS neurons. In addition, the discharge of four neurons actually decreased in response to increases in CSP and thus baroreceptor input (FIG. 4). For all baroreceptor-sensitive neurons studied, only one was found to display an obvious pulse-related discharge that tracked pulsatile changes in CSP. Long-term averaging to determine if any other correlations to CSP pulses could be observed were not performed. The mechanisms for the types of firing patterns observed in our study in the dog are not known but may be due in part to the type of baroreceptor input each neuron receives, the extent of convergence of inputs from more than one baroreceptor or type of baroreceptor, or the type(s) of neurotransmitter receptors present on the neuron.

## CARDIAC MECHANORECEPTOR-MODULATED NTS NEURONS

Unlike baroreceptor-modulated neurons, some cardiac receptor-modulated neurons have been found to reflect a cardiac-related discharge. In a recent study,[19] we examined discharge of pulse-synchronous NTS neurons and found that most re-

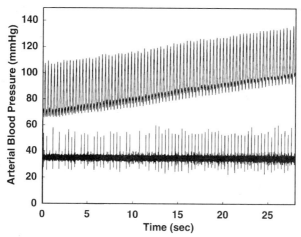

**FIGURE 5.** Tracings of arterial pressure *(upper trace)* and raw neuronal activity of a pulse-synchronous NTS neuron *(lower trace)* with left vagal afferent input, demonstrating the pressure sensitivity of the neuronal discharge. Firing of the neuron was found to increase with a small increase (about 30 mmHg) in mean arterial pressure. (Reprinted with permission from Seagard *et al.*[19])

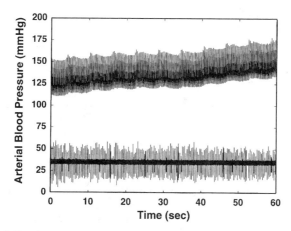

**FIGURE 6.** Tracings of arterial pressure *(upper trace)* and raw neuronal activity *(lower trace)* of the single neuron recorded with afferent input transmitted via the right vagus. The neuron discharged synchronously with each heart beat but did not respond to a 25-mmHg increase in arterial pressure, unlike the pressure-sensitive neurons with left vagal afferents, an example of which is shown in FIG. 5. (Reprinted with permission from Seagard *et al.*[19])

ceived input from putative cardiac mechanoreceptors with left vagal afferents. In response to small increases in arterial BP, 28 of 31 pulse-synchronous neurons increased discharge to reflect the increase in pressure (FIG. 5). However, in 3 of the 31 neurons recorded, the neurons were found to track heart rate but were insensitive to BP changes (FIG. 6).

Somewhat different results were found in an earlier study,[10] in which it was found that NTS neuronal activity evoked through activation of cardiac mechanoreceptors by bolus saline injections demonstrated a volume threshold, with no further increases in discharge despite larger saline injections. However, the number of neurons excited by the saline injections increased with increasing injectate volume. Investigators suggested that increased reflex responses due to mechanoreceptor activation resulted from recruitment of more NTS neurons at larger volumes, not to increases in discharge of individual neurons. A related type of integration may also be operative with the pressure-sensitive neurons recorded in our study. While the individual neurons did demonstrate some increases in activity to increases in arterial pressure, the peak discharge rates (1–12 spikes/cardiac cycle) never approached peak rates reported for peripheral afferent activity from the cardiac receptors (14–200 spikes/s).[20,21] However, possible recruitment and central convergence of more neurons at higher arterial pressures may lead to enhanced reflex responses reported for increasing activation of cardiac mechanoreceptors as a group. The possibility of recruitment or convergence of afferent inputs is an area of future investigation.

## ROLE OF GLUTAMATE AS A NEUROTRANSMITTER FOR BAROSENSITIVE INPUT

Many studies have pointed to GLU as the primary baroreceptor neurotransmitter within the NTS.[8,22,23] However, the mechanisms of GLU activation of second-order NTS baroreceptor neurons are not completely understood. There is evidence from whole animal,[24–27] brain slice,[26–28] and isolated cell studies[29,30] that different types of GLU receptors activate NTS neurons, although there is some controversy as to the extent of these individual contributions. Studies have suggested that NMDA,[24,28–30] non-NMDA,[22,25,28,29] or metabotropic GLU receptors[31–33] and various combinations of each[24–26,28,34] may be involved in the NTS transmission of baroreceptor afferent input. Studies from this laboratory examining the contributions of ionotropic receptors have found that both NMDA and nonNMDA receptor antagonists alter baroreceptor-modulated NTS neuronal discharge,[35,36] suggesting that each type of GLU ionotropic receptor may contribute to excitation of the neurons. However, in most neurons, blockade of non-NMDA receptors had the greatest attenuating effect on neuronal activity, suggesting a greater role for the non-NMDA receptors. In all neurons examined ($n = 8$), NBQX decreased or eliminated discharge of the baroreceptor-modulated neurons. Examples of the effects of NMDA versus non-NMDA receptor blockade on the discharge of baroreceptor-modulated neurons are shown in FIGURES 7 and 8. In five of eight neurons, blockade of the non-NMDA receptors with NBQX was found to abolish discharge in the neuron (FIG. 7). However, in three of eight neurons, additional blockade of the NMDA receptors with AP5 was also necessary to eliminate neuronal activity in combination with NBQX (FIG. 8). In two of the neurons in which NBQX alone was found to abolish neuronal activity, AP5 given first was found to decrease but not eliminate activity. This suggests that NMDA receptors contributed to some degree to the transmission of baroreceptor input in these neurons, but that non-NMDA receptor activation was necessary to maintain firing of the neurons.

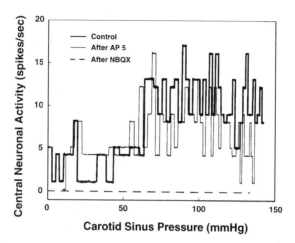

**FIGURE 7.** Effects of picoejection of AP5 and NBQX on integrated activity of a baroreceptor-modulated NTS neuron, which responded with an increase in discharge to an increase in carotid sinus pressure. Picoejection of 15 nL of AP5 (5 mM) had no significant effect on either spontaneous or pressure-induced discharge of the neuron. Picoejection of NBQX (100 µM) alone eliminated both spontaneous and pressure-related increases in neuronal discharge. Picoejection of vehicle had no effect.

The contribution of GLU receptor subtypes to the transmission of cardiac vagal afferent input has been less studied than the roles of the receptors in the transmission of baroreceptor afferent input, but the respective roles of NMDA versus non-NMDA receptors appear to be similar to those proposed for the transmission of baroreceptor input. Blockade of excitatory amino acid receptors with the broad antagonist kynurenate was found to eliminate discharge in NTS neurons evoked by either vagal or carotid sinus nerve stimulation in rats.[8] Neurons with monosynaptic and polysynaptic inputs were similarly attenuated, but antagonists for specific ionotropic GLU receptor subtypes were not used in the study. In a study that examined the transmission of vagal C-fiber chemosensitive cardiac input to the NTS, it was found that blockade of non-NMDA but not NMDA receptors significantly decreased synaptic activation of neurons primarily located in the commissural NTS.[12] However, this afferent input originated from chemosensitive c-fiber cardiac receptors, not mechanoreceptors; and the NTS neurons did not demonstrate any pulse-synchronous activity. In a recent study from this laboratory,[19] both non-NMDA and NMDA receptor antagonists were found to decrease discharges of NTS neurons receiving left vagal cardiac mechanoreceptor input. While both GLU receptor subtypes were found to be involved in activation of these neurons, blockade of non-NMDA receptors in 14 of 18 neurons was found to eliminate activity in the majority of neurons, suggesting a greater role for this GLU receptor subtype (FIG. 9). However, in 4 of 18 neurons, AP5 was also required to eliminate neuronal activity in cardiac mechanoreceptor-modulated neurons (FIG. 10). As found with baroreceptor-modulated neurons, in four of the neurons in which NBQX when given first eliminated activity, if AP5 was given first, it could decrease but not eliminate neuronal activity. This again

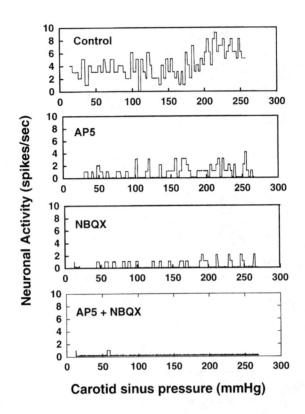

**FIGURE 8.** Effects of picoejection of AP5 and NBQX on integrated activity of a baroreceptor-modulated NTS neuron, which responded with an increase in discharge to an increase in carotid sinus pressure. Picoejection of 15 nL of either AP5 (5 mM) or NBQX (100 μM) decreased both spontaneous and pressure-related increases in neuronal discharge, with greater decreases seen in response to NBQX. Exposure to the combined NBQX and AP5 eliminated all activity of the neuron. Picoejection of vehicle had no effect.

suggests that NMDA receptors may contribute to cardiac mechanoreceptor-modulated neuronal firing, but this input is not sufficient by itself to activate the neurons.

## EFFECTS OF NEURONAL ORDER AND DEPOLARIZATION ON NMDA RECEPTOR ACTIVITY

The extent of involvement of each GLU receptor subtype may depend on the level of the neuron in the baroreflex arc. Some studies suggest that second-order neurons, which monosynaptically receive baroreceptor innervation, are activated primarily via non-NMDA receptors, while activation of higher-order neurons with polysynaptic inputs involves both non-NMDA and NMDA receptors.[22,25] However, other studies have suggested that NMDA receptors may also be involved in the activation of second-order neurons.[26,27] The possibility exists that increased excitation of

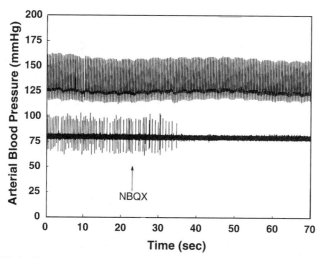

**FIGURE 9.** Tracings of arterial pressure *(upper trace)* and raw neuronal activity *(lower trace)* of a pulse-synchronous NTS neuron in the nucleus tractus solitarius before and after blockade of nonNMDA glutamate receptors by local exposure to NBQX. The cardiac-related discharge of the neuron was eliminated by picoejection of 7 nL of NBQX (100 μM). (Reprinted with permission from Seagard *et al.*[19])

barosensitive NTS neurons will enhance the central contribution of NMDA receptors, due to removal of the $Mg^{2+}$ block of the channel with neuronal depolarization. Thus, the role of NMDA receptors may be greater during periods of increased barosensitive afferent input, since some degree of neuronal depolarization increases the activation of NMDA receptors.[26,37]

The effect of neuronal depolarization on enhancing the activation of NMDA receptors has been described in other systems. In the hippocampus, high-frequency stimulation has been found to lead to depolarization of the postsynaptic membrane that removes the $Mg^{2+}$ block for NMDA channels, allowing $Ca^{2+}$ influx. This calcium, acting as a second messenger, is thought to lead to long-term potentiation of discharge of the neuron.[38,39] Conversely, some studies have found a desensitization or adaptation to the continued administration of either NMDA or AMPA[40] [non-NMDA receptor agonist, (±)-a-amino-3-hydroxy-5-methyl-isoxazole-4-proprionic acid]. Long-term depression via NMDA receptors has been reported following low-frequency stimulation in the hippocampus.[41] It is proposed that high-frequency stimulation may lead to a higher intracellular $Ca^{2+}$, which induces potentiation; while low intracellular $Ca^{2+}$ resulting from low-frequency stimulation may lead to depression. It is therefore possible that the phosphorylation state of the NMDA receptor influences whether hippocampal synapses are potentiated or depressed.[42] A similar mechanism may be active at NTS synapses. It is possible that frequency-dependent effects of the NMDA receptor may lead to variable levels of barosensitive neuronal activation. Long-term potentiation, long-term depression, accommodation, and other nonlinear responses to depolarization have been reported for NTS neurons thought to receive barosensitive inputs.[37,43,44] The role of NMDA receptors in initi-

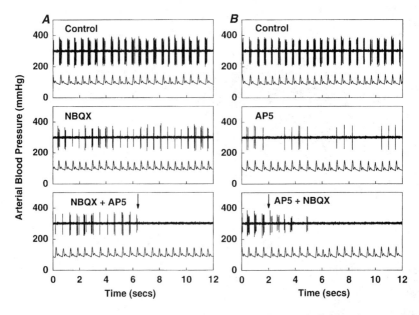

**FIGURE 10.** Tracings of arterial pressure *(upper trace in each panel)* and raw neuronal activity *(lower trace in each panel)* of a pulse-synchronous NTS neuron the discharge of which was decreased by both NBQX (100 μM), a non-NMDA receptor antagonist, and AP5 (5 mM), a NMDA receptor antagonist. Picoejection of 15 nL of either NBQX **(A)** or AP5 **(B)** decreased discharge of the neuron *(middle panels)*, with activity completely abolished by additional administration of the other antagonist *(lower panels)*. Thus, cardiac-related discharge of the neuron was eliminated only after local picoejection of both ionotropic glutamate receptor blockers. (Reprinted with permission from Seagard *et al.*[19])

ation of these responses has not been well defined, and the extracellular responses of the neurons to different levels of physiological activation by pressure stimulations of afferent inputs has not been described. In the above studies, the respective roles of the glutamate receptors in the transmission of vagal input at lower versus higher arterial pressures—and thus at lower versus higher levels of afferent input and neuronal activation—were not tested. It was not possible to determine if NMDA receptors could play a greater role at higher pressures. This aspect of the possible role of NMDA receptors has now been examined in our laboratory, as described below.

A preliminary study has been performed to examine whether the degree of barosensitive NTS neuronal excitation, due to different amounts of afferent input from barosensitive peripheral receptors, alters the role of GLU receptor subtypes in the transmission of afferent input. Careful changes in BP were performed to induce changes in afferent input from barosensitive cardiac mechanoreceptors. Blood pressure was set at either a high (mean 145 mmHg) or low (mean 95 mmHg) level, through changes in i.v. infusion of phenylephrine (1 mg%) or nitroprusside (1 mg%) for control and during picoejection of NMDA to examine any pressure-related differences in NMDA receptor transmission. In 7 of 11 neurons, NMDA induced a greater increase in discharge at the higher versus lower BP (FIG. 11). This data sug-

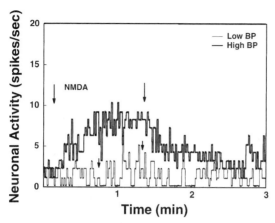

**FIGURE 11.** The response of a cardiac mechanoreceptor-modulated neuron to picoejection of NMDA (100 µM, between *arrows*) during low (mean 95 mmHg) and high (mean 134 mmHg) BP stimulation of the cardiac mechanoreceptor. Administration of NMDA during the higher-pressure stimulation, which resulted in increased afferent input from the peripheral receptor, produced a greater increase in neuronal discharge as compared to the NMDA response at the lower-pressure stimulation level. This suggests a greater availability of NMDA receptors when activation of the neuron was increased.

gests that the role played by NMDA receptors is greater at the higher level of pressure, possibly due to a greater availability of NMDA receptors through removal of the $Mg^{2+}$ block by the enhanced excitability of the neuron produced by the higher amount of synaptic excitation. However, the order of the neurons was not determined in these studies, and therefore it is not known if second- or higher-order neurons were studied. This factor may also be important, based on earlier studies.

## CONCLUDING REMARKS

The studies described above indicate that NTS neurons that receive barosensitive input can have a variety of firing patterns, suggesting that they do not simply serve as relays in the transmission of barosensitive input to the central reflex arc. The mechanisms behind the integration and encoding of afferent activity are not known, but evidence suggests that in many baromodulated NTS neurons, both non-NMDA and NMDA receptors can contribute in varying degrees to the transmission of afferent input. The importance of each receptor subtype may depend on order of the neuron studied or level of afferent input, which may alter the excitability of the NTS neurons and unmask a greater role for NMDA receptors.

## ACKNOWLEDGMENTS

This research was supported by NIH Grant HL 55490 and VA Medical Research Funds.

The authors would like to acknowledge the valuable assistance of Claudia Hermes; Maja Bago, M.D.; Ann Cowan, B.S.; and Sarah Botsford, B.S.

## REFERENCES

1. BROWN, A.M. 1979. Cardiac reflexes. In Handbook of Physiology, The Cardiovascular System, Section 2, Vol. 1, The Heart. R.M. Berne, N. Sperelakis & S.R. Geiger, Eds.: 670–689. American Physiological Society (Williams and Wilkins). Bethesda, MD.
2. DONALD, D.E. & J.T. SHEPHERD. 1978. Reflexes from the heart and lungs: physiological curiosities or important regulatory mechanisms. Cardiovas. Res. 12: 449–469.
3. THOREN, P. 1979. Reflex effects of left ventricular mechanoreceptors with afferent fibres in the vagal nerves. In Cardiac Receptors. R. Hainsworth, C.Kidd & R.J. Linden, Eds.: 259–278.Cambridge University Press. Cambridge.
4. CIRIELLO, J., A.W. HRYCYSHYN & F.R. CALARESU. 1981. Glossopharyngeal and vagal afferent projections to the brain stem of the cat: a horseradish peroxidase study. J. Auton. Nerv. Syst. 4: 63–79.
5. RUIZ-PESINI, P., E. TOME, L. BALAGUER, et al. 1995. The projections to the medulla of neurons innervating the carotid sinus in the dog. Brain Res.Bull. 37: 1–46.
6. KALIA, M. & M.-M. MESULAM. 1980. Brain stem projections of sensory and motor components of the vagus complex in the cat: 1. The cervical vagus and nodose ganglion. J. Comp. Neurol. 193: 435–465.
7. MIFFLIN, S.W., K.M. SPYER & D.J. WITHINGTON-WRAY. 1988. Baroreceptor inputs to the nucleus tractus solitarius in the cat: postsynaptic actions and the influence of respiration. J. Physiol. (London) 399: 349–367.
8. ZHANG, W. & S.W. MIFFLIN. 1995. Excitatory amino-acid receptors contribute to carotid sinus and vagus nerve evoked excitation of neruons in the nucleus of the tractus solitarius. J. Auton. Nerv. Syst. 55: 50–56.
9. ROGERS, R.F., J.F.R. PATON & J.S. SCHWABER. 1993. NTS neuronal responses to arterial pressure and pressure changes in the rat. Am. J. Physiol. 265(34): R1355–R1368.
10. HINES, T., G.M. TONEY & S.W. MIFFLIN. 1994. Responses of neurons in the nucleus tractus solitarius to stimulation of heart and lung receptors in the rat. Circ. Res. 74: 1188–1196.
11. SILVA-CARVALHO, L., J.F.R. PATON, I. ROCHA, et al. 1998. Convergence properties of solitary tract neurons responsive to cardiac receptor stimulation in the anesthetized cat. J. Neurophysiol. 79: 2374–2382.
12. WILSON, C.G., Z. ZHANG & A.C. BONHAM. 1996. Non-NMDA receptors transmit cardiopulmonary C fibre input in nucleus tractus solitarii in rats. J. Physiol. 493: 773–785.
13. DEAN, C. & J.L. SEAGARD. 1995. Expression of c-fos protein in the nucleus tractus solitarius in response to physiological activation of carotid baroreceptors. Neuroscience 69: 249–257.
14. DEAN, C. & J.L. SEAGARD. 1997. Mapping of carotid baroreceptor subtypes projections to the nucleus tractus solitarius using c-fos immunohistochemistry. Brain Res. 758: 201–208.
15. SEAGARD, J.L., J.F.M. VAN BREDERODE, C. Dean, et al. 1990. Firing characteristics of single-fiber carotid sinus baroreceptors. Circ. Res. 66: 1499–1509.
16. LIPSKI, J., R.M. MCALLEN & K.M. SPYER. 1975. The sinus nerve and baroreceptor input to the medulla of the cat. J. Physiol. (London) 251: 61–78.
17. HAYWARD, L.F. & R.B. FELDER. 1995. Cardiac rhythmicity among NTS neurons and its relationship to sympathetic outflow in rabbits. Am. J. Physiol. 269: H923–H933.
18. SEAGARD, J.L., C. DEAN & F.A. HOPP. 1995. Discharge patterns of baroreceptor-modulated neurons in the nucleus tractus solitarius. Neurosci. Lett. 191: 13–18.
19. SEAGARD, J.L., C. DEAN & F.A. HOPP. 1999. Role of glutamate receptors in transmission of vagal cardiac input to neurones in the nucleus tractus solitarius. J. Physiol. 520.1: 243–253.

20. COLERIDGE, H.M., J.C.G. COLERIDGE & C. KIDD. 1964. Cardiac receptors in the dog, with particular reference to two types of afferent endings in the ventricular wall. J. Physiol. **174:** 323–339.
21. GUPTA, B.N. & M.D. THAMES. 1983. Behavior of left ventricular mechanoreceptors with myelinated and nonmyelinated afferent vagal fibers in cats. Circ. Res. **52:** 291–301.
22. ANDRESEN, M.C. & M. YANG. 1990. Non-NMDA receptors mediate sensory afferent synaptic transmission in medial nucleus tractus solitarius. Am. J. Physiol. (Heart Circ. Physiol.) **259**(8): H1307–H1311.
23. MEELEY, M.P., M.D. UNDERWOOD, W.T. TALMAN & D.J. REIS. 1989. Content and in vitro release of endogenous amino acids in the area of the nucleus of the solitary tract of the rat. J. Neurochem. **53:** 1807–1817.
24. OHTA, H. & W.T. TALMAN. 1994. Both NMDA and non-NMDA receptors in the NTS participate in the baroreceptor reflex in rats. Am. J. Physiol. **267:** R1065–R1070.
25. ZHANG, J. & S.W. MIFFLIN. 1998. Differential roles for NMDA and non-NMDA receptor subtypes in baroreceptor afferent integration in the nucleus of the solitary tract of the rat. J. Physiol. **511.3:** 733–745.
26. AYLWIN, M.L., J.M. HOROWITZ & A.C. BONHAM. 1997. NMDA receptors contribute to primary visceral afferent transmission in the nucleus of the solitary tract. J. Neurophysiol. **77:** 2539–2548.
27. CHEN, C-Y. & A.C. BONHAM. 1998. Non-NMDA and NMDA receptors transmit area postrema input to aortic baroreceptor neurons in NTS. Am. J. Physiol. (Heart Circ. Physiol.) **275:** H1695–H1702.
28. MILLER, B.D. & R.D. FELDER. 1988. Excitatory amino acid receptors intrinsic to synaptic transmission in nucleus tractus solitarii. Brain Res. **456:** 333–343.
29. DREWE, J.A., R. MILES & D.L. KUNZE. 1990. Excitatory amino acid receptors of guinea pig medial nucleus tractus solitarius neurons. Am. J. Physiol. (Heart Circ. Physiol.) **259**(28): H1389–H1395.
30. NAKAGAWA, T., T. SHIRASAKI, N. TATEISHI, *et al.* 1990. Effects of antagonists on N-methyl-D-aspartate response in acutely isolated nucleus tractus solitarii neurons of the rat. Neurosci. Lett. **113:** 169–174.
31. GLAUM, S.R. & R.J. MILLER. 1992. Metabotropic glutamate receptors mediate excitatory transmission in the nucleus of the solitary tract. J. Neurosci. **12:** 2251–2258.
32. PAWLOSKI-DAHM, C. & F.J. GORDON. 1992. Evidence for a kynurenate-insensitive glutamate receptor in nucleus tractus solitarii. Am. J. Physiol. **262:** H1611–H1615.
33. FOLEY, C.M., H.W. VOGL, P.J. MUELLER, *et al.* 1999. Cardiovascular response to group I metabotropic glutamate receptor activation in NTS. Am. J. Physiol. **276:** R1469–R1478.
34. FOLEY, C.M., J.A. MOFFITT, M. HAY & E.M. HASSER. 1998. Glutamate in the nucleus of the solitary tract activates both ionotropic and metabotropic glutamate receptors. Am. J. Physiol. **275:** R1858–R1866.
35. SEAGARD, J.L., C. DEAN & F.A. HOPP. 2000. Neurochemical transmission of baroreceptor input in the NTS. Brain Res. Bull. **51:** 111–118.
36. SEAGARD, J.L., C. DEAN & F.A. HOPP. 1997. Glutamate receptor subtypes involved in transmission of baroreceptor input to NTS neurons. Soc. Neurosci. Abstr. **23:**722.
37. MIFFLIN, S.W. & R.B. FELDER. 1990. Synaptic mechanisms regulating cardiovascular afferent inputs to solitary tract nucleus. Am. J. Physiol. (Heart Circ. Physiol.) **259**(28):H653–H661.
38. BASHIR, Z, S. ALFORD, S. DAVIES, *et al.* 1991. Long-term potentiation of NMDA receptor–mediated synpatic transmission in the hippocampus. Nature 349: 156–158.
39. XIE, X., T. BERGER, & G. BARRIONUEVO. 1992. Isolated NMDA receptor–mediated synaptic responses express both LTP and LTD. J. Neurophysiol. **67:** 1009–1013.
40. OTIS, T.S., S. ZHANG & L.O. TRUSSEL. 1996. Direct measurement of AMPA receptor desensitization induced by glutamatergic synaptic transmission. J. Neurosci. **16:** 7496–7504.
41. KIRKWOOD, A., S. DUDEK, J. GOLD, *et al.* 1993. Common forms of synaptic plasticity in the hippocampus and neocortex in vitro. Science **260:** 1518–1521.

42. MAMMEN, A.T. & R.L. HUGANIR. 1997. Regulation of NMDA receptors by protein phosphorylation. *In* The Inotropic Glutamate Receptors. D.T. Monaghan & R.J. Wenthold, Eds.: 135–148. Humana Press. Totowa, NJ.
43. MIFFLIN, S.W. 1997. Short-term potentiation of carotid sinus nerve inputs to neurons in the nucleus of the solitary tract. Respir. Physiol. **110:**2 29–236.
44. FELDER, R.B. & S.W. MIFFLIN. 1993. Baroreceptor and chemoreceptor afferent processing in the solitary tract nucleus. *In* Nucleus of the Solitary Tract. I.R.A. Barraco, Ed.: 169–186. CRC Press. Boca Raton, FL.

# Response Properties of Baroreceptive NTS Neurons

JULIAN F. R. PATON,[a] YU-WEN LI,[b] AND JAMES S. SCHWABER[c]

[a]Department of Physiology, School of Medical Sciences, University of Bristol, Bristol BS8 1TD, UK

[b]CNS Diseases Research, DuPont Pharmaceuticals Company, G-009, 500 S. Ridgeway Avenue, Glenolden, Pennsylvania 19036, USA

[c]Department of Pathology, Anatomy, and Cell Biology, Thomas Jefferson Medical School, Philadelphia, Pennsylvania 19107, USA

ABSTRACT: Neurons in the nucleus of the solitary tract (NTS) responding to activation of arterial baroreceptors were recorded intracellularly using patch pipettes in an *in situ* arterially perfused working heart–brain stem preparation of rat. Seven of 15 (i.e., 46%) of NTS neurons showed adaptive (nonlinear) excitatory synaptic response patterns during baroreceptor stimulation followed by an "evoked hyperpolarization." This evoked hyperpolarization was stimulus intensity dependent and capable of shunting out a subsequent baroreceptor input. We suggest that this adaptive response behavior may be mediated, in part, by calcium-dependent potassium currents ($IK_{Ca}$) since neurons showed spike frequency adaptation during step depolarizations and an after-hyperpolarization after repetitive firing. Furthermore, in *in vivo* anesthetized rats, NTS microinjections of either charybdotoxin (225 fmol) or apamin (4.5 pmol) to block $IK_{Ca}$ increased the baroreceptor reflex gain. Our data purport that the responsiveness of baroreceptive NTS neurons can be regulated by intrinsic membrane conductances such as $IK_{Ca}$. Modulation of such conductances during either physiological (exercise) or pathophysiological (essential hypertension) conditions may lead to changes in both the operating point and gain of the baroreceptor reflex.

KEYWORDS: Carotid sinus; Calcium-dependent potassium currents; Charybdotoxin; Apamin; $GABA_A$ receptors

## INTRODUCTION

The petrosal and nodose baroreceptor afferent neurons project to the nucleus of the solitary tract (NTS), where they terminate at rostrocaudal levels corresponding to area postrema in both dorsal and dorsomedial subdivisions (for recent review, see Ref. 1). The neurons innervated by primary baroreceptor afferents (i.e., second-order neurons) may play a major role in governing the sensitivity and operating point of the arterial baroreceptor reflex. Since this changes during both physiological (e.g.,

Address for correspondence: Julian F. R. Paton, Department of Physiology, School of Medical Sciences, University of Bristol, Bristol BS8 1TD, UK. Voice: 44-(0)-117-928-7818; fax: 44-(0)-117-928-8923.

Julian.F.R.Paton@Bristol.ac.uk

exercise) and pathological-disease states (i.e., essential hypertension), an understanding of the factors controlling the excitability of baroreceptive NTS neurons is pivotal for revealing plausible mechanisms underlying reflex resetting.

It is generally accepted that the excitability of NTS neurons responding to baroreceptor inputs is tightly regulated such that these neurons rarely show pulse modulation on a beat-by-beat basis in a range of species.[2–6] We reported previously that stimulation of arterial baroreceptors by raising systemic pressure produced a nonlinear firing response in some neurons recorded extracellulary from the nucleus of the solitary tract (NTS) of the *in vivo* anesthetized rat.[6,7] These neurons exhibited a maximal firing response during the rising phase of a pressure stimulus; the discharge frequency then became reduced as the peak of the pressor stimulus was reached. We termed this response pattern-*adaptive*. Other studies revealed a comparable pattern.[2,8,9] The mechanism(s) underlying this adaptive behaviour could be important for controlling reflex sensitivity. Thus, the present study sought to determine plausible mechanisms, both intrinsic and synaptic, that may account for the nonlinear behavior of adaptive baroreceptive NTS neurons[10] in an arterially perfused preparation and in anesthetized *in vivo* rats.

## TECHNIQUES EMPLOYED TO STUDY THE BAROREFLEX AND BARORECEPTIVE NTS NEURONS

### In Vivo *Experiments*

Rats (Sprague Dawley, 220–270 g) were anesthetized with α-chloralose-urethane-pentobarbital mixture (69, 690, and 30 mg/kg, respectively[11]) and the arterial baroreceptor reflex stimulated by raising systemic pressure with phenylephrine (1–3 μg bolus i.v.). Multibarreled microelectrodes (tip diameter 35–40 μm) were placed into the caudal NTS for 45 nL pressure injections of calcium-dependent potassium channel blockers (apamin, 100 μM; charybdotoxin, 5 μM) and pontamine sky blue dye (2%) to mark injection sites. Injection sites were histologically verified and located in areas dorsal and medial to the solitary tract at the level of the area postrema.

### In Situ *Studies*

We applied whole-cell intracellular recording techniques with patch pipettes to the NTS while activating arterial baroreceptors with physiological pressure stimuli in an *in situ* arterially perfused working heart–brain stem preparation (WHBP) of rat. This approach has helped in circumventing the technical problems relating to small neuronal size and mechanical instability of the brain stem. This preparation was developed by us[12] to study NTS neurons responding to visceral afferent inputs such as peripheral chemoreceptors,[13] abdominal vagal afferents,[14] and pharyngoesophageal receptors[15] using whole-cell patch pipettes. This is possible *in situ* since cardiac pulsing is reduced, thereby enhancing mechanical stability of the brain stem.

WHBPs of mature rats (Sprague-Dawley; 90–140 g) was based on techniques described originally in mice.[12] Preparations were perfused via the left ventricle with a Ringer's solution containing 2.2% dextran at 31°C. Arterial baroreceptors were stimulated by either distending the aortic arch with a balloon-tipped catheter, inserted retrogradely via the descending aorta, and/or by inflation of the ipsilateral carotid sinus using injections of perfusate via one lumen of a double-lumen cannula placed into the common carotid artery. The second lumen of this cannula was used to monitor pressure. Note the carotid sinus was perfused continuously via a separate circuit to ensure viability of the carotid sinus. Freshly carbogenated perfusate was injected into the sinus to avoid coactivation of carotid body chemoreceptors. Preparations were paralyzed using vecuronium bromide (0.04 μg/mL), which does not interrupt vagal efferent traffic to the heart. The NTS was exposed by peeling away the dorsal column nuclei using fine watchmaker's forceps. This had no effect on the baroreceptor reflex gain. Once exposed, the solitary tract was clearly visible and stimulated electrically using a bipolar tungsten steel microelectrode distanced 2–2.5 mm from the recording site. This technique was adopted to assess whether NTS neurons received relatively direct or indirect synaptic inputs from primary afferent fibers. Neurons were recorded with patch pipettes (4–6 MΩ) that were filled with (in mM): 140 K gluconate, 10 Hepes, 0.2 EGTA, 7.7 NaCl, 0.05 cAMP, 4 MgATP, 0.5 GTP. In some experiments the patch pipette contained 0.5% neurobiotin for intracellular labeling. Patch pipettes were pressurized (40–60 mmHg) and advanced into the NTS. Current pulses were delivered (1 Hz) and changes in input resistance measured continuously as the pipette approached a neuron. This was evident from an increase in input resistance. At this time intrapipette pressure was reduced and a gigohm seal formed. Access to the cell was made with negative pressure.

## ELECTROPHYSIOLOGICAL PROPERTIES OF BARORECEPTIVE NTS NEURONS

In 15 baroreceptive NTS neurons resting membrane potential was −54 ± 1 mV, and membrane input resistance was 198 ± 13 MΩ (mean ± SEM.). Recordings lasted for up to 25 minutes. Of these 15 neurons 12 had ongoing discharge (2.8 ± 0.7 Hz) and were driven by excitatory postsynaptic potentials (EPSPs); there was no sign of autoactive firing behavior (i.e., intrinsically active or pacemaker-like) as reported in some NTS neurons *in vitro*.[16] Action potential height was 62 ± 4.2 mV, and its duration at half action potential height was 1.46 ± 0.4 ms. After-hyperpolarizations following a single action potential were small when measurable (i.e., 1.7 ± 2.33 mV). Electrical stimulation of the ipsilateral solitary tract evoked an EPSP and/or spike (latency: 4.2 ± 0.4 ms; *n* = 6). Increases in pressure within either the aortic arch or ipsilateral carotid sinus evoked an increase in the frequency of fast EPSPs that summated, leading to action potential generation in most cases.

## LOCATION AND MORPHOLOGY OF BARORECEPTIVE NTS NEURONS

The location, morphology, and axonal projection of typical baroreceptive neurons were described previously by us (see Ref. 17 for details). We found that somata of labeled baroreceptive NTS neurons had dimensions of 26 × 14 μm and contained 3–8 primary dendrites. They were located in dorsal, dorsomedial, and medial regions of the NTS at rostrocaudal levels from the commissural subdivision to the rostralmost point of the area postrema. These neurons projected both locally within the

NTS but also to the ventrolateral medulla. Axons were mostly unmyelinated with boutons of the en passant variety. These labeled neurons received a short, invariant synaptic excitatory response following activation of the solitary tract at a latency of $3.95 \pm 0.3$ ms (at $31°C$; $n = 6$), indicative of a relatively direct synaptic contact from primary afferent fibers. Overall, baroreceptive NTS neurons showed no consistent morphological characteristics and were heterogeneous.

## SYNAPTIC RESPONSE PATTERNS OF BARORECEPTIVE NTS NEURONS

Three firing patterns of response were found and included adaptive (FIG. 1A), nonadaptive (FIG. 1B), and prolonged excitatory responses. The adaptive pattern was found in approximately 46% of baroreceptive neurons studied. The properties of adaptive baroreceptive neurons are described below.

### Characteristics of the Adaptive Response to Increases in Carotid Sinus Pressure

It was possible to closely examine the firing response and membrane potential trajectories of adaptive baroreceptive NTS neurons ($n = 7$) during ramp increases in ipsilateral carotid sinus pressure. The pattern of response evoked consisted of either an increase in amplitude and frequency of EPSPs or spiking as pressure was elevated. However, during the pressure excursion, EPSPs/firing reached a maximum and decreased as pressure continued to rise (FIG. 1A). After cessation of the baroreceptor

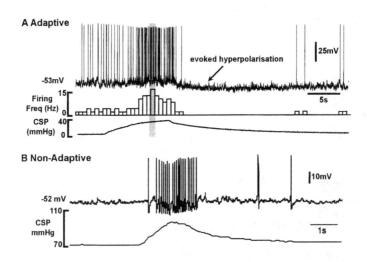

**FIGURE 1.** Baroreceptive NTS neurons exhibited adaptive (**A**) and nonadaptive (**B**) firing responses to baroreceptor stimulation evoked by increasing ipsilateral carotid sinus pressure in the WHBP. The adaptive response was characterized by the peak firing response occurring during the rising phase of the pressure stimulus and not its peak. The adaptive response was followed by a hyperpolarization (termed *evoked hyperpolarization*; see text).

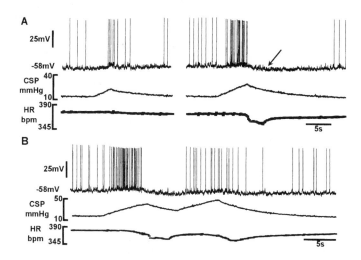

**FIGURE 2.** (**A**) shows that the magnitude and duration of the evoked hyperpolarization was stimulus intensity dependent. Note that a baroreceptor-evoked excitatory synaptic response failed if it was timed to be coincident with the evoked hyperpolarization (**B**). Thus, the evoked hyperpolarization was functionally capable of shunting repeated inputs.

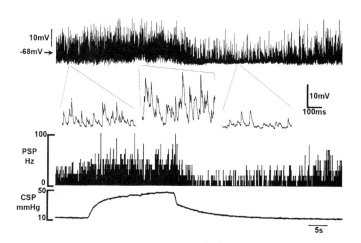

**FIGURE 3.** A mechanism to explain the evoked hyperpolarization in adaptive baroreceptive NTS neurons is disfacilitation. This baroreceptive NTS neuron was hyperpolarized relative to resting membrane potential to prevent spiking. Ipsilateral carotid sinus pressure was elevated and evoked an increase in the frequency and amplitude of EPSPs. Note that during the evoked hyperpolarization, there was a reduction in the frequency and amplitude of PSPs.

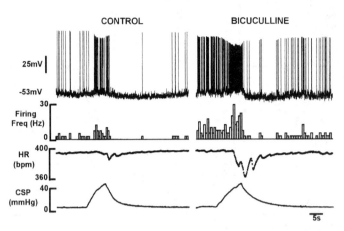

**FIGURE 4.** Both ongoing firing and the evoked excitatory response of a baroreceptive adaptive NTS neuron were elevated after blockade of $GABA_A$ receptors. However, the evoked hyperpolarization persisted.

stimulus the membrane potential hyperpolarized by $5.0 \pm 1$ mV below resting membrane potential, and there was a reduction in ongoing EPSPs that lasted 10–15 s (FIGS. 1A, 2A); we term this an *evoked hyperpolarization*. The magnitude and duration of both the excitatory synaptic response and the evoked hyperpolarization were dependent upon the intensity and/or duration of the pressure stimulus (FIG. 2A). Further, repeated activation of baroreceptors coincident with the evoked hyperpolarization resulted in a greatly reduced excitatory synaptic effect (FIG. 2B). FIGURE 3 shows that the evoked hyperpolarization was associated with a reduction in the amplitude of PSPs; this may indicate a reflexly induced disfacilitation in adaptive baroreceptive neurons.

### Role of GABA_A Receptors for Mediating the Evoked Hyperpolarization

There are a number of possible mechanisms that could account for the evoked hyperpolarization. We tested the role of $GABA_A$ receptors by applying bicuculline focally around the patch pipette using a perfusable well device as described previously.[18] As FIGURE 4 shows, the post-excitatory hyperpolarization was resistant to $GABA_A$ receptor blockade. However, FIGURE 4 does indicate that, following blockade of $GABA_A$ receptors, both the basal firing discharge and the response to an increase in carotid sinus pressure were increased.

### Role of Intrinsic Membrane Properties

Injection of positive current in adaptive baroreceptive neurons led to spike frequency adaptation (FIG. 5). At the end of the injection of current and repetitive firing there was a marked after-hyperpolarization of $4.8 \pm 1$ mV lasting up to 1–2 s (FIG. 5); this was considerably shorter than the evoked hyperpolarization observed after a baroreceptor stimulus (10–15 s; see above). Both the spike frequency adaptation and

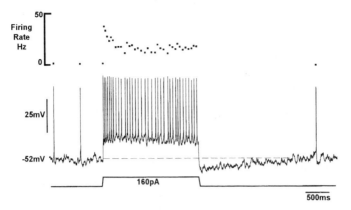

**FIGURE 5.** Adaptive baroreceptive NTS neurons exhibit spike frequency adaptation to depolarizing current injection and an after-hyperpolarization. This cell is the same as that in FIG. 2A.

the after-hyperpolarization following repetitive firing are consistent with activation of a calcium-dependent potassium channel(s).

## Effect of Blocking Calcium-Dependent Potassium Channels in the NTS on the Baroreflex *in* Vivo

Calcium-dependent potassium conductances (both SK and BK types) are found in some NTS neurons *in vitro* (see Refs. 19–21). Their blockade increased the firing response and excitability of neurons. Thus, could blockade of calcium-dependent potassium channels in NTS alter the gain of the baroreceptor reflex? In *in vivo* anesthetized rats, bilateral microinjection of either apamin (4.5 pmol) or charybdotoxin (225 fmol), selective calcium-dependent potassium channel antagonists of the SK and BK type conductances, respectively, potentiated significantly the baroreceptor reflex-mediated vagal bradycardia by approximately 50% (FIG. 6; $n = 6$; $p < 0.05$; see Ref. 11).

## The Origin of Ongoing Excitatory Postsynaptic Potentials

We noted that fast EPSPs continuously bombarded many adaptive baroreceptive NTS neurons (FIGS. 3 and 7). In three cells membrane input resistance was relatively low, measuring 170, 174, and 190 MΩ. To assess the role of baroreceptor afferent activity in contributing to this pronounced excitatory synaptic input we lowered systemic arterial pressure by ~20 mmHg. We found that the amplitude of incoming EPSPs was reduced as arterial pressure was lowered (FIG. 7). Further, neurons became hyperpolarized (~3 mV) at reduced perfusion pressure levels (FIG. 7). Thus, membrane potential and the amount of excitatory synaptic drive is partly dependent on the level of baroreceptor afferent input and therefore the absolute level of arterial pressure in adaptive neurons.

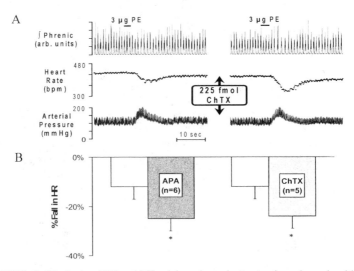

**FIGURE 6.** Blockade of SK and BK calcium-dependent potassium channels with apamin (APA) and charybdotoxin (ChTX) potentiates the bradycardic component of the baroreceptor reflex *in vivo*. (**A**) shows the reflex response in integrated phrenic nerve activity and heart rate to a phenylephrine-induced pressor effect before and after ChTX microinjection into the NTS. Below (**B**) indicates the baroreflex bradycardic response as a percentage of baseline heart rate in control (*open bars*) and after bilateral microinjection of calcium-dependent potassium channel blockers. (Data from Butcher & Paton,[11] used with permission.)

## DISCUSSION

We report that a substantial number of baroreceptive NTS neurons exhibit a nonlinear, adaptive firing response to ramp increases in pressure within the ipsilateral carotid sinus. Our data indirectly support the notion that adaptive baroreceptive NTS neurons exhibit intrinsic membrane conductances, such as calcium-dependent potassium currents, which could contribute to this nonlinear, adaptive behavior.

### The WHBP as a Model for Studying Baroreceptor Control

The WHBP permitted us to make the first whole-cell recording of baroreceptive NTS neurons as defined by their response to increases in arterial pressure within barosensitive sites. We acknowledge that pulsatile pressure would more accurately mimic a physiological stimulus. The short latency synaptic response evoked following electrical stimulation of the solitary tract indicates a relatively direct input from primary afferents.

### Are the Properties of Baroreceptive NTS Neurons Unique?

Recently, we provided the first morphological details and axonal projection data of baroreceptive NTS neurons in the rat (see Ref. 17). Baroreceptive neuron morphology was heterogeneous and was not distinct from neurons receiving peripheral

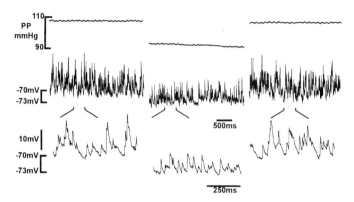

**FIGURE 7.** To determine whether the contribution of the ongoing PSPs in adaptive baroreceptive neurons was dependent on baroreceptor afferent input, these receptors were unloaded. Reducing perfusion pressure by approximately 20 mmHg reversibly reduced the amplitude of ongoing PSPs.

chemo-, pharyngoesophageal, or gastrointestinal receptor inputs.[13,14] Moreover, from our data the electrical properties (input resistance, response patterns to injected current) of baroreceptive neurons were not unique.[13,14,17]

Three distinct patterns of response to pressure stimuli were found, which included adaptive, nonadaptive, and prolonged excitation. These patterns may relate to their output targets such as vagal or sympathetic circuitry. Regarding the adaptive pattern, a possibility is that this response profile reflects adaptation of the baroreceptor afferents themselves. However, this is unlikely: (1) the time period in which we raised pressure is too short for baroreceptor adaptation; (2) we found neurons that did not adapt but showed a more linear encoding of the pressure signal over similar stimulation periods.

### Mechanisms Underlying the Adaptive Nature of NTS Baroreceptive Neurons

Unearthing the adaptive pattern of response of baroreceptive neurons may allow a greater understanding of the neuronal machinery governing reflex gain and operating point. There are a number of mechanisms that could contribute to this response. First, neurons displaying the adaptive property also showed spike frequency adaptation to constant current injection. This firing response has been associated with calcium-dependent potassium currents, which can be blocked by apamin and charybdotoxin.[19–21] This current limits the rate of firing of neurons and hence their responsiveness to incoming excitatory synaptic drive. Thus, blockade of this current would be expected to increase baroreflex performance. From our *in vivo* data this was the case: both charybdotoxin and apamin, calcium-dependent potassium channel antagonists, microinjected into the NTS augmented the baroreflex gain (see FIG. 6 and Ref. 11). Second, following the neuronal excitatory synaptic response to a baroreceptor stimulus, there was an evoked hyperpolarization. Its magnitude and duration were dependent upon the intensity of the pressure stimulus and therefore the degree of depolarization and calcium ion entry. Its function may act as a filter to dampen incoming excitatory baroreceptor drive and loss of the beat-by-beat neural energy characteristic of the primary afferents.

The mechanism for this evoked hyperpolarization is unknown but may in part reflect the slow time course of inactivation of a calcium-dependent potassium current. We emphasise that this may be only one contributing factor, since the after-hyperpolarization that followed repetitive firing (during current injection) lasted 1–2 s, whereas the evoked hyperpolarization following the baroreceptor evoked excitatory response lasted 10–15 s (compare FIGS. 1A and 2A with FIG. 5). The evoked hyperpolarization was powerful enough to shunt the excitatory response following a second baroreceptor challenge (FIG. 2B). Despite differences in the time interval, the latter finding has parallels to the frequency-dependent depression of synaptic input where paired electrical pulse stimulation was used.[22,23] In the latter studies the second evoked EPSP was attenuated relative to the first. We suggest that activation of calcium-dependent potassium currents could contribute to frequency-dependent depression in the NTS.

In addition to a slow time course of inactivation of a calcium-dependent potassium current, another possibility for the evoked hyperpolarization is disfacilitation as manifested via recurrent inputs. We found that there was a reduction in both the number and amplitude of EPSPs during the evoked hyperpolarization (FIG. 3). Alternatively, the evoked hyperpolarization may be due to evoked inhibitory synaptic feedback. We tested this by applying bicuculline to assess a role for $GABA_A$ receptors, but this was without effect. The possibility that the evoked hyperpolarization is in part mediated by $GABA_B$ or glycine receptors remains to be tested.

### Ongoing PSPs in Baroreceptive NTS Neurons: Relevance to Membrane Input Resistance

It is clear from FIGURES 3 and 7 that adaptive baroreceptive neurons are being bombarded by synaptic potentials below the threshold to induce action potentials. We attempted to determine whether these PSPs were of peripheral origin from arterial baroreceptors by reducing systemic pressure. Unloading baroreceptors reduced the magnitude of synaptic events arriving at the postsynaptic membrane of baroreceptive neurons. Since these were summated events, a reduction in magnitude may also reflect a decrease in number of PSPs. Thus, an origin for these synaptic inputs is the activity of the arterial baroreceptor afferents themselves. From our data, these ongoing PSPs may contain both IPSPs and EPSPs. However, ongoing IPSPs were difficult to see, and this may be due to the closeness of their reversal potential to resting membrane potential. Nevertheless, focal administration of bicuculline elevated both the ongoing activity and the responsiveness of neurons, suggesting a tonic $GABA_A$ receptor–mediated input (FIG. 4).

The presence of such high levels of PSP activity may account for the relatively low input resistance or high conductance state of the membranes in these adaptive baroreceptive neurons. Indeed, as baroreceptor afferent activity increases, so does input resistance fall (due to the greater arrival of EPSPs increasing the conductance state of the membrane) and the neuron becomes, paradoxically, less responsive. This intrinsic mechanism may also contribute to shunting incoming excitatory afferent inputs in dendrites and thus contribute to their adaptive behavior. It may provide a protective mechanism in neurons that receive high amounts of peripheral activity, thus preventing neurons from becoming overactive and energy depleted.

## CONCLUSIONS

The NTS provides a powerful site for modulation of the baroreceptor reflex. This study has emphasized the importance of intrinsic membrane conductances and input resistance of baroreceptive NTS neurons in governing their response patterns to incoming baroreceptor signals. Charybdotoxin and apamin enhanced baroreceptor reflex gain, and this suggests that both BK and SK conductances are involved. Modulation of these channels via G protein–coupled receptors may be important in controlling both the operating point and gain of the baroreceptor reflex in health and disease.

## ACKNOWLEDGMENTS

The financial support of the BBSRC (24/S11296), British Heart Foundation (BS 93003), E.I. Du Pont, NATO, and The Wellcome Trust (044994) is acknowledged.

## REFERENCES

1. BLESSING, W.W. 1997. Anatomy of the lower brainstem. *In* The Lower Brainstem and Bodily Homeostasis: 29–99. Oxford University Press. New York.
2. LIPSKI, J., R.M. MCALLEN & K.M. SPYER. 1975. The sinus nerve and baroreceptor input the medulla of the cat. J. Physiol. **251:** 61–78.
3. LIPSKI, J., R.M. MCALLEN & A. TRZEBSKI. 1976. Carotid baroreceptor and chemoreceptor inputs onto single medullary neurons. Brain Res. **107:** 133–136.
4. MIFFLIN, S.W. & R.B. FELDER. 1990. Synaptic mechanisms regulating cardiovascular afferent inputs to solitary tract nucleus. Am. J. Physiol. **259:** H653–H661.
5. PATON, J.F.R., L. SILVA-CARVALHO, G.E. GOLDSMITH & K.M. SPYER. 1990. Inhibition of barosensitive neurones evoked by lobule IXb of the posterior cerebellar cortex in the decerebrate rabbit. J. Physiol. **427:** 553–565.
6. ROGERS, R.F., J.F.R. PATON & J.S. SCHWABER. 1993. NTS neuronal responses to arterial pressure and pressure changes in the rat. Am. J. Physiol. **265:** R1355–R1368.
7. ROGERS, R.F., W.C. ROSE & J.S. SCHWABER. 1996. Simultaneous encoding of carotid sinus pressure and dP/dt by NTS target neurons of myelinated baroreceptors. J. Neurophysiol. **76:** 2644–2660.
8. LIPSKI, J. & A. TRZEBSKI 1975. Bulbo-spinal neurons activated by baroreceptor afferents and their possible role in inhibition of preganglionic sympathetic neurons. Pflüg. Arch. **356:** 181–192.
9. SEAGARD, J.L., C. DEAN & F.A. HOPP. 1995. Discharge patterns of baroreceptor modulated neurons in the nucleus tractus solitarius. Neurosci. Lett. **191:** 13–18.
10. PATON, J.F.R., Y-W. LI, J.S. SCHWABER & S. KASPAROV. 1998. Whole cell recordings and response properties of baroreceptive neurones located in the solitary tract nucleus of a working heart-brainstem preparation of mature rat. J. Physiol. **513.P:** 78P.
11. BUTCHER, J.W. & J.F.R. PATON. 1998. $K^+$ channel blockade in the NTS alters efficacy of two cardiorespiratory reflexes *in vivo.* Am. J. Physiol. **274:** R677–R685.
12. PATON, J.F.R. 1996. A working heart-brainstem preparation of the mouse. J. Neurosci. Meth. **65:** 63–68.

13. DEUCHARS, J., Y.-W. LI, S. KASPAROV & J.F.R. PATON. 2000. Morphology of neurones in the nucleus tractus solitarius (NTS) of the rat receiving afferent input from peripheral arterial chemoreceptors. J. Physiol. **523.P:** 265P.
14. PATON J.F.R , Y-W. LI, J. DEUCHARS & S. KASPAROV. 2000. Properties of solitary tract neurones receiving inputs from the sub-diaphragmatic vagus nerve. Neuroscience **95:** 141–153.
15. PATON, J.F.R., Y-W. LI & S. KASPAROV. 1999. Reflex response and convergence of pharyngoesophageal and peripheral chemo-receptors in the nucleus of the solitary tract. Neuroscience **93:** 143–154.
16. PATON, J.F.R., W.T. ROGERS & J.S. SCHWABER. 1991. Tonically rhythmic neurones within a cardiorespiratory region of the nucleus tractus solitarii of the rat. J. Neurophysiol. **66:** 824–838.
17. DEUCHARS, J., Y-W. LI, S. KASPAROV & J.F.R. PATON. 2000. Morphological and electrophysiological properties of physiologically characterised baroreceptive neurones in the dorsal vagal complex of the rat. J. Comp. Neurol. **417:** 233–249.
18. PATON, J.F.R. 1998. Importance of neurokinin-1 receptors in the nucleus tractus solitarii of mice for the integration of cardiac vagal inputs. Eur. J. Neurosci. **10:** 2261–2275.
19. BUTCHER, J.W., S. KASPAROV & J.F.R. PATON 1999. Differential effects of apamin on neuronal excitability in the nucleus tractus solitarius studied *in vitro*. J. Auton. Nerv. Sys. **77:** 90–97
20. MOAK, J.P. & D. KUNZE. 1993. Potassium currents of neurons isolated from the medial nucleus tractus solitarius. Am. J. Physiol. **265:** 1596–1602.
21. PATON, J.F.R., W.R. FOSTER & J.S. SCHWABER 1993. Characteristic firing behavior of cell types in the cardiorespiratory region of the nucleus tractus solitarii of the rat. Brain Res. **604:** 112–125.
22. MIFFLIN, S.W. & R.B. FELDER. 1988. An intracellular study of time dependent cardiovascular afferent interactions in nucleus tractus solitarius. J. Neurophysiol. **59:** 1798–1813.
23. MILES, R. 1986. Frequency dependence of synaptic transmission in nucleus of the solitary tract. J. Neurophysiol. **55:** 1076–1090.

# Nitroxidergic Influences on Cardiovascular Control by NTS: A Link with Glutamate

WILLIAM T. TALMAN, DEIDRE NITSCHKE DRAGON, HISASHI OHTA, AND LI-HSIEN LIN

*Laboratory of Neurobiology, Department of Neurology and Neuroscience Program, University of Iowa and Department of Veterans Affairs Medical Center, Iowa City, Iowa 52242, USA*

ABSTRACT: Glutamate (GLU) receptor activation, which is important in cardiovascular reflex transmission through the nucleus tractus solitarii (NTS), leads to release of nitric oxide (NO·) from central nitroxidergic neurons. Therefore, we hypothesized that GLU and NO· are linked in cardiovascular control by NTS. We first sought to determine if NO· released into NTS led to cardiovascular changes like those produced by GLU and found that the nitrosothiol S-nitrosocysteine, but not NO· itself or other NO· donors, elicited such responses in anesthetized rats. The responses were dependent on activation of soluble guanylate cyclase but, not being affected by a scavenger of NO·, likely did not depend on release of NO· into the extracellular space. Responses to ionotropic GLU agonists in NTS, like those to S-nitrosocysteine, were inhibited by inhibition of soluble guanylate cyclase. Inhibition of neuronal NO· synthase (nNOS) also inhibited responses to ionotropic GLU agonists. The apparent physiologic link between GLU and NO· mechanisms in NTS was further supported by anatomical studies that demonstrated frequent association between GLU-containing nerve terminals and neurons containing nNOS. Furthermore, GLU receptors were often found on NTS neurons that were immunoreactive for nNOS. The anatomical relationships between GLU and nNOS and GLU receptors and nNOS were more pronounced in some subnuclei of NTS than in others. While seen in subnuclei that are known to receive cardiovascular afferents, the association was even more prominent in subnuclei that receive gastrointestinal afferents. These studies support a role for nitroxidergic neurons in mediating cardiovascular and other visceral reflex responses that result from release of GLU into the NTS.

KEYWORDS: Baroreceptor; Blood pressure; Cardiovascular; Confocal microscopy; Glutamate; Heart rate; Immunohistochemistry; Nitric oxide; Nitric oxide synthase; NMDA; Nucleus tractus solitarii; Receptor

## INTRODUCTION

The nucleus tractus solitarii (NTS) is the primary site of termination of cardiovascular and visceral afferent fibers of the vagus and glossopharyngeal nerves.[1–3] As such it plays a critical role in regulation of blood pressure and peripheral blood flow.

Address for correspondence: William T. Talman, M.D., Department of Neurology, University of Iowa, Iowa City, IA 52242. Voice: 319-356-8750; fax: 319-356-4505.
william-talman@uiowa.edu

Stimulation of NTS leads to marked changes in arterial blood pressure and regional blood flow,[4,5] while lesions lead to acute hypertension in humans[6] as well as in experimental animals.[7,8]

Numerous studies have suggested that glutamate (GLU) is a neurotransmitter released from cardiovascular afferent terminals in NTS,[9] and others have suggested that nitric oxide (NO·) may similarly participate in central cardiovascular control by the NTS.[10] This review will focus on our own studies and those from other laboratories that have sought to establish whether there is a link between glutamatergic and nitroxidergic neurons in NTS.

Garthwaite first identified potential relationships between actions of GLU and NO·. Activation of GLU receptors in brain was shown to lead to synthesis and release of NO·.[11,12] Therefore, GLU might act through these effects on NO· synthesis and release to activate soluble guanylate cyclase and increase cyclic GMP, which might, in turn, contribute to cellular responses to GLU itself.[13,14] Some responses to GLU may depend on the link to NO· synthesis. For example, destruction of GLU receptors eliminates activation of soluble guanylate cyclase by GLU, even though the same neuronal pools of the enzyme could still be activated by an NO· donor acting "downstream" of the GLU receptor.[13] Although influences of NMDA receptor activation on NO· production were described first, it is now clear that kainate, metabotropic (ACPD responsive), and $\alpha$-amino-3-hydroxy-5-methylisoxozole-proprionic acid (AMPA) receptor agonists have similar influences on production of NO·.[15–18] On the other hand, antagonists of GLU receptors may themselves effect release of NO·;[19] and in some systems, NO·, which may act presynaptically as well as postsynaptically,[20,21] may provide a feedback mechanism influencing release of GLU.[22]

Thus, GLU and NO· may produce integrated responses in the brain. The two compounds may jointly play a role in such critical activities as long-term potentiation in the hippocampus[23] and long-term depression in the cerebellum.[24] While little is known of the physiological significance of their joint actions within the NTS, some studies now suggest that NO· release also may be linked with GLU receptor activation in that nucleus.[25,26] Inasmuch as nitroxidergic transmission may contribute to signal transduction effected by GLU transmission, studies of nitroxidergic neuronal transmission in NTS could yield important insights into integrative and transduction mechanisms both in NTS and other central sites.

The aforementioned studies support the potential in the central nervous system for integration of GLU and NO·. In some sites that integration may be intracellular and effected through a common transduction pathway that in part involves soluble guanylate cyclase; while in other sites the integration may be intercellular and involve activation of nitroxidergic neurons by glutamate receptor activation. Our own studies in NTS support direct and integrative effects of glutamatergic and nitroxidergic neurons on transmission of cardiovascular reflex signals within the NTS.

## VAGAL AFFERENTS CONTAIN NITRIC OXIDE SYNTHASE

Using histochemical, immunohistochemical, and in situ hybridization techniques, we[27] and others[28–30] have demonstrated that neuronal NO· synthase (nNOS) is expressed in neurons and terminals in the dorsal vagal complex and NTS. Various degrees of reduction in NOS staining in terminal fields of the NTS are demonstrable after deafferentation of vagus fibers.[28,30,31] Studies from our lab confirm that nNOS is present in vagal afferents and their terminals in NTS.[27] These studies support the possibility that NO· may be released from terminals of the vagus nerve in NTS.

In our study,[27] biotinylated dextran amine (BDA) was injected into the nodose ganglion of anesthetized rats to anterogradely label vagus nerve axon terminals in the NTS. The projections were studied at the light microscopic level, and terminations were compared with neurons and neuritic processes stained for nNOS immunoreactivity (IR). BDA-labeled terminals and nNOS-IR were concentrated in homologous regions of NTS. We then sought to determine if vagus nerve terminals that were degenerating as a result of removal of a nodose ganglion contained nNOS.[27] We found that 20–30% of the neurons in the nodose ganglia that had been removed were immunopositive for nNOS. After a three-day recovery that allowed for degeneration of centrally projecting vagus nerve axons, we observed that degenerating terminals in NTS contained nNOS. It is important to note that removal (or death) of the ganglion cells would preclude further production of nNOS at the terminal, and thus our data would, if anything, tend to underestimate the concentration of the enzyme at degenerating afferent terminals.

In other studies[31] we assessed the density of staining for nNOS and for nNOS mRNA with a cDNA probe provided by Dr. David Bredt. We compared staining on the deafferented side with that on the control side and on both sides in control animals. There was minimal (approximately 15% by quantitative image analysis) reduction of nNOS-IR and mRNA in the NTS of the lesioned side, but there was a marked increase in nNOS-IR and mRNA both in the dorsal motor nucleus of the vagus and in the nucleus ambiguus. The findings in NTS were fully consistent with our immunoelectron microscopic studies, in which 68% of degenerating vagus nerve axon terminals from the nodose ganglion were positive for nNOS-IR.[27] However, not all nNOS in NTS is present in vagus nerve afferents. A large proportion of the nNOS in NTS is either found in intrinsic structures or within nonvagal afferents (glossopharyngeal, trigeminal, etc.) that also terminate in NTS. There are no data that address contributions of nonvagal afferents to the pool of nNOS in NTS, but an additional observation from our studies suggests that intrinsic structures make major contributions. Specifically, we found many immunopositive dendrites, some immunopositive neurons, and some nondegenerating immunopositive axons in NTS. The abundance of labeled dendrites makes it unlikely that nonvagal afferent axons are solely responsible for residual immunoreactivity seen in NTS after removal of the nodose ganglion.

## PHARMACOLOGY OF NITRIC OXIDE IN NTS

Other studies have suggested that the nitroxidergic input to NTS may alter cellular activity in the nucleus. Activity of neurons in NTS may be tonically influenced by NO· released from those terminals in that their activity is diminished when the neurons are exposed to an inhibitor of NOS.[32] Furthermore, in anesthetized rats microinjection of S-nitrosothiols, which may act as donors of NO·, elicits depressor and bradycardic responses like those produced by GLU.[33] Unlike GLU, which produces depressor responses in anesthetized animals and pressor responses in awake animals, injection of S-nitrosothiols in the NTS elicits depressor responses in either animal model.[34] Our studies suggest that responses to S-nitrosothiols are dependent on the presence of NO· within the S-nitrosothiol. However, responses may not be a result of NO· itself in that S-nitrosothiols elicited cardiovascular responses even in the presence of hemoglobin, which would scavenge NO· released into the extracellular space. Furthermore, cardiovascular responses occurred with injection of S-nitrosocysteine and not with injection of other NO· donors or NO· itself.

Actions of the S-nitrosothiols, like those produced by NO·, may be mediated, at least in part, through activation of soluble guanylate cyclase in that effects of the S-nitrosothiols are blocked by methylene blue,[35] commonly used to block activation of soluble guanylate cyclase by NO·.[11] The biological relevance of this blockade has been supported by studies showing that methylene blue also blocks the cardiopulmonary (Bezold Jarisch) reflex.[36] The role played in the baroreflex by NO· in the NTS is not fully established, and results of studies of more selective blockers of guanylate cyclase that have recently begun to appear do not directly address reflex transmission.[26] Peripheral inhibition of NOS may contribute to resetting of baroreflex responses to hypertension,[37] but others have reported that blocking synthesis of NO· in NTS may increase arterial pressure without affecting baroreflex modulation of sympathetic nerve activity.[38] Blockade of GLU receptors, on the other hand, alters both basal arterial pressure and the gain of the baroreflex.[39] As with the baroreflex, it is not known whether effects of NO· relate to its participation in arterial chemoreflexes. However, that possibility is supported by the presence of NOS in the carotid body and alteration of chemoreflex activity after peripheral administration of a NOS inhibitor.[40,41]

## EVIDENCE FOR A LINK BETWEEN GLUTAMATE AND NITRIC OXIDE IN NTS

### An Anatomical Link between Glutamatergic and Nitroxidergic Neurons in NTS

The similarity between the physiological responses to GLU and nitrosothiols and in the distribution of GLU and NO· terminals in NTS suggests a possible link between the actions of the two putative transmitter mechanisms. One study even suggests that the two may act on the same neurons in NTS.[10] In an effort to provide anatomical definition of the possible link between GLU and NO·, we performed a series of immunohistochemical, confocal microscopic studies. In the first of these studies[42] we found that antibodies to glutamate and to nNOS identified NTS neurons that colocalized both markers and others that contained only one (FIG. 1). Neuronal NOS-IR was present in neurons throughout NTS, but it was not uniformly distributed among the subnuclei. Likewise, neurons that colocalized GLU-IR and nNOS-IR were unevenly distributed among NTS subnuclei. The highest density of double-labeled neurons was found in the central subnucleus, which receives afferents from stomach, mouth, and esophagus;[43] but subnuclei that receive cardiovascular afferents also contained neurons that prominently colocalized GLU-IR and nNOS-IR. Some fibers traversing NTS also contained both immunolabels; some fibers that lay in close apposition contained one or both markers. Rotation of confocal images revealed that some apparent contacts that were appreciated in one visual plane were

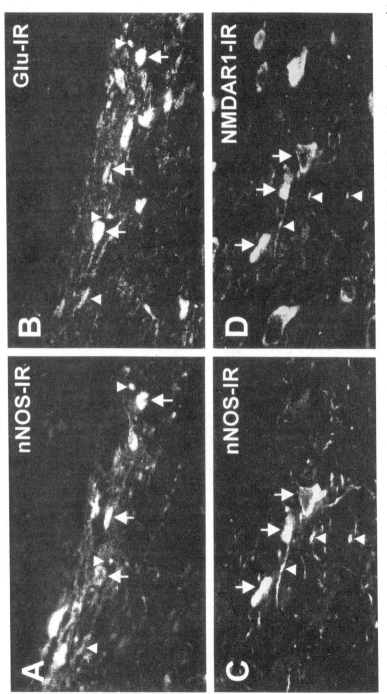

**FIGURE 1.** Colocalization of nNOS and glutamate (**A,B**) and of nNOS and NMDAR1 (**C,D**) in the NTS. A,B: Confocal images (in *gray scale*) of nNOS immunoreactivity (nNOS-IR) (shown in **A**) and glutamate immunoreactivity (Glu-IR) (shown in B) in the dorsolateral subnucleus of the NTS of the same section. *Arrows and arrowheads* indicate examples of double-labeled neurons and fibers, respectively. C,D: Confocal images of nNOS-IR (shown in C) and NMDAR1 immunoreactivity (NMDAR1-IR) (shown in D) in the dorsolateral subnucleus of the NTS of the same section. *Arrows and arrowheads* indicate examples of double-labeled neurons and fibers, respectively. *Scale bar* = 10 μm.

clearly separated in another plane, while some apparent contacts remained regardless of the visual plane. The persistent apposition supported the possibility that GLU- and nNOS-containing fibers make synaptic contact in NTS.

As a result, we sought to determine if nNOS-containing neuronal elements in NTS also contained specific GLU receptors or made contact with other elements in which the receptors could be identified immunohistochemically. Using antibodies to the NMDAR1 receptor subunit and nNOS,[44] we found the same wide, but heterogeneous, distribution of nNOS in NTS as in the first study. We were able to identify very few neurons that contained nNOS but did not contain NMDAR1-IR, but we did find neurons that contained only NMDAR1-IR (FIG. 1). Neurons that contained both types of immunoreactivity were present in cardiovascular regions of NTS but again were more prominent in subnuclei that may subserve gastrointestinal functions. We have now begun electron microscopic analysis of contacts between NMDAR1-IR and nNOS containing neuronal elements. Within NTS we have identified synapses formed by nNOS-containing terminals and NMDAR1-IR postsynaptic dendritic membranes, as well as other terminals that do not contain nNOS-IR but also synapse with NMDAR1-IR-containing dendrites.

Our recent confocal microscopic analysis of nNOS and non-NMDA receptors labeled with an antibody to GLUR1[45] has demonstrated that the distribution of GLUR1-IR is quite similar to that of NMDAR1-IR in the earlier study. Furthermore, like NMDAR1-IR, GLUR1-IR is found in virtually every NTS neuron that contains nNOS-IR.

### A Pharmacological Link between Glutamate and Nitric Oxide in NTS

Pharmacological studies provide additional evidence for a possible link between NO· and GLU neurons in NTS. Because soluble guanylate cyclase plays an important role in transduction of signals initiated by NO·,[46] we first studied whether cardiovascular responses elicited by microinjection of GLU into NTS were affected by inhibition of the enzyme. Responses to GLU and GLU agonists that act at ionotropic receptors were blocked by prior administration into NTS of the guanylate cyclase inhibitor methylene blue (TABLE 1).[47] Doses for each agonist were approximately the $ED_{50}$ for each, so that detection of inhibitory effects on their actions would be maximized. In contrast, actions of acetylcholine, glycine, and quisqualic acid, which acts both at metabotropic as well as ionotropic receptors, were not attenuated. Therefore, methylene blue selectively attenuated responses to ionotropic receptor activation but did not affect agonists that act at metabotropic receptors. Attenuation of responses to GLU agonists by methylene blue also occurred when the experiments were repeated with injection of superoxide dismutase simultaneously with injection of methylene blue in the NTS. Thus, effects of methylene blue were not likely the result of formation of oxygen radicals. We have repeated the studies with more selective inhibitors of soluble guanylate cyclase and have seen similar results. For example, depressor and bradycardic responses to NMDA were reduced in a dose-dependent manner by prior injection of LY83583. Effects of LY83583 on responses to injection of GLU into NTS were similar to effects on responses to NMDA. Current studies are aimed at determining if effects of selective blockade of soluble guanylate cyclase with LY83583 or a still more selective inhibitor like 1H-[1,2,4]oxadiazolo[4,3,-a] quinoxalin-1-one (ODQ)[48] are limited to ionotropic agonists as they were when me-

**TABLE 1.** Effect of methylene blue (500 pmol) on depressor responses produced by GLU: receptor agonists and acetylcholine (ACh) injected into NTS

| Agents | $n$ | Baseline | Control | 10 min | 20 min | 30 min |
|---|---|---|---|---|---|---|
| GLU (50 pmol) | 6 | $95 \pm 4$ | $-31 \pm 5$ | $-20 \pm 6$ | $-14 \pm 4^*$ | $-11 \pm 4^*$ |
| NMDA (0.5 pmol) | 6 | $99 \pm 4$ | $-31 \pm 3$ | $-14 \pm 4^*$ | $-12 \pm 6^*$ | $-10 \pm 3^*$ |
| KA[a] (0.2 pmol) | 6 | $105 \pm 2$ | $-41 \pm 6$ | $-21 \pm 5^*$ | | $-12 \pm 5^*$ |
| AMPA (0.2 pmol) | 4 | $93 \pm 3$ | $-42 \pm 4$ | $-19 \pm 6$ | $-8 \pm 4^*$ | $-3 \pm 1^*$ |
| QUIS (2 pmol) | 6 | $96 \pm 5$ | $-31 \pm 5$ | $-29 \pm 5$ | $-28 \pm 5$ | $-21 \pm 5$ |
| ACh (250 pmol) | 4 | $116 \pm 11$ | $-33 \pm 11$ | $-37 \pm 9$ | $-34 \pm 10$ | $-37 \pm 8$ |

$^*p < 0.05$.
[a]GLU agonists tested at 10, 20, and 30 min after injection of methylene blue, except KA, which was tested 15 and 30 min after injection of methylene blue.

thylene blue was used. While selective blockade of ionotropic agonists has not been established for agents other than methylene blue, others have suggested that ODQ is an effective inhibitor of glutamate and agonists for glutamate receptors.[26]

A second series of studies[49] focused on responses to GLU agonists after inhibition of NO· synthesis. Responses to NMDA microinjected unilaterally into NTS of anesthetized rats were significantly attenuated in a dose-dependent manner by prior intraperitoneal injection of the nNOS inhibitor 7-nitroindazole (7-NI). The attenuation of responses elicited by NMDA was reversed by administration of L-arginine, the precursor for synthesis of NO· by nNOS. D-arginine did not alter effects of 7-NI.

There are two limitations to our 7-NI studies and to those that have been published.[26] First, intraperitoneal injection of 7-NI could have affected responses to GLU agonists administered into NTS by inhibiting nNOS outside NTS. Second, injection of this highly hydrophobic agent into NTS requires use of solvents that may either alter its specificity for nNOS or may themselves effect neuronal dysfunction. Therefore, studies are needed to determine if selective, aqueous soluble nNOS inhibitors injected into NTS will attenuate responses to glutamate agonists injected at the same sites.

## SUMMARY

Recent studies indicate that other putative neuronal messengers may participate in generating responses elicited by GLU. One such messenger is NO·, which may exert both pre- and postsynaptic effects and has been found also to play a role in cardiovascular regulation at the level of NTS.[10] Responses to injection of NO· donors into NTS, both in anesthetized and awake animals, mimic those elicited by injection of GLU agonists in anesthetized rats.[33,34,50] Furthermore, close apposition and synaptic contacts between glutamatergic and nitroxidergic fiber as well as colocalization of GLU and nnOS in neurons of NTS provide an anatomical basis for a potential physiologically relevant link between the two. However, it is not clear that NO· or NO·-containing compounds[33] contribute to cardiovascular signal transduction in NTS[38,51] or, if they do,[36] to what extent their contribution is dependent upon actions of GLU in the nucleus.

## ACKNOWLEDGMENTS

This work was funded in part by NIH Grant R01 HL59593 and an American Heart Association Grant in Aid.

## REFERENCES

1. PANNETON, W.M. & A.D. LOEWY. 1980. Projections of the carotid sinus nerve to the nucleus of the solitary tract in the cat. Brain Res. **191:** 239–244.
2. WALLACH, J.H. & A.D. LOEWY. 1980. Projections of the aortic nerve to the nucleus tractus solitarius in the rabbit. Brain Res. **188:** 247–251.
3. KALIA, M. & M.-M. MESULAM. 1980. Brain stem projections of sensory and motor components of the vagus complex in the cat: II. laryngeal, tracheobronchial, pulmonary, cardiac, and gastrointestinal branches. J. Comp. Neurol. **193:** 467–508.
4. YIN, M. et al. 1994. Hemodynamic effects elicited by stimulation of the nucleus tractus solitarii. Hypertension **23**(Suppl.): I73–I77.
5. COLOMBARI, E. et al. 1998. Hemodynamic effects of L-glutamate in NTS of conscious rats: a possible role of vascular nitrosyl factors. Am. J. Physiol. **274:** H1066–H1074.
6. MONTGOMERY, B.M. 1961. The basilar artery hypertensive syndrome. Arch. Intern. Med. **108:** 559–569.
7. DOBA, N. & D.J. REIS. 1973. Acute fulminating neurogenic hypertension produced by brainstem lesions in the rat. Circ. Res. **32:** 584–593.
8. TALMAN, W.T. et al. 1981. Acute hypertension after the local injection of kainic acid into the nucleus tractus solitarii of rats. Circ. Res. **48:** 292–298.
9. GORDON, F J. & W.T. TALMAN. 1992. Role of excitatory amino acids and their receptors in bulbospinal control of cardiovascular function. In Central Neural Mechanisms in Cardiovascular Regulation, Vol. 2. G. Kunos & J. Ciriello, Eds.: 209–225. Birkhauser. New York.
10. TAGAWA, T. et al. 1994. Nitric oxide influences neuronal activity in the nucleus tractus solitarius of rat brainstem slices. Circ. Res. **75:** 70–76.
11. GARTHWAITE, J. et al. 1988. Endothelium-derived relaxing factor release on activation of NMDA receptors suggests role as intercellular messenger in the brain. Nature **336:** 385–388.
12. GARTHWAITE, J. et al. 1989. NMDA receptor activation induces nitric oxide synthesis from arginine in rat brain slices. Eur. J. Pharmacol. **172:** 413–416.
13. GARTHWAITE, J. & G. GARTHWAITE. 1987. Cellular origins of cyclic GMP responses to excitatory amino acid receptor agonists in rat cerebellum in vitro. J. Neurochem. **48:** 29–39.
14. DE VENTE, J. et al. 1990. Immunocytochemistry of cGMP in the cerebellum of the immature, adult, and aged rat: the involvement of nitric oxide. A micropharmacological study. Eur. J. Neurosci. **2:** 845–862.
15. GARTHWAITE, J. et al. 1989. A kainate receptor linked to nitric oxide synthesis from arginine. J. Neurochem. **53:** 1952–1954.
16. KIEDROWSKI, L. et al. 1992. Glutamate receptor agonists stimulate nitric oxide synthase in primary cultures of cerebellar granule cells. J. Neurochem. **58:** 335–341.

17. SOUTHAM, E. *et al.* 1991. Excitatory amino acid receptors coupled to the nitric oxide/cyclic GMP pathway in rat cerebellum during development. J. Neurochem. **56:** 2072–2081.
18. OKADA, D. 1992. Two pathways of cyclic GMP production through glutamate receptor–mediated nitric oxide synthesis. J. Neurochem. **59:** 1203–1210.
19. MARIN, P. *et al.* 1993. Non-classical glutamate receptors, blocked by both NMDA and non-NMDA antagonists, stimulate nitric oxide production in neurons. Neuropharmacology **32:** 29–36.
20. LARKMAN, A.U. & J.J. JACK. 1995. Synaptic plasticity: hippocampal LTP (review). Curr. Opin. Neurobiol. **5:** 324–334.
21. HAWKINS, R.D. *et al.* 1994. Nitric oxide and carbon monoxide as possible retrograde messengers in hippocampal long-term potentiation. J. Neurobiol. **25:** 652–665.
22. SEGIETH, J. *et al.* 1995. Nitric oxide regulates excitatory amino acid release in a biphasic manner in freely moving rats. Neurosci. Lett. **200:** 101–104.
23. IZUMI, Y. *et al.* 1992. Inhibition of long-term potentiation by NMDA-mediated nitric oxide release. Science **257:** 1273–1276.
24. SHIBUKI, K. & D. OKADA. 1991. Endogenous nitric oxide release required for long-term synaptic depression in the cerebellum. Nature **349:** 326–328.
25. DI PAOLA, E. D. *et al.* 1991. L-Glutamate evokes the release of an endothelium-derived relaxing factor–like substance from the rat nucleus tractus solitarius. J. Cardiovasc. Pharmacol. **17**(Suppl. 3): S269–S272.
26. LIN, H. C. *et al.* 1999. Modulation of cardiovascular effects produced by nitric oxide and ionotropic glutamate receptor interaction in the nucleus tractus solitarii of rats. Neuropharmacology **38:** 935–941.
27. LIN, L-H. *et al.* 1998. Direct evidence for nitric oxide synthase in vagal afferents to the nucleus tractus solitarii. Neuroscience **84:** 549–558.
28. RUGGIERO, D.A. *et al.* 1996. Central and primary visceral afferents to nucleus tractus solitarii may generate nitric oxide as a membrane-permeant neuronal messenger. J. Comp. Neurol. **364:** 51–67.
29. KRISTENSSON, K. *et al.* 1994. Co-induction of neuronal interferon-gamma and nitric oxide synthase in rat motor neurons after axotomy: a role in nerve repair or death? J. Neurocytol. **23:** 453–459.
30. LAWRENCE, A.J. *et al.* 1998. The distribution of nitric oxide synthase-, adenosine deaminase- and neuropeptide Y-immunoreactivity through the entire rat nucleus tractus solitarius: effect of unilateral nodose ganglionectomy. J. Chem. Neuroanat. **15:** 27–40.
31. LIN, L-H. *et al.* 1997. Up-regulation of nitric oxide synthase and its mRNA in vagal motor nuclei following axotomy in rat. Neurosci. Lett. **221:** 97–100.
32. MA, S. *et al.* 1995. Effects of L-arginine–derived nitric oxide synthesis on neuronal activity in nucleus tractus solitarius. Am. J. Physiol. Regul. Integr. Comp. Physiol. **268:** R487–R491.
33. OHTA, H. *et al.* 1997. Actions of s-nitrosocysteine in the nucleus tractus solitarii are unrelated to release of nitric oxide. Brain Res. **746:** 98–104.
34. MACHADO, B.H. & L.G.H. BONAGAMBA. 1992. Microinjection of S-nitrosocysteine into the nucleus tractus solitarii of conscious rats decreases arterial pressure but L-glutamate does not. Eur. J. Pharmacol. **221:** 179–182.
35. LEWIS, S.J. *et al.* 1991. Microinjection of S-nitrosocysteine into the nucleus tractus solitarii decreases arterial pressure and heart rate via activation of soluble guanylate cyclase. Eur. J. Pharmacol. **202:** 135–136.
36. LEWIS, S.J. *et al.* 1991. Processing of cardiopulmonary afferent input within the nucleus tractus solitarii involves activation of soluble guanylate cyclase. Eur. J. Pharmacol. **203:** 327–328.
37. VARGAS DA SILVA, S. *et al.* 1994. Blockers of the L-arginine–nitric oxide–cyclic GMP pathway facilitate baroreceptor resetting. Hypertension **23**(Suppl.): I60–I63.
38. ZANZINGER, J. *et al.* 1995. Effects of nitric oxide on sympathetic baroreflex transmission in the nucleus tractus solitarii and caudal ventrolateral medulla in cats. Neurosci. Lett. **197:** 199–202.
39. OHTA, H. & W.T. TALMAN. 1994. Both NMDA and non-NMDA receptors in the NTS participate in the baroreceptor reflex in rats. Am. J. Physiol. **267:** R1065–R1070.

40. GRIMES, P.A. *et al.* 1994. Nitric oxide synthase occurs in neurons and nerve fibers of the carotid body. Adv. Exp. Med. Biol. **360:** 221–224.
41. TRZEBSKI, A. *et al.* 1994. Carotid chemoreceptor activity and heart rate responsiveness to hypoxia after inhibition of nitric oxide synthase. Adv. Exp. Med. Biol. **360:** 285–288.
42. LIN, L-H. *et al.* 2000. Apposition of neuronal elements containing nitric oxide synthase and glutamate in the nucleus tractus solitarii of rat: a confocal microscopic analysis . Neuroscience **96:** 341–350.
43. ALTSCHULER, S.M. *et al.* 1989. Viscerotopic representation of the upper alimentary tract in the rat: sensory ganglia and nuclei of the solitary and spinal trigeminal tracts. J. Comp. Neurol. **283:** 248–268.
44. LIN, L-H. & W.T. TALMAN. 2000. N-methyl-D-aspartate receptors on neurons that synthesize nitric oxide in rat nucleus tractus solitarii. Neuroscience **100:** 581–588.
45. LIN, L-H. & W.T. TALMAN. 2000. AMPA receptor subunit GLUR1 and neuronal nitric oxide synthase are colocalized in the nucleus tractus solitarii (abstr.). FASEB J. **14:** A628.
46. MONCADA, S. 1992. The 1991 Ulf von Euler Lecture. The L-arginine:nitric oxide pathway. Acta Physiol. Scand. **145:** 201–227.
47. OHTA, H. & W.T. TALMAN. 1992. Excitatory amino acids activate guanylate cyclase in nucleus tractus solitarii of rat (abstr.). FASEB J. **6:** A1164.
48. ABI-GERGES, N. *et al.* 1997. A comparative study of the effects of three guanylyl cyclase inhibitors on the L-type Ca2+ and muscarinic K+ currents in frog cardiac myocytes. Br. J. Pharmacol. **121:** 1369–1377.
49. TALMAN, W.T. *et al.* 1998. Cardiovascular responses to glutamate linked to neuronal nitric oxide synthesis (abstr.). Soc. Neurosci. Abstr. **24:** 1028.
50. TALMAN, W.T. 1989. Kynurenic acid microinjected into the nucleus tractus solitarius of rat blocks the arterial baroreflex but not responses to glutamate. Neurosci. Lett. **102:** 247–252.
51. HARADA, S. *et al.* 1993. Inhibition of nitric oxide formation in the nucleus tractus solitarius increases renal sympathetic nerve activity in rabbits. Circ. Res. **72:** 511–516.

# Neurotransmission of the Cardiovascular Reflexes in the Nucleus Tractus Solitarii of Awake Rats

BENEDITO H. MACHADO

*Department of Physiology, School of Medicine of Ribeirão Preto, University of São Paulo, 14049-900, Ribeirão Preto, SP, Brazil*

ABSTRACT: Chemoreflex activation with potassium cyanide (i.v.) produces pressor and bradycardic responses in awake rats. Microinjection of AP-5, a selective NMDA receptor antagonist, into the nucleus tractus solitarii (NTS) produced a dose-dependent blockade of the bradycardic response; while microinjection of DNQX, a selective non-NMDA receptor antagonist, or kynurenic acid, a nonselective ionotropic receptor antagonist, produced only a partial reduction in the pressor response, indicating that the bradycardic component of the chemoreflex is mediated by NMDA receptors and that the sympathoexcitatory component may involve neurotransmitters other than excitatory amino acids. With respect to the baroreflex, we verified that the gain of baroreflex bradycardia in response to phenyleprine (Phe) infusion was significantly reduced in a dose-dependent manner by microinjection of AP-5 into the NTS, indicating that the parasympathetic component of the baroreflex is mediated mainly by NMDA receptors. However, in a series of experiments involving the electrical stimulation of the aortic depressor nerve (ADN) we observed that the maximal bradycardic response was almost blocked by the combination of microinjection of NMDA and non-NMDA receptor antagonists into the NTS, while the depressor response was only partially reduced. These data indicate that the bradycardic response produced by the activation of the baroreflex with Phe is mediated by mechanisms differing from those in response to the electrical stimulation of the ADN because phenylephrine also activates carotid and aortic baroreceptors, while unilateral electrical stimulation of the ADN involves only one specific set of baroreceptor afferents. These data also indicate that the sympatho inhibitory component of this response may involve neurotransmitters other than L-glutamate. We discuss the possibility that two different afferent systems of arterial baroreceptors are involved in the modulation of parasympathoexcitation and sympathoinhibition: one activated within the normal range of pulsatile arterial pressure (on a pulse-to-pulse basis) and the other acting under circumstances of challenge to the pulsatile arterial pressure above the normal range.

KEYWORDS: Chemoreflex; Baroreflex; Aortic depressor nerve; Cardiovascular regulation; Autonomic regulation; Excitatory amino acid receptors; L-Glutamate; Substance P; Adenosine; ATP; Ionotropic receptors; Metabotropic receptors

Address for correspondence: Benedito H. Machado, Department of Physiology, School of Medicine of Ribeirão Preto, University of São Paulo, 14049-900, Ribeirão Preto, SP, Brazil. Voice: 55-16-602-3015; fax: 55-16-633-0017.
bhmachad@fmrp.usp.br

## INTRODUCTION

The nucleus tractus solitarii (NTS) is the site in the brain stem in which the first synapses of the baro-, chemo-, and cardiopulmonary reflex afferents occur in the central nervous system.[1,2] There is evidence indicating that the excitatory amino acid L-glutamate is the neurotransmitter released by the afferents of the different cardiovascular reflexes in the NTS,[3–5] and the different subtypes of ionotropic receptors (NMDA and non-NMDA) play an important role in this neurotransmission.[6–13] In our laboratory we are currently evaluating the involvement of the different subtypes of ionotropic (NMDA and non-NMDA) and metabotropic receptors in the processing of each autonomic component of the cardiovascular reflexes at the NTS level. We performed our experiments on awake rats because anesthetics may affect the processing of the glutamatergic neurotransmission in the NTS, as we verified previously.[14] In the experiments performed in our laboratory we used the technique developed by Michelini and Bonagamba,[15] which permits microinjections into the NTS of awake rats in a reliable manner.

## CHEMOREFLEX

To study the chemoreflex in awake rats we used the method described by Franchini and Krieger,[16] which consists of intravenous (i.v.) injection of potassium cyanide (KCN). KCN (i.v.) produces a tachypneic response and increases arterial pressure and bradycardia. The bradycardic response was not of baroreflex origin because blockade of the pressor response with prazosin, an alpha adrenergic antagonist, produced no effect on the bradycardic response, which was abolished after methylatropine. Therefore, these data indicate that chemoreflex activation in awake rats produces two independent cardiovascular responses—an increase in arterial pressure (sympathoexcitation) and bradycardia (parasympathoexcitation).[16–17] In a series of experiments reported here, we tried to determine the ionotropic and metabotropic mechanisms involved in the processing of these two autonomic components of the chemoreflex at the NTS level.

Initially, we evaluated the role of NMDA receptors in the processing of the chemoreflex at the NTS level. To this end, we activated the chemoreflex before and after bilateral microinjection of AP-5, a selective NMDA receptor antagonist, into the NTS.[17] FIGURE 1 illustrates this experimental protocol and shows that increasing doses of AP-5 (0.5, 2, and 10 nmol/100 nL) produced a dose-dependent blockade of the bradycardic response and no changes in the pressor response to chemoreflex activation. These data indicate that NMDA receptors are involved mainly in the bradycardic response but not in the neurotransmission of the sympathoexcitatory component (pressor response) of the chemoreflex activation in the NTS. The possible involvement of NMDA receptors in the parasympathetic component of the chemoreflex is also supported by findings of another study from our laboratory,[18] in which the blockade of the bradycardic response to chemoreflex activation was effective only when kynurenic acid was microinjected into the lateral aspect of the commissural NTS. In this case, the microinjection of kynurenic acid into the medial aspect of the commissural NTS produced no effect on the bradycardic response, in-

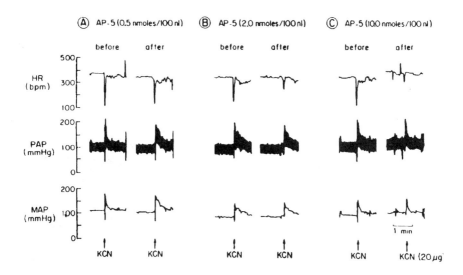

**FIGURE 1.** Changes in heart rate (HR), pulsatile arterial pressure (PAP), and mean arterial pressure (MAP) in response to injection of KCN (20 μg · rat$^{-1}$ · 0.1 mol$^{-1}$ i.v.) before and after bilateral microinjection of phosponovaleric acid (AP-5) at 0.5 **(A)**, 2.0 **(B)**, and 10.0 nmol/100 nL **(C)** into the nucleus tractus solitarii of three different rats. (Data reprinted with permission from Haibara et al.[17])

dicating that the processing of the parasympathetic component of the chemoreflex is restricted to the lateral aspect of the NTS.

With respect to these experiments, the data also suggest that NMDA receptors are not involved in the processing of the sympathoexcitatory component of the chemoreflex in the NTS because the pressor response was not affected by bilateral microinjection of AP-5. The possible involvement of non-NMDA receptors in the processing of the sympathoexcitatory component of the chemoreflex was explored in another experimental protocol, as shown in FIGURE 2. In this case, we activated the chemoreflex before and after bilateral microinjection of increasing doses of DNQX, a selective non-NMDA receptor antagonist, into the NTS. It is important to note that bilateral microinjection of DNQX into the NTS produced a significant increase in baseline mean arterial pressure (MAP). We may suggest that this increase in baseline MAP is related to the blockade of non-NMDA receptors located in the neurons of the NTS involved in the sympathoinhibitory projections from the NTS to the rostral ventrolateral medulla (RVLM), via the caudal ventrolateral medulla (CV-LM), which is integral to the baroreflex pathways. The blockade of this sympathoinhibitory projection by DNQX may increase the activity of RVLM neurons and consequently increase baseline MAP. The pressor response to chemoreflex activation after DNQX was reduced but not abolished. This reduction may have been related to the increase in baseline MAP; nevertheless, DNQX was not able to block the pressor response to the chemoreflex, suggesting that the neurotransmission of the sympathoexcitatory component of the chemoreflex at the NTS level may involve a

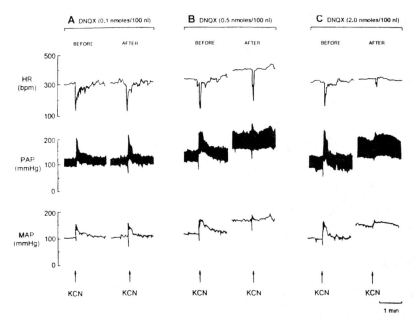

**FIGURE 2.** Changes in heart rate (HR), pulsatile arterial pressure (PAP), and mean arterial pressure (MAP) in response to KCN (20 μg · rat$^{-1}$ · 0.1 mol$^{-1}$ i.v.) before and 10 min after bilateral microinjection of increasing doses of 6,7-dinitroquinoxaline-2,3-dione (DNQX) [0.1 (**A**), 0.5 (**B**), and 2.0 nmol/100 nL (**C**)] into the lateral portion of the commissural nucleus of the solitary tract (NTS$_{lat}$) of three different rats representative of their respective groups. bpm, beats/min. (Data reprinted with permission from Haibara et al.[18])

neurotransmitter other than L-glutamate. It is important to note that the dose of DNQX selective for non-NMDA receptors (0.5 nmol/100 nL) produced no effect on the bradycardic response. The dose of 2.0 nmol/50 nL presented in FIGURE 2 was not selective for non-NMDA receptors, and for this reason the bradycardic response was also affected. Although this dose was not selective for non-NMDA receptors, the pressor response to chemoreflex activation was not blocked.[18]

For a better evaluation of the role of excitatory amino acid receptors in the processing of the sympathoexcitatory component of the chemoreflex, we evaluated the effect of microinjections of kynurenic acid, a nonselective EAA receptor antagonist, into the lateral and medial aspect of the commissural NTS, considering that several experimental lines of evidence suggest that the processing of the chemoreflex afferents occurs mainly at the medial aspect of the commissural NTS.[2,19,20] Therefore, in the next step kynurenic acid was microinjected into the lateral commissural NTS or into the midline portion of the commissural NTS or simultaneously at three sites into the NTS (lateral and medial aspect of the commissural NTS) in order to block all ionotropic receptors in this area, as shown in FIGURE 3. In spite of these procedures, the data summarized in FIGURE 4 show that kynurenic acid produced a reduction of only approximately 50% of the pressor response of the chemoreflex. The involvement of metabotropic receptors in this processing in the NTS was also eval-

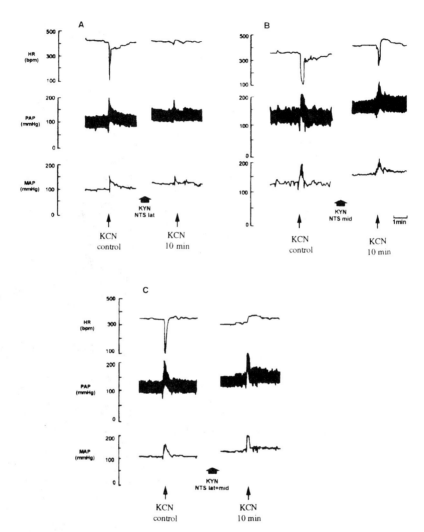

**FIGURE 3.** Changes in heart rate (HR), pulsatile arterial pressure (PAP), and mean arterial pressure (MAP) in response to KCN (20 μg · rat$^{-1}$ · 0.1 mol$^{-1}$ i.v.) before and 10 min after bilateral microinjection of kynurenic acid (kyn, 10 nmol/100 nL) into the NTS$_{lat}$ (**A**), midline portion of the commissural NTS (NTS$_{mid}$, **B**), or NTS$_{lat+mid}$ (**C**) of three different rats representative of their respective groups. (Data reprinted with permission from Haibara *et al.*[18])

uated using MCPG, a metabotropic receptor antagonist. We verified that bilateral microinjection of MCPG into the NTS produced no effect on the pressor or bradycardic responses to chemoreflex activation, indicating that metabotropic receptors also play no major role in the neurotransmission of the sympathoexcitatory component of the chemoreflex at the NTS level. Taken together, these data show that the

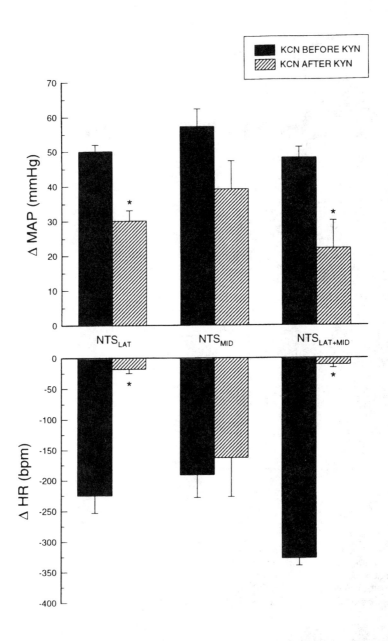

**FIGURE 4.** Changes in pulsatile arterial pressure (PAP), mean arterial pressure (MAP), and heart rate (HR) in response to KCN (20 μg · rat$^{-1}$ · 0.1 mol$^{-1}$ i.v.) before and 10 min after bilateral microinjection of kynurenic acid (kyn, 10 nmol/100 nL) into NTS$_{lat}$, midline portion of the commissural NTS (NTS$_{mid}$), or NTS$_{lat+mid}$ of three different rats representative of their respective groups. (Data reprinted with permission from Haibara *et al.*[18])

neurotransmission of the sympathoexcitatory component of the chemoreflex in the NTS is only partially affected by microinjection of an excitatory amino acid receptor antagonist into different subregions of the NTS simultaneously, suggesting that other neurotransmitters or cotransmitters may also participate in this processing. However, before ruling out the involvement of EAA receptors in the processing of the full sympathoexcitatory component of the chemoreflex it will be necessary to perform the microinjection of ionotropic and metabotropic receptor antagonists simultaneously into the different subregions of the NTS.

With respect to the inhibitory neuromodulation of the sympathoexcitatory component of the chemoreflex, we verified that microinjection of muscimol or baclofen into the lateral aspect of the commissural NTS produced an increase in baseline MAP. In the case of baclofen the magnitude of the pressor response to chemoreflex activation was reduced but not abolished, similarly to the findings with microinjections of kynurenic acid; while microinjection of muscimol into the NTS produced no changes in the pressor response.[21] In this case we also suggest that the attenuation of the pressor response of the chemoreflex by a $GABA_B$ receptor agonist (baclofen) may be the consequence of the blockade of the sympathoexcitatory neurons in the NTS involved in the chemoreflex pathways or to the large increase in baseline MAP secondary to the blockade of sympathoinhibitory neurons of the NTS involved in the baroreflex pathways.

The possible role of substance P in the neurotransmission of the sympathoexcitatory component of the chemoreflex in the NTS was also evaluated, considering that previous studies have shown an increase of substance P in the NTS during hypoxia.[22] The bilateral microinjection of an NK-1 receptor antagonist into the NTS (WIN) produced no changes in the cardiovascular responses to chemoreflex activation. We also evaluated the possible role of adenosine and adenosine receptors in this neurotransmission. For this purpose the chemoreflex was activated before and after bilateral microinjection of DPCPX, a nonselective A1 and A2 receptor antagonist. In these experiments the data also showed that the cardiovascular responses to chemoreflex activation were not affected, indicating that adenosine and adenosine receptors are also not involved in this neurotransmission in the NTS (de Paula and Machado, unpublished data from our laboratory).

In a current series of experiments we are exploring the possibility that ATP may act as a neurotransmitter of the sympathoexcitatory component of the chemoreflex in the NTS. Microinjection of ATP into the NTS produced cardiovascular responses similar to those obtained after chemoreflex activation.[23] In addition, microinjection of suramin, a nonselective P2x and P2y receptor antagonist, into the medial aspect of the commissural NTS produced a significant reduction in the pressor response of the chemoreflex. In this case, we are considering the possibility that ATP may act as a cotransmitter of L-glutamate because kynurenic acid, a nonselective ionotropic receptor antagonist, produced a significant reduction in the cardiovascular responses to microinjection of ATP into the NTS.[23] Another important aspect of the sympathoexcitatory component of the chemoreflex that we are exploring is the involvement of other areas of the brain that may play some role in its generation and/or modulation. There is evidence in favor of a direct projection from the NTS to the rostral ventrolateral medulla (RVLM), which could be part of the sympathoexcitatory component of the chemoreflex.[24–27] However, in a recent study we verified that these projections do not seem to be essential to the sympathoexcitatory response to

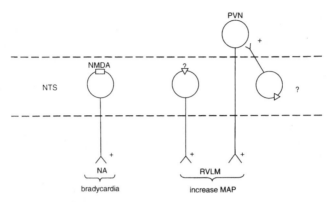

**FIGURE 5.** Schematic drawing showing a neuron of the parasympathetic component of the chemoreflex containing NMDA receptors and projecting to the nucleus ambiguus (NA) and two possible neurons of the sympathoexcitatory component of the chemoreflex projecting from NTS to RVLM or from NTS to PVN. In both cases these neurons may not contain excitatory amino acid receptors.

chemoreflex activation in awake rats (Mauad and Machado, unpublished data). On the other hand, there is anatomical and electrophysiological evidence of connections between the NTS and the paraventricular nucleus of the hypothalamus (PVN),[28–31] as well as projections from the PVN to the RVLM[32–34] and to the spinal cord.[32,35] In addition, the PVN seems to play an important role in the modulation of sympathetic activity[36–40] and is also involved in the cardiovascular responses to chemoreflex activation in anesthetized rats.[41] Recent studies from our laboratory[42,43] have documented that the pressor response of the chemoreflex is partially dependent on the integrity of the paraventricular nucleus of the hypothalamus. Therefore, it is plausible to suggest that the projection from NTS to PVN uses L-glutamate and ATP as cotransmitters, but this possibility is still under investigation. FIGURE 5 is a schematic drawing showing the possible mechanisms involved in the neurotransmission of the chemoreflex at the NTS level.

## BAROREFLEX

The activation of the baroreceptor afferents produces reflex bradycardia by excitation of NTS neurons involved in projections to parasympathetic preganglionic neurons in the nucleus ambiguus or in the dorsal motor nucleus of the vagus; and hypotension by excitation of the neurons projecting from NTS to CVLM, which, when excited, inhibit the sympathetic vasomotor neurons located in the RVLM.[44–46] Conventionally the autonomic baroreflex responses have been studied by means of injection or infusion of phenylephrine (i.v.), which produces vasoconstriction and a consequent increase in MAP. This increase in MAP activates the arterial baroreceptors, and the reflex bradycardia can easily be evaluated. However, with this procedure the sympathoinhibition resulting in vasodilation cannot be evaluated, due to the direct effect of phenylephrine on vascular smooth muscle. In this case, it is necessary

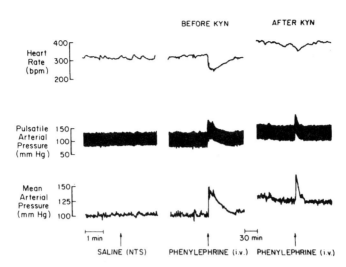

**FIGURE 6.** Typical tracing showing the effect of kynurenic acid (kyn: 10 nmol/ 100 nL) microinjected bilaterally into the NTS on the reflex bradycardia induced by pressor doses of phenylephrine (3 µg/kg i.v.). Saline (vehicle) was microinjected into the NTS as a volume control. The time interval between the first injection of phenylephrine (before kyn) and the microinjection of kyn was 10 min, and the second injection of phenylephrine was performed 20 min after bilateral microinjection of kynurenic acid into the NTS (after kyn). *Arrows* indicate the injections. (Data reprinted with permission from Colombari *et al.*[47])

to record the sympathetic nerve discharge; but this approach is quite difficult, particularly in conscious, freely moving animals. In a study from our laboratory, illustrated in FIGURE 6, we activated the baroreflex with a phenylephrine injection before and after bilateral microinjection of kynurenic acid into the NTS, and we observed that the reflex bradycardia was blocked, indicating that the processing of the parasympathetic component of the baroreflex at the NTS level involves EAA receptors. The microinjection of kynurenic acid into the NTS produced a significant change in baseline MAP and HR, demonstrating that the pulse-to-pulse regulation of baseline MAP and HR involves EAA receptors.[47]

In order to study the role of each EAA receptor subtype in the processing of the parasympathetic component of the baroreflex, in the next step we evaluated the gain of the baroreflex before and after bilateral microinjection of AP-5, a selective NMDA receptor antagonist, into the NTS.[48] In this case the gain of the baroreflex bradycardia was determined by assessing blood pressure and heart rate responses to a short-duration (20-s) intravenous infusion of phenylephrine. In these experiments we first observed that bilateral microinjection of AP-5 into the NTS produced no changes in baseline MAP or HR. However, the gain of the reflex bradycardia was significantly reduced 2 minutes after AP-5,[48,49] as shown in FIGURE 7. These findings may have several implications; our interpretation of these data is as follows: (1) NMDA receptors apparently are not involved in the processing of the parasympathetic component of the baroreflex afferents on a pulse-to-pulse basis, because basal

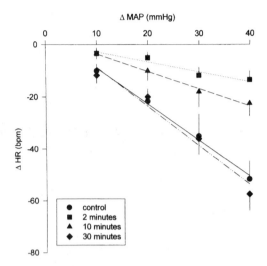

**FIGURE 7.** Gain of the baroreflex before (control) and 2, 10, and 30 min after bilateral microinjection of AP-5 (10 nmol/50 nL, $n = 6$) into the NTS. (Data reprinted with permission from Frigero et al.[48])

heart rate was not affected after AP-5; in this case we may suggest that non-NMDA receptors are relatively more important in the regulation of heart rate on a pulse-to-pulse basis. (2) NMDA receptors apparently are also not involved in the processing of the sympathoinhibitory component of the baroreflex because no change in baseline MAP was observed. (3) NMDA receptors seem to play a key role in the processing of the parasympathetic component of the baroreflex when the baroreceptor afferents are submitted to a MAP challenge in response to phenylephrine infusion, for example, or in any other situation in which the arterial pulse pressure is increased above the normal level of the pulsatile range (80–120 mmHg). If this hypothesis is correct, we may suggest that there are two different parasympathetic pathways from the NTS to the preganglionic parasympathetic neurons in the nucleus ambiguus or in the dorsal motor nucleus of the vagus: one activated on a pulse-to-pulse basis, in which neurons do not contain NMDA receptors; and the other activated during challenges to arterial pressure, in which neurons contain NMDA receptors, as shown in the schematic drawing in FIGURE 8. This possibility is valid if we consider the challenges in MAP in response to the short-duration infusion of phenylephrine, which produces activation of all sets of arterial baroreceptors. This interpretation was not necessarily the same in the experiments in which we produced a challenge in the baroreceptor afferents by unilateral electrical stimulation of the aortic depressor nerve, as we will discuss later.

It is important to note that the dose of AP-5 used in these experiments was selective for NMDA receptors because it produced no effect on the cardiovascular responses to microinjection of AMPA, a non-NMDA receptor agonist, into the NTS.[48] The reflex bradycardia in response to phenylephrine infusion was not tested after blockade of non-NMDA receptors because the selective antagonism of these recep-

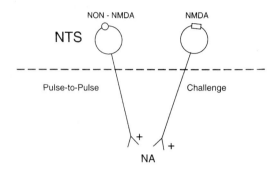

**FIGURE 8.** Schematic drawing showing two different neurons with different subtypes of excitatory amino acid receptors [pulse-to-pulse (non-NMDA) and challenge (NMDA)] projecting from NTS to nucleus ambiguus.

tors with DNQX, for example, produced a significant increase in baseline MAP, which may affect the gain of the baroreflex. With respect to this problem, we verified in a recent study that changes in baseline arterial pressure produce an important autonomic imbalance to the heart, with consequences for the correct evaluation of the gain of the baroreflex.[50] In order to avoid this potential problem and also to evaluate the hypotension (sympathoinhibition) in response to baroreflex activation, which is not possible with the use of phenylephrine infusion, we developed the technique for electrical stimulation of the ADN, which will be described and discussed later.

Using the phenylephrine infusion approach we also evaluated the possible involvement of L-glutamate metabotropic receptors in the neurotransmission of the parasympathoexcitatory component of the baroreflex in the NTS.[51] The data showed that bilateral microinjection of MCPG, a metabotropic receptor antagonist, into the lateral aspect of the commissural NTS had no effect on the gain of the baroreflex bradycardia and also produced no changes in baseline MAP or HR, indicating that metabotropic receptors are not involved in neurons of the NTS participating in the pulse-to-pulse regulation or in the challenge regulation (additional increase in the pulsatile arterial pressure) of the HR (parasympathoexcitation); and that this class of receptors is not involved in the pulse-to-pulse regulation of the sympathoinhibitory pathway of the baroreflex at the NTS level. However, the involvement of metabotropic receptors in sympathoinhibition during the challenge to baroreceptor activity is still a matter for further investigation.

In order to explore in more detail the parasympathoexcitatory and sympathoinhibitory components of the baroreceptor afferents in the NTS without major previous changes in baseline MAP, we developed a technical approach that permitted us to perform electrical stimulation of the aortic depressor nerve (ADN) in awake rats. To study the neurotransmission of the ADN afferents in the NTS this technique was combined with the implant of the guide cannulas in the direction of the NTS in order to perform microinjections of different antagonists into the NTS. With this approach, our intention was to evaluate the processing of both the parasympathoexcitatory and the sympathoinhibitory component of the baroreceptor afferents in awake rats by measuring the bradycardic and hypotensive responses, respectively. The method for

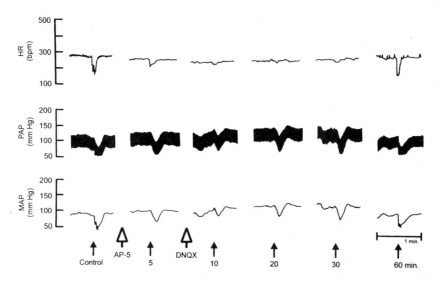

**FIGURE 9.** Changes in heart rate (HR), pulsatile arterial pressure (PAP), and mean arterial pressure (MAP) in response to electrical stimulation (*black-headed arrows*) of the aortic depressor nerve before (control) and 5 (after AP-5), 10 (5 min after DNQX), 20, 30, and 60 min after sequential microinjection of AP-5 (10 nmoles/50 nL) and DNQx (0.5 nmoles/50 nL) into the NTS (*white-headed arrows*). (Data reprinted with permission from Machado et al.[53])

electrical stimulation of the aortic depressor nerve in awake rats was previously standarized in a study from our laboratory,[52] in which we verified that the fall in MAP was dependent on the intensity as well as the frequency of the stimulus. In a study combining microinjections of an EAA receptor antagonist into the NTS with electrical stimulation of the ADN,[53] we used an intensity of 4 V and a frequency of 50 Hz in an experimental protocol consisting of electrical stimulation of the ADN before and after sequential microinjection of NMDA and non-NMDA receptor antagonists into the NTS. The opposite sequence of microinjections was also used.

The control electrical stimulation of the ADN produced significant and consistent bradycardic and hypotensive responses. Bilateral microinjection of AP-5 into the NTS produced mainly a reduction in the bradycardic response to electrical stimulation of the ADN, as documented in FIGURE 9. After the subsequent microinjection of DNQX into the NTS we verified that the bradycardic response was almost blocked, while the hypotensive response presented only a partial reduction. After DNQX an increase in baseline MAP was observed, similarly to previous experiments in which DNQX[18] or kynurenic acid[47] was microinjected into the NTS. In the protocol in which DNQX was microinjected before AP-5, illustrated in FIGURE 10, we also observed a significant reduction in the bradycardic response to electrical stimulation of the ADN. After the subsequent microinjection of AP-5 we verified that the bradycardic response was blocked, while the hypotensive response was only partially reduced, similarly to the experimental protocol in which AP-5 was microinjected first (FIG. 9). It is also important to mention that in both experimental pro-

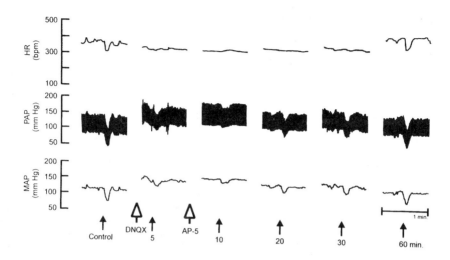

**FIGURE 10.** Changes in heart rate (HR), pulsatile arterial pressure (PAP), and mean arterial pressure (MAP) in response to electrical stimulation (*black-headed arrows*) of the aortic depressor nerve before (control) and 5 (after DNQX), 10 (5 min after AP-5), 20, 30, and 60 min after sequential microinjection of DNQX (0.5 nmoles/50 nL) and DNQx (10 nmoles/50 nL) into the NTS (*white-headed arrows*). (Data reprinted with permission from Machado *et al.*[53])

tocols the cardiovascular responses to electrical stimulation of the ADN returned to control levels 60 min after microinjection of the antagonists into the NTS, showing the reversibility of the blockade.

The data of the first protocol showing that AP-5 produced no changes in baseline HR give additional support to the idea that the pulse-to-pulse activity of the baroreceptor afferents on the parasympathetic component in the NTS is not mediated by NMDA receptors. As mentioned before, NMDA receptors seem to play an important role only when the baroreceptors are submitted to a challenge such as the electrical stimulation of the ADN or the increase in baseline pulsatile arterial pressure produced by phenylephrine infusion. The sequential microinjection of DNQX produced an additional reduction in the bradycardic response, indicating that during the challenge produced by the electrical stimulation of the ADN both NMDA and non-NMDA receptors participate in the processing of the parasympathetic component in the neurons of the NTS projecting to the nucleus ambiguus or dorsal motor nucleus of the vagus. These findings were supported by the results of the second protocol, in which sequential microinjection of DNQX and AP-5 produced a similar blockade of the bradycardic response.

We have previously reported that bilateral microinjection of kynurenic acid into the NTS produced a significant increase in baseline HR,[47] while microinjection of AP-5 into the NTS produced no changes in baseline HR.[48] These data, as previously mentioned, suggest that the pulse-to-pulse regulation of HR involves only non-NMDA receptors because an increase in HR was observed after kynurenic acid, a nonselective receptor antagonist, but not after AP-5, an NMDA receptor antagonist.

However, microinjection of DNQX into the NTS produced no significant increase in baseline HR (FIG. 10). In this case two possible alternatives can be proposed to explain these findings: (1) The regulation of the parasympathoexcitatory component of the baroreflex, on a pulse-to-pulse basis, used both non-NMDA and NMDA receptors, and only the simultaneous blockade of these EAA receptors, as observed with microinjection of kynurenic acid, may result in the blockade of the parasympathoexcitatory component of the baroreflex. (2) The significant increase in baseline MAP after bilateral microinjection of DNQX may activate baroreceptor afferents and prevent the increase in basal HR. In the second case the challenge produced by the increase in pulsatile arterial pressure activated the branch of the parasympathetic component of the baroreflex, which is mediated by NMDA receptors and is not affected by DNQX. In this case, the apparent normal HR observed after DNQX may correspond to a bradycardic response secondary to the increase in baseline MAP. This second possibility does not seem to be valid, because the sequential microinjection of AP-5 into the NTS to block the NMDA receptors produced no additional increase in basal HR. Therefore, it is possible that only the simultaneous double blockade of NMDA and non-NMDA receptors using AP-5 and DNQX could be effective in blocking the pulse-to-pulse regulation of the parasympathoexcitatory component and sympathoinhibitory component to the heart. This hypothesis is supported by previous experiments in which bilateral microinjection of kynurenic acid into the NTS produced a large increase in baseline heart rate (FIG. 6).

Similarly to the processing of the parasympathoexcitatory component, we may also suggest that the sympathoinhibitory component of baroreceptor afferents in the NTS contains two subsystems involved in the modulation of sympathetic activity, illustrated in FIGURE 11: (1) an afferent system, which regulates efferent sympathetic activity on a pulse-to-pulse basis and is observed after bilateral microinjection of kynurenic acid or DNQX into the NTS when baseline MAP increases and which seems to be mediated by non-NMDA receptors; (2) a system that is activated during a challenge, which in our experiments consisted of electrical stimulation of the ADN; apparently ionotropic receptors are not the only class of receptors involved in

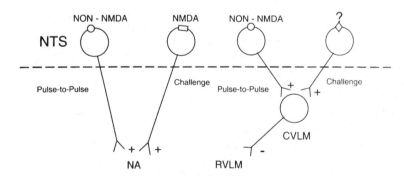

**FIGURE 11.** Schematic drawing showing different projections from the NTS to the nucleus ambiguus [pulse-to-pulse (non-NMDA) and challenge (NMDA)] and from NTS to CVLM [pulse-to-pulse (non-NMDA) and challenge [unknown receptors(?)].

the mediation of this sympathoinhibitory response, because the fall in arterial pressure was only partially reduced (approximately 50%) by sequential microinjection of AP-5 and DNQX into the NTS. These hypotheses are supported by two recent studies by Seagard et al.[54,55] showing that (1) vagal pressure-sensitive afferent input from cardiac mechanoreceptors is transmitted primarily via non-NMDA receptors to neurons in the NTS; (2) NMDA and non-NMDA receptors contribute to the discharge in barosensitive neurons; and (3) the role of each subtype of ionotropic receptors can vary for different neurons in the NTS.

The data from our studies indicate that the ionotropic receptor antagonists of EAA receptors, when microinjected into the specific subregions of the lateral aspect of the commissural NTS, were not effective in blocking the sympathoinhibitory component of the baroreceptor afferents. Several possibilities may be raised to explain these findings. Initially, we cannot rule out the possibility that part of the neurons involved with this sympathoinhibitory pathway in the NTS were not reached by the volume of antagonists microinjected. Second, we also cannot rule out the possible involvement of metabotropic receptors in this processing, considering that experiments using simultaneous microinjection of ionotropic and metabotropic antagonists into the NTS were not performed. Alternatively, we may also consider the possibility that the remaining hypotensive response is mediated by a neurotransmitter other than L-glutamate. Further experiments are required to verify all these possibilities.

## CONCLUSIONS

With respect to the neurotransmission of the chemoreflex in the NTS, the data showed that the parasympathoexcitatory component was blocked by NMDA receptor antagonists while the sympathoexcitatory component was only partially reduced by non-NMDA receptor antagonists, suggesting that neurotransmitters other than L-glutamate may participate in the processing of this component of the chemoreflex.

The data of several experiments suggest that both the sympathoinhibitory and the parasympathoexcitatory components of the baroreceptor afferents are mediated by different subtypes of ionotropic receptors of L-glutamate in the two physiological conditions in which they are activated: (1) on a pulse-to-pulse basis or (2) during the challenge in pulsatile arterial pressure produced by any physiological stimulus that may recruit a different population of baroreceptor afferent fibers. The origin of these afferent fibers in relation to the aortic or carotid sinus as well as the possibility that different afferent fibers regulate distinct branches of the autonomic nervous system remain as important questions to be further investigated.

## ACKNOWLEDGMENTS

The studies performed in our laboratory were supported by grants from Fundação de Amparo à Pesquisa do Estado de São Paulo (FAPESP), Conselho Nacional de Desenvolvimento Científico e Tecnológico (CNPQ), and Programa de Apoio aos Núcleos de Excelência (PRONEX).

## REFERENCES

1. PALKOVITZ, M. & L. ZABORSKY. 1977. Neuroanatomy of central cardiovascular control. Nucleus tractus solitarii: afferent and efferent neuronal connections in relation to the baroreceptor reflex arc. Prog. Brain Res. **47:** 9–31.

2. CIRIELLO, J., S.L. HOCHSTENBACH & S. RODER. 1994. Central projections of baroreceptor afferent fibres in the rat. *In* Nucleus of Solitary Tract. I. Robin A. Barraco, Ed.: 35–50. CRC Press. London.

3. TALMAN, W.T., M.H. PERRONE & D.J. REIS. 1980. Evidence of L-glutamate as the neurotransmitter of baroreceptor afferent nerve fibers. Science **209:** 813–815.

4. GORDON, F.J. & W.T. TALMAN. 1992. Role of excitatory amino acids and their receptors in bulbospinal control of cardiovascular function. *In* Central Neural Mechanisms in Cardiovascular Regulation, Vol. 2. G. Kunos & J. Ciriello, Eds.: 209–225. Birkauser. Boston.

5. MACHADO, B.H., H. MAUAD, D.A. CHIANCA, JR., A.S. HAIBARA & E. COLOMBARI. 1997. Autonomic processing of the cardiovascular reflexes in the nucleus tractus solitarii. Braz. J. Med. Biol. Res. **30:** 533–544.

6. MACHADO, B.H. & L.G.H. BONAGAMBA. 1992. Microinjection of L-glutamate into the nucleus tractus solitarii increases arterial pressure in conscious rats. Brain Res. **576:** 131–138.

7. MICHELINI, L.C. & L.G.H. BONAGAMBA. 1988. Baroreceptor reflex modulation by vasopressin microinjected into the nucleus tractus solitarii of conscious rats. Hypertension **11:** 75–79.

8. ANDRESEN, M. C. & M. YANG. 1990. Non-NMDA receptors mediate sensory afferent synaptic transmission in medial nucleus tractus solitarius. Am. J. Physiol. **259** (Heart Circ. Physiol. **28**): H1307–H1311.

9. ANDRESEN, M.C. & D.L. KUNZE. 1994. Nucleus tractus solitarius; gateway to neural circulatory control. Annu. Rev. Physiol. **56:** 93–116.

10. AYLWIN, M.L., J.M. HOROWITZ & A.C. BONHAM. 1997. NMDA receptors contribute to primary visceral afferent transmission in the nucleus of the solitary tract. J. Neurophysiol. **77:** 2539–2548.

11. COLOMBARI, E., L.G.H. BONAGAMBA & B.H. MACHADO. 1997. NMDA receptor antagonist blocks the bradycardic but not the pressor response to L-glutamate microinjected into the NTS of anesthetized rats. Brain Res. **749:** 209–213.

12. LEONE, C., & F.J. GORDON. 1989. Is L-glutamate a neurotransmitter of baroreceptor information in the nucleus of the tractus solitarius? J. Pharmacol. Exp. Ther. **250:** 953–962.

13. OHTA, H., & W.T. TALMAN. 1997. Both NMDA and non-NMDA receptor in the NTS participate in the baroreceptor reflex in rats. Am. J. Physiol. **267:** R1065–R1070.

14. ZHANG, W. & S.W. MIFFLIN. 1995. Excitatory amino-acid receptors contribute to carotid-sinus and vagus nerve evoked excitation of neurons in the nucleus of the tractus-solitarius. J. Auton. Nerv. Syst. **55:** 50–56.

15. ZHANG, W. & S.W. MIFFLIN. 1998. Differential roles for NMDA and non-NMDA receptor subtypes in baroreceptor afferent integration in the nucleus of the solitary tract of the rat. J. Physiol. **511:** 733–745.

16. FRANCHINI, K.G. & E.M. KRIEGER. 1993. Cardiovascular responses of conscious rats to carotid body chemoreceptor stimulation by intravenous KCN. J. Auton. Nerv. Syst. **42:** 63–70.

17. HAIBARA, A.S., E. COLOMBARI, D.A. CHIANCA-JR., L.G. H BONAGAMBA & B.H. MACHADO. 1995. NMDA receceptors in NTS are involved in bradycardic but not in pressor response of chemoreflex. Am. J. Physiol. **269** (Heart Circ. Physiol. **38**): H1421–H1427.

18. HAIBARA, A.S., L.G.H. BONAGAMBA & B.H. MACHADO. 1999. Neurotransmission of the sympatho-excitatory component of chemoreflex in the nucleus tractus solitarii of unanesthetized rats. Am. J. Physiol. **276** (Regul. Integr. Comp. Physiol. **45**): R69–R80.

19. ZHANG, W. & S.W. MIFFLIN. 1993. Excitatory amino acid receptors within NTS mediate arterial chemoreceptor reflexes in rats. Am. J. Physiol. **265** (Heart Circ. Physiol. **34**): H770–H773.

20. VARDHAN, A., A. KACHROO & H.N. SAPRU. 1993. Excitatory amino acid receptors in the commissural nucleus of the NTS mediate carotid chemoreceptors responses. Am. J. Physiol. **264:** R41–R50.
21. CALLERA, J.C., L.G.H. BONAGAMBA, A. NOSJEAN, R. LAGUZZI & B.H. MACHADO. 1999. Activation of GABAA but not GABAB receptors in the NTS blocked bradycardia of chemoreflex in awake rats. Am. J. Physiol. **276:** H1902–H1910.
22. ZHANG, C.H., L.G.H. BONAGAMBA & B.H. MACHADO. 2000. Blockade of NK-1 receptors in the nucleus tractus solitarii of awake rats produced no effect on the cardiovascular responses to chemoreflex activation. Braz. J. Med. Biol. Res. **33:** 1379–1385.
23. DE PAULA, P.M., L.G.H. BONAGAMBA & B.H. MACHADO. 2000. Involvement of purinergic mechanisms in the neurotransmission of the chemoreflex in the nucleus tractus solitarius of awake rats (abstr.). Auton. Neurosci.: Basic Clin. **82:** 55.
24. AICHER, S.A., R.H. SARAVAY, S. CRAVO, I. JESKE, S.F. MORRISON, D.J. REIS & T.A. MILNER. 1996. Monosynaptic projections from the nucleus tractus solitarii to C1 adrenergic neurons in the rostral ventrolateral medulla: comparison with input from caudal ventrolateral medulla. J. Comp. Neurol. **373:** 62–75.
25. GUYENET, P.G. & N. KOSHIYA, 1992. Respiratory-sympathetic integration in the medulla oblongata. *In* Central Neural Mechanisms in Cardiovascular Regulation. G. Kunos & J. Ciriello, Eds.: 226–247. Birkhauser. Boston.
26. ROSS, C.A., D.A. RUGGIERO & D.J. REIS. 1985. Projections from the nucleus tractus solitarii to the rostral ventrolateral medulla, J. Comp. Neurol. **242:** 511–534.
27. URBANSKI, R.W. & H.N. SAPRU. 1988. Evidence for a sympathoexcitatory pathway from the nucleus tractus solitarii to the ventromedullary pressor area, J. Auton. Nerv. Syst. **23:** 161–174.
28. CIRIELLO, J. & F.R. CALARESU. 1980. Monosynaptic pathway from cardiovascular neurons in the nucleus tractus solitarii to the paraventricular nucleus in the cat. Brain Res. **193:** 529–533.
29. RICARDO, J. & E.T. KOH. 1978. Anatomical evidence of direct projections from the nucleus of the solitary tract to the hypothalamus, amygdala, and other forebrain structures in the rat. Brain Res. **153:** 1–26.
30. SILVA-CARVALHO, L., M. DAWID-MILNER & K.M. SPYER. 1995. The pattern of excitatory inputs to the nucleus tractus solitarii evoked on stimulation in the hypothalamic defence area in the cat. J. Physiol. **487:** 727–737.
31. SILVA-CARVALHO, L., M.S. DAWID-MILNER & K.M. SPYER. 1995. Hypothalamic modulation of the arterial chemoreceptor reflex in the anaesthetized cat: role of the nucleus tractus solitarii. J. Physiol. **487:** 751–760.
32. PYNER, S. & J.H. COOTE. 1997. The organization of the PVN projection to the RVLM and sympathetic preganglionic neurones in the spinal cord of rats. J. Physiol. **501P:** P82–P83.
33. PYNER, S. & J.H. COOTE. 1999. Identification of an efferent projection from the paraventricular nucleus of the hypothalamus terminating close to spinally projecting rostral ventrolateral medulla neurons. Neuroscience **88:** 949–957.
34. YANG, Z. & J.H. COOTE. 1998. Influence of the hypothalamic paraventricular nucleus on cardiovascular neurones in the rostral ventrolateral meudulla of the rat. J. Physiol. **513:** 521–530.
35. HOSOYA, Y., Y. SUGIURA, N. OKADO, A.D. LOEWY & K. KOHNO. 1991. Descending input from the hypothalamic paraventricular nucleus to sympathetic preganglionic neurons in the rat. Exp. Brain Res. **85:** 10–20.
36. BADOER, E. & J. MEROLLI. 1998. Neurons in the hypothalamic paraventricular nucleus that project to the rostral ventrolateral medulla are activated by haemorrhage. Brain Res. **791:** 317–320.
37. COOTE, J.H., Z. YANG, S. PYNER & J. DEERING. 1998. Control of sympathetic outflows by the hypothalamic paraventricular nucleus. Clin. Exp. Pharmacol. Physiol. **25:** 461–463.
38. KATAFUCHI, T., Y. OOMURA & M. KUSOWA. 1988. Effects of chemical stimulation of the paraventricular nucleus on adrenal and renal nerve activity in rats. Neurosc. Lett. **86:** 195–200.
39. MARTIN, D.S. & J.R. HAYWOOD. 1992. Sympathetic nervous system activation by glutamate injections into the paraventricular nucleus. Brain Res. **577:** 262–267.

40. PORTER, J.P. & M.J. BRODY. 1986. A comparison of the hemodynamic effects produced by electrical stimulation of subnuclei of the paraventricular nucleus. Brain Res. **375:** 20–29.
41. KUBO, T., Y. YANAGIHARA, H. YAMAGUCHI & R. FUKUMORI. 1997. Excitatory amino acid receptor in the paraventricular hypothalamic nucleus mediate pressor response induced by carotid body chemoreceptor stimulation in rats. Clin. Exp. Hypertens. **19:** 1117–1134.
42. MACHADO, B.H., E. TAMASHIRO, L.G.H. BONAGAMBA, A.S. HAIBARA & M.V. OLIVAN. 2000. Involvement of paraventricular nucleus of hypothalamus and parabrachial nucleus in the cardiovascular responses of chemoreflex in awake rats (abstr.). FASEB J. **14:** A66.
43. OLIVAN, MV., L.G.H. BONAGAMBA & B.H. MACHADO. 2001. Involvement of the paraventricular nucleus of the hypothalamus in the pressor response to chemoreflex activation in awake rats. Brain Res. **895:** 167–172.
44. URBANSKI, R.W. & H.N. SAPRU. 1988. Evidence for a sympathoexcitatory pathway from the nucleus tractus solitarii to the ventrolateral medullary pressor area. J. Auton. Nerv. Syst. **23:** 161–174.
45. GUYENET, P.G.. 1990. Role of the ventral medulla oblongata in blood pressure regulation. *In* Central Regulation of Autonomic Functions. A.D. Loewy & K.M. Spyer, Eds.: 145–167. Oxford University Press. New York.
46. SPYER, K.M. 1990. The central nervous organization of reflex circulatory control. *In* Central Regulation of Autonomic Functions. A.D. Loewy & K.M. Spyer, Eds.: 168–188. Oxford University Press. New York.
47. Colombari, E., L.G.H. Bonagamba & B.H. Machado. 1994. Mechanisms of pressor and bradycardic responses to L-glutamate microinjected into the NTS of conscious rats. Am. J. Physiol. **266** (Regul. Integr. Comp. Physiol. **35**): R730–R738.
48. FRIGERO, M., L.G.H. BONAGAMBA & B.H. MACHADO. 2000. The gain of the baroreflex bradycardia is reduced by microinjection of NMDA receptor antagonists into the NTS of awake rats. J. Auton. Nerv. Syst.**79:** 28–33.
49. CANESIN, R.O., L.G.H. BONAGAMBA & B.H. MACHADO. 2000. Bradycardic and hypotensive responses to microinjection of L-glutamate into the lateral aspect of the commissural NTS are blocked by an NMDA receptor antagonist. Brain Res. **852:** 68–75.
50. CALLERA, J.C., L.G.H. BONAGAMBA, A. NOSJEAN, et al. 2000. Activation of GABA receptors in the NTS of awake rats reduces the gain of baroreflex bradycardia. Autonom. Neurosci.: Basic Clin. **84:** 58–67.
51. ANTUNES, V.R. & B.H. MACHADO. 2000. Evaluation of the gain of baroreflex after blockade of metabotropic receptors in the nucleus tractus solitary of awake rats (abstr.). FASEB J. **14:** A628.
52. DE PAULA, P.M., J.A. CASTANIA, H.C. SALGADO & B.H. MACHADO. 1999. Hemodynamic responses to electrical stimulation of the aortic depressor nerve in awake rats. Am. J. Physiol. **277** (Regul. Integr. Comp. Physiol. **46**): R31–R38.
53. MACHADO, B.H., J.A. CASTANIA, L.G.H. BONAGAMBA & H.C. SALGADO. 2000. Neurotransmission of autonomic components of aortic baroreceptor afferents in the NTS of awake rats. Am. J. Physiol. **279:** H67–H75.
54. SEAGARD, J.L., C. DEAN & F.A. HOPP. 1999. Role of glutamate receptors in transmission of vagal cardiac input to neurones in the nucleus tractus solitarii in dogs. J. Physiol. **520:** 243–253.
55. SEAGARD, J.L., C. DEAN & F.A. HOPP. 2000. Neurochemical transmission of baroreceptor input in the nucleus tractus solitarius. Brain Res. Bull. **51:** 111–118.

# Adenovirus-mediated Gene Transfer into the NTS in Conscious Rats

## A New Approach to Examining the Central Control of Cardiovascular Regulation

YOSHITAKA HIROOKA, KOJI SAKAI, TAKUYA KISHI, AND AKIRA TAKESHITA

*Department of Cardiovascular Medicine, Cardiovascular Science, Graduate School of Medical Sciences, Kyushu University, Fukuoka 812-8582, Japan*

ABSTRACT: The nucleus tractus solitarii (NTS) is an important site for the regulation of sympathetic nerve activity. It receives the signals through afferent fibers from arterial baroreceptors, chemoreceptors, cardiopulmonary receptors, and other visceral receptors. Many studies have examined the role of nitric oxide (NO) in the NTS in cardiovascular regulation. However, most of these studies were conducted in an acute state with anesthesia. We have developed a novel technique of endothelial nitric oxide synthase (eNOS) gene transfer into the NTS *in vivo*. Adenovirus vectors encoding either the β-galactosidase gene (Adβgal) or the endothelial nitric oxide synthase gene (AdeNOS) gene were transfected into the NTS. In the Adβgal-treated rats, the local expression of β-galactosidase was confirmed by X-Gal staining, and β-galactosidase activity was quantified using a colorimetric assay. In the AdeNOS-treated rats, the local expression of eNOS protein was confirmed by immunohistochemistry, and eNOS production was measured by *in vivo* microdialysis. Blood pressure and heart rate were monitored by a radiotelemetry system in a conscious state. The expression of each gene was observed from day 5 to day 10 after the gene transfer. In the AdeNOS-treated rats, blood pressure and heart rate significantly decreased from day 5 to day 10, and then thereafter gradually recovered over time. Our method may be useful in examining the local effect of a particular substance produced by a specific gene in the brain on cardiovascular function.

KEYWORDS: Sympathetic nervous system; Brain; Nitric oxide; Blood pressure; Gene transfer

## INTRODUCTION

The nucleus tractus solitarii (NTS) receives signals through afferent fibers from arterial baroreceptors, chemoreceptors, cardiopulmonary receptors, and other visceral receptors.[1–4] Thus the NTS plays an important role in the integration of the cardiovascular system.[1–6] The major neurotransmitter in the NTS is thought to be L-

Address for correspondence: Yoshitaka Hirooka, M.D., Ph.D., Department of Cardiovascular Medicine, Cardiovascular Science, Graduate School of Medical Sciences, Kyushu University, 3-1-1 Maidashi, Higashi-ku, Fukuoka 812-8582, Japan. Voice: +81-92-642-5360; fax: +81-92-642-5374.

hyoshi@cardiol.med.kyushu-u.ac.jp

glutamate, although many other substances are also acting as neurotransmitters or neuromodulators in this region.[2,3] In addition, substances such as γ-amino butyric acid (GABA), angiotensin II, nitric oxide (NO), and endothelin-1 may contribute to pathological states such as hypertension or heart failure.[2–5] However, most of this evidence is derived from studies that were performed in anesthetized animals using acute experiments.

Neuronal NO synthase (nNOS) is expressed in specific regions of the brain stem, including the NTS and the ventrolateral medulla (VLM).[3,7] Our laboratory and others have demonstrated that NO in the brain stem contributes to blood pressure regulation through the sympathetic nervous system.[8–13] For example, microinjection of an NOS inhibitor into the NTS increased blood pressure and sympathetic nerve activity.[8,12] However, conflicting results have also been reported.[13]

Experiments using animals in a conscious state examining more chronic effects on cardiovascular responses are preferable. Therefore, we have developed a technique of gene transfer locally into the NTS to examine the effects of increased production of substances such as NO for a much longer period in a conscious state. Some portions of this study were originally published elsewhere.[14]

## METHODS

The study was reviewed and approved by the Committee on Ethics of Animal Experiments, Faculty of Medicine, Kyushu University, and was conducted according to the Guidelines for Animal Experiments of the Faculty of Medicine, Kyushu University.

### Gene Transfer and Expression in the NTS

We used adenoviral vectors encoding either the bacterial β-galactosidase gene or the bovine endothelial NOS (eNOS) gene. These adenoviral vectors were constructed in the Gene Transfer Vector Core Laboratory at the University of Iowa.[15,16]

Adult male Wistar Kyoto rats were used in this study. For gene transfer, the rats were anesthetized with sodium pentobarbital (50 mg/kg, ip) and placed in a stereotaxic frame. Microinjections were performed at six sites in the bilateral NTS defined according to an atlas of the rat brain (See Fig. 1 in Ref. 14).[17] An adenoviral suspension containing $1 \times 10^8$ plaque forming unit (pfu)/mL was injected into each injection site over a 5-minute period (800 nL for each site, infusion rate >0.2 μl/min). After the injection, all rats recovered from anesthesia and were kept unrestrained and free to move in their cages.

At day 7 after the gene transfer, animals were deeply anesthetized with an overdose of pentobarbital. Sections of the medulla (50 μm) were evaluated for either β-galactosidase expression by X-Gal staining or eNOS expression by immunohistochemistry. For eNOS immunohistochemistry, the sections were incubated in mouse IgG monoclonal antibody to human eNOS (1:200) (Transduction Laboratories). After incubation in biotinylated horse anti-mouse IgG (1:1000, Vector Laboratories) as a secondary antibody, the sections were incubated in a mixture of streptavidin-conjugated fluorescein isothiocyanate (1:100, Vector Laboratories) and propidium iodide (PI, 10 μg/mL).

## Quantification of β-Galactosidase Activity

We quantified β-galactosidase activity in the rats transfected with Adβgal by a colorimetric assay using o-nitrophenyl-β-D-galactophyranosidase (ONPG, Boehringer Manhein Biomica, Manheim, Germany) as described previously, but with some modifications. The β-galactosidase activity was assayed before and at 7, 14, and 21 days after the gene transfer of β-galactosidase.[18] The rats were deeply anesthetized with sodium pentobarbital and perfused transcardially with PBS, followed by 4% paraformaldehyde in PBS. The brain was removed and a coronal block of the brain, weighing 0.2 g (approximately 3 mm thick) and containing the injected sites within the NTS, weighing 0.2 g, was excised and placed in ice-cold PBS containing 1 mM phenylmethanesulfonyl fluoride (PMSF). The brain blocks were homogenized for 60 seconds in 3 mL lysis buffer containing 40 mM HEPES, 1% Triton X-100, 10% glycerol, and 1 mM PMSF. Thirty μL of each lysate was assayed in a 270-μL reaction mixture containing 80 mM PBS (pH 7.3), 102 mM 2-mercaptoethanol, 9 mM $MgCl_2$, and 8 mM ONPG, and was incubated for 30 min at 37°C. The absorbance at 420 nm was measured using a spectrophotometer. Purified bacterial β-galactosidase (Boehringer Manheim Biochemica, Manheim, Germany) was used to generate a standard curve for a qualitative analysis. By definition, 1 unit is the amount of enzyme that hydrolyzes 1 μmol of ONPG per min at 37°C. The β-galactosidase activity was normalized with respect to the protein content as determined by a dye-binding assay.

## Microdialysis and Measurement of Total NO Metabolites

We measured the production of NO in the NTS before and at day 7 after the gene transfer as nitrite and nitrate (NOx) using *in vivo* microdialysis as described previously with some modification.[19] (See details in Methods section in Ref. 14). Animals were anesthetized with pentobarbital (50 mg/kg, ip), mechanically ventilated with room air supplemented with oxygen, and placed in a stereotaxic frame. A microdialysis probe [A-I-12-01 (1 mm length)]; Eicom, Kyoto, Japan] was inserted into the medial NTS and perfused with Ringer's solution at a constant flow rate of 2 μL/min. The perfused dialysates were corrected every 10 minutes in a sample loop of an automated sample injector connected to an automated NO detector high-performance liquid chromatography system (ENO-10, Eicom), which was based on a Griess reaction. The test agents were administered after three consecutive stable samples had been collected (basal levels). The basal NOx levels were measured by averaging three consecutive stable dialysate samples, which were obtained approximately 1 hour or more after starting perfusion with Ringer's solution via the microdialysis probe.

## Monitoring Blood Pressure and Heart Rate in a Conscious State

We measured blood pressure and heart rate in a conscious state using a radio-telemetry system (UA-10; Data Science International, St. Paul, Minnesota).[20] In brief, the monitoring system consisted of a transmitter (radio frequency transducer model; TA11PA-C40 or TL11M2-C50-PXT), receiver panel, consolidation matrix, and personal computer with MacLab System (AD Instruments, Milford, Massachusetts). Calibrations were verified to be accurate within the flexible catheter of the

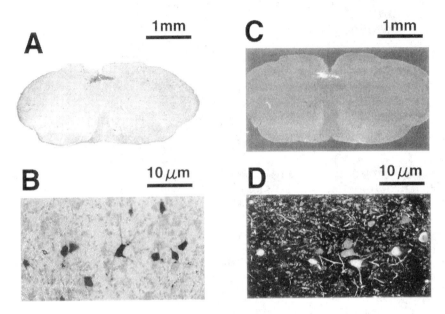

**FIGURE 1.** Photomicrographs demonstrating the expression of β-galactosidase using X-Gal staining **(A,B)** and expression of eNOS by immunohistochemistry **(C,D)** in the NTS. Each procedure was performed at day 7 after the gene transfer.

transmitter, and the device was surgically secured in the abdominal aorta just below the renal arteries while pointing upstream (against the flow). The transmitter was sutured to the abdominal wall. Each rat was housed in an individual cage after the operation, which was placed over the receiver panel that was connected to the personal computer for data acquisition. The rats were unrestrained and free to move in their cages. Blood pressure and heart rate were recorded using a multichannel amplifier and a signal converter.

### Statistical Analysis

Values are expressed as mean ± SE. One-way ANOVA was used to analyze the values of β-galactosidase activity. Two-way ANOVA was used to compare the values between the two groups. Differences were considered to be significant when $p < 0.05$.

## RESULTS

### Gene Expression in the NTS

As shown in FIGURE 1, β-galactosidase activity was detected locally in the NTS and was noted in the section of the medulla at day 7 after transfection with Adβgal.

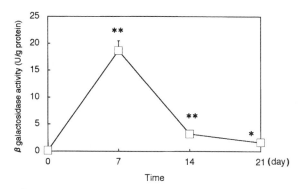

**FIGURE 2.** β-Galactosidase activity in the NTS of rats transfected with Adβgal. Rats were sacrificed with an overdose of pentobarbital at the indicated days after the gene transfer, and β-galactosidase activity was quantified using the colorimetric assay described in the text (at each point, $n = 5$). *$p < 0.05$, **$p < 0.01$ compared with the values at day 0.

In addition, eNOS protein immunoreactivity was observed locally in the NTS at day 7 after transfection with AdeNOS (FIG. 1 C,D).

### *Quantification of β-Galactosidase Activity*

FIGURE 2 shows the time course of β-galactosidase activity before and after transfection with Adβgal. The β-galactosidase activity in the medulla peaked at day 7 after transfection and, thereafter, declined over time. No β-galactosidase activity was detected at day 7 after the AdeNOS transfer ($n = 5$).

### *NOx Production in the NTS*

We measured the production of NO in the NTS as NOx before and after the gene transfer using *in vivo* microdialysis ($n = 5$). The basal level and the level at 1 mm deeper from the NTS of NOx was significantly higher at day 7 in rats transfected with AdeNOS than in the Adβgal-transfected rats (FIG. 3). We also measured NOx levels at a further 3 mm deeper from the NTS. At that site, there were no significant differences between the two treated groups.

### *Blood Pressure and Heart Rate Changes*

We monitored blood pressure and heart rate before and after the gene transfer. FIGURE 4 shows an original recording of blood pressure, electrocardiogram, body temperature, and heart rate in a conscious rat. In the rats transfected with Adβgal, the parameters did not change. In the rats transfected with AdeNOS, however, blood pressure and heart rate decreased at day 5 to day 10 after the gene transfer (see Fig. 2 in Ref. 14). The maximal changes in blood pressure ($-17 \pm 5$ mmHg) and heart rate ($-63 \pm 11$ bpm) were observed at day 7 after gene transfer ($p < 0.05$ compared the values of Adβgal-treated rats). In addition, we observed no change in body temperature and respiration before versus after the gene transfer.

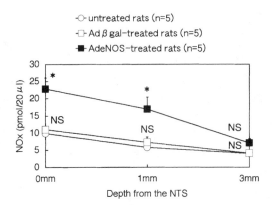

**FIGURE 3.** The levels of NOx in the dialysate obtained at the NTS and at 1 mm and 3 mm deeper from the NTS (each group, $n = 5$). *$p < 0.05$ compared with the values of AdeNOS-treated rats.

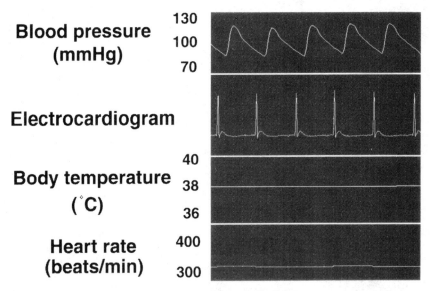

**FIGURE 4.** Examples of original recordings of blood pressure, an electrocardiogram, body temperature, and heart rate using the radiotelemetry system.

## DISCUSSION

The purpose of our study was to deliver a specific gene locally into the NTS and to determine whether the delivered gene produces the specific, active protein. Our results clearly demonstrate that we were able to deliver either the β-galactosidase gene or the eNOS gene into the NTS.

In experiments using adenovirus as a vector, it is important to check the extent of inflammation resulting from the adenovirus infection[21] and whether the inflammation might have affected the results. We used a relatively low titer of adenovirus ($1 \times 10^8$ pfu/mL) that is not cytotoxic. In preliminary experiments, we applied a high titer of the vector ($1 \times 10^9$ pfu/mL). In that experiment, we observed a marked inflammation in the NTS, although the animals survived. Previous studies have shown that cultured cells treated with a high titer of adenovirus do not survive as long as those treated with lower viral titers.[22] In addition, we quantitated ED-1–positive cells, which are a marker of inflammation, and found that their numbers did not differ between rats treated with Adβgal and those treated with AdeNOS. In the Adβgal-treated rats, blood pressure, heart rate, and NOx production did not change after the gene transfer.

We used eNOS instead of neuronal NOS (nNOS), which is normally abundant in the central nervous system. The purpose of our study was to increase the NO production locally in the NTS by overexpression of NOS. In addition, eNOS was more useful in discrimination of de novo production resulting from gene transfer from endogenous production, since we were unable to detect eNOS-positive neurons in the medulla by immunohistochemistry at least under usual microscopic examination.

Experiments using adenovirus vectors as a retrograde transporter provide unique perspective.[23] Adenovirus vector can be taken up by axon terminals in the vicinity of the injection site and retrogradely transported to the cell soma. Vasquez *et al.* have shown that the β-galactosidase gene injected to the pituitary gland was transported to the neurohypophysis, supraoptic nucleus, and paraventricular nucleus of the hypothalamus.[22] However, at least in our experiments, we could not see X-Gal–positive neurons or eNOS-positive neurons in the VLM or hypothalamus. The reasons for this are unclear; however, when we transfected with a much higher titer of adenovirus, we were able to observe retrogradely labeled neurons in other areas of the brain.

Previous studies have used other vectors for *in vivo* transfection of specific genes into the brain. For example, the intracerebroventricular administration of angiotensin-converting enzyme (ACE) gene was accomplished using the hemagglutinating virus of Japan-liposome complex as a vector.[24] In that study, the ACE gene was delivered to supraoptic nucleus, paraventricular hypothalamus, and the rostral VLM, which are located at the surface of the brain.[24] In addition, this study showed that the transfected ACE gene caused the pressor response.[24] Currently, we are not able to determine which vector is better suited for these types of experiments. This vector may be used for local administration into specific nuclei, since the intraparenchymal administration of vectors is thought to be more effective than intracerebroventricular administration. This advantage was clearly demonstrated in the case of the spinal cord.[25]

With regard to the physiological parameters, blood pressure and heart rate decreased after the gene transfer of AdeNOS only. These results suggest that the increased production of NO in the NTS results in hypotension and bradycardia for several days. In addition, our results suggest that the adenovirus transfection itself does not alter these parameters. Interestingly, we observed an increased level of NOx at 1 mm deeper within the NTS, although we did not observe immunohistochemical eNOS-positive neurons in this area. Local NO produced by transfected eNOS in the NTS may diffuse beyond the injection areas in the NTS. In addition, we did not observe changes in respiration after the gene transfer, although we did not measure respiration rate and volume by a precise method such as plethysmography. Further studies will be needed to examine the precise changes in respiration rate and arterial blood gas changes after the eNOS gene transfer.

The role of NO within the brain in the control of the sympathetic nervous system is complex. In general, NO decreases sympathetic nerve activity, which in turn decreases blood pressure.[26] However, NO acts on many sites within the brain nuclei that are important in controlling the sympathetic nerve activity.[26] The approach described here will be useful in examining the role of NO in other areas of the brain such as the VLM or the hypothalamus. Recently, we applied this technique to the rostral VLM to examine the role of NO in cardiovascular regulation.[27]

In summary, we have developed a novel technique of gene transfer into the NTS *in vivo*. Using this technique, we were able to demonstrate that overexpression of eNOS in the NTS, at least for several days, decreases blood pressure and heart rate in conscious rats. These methods will be useful in the study of the role of specific genes in the particular areas within the brain that regulate blood pressure.

## ACKNOWLEDGMENTS

This work was supported by a Grant-in-Aid for Encouragement of Young Scientists (09770489) and a Grant-in-Aid for Scientific Research (C11670689) from the Ministry of Education, Science, Sports and Culture, and the Japan Society for the Promotion of Science.

The authors thank Drs. D. D. Heistad, B. L. Davidson, and R. D. Anderson (The University of Iowa Gene Transfer Vector Core, supported by National Institute of Health Grants and the Carver Foundation, for the preparation of vectors). We also thank Dr. T. Kosaka for the immunohistochemical analysis for eNOS.

## REFERENCES

1. ANDRESEN, M.C. 1994. Nucleus tractus solitarius: gateway to neural circulatory control. Annu. Rev. Physiol. **56:** 93–116.
2. VAN GIERSBERGEN, P.L.M., M. PALKOVITS & W. DE JONG. 1992. Involvement of neurotransmitters in the nucleus tractus solitarii in cardiovascular regulation. Physiol. Rev. **72:** 789–824.
3. LAWRENCE, A.J. & B. JARROTT. 1996. Neurochemical modulation of cardiovascular control in the nucleus tractus solitarius. Prog. Neurobiol. **48:** 21–53.
4. Paton, J.F.R & S. Kasparov. 2000. Sensory channel specific modulation in the nucleus of the solitary tract. J. Auton. Nerv. Syst. **80:** 117–129.
5. KUMADA, M., N. TERUI & T. KUWAKI. 1990. Arterial baroreceptor reflex: its central and peripheral neural mechanisms. Prog. Neurobiol. **35:** 331–361.
6. DAMPNEY, R.A.L. 1994. Functional organization of central pathways regulating the cardiovascular system. Physiol. Rev. **74:** 323–364.
7. VINCENT, S R. & H. KIMURA. 1992. Histochemical mapping of nitric oxide synthase in the rat brain. Neuroscience **46:** 755–784.
8. HARADA, S., S. TOKUNAGA, M. MOMOHARA, *et al.* 1993. Inhibition of nitric oxide formation in the nucleus tractus solitarius increases renal sympathetic nerve activity in rabbits. Circ. Res. **72:** 511–516.
9. TAGAWA, T., T. IMAIZUMI, S. HARADA, *et al.* 1994. Nitric oxide influences neuronal activity in the nucleus tractus solitarius of rat brain stem slices. Circ. Res. **75:** 70–76.

10. HIRONAGA, K., Y. HIROOKA, I. MATSUO, *et al.* 1998. Role of endogenous nitric oxide in the brain stem on rapid adaptation of barorefelex. Hypertension **31**: 27–31.
11. ESHIMA, K., Y. HIROOKA, H. SHIGEMATSU, *et al.* 2000. Angiotensin in the nucleus tractus solitarii contributes to neurogenic hypertension caused by chronic nitric oxide synthase inhibition. Hypertension **36**: 259–263.
12. TSENG, C-J., H-Y. LIU, L-P. GER, *et al.* 1996. Cardiovascular effects of nitric oxide in the brain stem nuclei of rats. Hypertension **27**: 36–42.
13. MATSUMURA, K., T. TSUCHIHASHI, S. KAGIYAMA, *et al.* 1998. Role of nitric oxide in the nucleus of the solitary tract of rats. Brain Res. **798**: 232–238.
14. SAKAI, K., Y. HIROOKA, I. MATSUO, *et al.* 2000. Overexpression of eNOS in NTS causes hypotension and bradycardia in vivo. Hypertension **36**: 1023–1028.
15. DAVIDSON, B.L., E.D. ALLEN, K.F. KOZARSKY, *et al.* 1993. A model system for in vivo gene transfer into the central nervous system using an adenoviral vector. Nat. Genet. **3**: 219–223.
16. OOBOSHI, H., M.J. WELSH, C.D. RIOS, *et al.* 1995. Adenovirus-mediated gene transfer in vivo to cerebral blood vessels and perivascular tissue. Circ. Res. **77**: 7–13.
17. PAXINOS, G. & C. WATSON. 1998. The rat brain in stereotaxic coordinates. *In* The Rat Brain in Stereotaxic Coordinates. Academic Press. New York.
18. UENO, H., J.J. LI, H. TOMITA, *et al.* 1995. Quantitative analysis of repeat adenovirus-mediated gene transfer into injured canine femoral arteries. Arterioscler. Thromb. Vasc. Biol. **15**: 2246–2253.
19. YAMADA, K. & T. NABESHIMA. 1997. Simultaneous measurement of nitrite and nitrate levels as indices of nitric oxide release in the cerebellum of conscious rats. J. Neurochem. **68**: 1234–1243.
20. ANDERSON, N.H., A.M. DEVLIN, D. GRAHAM, *et al.* 1999. Telemetry for cardiovascular monitoring in a pharmacological study: new approaches to data analysis. Hypertension **33**: 248–255.
21. BYRNES, A.P., J.E. RUSBY, M.J.A. WOOD & H.M. CHARLTON. 1995. Adenovirus gene transfer causes inflammation in the brain. Neuroscience **66**: 1015–1024.
22. VASQUEZ, E.C., T.G. BELTZ, S.S. MEYRELLES & A.K. JOHNSON. 1999. Adenovirus-mediated gene delivery to hypothalamic magnocellular neurons in mice. Hypertension **34**: 756–761.
23. KUO, H., D.K. INGRAM, R.G. CRYSTAL & A. MASTRANGELI. 1995. Retrograde transfer of replication deficient recombinant adenovirus vector in the central nervous system for tracing studies. Brain Res. **705**: 31–38.
24. NAKAMURA, S., A. MORIGUCHI, R. MORISHITA, *et al.* 1999. Activation of the brain angiotensin system by in vivo human angiotensin-converting enzyme gene transfer in rats. Hypertension **33**: 302–308.
25. MANNES, A.J., R.M. CAUDLE, B.C. O'CONNEL & M.J. IADAROLA. 1998. Adenoviral gene transfer to spinal cord neurons: intrathecal vs. intraparenchymal administration. Brain Res. **793**: 1–6.
26. PERSSON, P.B. 1996. Modulation of cardiovascular control mechanisms and their interaction. Physiol. Rev. **76**: 193–244.
27. KISHI, T., Y. HIROOKA, K. SAKAI, *et al.* 2001. Overexpression of eNOS in the RVLM causes hypotension and bradycardia via GABA release. Hypertension. In press.

# Oxytocin in the NTS

## A New Modulator of Cardiovascular Control during Exercise

LISETE COMPAGNO MICHELINI

*Department of Physiology and Biophysics, ICB, University of São Paulo, 05508-900, São Paulo, SP, Brazil*

ABSTRACT: The role of brain stem oxytocinergic projections in the modulation of heart rate control during exercise is discussed on the basis of both changes in endogenous peptide content and heart rate changes observed during exercise. Running on a treadmill caused an increase in oxytocin content in dorsal/ventral brain stem areas and spinal cord, specifically in trained rats. Trained rats pretreated with a specific oxytocin receptor antagonist into the dorsal brain stem area (corresponding to the nucleus tractus solitarii and dorsal motor nucleus of the vagus, or NTS/DMV) showed a significant potentiation of exercise tachycardia with no change in the blood pressure response. The same treatment in sedentary rats was without effect. On the other hand, administration of exogenous oxytocin into this area caused significant blunting of exercise tachycardia in both groups, with no change in the pressure response. It is proposed that long-descending oxytocinergic pathways from the hypothalamus to the NTS/DMV area serve as a link between the two main neural controllers of the circulation—that is, the central command and feedback control mechanisms driven by the peripheral receptor signals. Our results strongly suggest that oxytocinergic input to NTS/DMV, by restraining the tachycardic response of trained individuals, contributes to the smaller response observed after training, without compromising cardiac output adjustment and the circulatory demand during exercise.

KEYWORDS: OT receptors; Nucleus tractus solitarii; Dorsal motor nucleus of the vagus; Peptides; Blood pressure; Sedentary and trained rats

## CIRCULATORY CONTROL AT REST AND DURING DYNAMIC EXERCISE

It is well known that cardiac output, total peripheral resistance, and venous capacitance are neurally regulated (on a moment-to-moment basis) to keep blood pressure and volume in a narrow range, maintaining adequate blood supply to different vasculatures. To maintain blood pressure and efficiently adjust flow to several territories in different environmental situations, the central nervous system (CNS) processes peripheral information on such parameters as pressure, blood gases, pH, volume, and temperature, conveyed by different sets of receptors such as barorecep-

Address for correspondence: Lisete C. Michelini, Ph.D., Dep. Fisiologia e Biofísica, ICB-USP, Av. Prof. Lineu Prestes, 1524, 05508-900, São Paulo, SP, Brasil. Voice/fax: 55-11-3818-7213.
michelin@usp.br

tors, chemoreceptors, cardiopulmonary receptors, and others.[1–3] The peripheral information is integrated in different areas and at different levels of the CNS to provide adequate changes in sympathetic and parasympathetic tone to the heart and blood vessels, the main effectors of circulatory control.[3]

Among the neural mechanisms, the baroreceptors are the major controllers of blood pressure.[2–4] Baroreceptor afferents or arterial mechanoreceptors are tonically active and stimulated by the stretch of the vessel during the systolic phase of each cardiac cycle. The firing rate of afferents can be increased or decreased instantaneously according to the larger or smaller stretch of the wall, proportional to the transient increase or decrease in pressure from control levels. The afferents, conveying peripheral information to integrative centers, first project to the nucleus tractus solitarii (NTS) in the brain stem, a heterogeneous cell group. Following pressure increases, second-order neurons in the NTS are stimulated and excite both the parasympathetic preganglionic neurons (in the nucleus ambiguus and dorsal motor nucleus of the vagus—DMV, resulting in an increased vagal outflow to the heart and bradycardia) and the inhibitory GABAergic neurons in the caudal ventrolateral medulla that project to the rostral ventrolateral medulla (RVLM). This inhibition results in a simultaneous reduction of sympathetic tone to the heart (with a further increase of the bradycardic response and reduction of cardiac output) and blood vessels (resulting in an increase in venous capacitance and a decrease in total peripheral resistance), thus contributing to antagonizing the initial pressure increase. Opposite responses—a decrease in venous capacitance (with an increase in venous return) and an increase in both total peripheral resistance and cardiac output—are observed during a transient pressure decrease. Therefore, at resting condition, by stimulating bulbar baroreceptor-mediated mechanisms, pressure challengers always result in a strong reflex bradycardia.

During dynamic exercise, however, there is a moderate increase in pressure maintained throughout the exercise (average of 10–20 mmHg), accompanied not by bradycardia, but by a marked tachycardic response.[5–7] Tachycardia is essential to maintain increased cardiac output (and pressure) in order to provide appropriate flow for exercising muscles. This does not mean that baroreceptors are not working properly during exercise. It has been shown that normal blood pressure, heart rate, cardiac output, and systemic vascular resistance responses to exercise require functional arterial baroreceptors.[5,6,8,9] Experimental evidence also demonstrates that baroreceptors are active during exercise. In rats, loading of baroreceptors during running on a treadmill produces reflex bradycardia;[10] the sensitivity of the bradycardic response after an acute bout of exercise is similar to that seen during rest.[11] It has been proposed that reflex sensitivity is maintained during exercise because the operating point of the arterial baroreflex is reset to higher pressures.[9,12] However, the mechanism(s) that would permit the coexistence of marked tachycardia with a moderate increase in blood pressure during exercise without changing the bradycardic protective response in the case of a further pressure challenge is (are) not known.

## PROPOSED MECHANISMS TO MAINTAIN CIRCULATORY CONTROL DURING EXERCISE

FIGURE 1 summarizes the current knowledge of circulatory control during exercise. It is governed by two main neural mechanisms: a "central command," a feed-

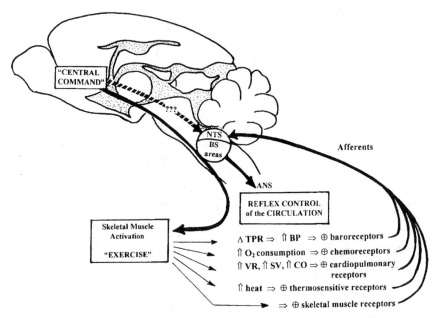

**FIGURE 1.** Schematic representation of the two neural mechanisms that control circulation during exercise: the "central command" and the feedback control mechanisms, driven by different receptors from cardiovascular areas and active muscles. The hypothetic pathway integrating the two mechanisms is represented by the *dashed line*. ANS = autonomic nervous system, BP = blood pressure; BS = brain stem; CO = cardiac output; NTS = nucleus tractus solitarii; SV = stroke volume; TPR = total peripheral resistance; VR = venous return. (Reprinted with permission from Michelini & Morris.[14])

forward control to set the basic pattern of motor activity for the skeletal muscles; and feedback control mechanisms driven by the receptors from cardiovascular areas and active muscles.[6,12–14] Skeletal muscle activation causes (directly and/or indirectly) changes in total peripheral resistance, leading to an increase in pressure that is accompanied by an increase in oxygen consumption, a reduction of venous capacitance with an increase in venous return, and heat production. As shown in FIGURE 1, these changes are continuously monitored by baroreceptors, chemoreceptors, cardiopulmonary receptors, and thermosensitive receptors, respectively. These receptors, together with the receptors located in active muscles, reflexly regulate the circulation, determining appropriate changes in the autonomic outflow to heart and blood vessels. Although it is likely that both feedforward and feedback controllers of circulation interact to regulate blood pressure and heart rate responses during exercise, very little is known about this interaction. An attractive hypothesis we have pursued for the last few years is that projections from central integrative areas, such as those from the hypothalamus to the cardiovascular relay areas in the brain stem would serve as links between the central command and the feedback control driven by peripheral receptors (dashed arrow in the FIG. 1).

Among the modulatory centers in the hypothalamus, the paraventricular nucleus (PVN), an important integrative forebrain area, is of great importance in cardiovascular control. It comprises two distinct regions:[15,16] the magnocellular neurons, which synthesize and release vasopressin and oxytocin into the blood via the neurohypophysis;[17] and the neurons of the parvocellular region, which project to brain stem areas (NTS, DMV, VLM) and to the intermediolateral column of the spinal cord and are involved in autonomic control of heart and vessels.[18–23] The NTS in the brain stem is an important candidate site for the proposed interaction between feedforward and feedback controllers of the circulation during exercise because: (1) it is the first synaptic relay of all peripheral afferents in the central nervous system;[4,23,24] (2) it projects to brain stem areas controlling parasympathetic and sympathetic outflow;[2,4] (3) it projects directly (and indirectly via bulbar, pontine, and midbrain groups) to PVN and other hypothalamic nuclei, amygdala, and cortex;[4,25–27] and (4) it receives monosynaptic projections from the PVN.[18–21] The reciprocal direct NTS $\rightarrow$ PVN and PVN $\rightarrow$ NTS innervation provides anatomic support for a prompt feedback control loop through which the PVN, besides the autonomic and neuroendocrine control, could also modulate cardiovascular control at NTS level.[14,27]

The long-descending monosynaptic projections from the PVN to the NTS have been shown to contain vasopressin, oxytocin, enkephalins, and somatostain.[21–23] Since vasopressin (VP) and VP receptors are present in the NTS[28–32] and the PVN has been shown to be the only source of vasopressinergic projections to the NTS,[20,21] we first investigated the effects of VP on baroreceptor reflex control of the heart. VP restricted to the NTS displaced reflex bradycardia toward high heart rate values, thus reducing the bradycardic response during loading of baroreceptors.[33] The occlusional bradycardic response is an important adaptive response to dynamic exercise because of the maintenance of blood pressure at a moderately elevated level. Next we investigated the role of vasopressinergic projections as possible links between the central command and the reflex control of the circulation during exercise. Our studies, focusing on the role of PVN vasopressinergic input to the NTS in the modulation of cardiovascular control, do confirm this hypothesis.[14,34] We showed that these projections are activated during dynamic exercise in both sedentary (S) and trained (T) rats, as demonstrated by the increase in VP content into dorsal brain stem areas and by the blunting of exercise tachycardia following VP antagonist pretreatment in the NTS.[14,34] We also showed that exogenous VP administered into the NTS, mimicking a strong stimulation of vasopressinergic projections, significantly potentiated exercise tachycardia in both S and T rats.[14,34] However, endogenous VP does not account for the entire tachycardic effect, since pretreatment with a specific receptor antagonist blunted, but did not block, the exercise-induced tachycardia.[34] Furthermore, the difference in the tachycardic response between trained (smaller heart rate increase) and sedentary individuals (higher heart rate response for similar submaximal exercise intensity, depicted in Fig. 2) was not correlated with changes in central VP content.[34] Actually, training did not change the maximal heart rate response to dynamic exercise (attained at higher exercise loads), but significantly reduced the magnitude of exercise-induced tachycardia at similar submaximal exercise intensities, when compared to S individuals.[35,36] This characteristic adaptive effect of training has been shown to be accompanied by changes in vagal and sympathetic tone to the heart[36–39] and by alterations in the central oxytocinergic system.[40]

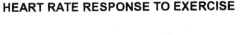

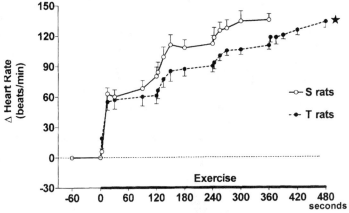

**FIGURE 2.** Comparison of heart rate responses to graded exercise in groups of sedentary (S) and trained rats (T). Dynamic exercise tests (slope = 0%) were performed on a treadmill up to the achievement of maximal response, with intensity increasing every 2 min (0.4, 0.8, 1.1, and 1.4 km/h). *($p < 0.05$) means a different response at similar exercise load.

## ARE OXYTOCINERGIC PROJECTIONS TO THE NTS ALSO INVOLVED IN THE MODULATION OF CARDIOVASCULAR CONTROL DURING EXERCISE?

Besides the well-known effects of oxytocin (OT) on uterine contraction and milk ejection in females, OT is universally important in complex physiological functions such as behavioral, gastrointestinal, renal, and cardiovascular.[41] OT is present in males and females in similar levels and is secreted in response to stress, volume, osmotic, and satiety stimuli.[42–45] OT is structurally similar to VP, with which it shares several stimuli for release. However, different from VP, the role of OT in cardiovascular regulation has been the subject of limited investigation. Although being a weaker vasoconstrictor than VP, OT has significant effects on blood pressure, vascular tone, and renal function.[46–48] There is also evidence for central effects of OT on cardiovascular function. OT is present in brain stem integrative centers, the result of projections from parvocellular neurons of the PVN.[18–21] Manipulation of PVN OT systems with antisense oligonucleotides, antagonists, or lesions results in prominent alterations in cardiovascular responses to stress and peptidergic stimulation and alterations in salt consumption.[45,49,50] OT receptors are densely present in dorsal brain stem areas.[31,51] Brain stem administration of OT or OT receptor antagonist changed local neuronal activity[52,53] and autonomic control of the heart.[54] Nevertheless, there are some controversies concerning the nature of OT regulation of cardiac function. OT has been shown to have no effect or to decrease basal heart rate[46,55] and to enhance or reduce baroreceptor reflex gain.[56,57]

OXYTOCIN

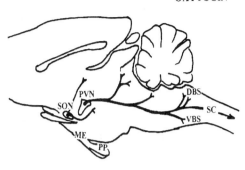

BRAIN / PLASMA OXYTOCIN CONTENT

|  | at rest<br>T x S | exercise x rest<br>S rats | exercise x rest<br>T rats |
|---|---|---|---|
| PVN | + 72% | ~ | ~ |
| SON | ~ | ~ | ~ |
| ME | ~ | ~ | ~ |
| PP | ~ | ~ | ~ |
| DBS | ~ | ~ | + 355 % |
| VBS | ~ | ~ | + 176 % |
| SC | ~ | ~ | + 228 % |
| plasma | + 37% | ~ | - 50 % |

**FIGURE 3.** Schematic representation of extrahypothalamic oxytocinergic pathways arising from parvicellular regions of the supraoptic (SON) and paraventricular (PVN) nuclei in the hypothalamus and of the other central areas in which oxytocin content was measured. In the table, OT content changes are compared between trained (T) and sedentary (S) rats at rest (T × S) and between exercise and resting conditions in each group (exercise × rest). Basal content of oxytocin was not changed by training, except for increases in PVN and plasma; immediately after dynamic exercise, marked increases in oxytocin content in the DBS, VBS, and SC, accompanied by decrease in plasma levels, were observed only in trained rats. DBS = dorsal brain stem; ME = median eminence; PP = posterior pituitary; SC = spinal cord; VBS = ventral brain stem. (Modified from Braga *et al.*[40])

To elucidate, if central OT is also involved in modulation of cardiovascular control during exercise, our first approach was to determine OT content in different CNS areas and plasma. Sedentary and trained rats were sacrificed at rest or after an exercise protocol on a treadmill resulting in maximal exercise tachycardia.[40] The results of the T and S groups[40] are summarized in FIGURE 3, showing a schematic drawing of main central areas (and some oxytocinergic projections) involved in cardiovascular control. Regional brain OT (nuclear and terminal projection areas) and plasma OT content showed no significant differences between S and T rats under resting conditions. However, a close observation on OT levels revealed that after training resting PVN content was increased by 72% (group effect, $p < 0.05$), while plasma level was increased by 37% (group x condition interaction, $p < 0.05$). Immediately after dynamic exercise OT content was not changed in the biosynthetic areas (PVN,

SON) or in the areas corresponding to magnocellular pathways (PP, ME), but there was a marked increment in the dorsal brain stem OT content (DBS = 4.5-fold increase), accompanied by significant increases in ventral brain stem and spinal cord OT content (VBS = 2.7-fold increase; SC = 3.4-fold increase) only in the T group. In this group plasma OT was reduced by 50% immediately after the treadmill exercise. No changes were observed in the S group after dynamic exercise on the treadmill (vs. resting condition, FIG. 3).

These results demonstrated that oxytocinergic projections to the NTS are stimulated when rats exercise, but this stimulation occurs only in the trained animals. Furthermore, the specific increases of OT content in parvocellular pathways projecting to brain stem areas and spinal cord, without any detectable change in the biosynthetic areas or in the magnocellular pathways to neurohypophysis, suggested that the central oxytocinergic system does not act as a whole, but responds differentially to different stimuli. As we have shown here, dynamic exercise stimulates specifically the parvocellular oxytocinergic pathways modulating autonomic outflow, while decreasing plasma OT content in the trained rats. Our next question was: what is the functional significance of differential oxytocinergic input to brain stem areas during dynamic exercise?

## OXYTOCINERGIC INPUT TO THE DORSAL BRAIN STEM MODULATES EXERCISE TACHYCARDIA

To determine whether changes in OT content in the dorsal brain stem (NTS/DMV area) are associated with cardiovascular responses to dynamic exercise, we investigated blood pressure and heart rate responses to treadmill exercise. Studies employed a technique we developed for microinjection of peptides into dorsal brain stem areas of conscious rats.[33] S and T rats were pretreated with a specific blocker of OT receptors into the NTS/DMV. In both groups, injection of a small dose of OT antagonist into this area (20 pmol/200 nL) did not change baseline values of arterial pressure and heart rate.[40] As shown in FIGURE 4, mean arterial pressure response to the treadmill exercise was not changed in either group, but OT receptor blockade restricted to the NTS/DMV area significantly potentiated the exercise tachycardia only in the trained group. In this group maximal heart rate response was increased by 26% over the maximal value observed after VEH treatment. On the other hand, exercise tachycardia in S rats was not changed by OT receptor blockade in the NTS/DMV (FIG. 4).

Curiously, when the agonist OT was administered in the NTS/DMV, a significant and similar reduction of exercise tachycardia was observed in both groups: maximal heart rate response (vs. respective VEH control) was reduced by 23% and 26% in the T and S groups, respectively, with no change in the pressure response.[40] A comparison between the facilitatory/inhibitory effects of oxytocinergic synapses at NTS/DMV in T versus S rats (FIG. 5) shows clearly that the effect of OT receptor blockade on exercise tachycardia differs dramatically between groups (marked improvement vs. no change), while the effect of OT was exactly the same in both groups. This inhibitory effect of exogenous OT upon exercise tachycardia indicate that the differential response is not due to the presence/absence of functional OT receptors in the NTS/DMV, but that brain stem OT input is not activated when S rats exercise. There-

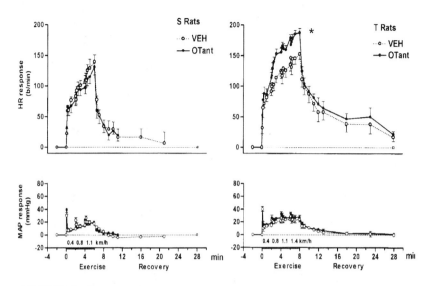

**FIGURE 4.** Heart rate (HR, *top*) and mean arterial pressure responses (MAP, *bottom*) during different exercise intensities and recovery in groups of sedentary (S, *left*) and trained rats (T, *right*) pretreated with vehicle (VEH, saline) and oxytocin receptor antagonist (OTant) into the solitary-vagal complex (NTS/DMV). *Significance $p < 0.05$ vs. VEH. (Reprinted with permission from Braga et al.[40])

fore, the functional responses (FIG. 5) are very consistent with the measured changes in OT content following exercise that we described above (FIG. 3), indicating a specific stimulation of the parvocellular oxytocinergic pathway during exercise only in T rats.

Previous work actually demonstrated that the PVN is the primary source of OT in the brain stem and spinal cord,[18–21] and the present results indicate that these parvocellular projections to DBS are involved in the modulation of exercise tachycardia. It should be noted that immediately after the treadmill exercise, OT content was also increased in VBS and SC (FIG. 3). Although it is possible that these regions could act together to modulate heart rate response via combined effects on afferent input plus vagal and sympathetic output, the functional effects of OT in the ventral brain stem (corresponding to VLM) and spinal cord during exercise remain to be determined.

Support for a brain stem–centered modulation of cardiovascular control by oxytocinergic synapses was also provided by the study of fourth ventricular injections.[40] Intracerebroventricular administration of OT or OTant produced no effect on the cardiovascular responses to exercise, suggesting that OT in the cerebrospinal fluid is not involved in this response .

And what is the functional meaning of the differential oxytocinergic stimulation in sedentary and trained individuals? Speculating on the possible significance, one should consider that trained individuals presented increased maximal oxygen uptake, which is accompanied by cardiovascular adaptations such as increased myocar-

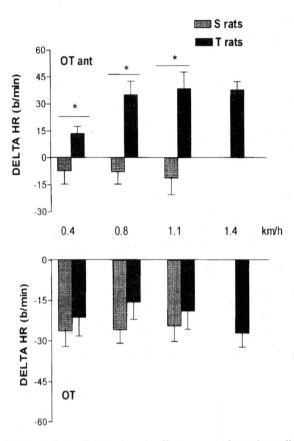

**FIGURE 5.** Comparison of oxytocinergic effects on exercise tachycardia between sedentary (S) and trained (T) rats pretreated with the peptides into the NTS/DMV. *Bars* represent the differential heart rate effect of both antagonist (OTant response minus VEH response) and agonist (OT response minus VEH response) at different workloads. All heart rate changes (DHR) were significant, except those after OTant treatment in the S group. *Indicates a significant difference ($p < 0.05$) between S and T rats. (Reprinted with permission from Braga *et al.*[40])

dium contractility and cardiac output, increased capillary supply with larger flow, and increased oxygen extraction by the exercising muscles.[35,36,58,59] These cardiac and skeletal muscle adaptations occur without alterations in resting blood pressure. It is also well established that during exercise trained individuals show maximal heart rate responses, which are similar to those of sedentary individuals (FIG. 2). Compared to sedentary controls, however, the maximal responses are attained at a higher exercise load, with smaller tachycardic responses seen at similar submaximal exercise intensities.[35,60] It is also known that trained and sedentary individuals exhibited differential parasympathetic withdrawal and sympathetic activation,[39,60,61] but the central mechanism(s) responsible for these training-induced changes have not been identified. On the basis of our data, we hypothesize that OT released specifically into the dorsal brain stem of trained rats acts to reduce exercise tachycardia, and the resulting energy expense, without changing the blood pressure response. Therefore, activation of oxytocinergic pathways to NTS/DMV could be the main central mechanism to explain the smaller exercise tachycardia of trained individuals without compromising an adequate cardiac output and blood flow to active muscles.

The modulation of exercise tachycardia by OT into the NTS/DMV is an original observation with two new implications: (1) it points to the NTS as an important area for modulation of afferent cardiovascular inputs (level? type? distribution?) coming from the periphery; (2) it uncovers the importance of oxytocin as a central cardiovascular modulatory peptide. Actually, recent studies in our laboratory showed that oxytocinergic receptors in the NTS do modulate baroreceptor reflex control of heart rate by facilitating the bradycardic response to pressure challenges.[62] We also observed prominent differences in autonomic control of the heart and altered baroreflex function in OT knockout mice.[63]

## CONCLUSIONS

Specific modulation of the heart rate response (and thus cardiac output) during exercise constitutes a very precise and selective mechanism for maintaining adequate blood supply to the brain, heart, skin, and active muscles. In this condition the central control of heart functions (rate, filling, contractility) is of paramount importance. During exercise, the "disconnection" between pressure increase and the baroreceptor reflex control of the heart, resulting in tachycardia rather than bradycardia, is a very important mechanism to guarantee cardiovascular homeostasis. It is our working hypothesis that projections from integrative hypothalamic centers (as the PVN) to cardiovascular relay areas in the brain stem (NTS/DMV) act as links between the central command and reflex control of the circulation. Activation of these projections would adjust cardiovascular control to many different situations, thus keeping its efficiency.

Actually, our previous data with stimulation of central vasopressinergic projections[14,27,33,34] and the recent results on OT content changes and functional responses following activation/inhibition of oxytocinergic input during dynamic exercise[40] provided experimental evidence that does confirm our hypothesis. As illustrated in FIGURE 6, we proposed that OT pathways from PVN to the dorsal brain stem, as well as the vasopressinergic projections we showed before,[14] also serve as links between the central command and the autonomic control of circulation. VP facilitates the tachycardic response (without changing baroreflex sensitivity) in both S and T rats, while OT facilitates the slow down of the heart in the T group, protecting against sharp and perhaps detrimental heart rate increases. In addition we showed that exogenous OT given into the NTS depresses exercise tachycardia in both S and T groups,[40] and it also facilitates reflex bradycardia during transient hypertension.[62]

It should be stressed that when trained individuals exercise, VP and OT are released in the DBS, showing specific and opposite effects upon heart rate control. These opposite effects are not unusual. Similar "arrangements" in which two closely related substances have opposite effects are present in other biological systems, such as the renin-angiotensin (angiotensin II × angiotensin 1–7[64,65]) and the endothelium-

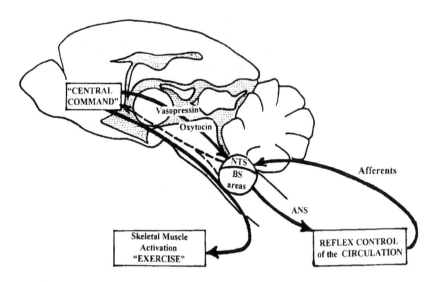

**FIGURE 6.** Proposed vasopressinergic and oxytocinergic links to adjust the feedforward (central command) and feedback controllers of the circulation during exercise. *Dashed line* represents afferent-encoded information from cardiovascular receptors conveyed by the NTS (and other brain stem areas, = BS) to suprabulbar integrative centers. ANS = autonomic nervous system.

derived factors (EDRFs × EDCFs[66]). A balance between excitatory (VP) and inhibitory (OT) stimuli improves efficiency of the system in trained individuals to better adjust physiological responses to momentary requirements. It is important to note that training also triggers several peripheral adaptations (for example, cardiac eccentric hypertrophy, larger capillary bed in myocardium and skeletal muscles, and increased oxygen extraction[35,36,59,67]) that help to maintain adequate cardiac output and tissue perfusion even with smaller exercise tachycardia. In sedentary individuals the absence of these adaptive responses is compensated for by higher tachycardic response, driven only by the vasopressinergic input to DBS areas. Therefore, at the NTS level of trained individuals OT and VP (or VP alone in the sedentary individuals) act as neurotransmitters to modulate heart rate response to exercise by blunting or potentiating, respectively, the tachycardia. It is apparent from our previous experiments[34,40] that the oxytocinergic input predominates after training.

We must emphasize that the vasopressinergic and oxytocinergic pathways to the DBS are not the only central mechanism involved in the genesis of exercise tachycardia (and/or central adaptations to training). Other peptides have been identified in the solitarii-vagal complex,[23] some of hypothalamic origin.[21] Kregel et al.[68] suggested that corticotropin releasing factor is important because a partial blunting of tachycardic response was observed after intracerebroventricular administration of its receptor antagonist.

Taken together, the anatomic, immunohistochemical, radioautographic, biochemical, and functional data summarized in this chapter indicate the NTS as an important modulatory site in the brain stem for cardiovascular control. They indicate also that the long-descending vasopressinergic and oxytocinergic projections from PVN to this area are part of the central mechanisms modulating baroreceptor reflex control of heart rate during pressure challenges and exercise, thus contributing to the adjustment of cardiac output (and pressure) to different environmental conditions.

## ACKNOWLEDGMENTS

This work was supported by Fundacao de Amparo a Pesquisa do Estado de Sao Paulo (FAPESP: 98/04891-5 and 99/08012-9) and Conselho Nacional de Desenvolvimento Científico e Tecnológico (CNPq: 451385/00-4 and 465209/00-9).

## REFERENCES

1. PALKOVITS, M. 1980. The anatomy of central cardiovascular neurons. In Central Adrenalin Neurons: Basic Aspects and Their Role in Cardiovascular Functions. K. Fuke, M. Goldstein, B. Hökfelt & T. Hökfelt, Eds.: 3–17. Pergamon Press. Oxford.
2. CHALMERS, J. & P. PILOWSKY. 1991. Brainstem and bulbospinal neurotransmitter systems in the control of blood pressure. J. Hypertens. **9:** 675–694.
3. DAMPNEY, R.A.L. 1994. Functional organization of central pathways regulating the cardiovascular system. Physiol. Rev. **74:** 323–364.
4. SVED A.F. & F.J. GORDON. 1994. Amino acids as central neurotransmitters in the baroreceptor reflex pathway. News Physiol. Sci. **9:** 243–246.
5. LUDBROOK, J. 1983. Reflex control of blood pressure during exercise. Annu. Rev. Physiol. **45:** 155–168.
6. ROWELL, L.B. 1992. Reflex control of the circulation during exercise. Int. J. Sports Med. **13**(Suppl. I): S25–S27.
7. AMARAL, S.L. & L.C. MICHELINI. 1997. Validation of transit-time flowmetry for chronic measurements of regional blood flow in resting and exercising rats. Braz. J. Med. Biol. Res. **30:** 897–908.
8. DICARLO, E. & V.S. BISHOP. 1990. Exercise training enhances cardiac afferent inhibition of baroreflex function. Am. J. Physiol. **258** (Heart Circ. Physiol. 27): H212–H220.
9. DICARLO, E. & V.S. BISHOP. 1992. Onset of exercise shifts operating point of arterial baroreflex to higher pressures. Am. J. Physiol. **262** (Heart Circ. Physiol. 31): H303–H307.
10. KRIEGER, E.M., P.C. BRUM & C.E. NEGRÃO.1999. Role of arterial baroreceptors during acute and chronic exercise. Biol. Res. In press.
11. SILVA, G.J., P.C. BRUM, C.E. NEGRÃO & E.M. KRIEGER. 1997. Acute and chronic effects of exercise on baroreflexes in spontaneously hypertensive rats. Hypertension **30** (Pt.2): 714–719.
12. ROWELL, L.B. & D.S. O'LEARY. 1990. Reflex control of the circulation during exercise: chemoreflexes and mechanoreflexes. J. Appl. Physiol. **69:** 407–418.
13. MITCHEL, J.H. 1990. Neural control of the circulation during exercise. Med. Sci. Sports Exerc. **22:** 141–154.
14. MICHELINI. L.C. & M. MORRIS. 1999. Endogenous vasopressin modulates the cardiovascular responses to exercise. Ann. N.Y. Acad. Sci. **897:** 198–211.
15. SWANSON, L.W. & H.G.J.M. KUYPERS. 1980. The paraventricular nucleus of the hypothalamus: cytoarchitectonic subdivisions and organization of projections to the pituitary, dorsal vagal complex and spinal cord as demonstrated by retrograde fluorescence double-labeling methods. J. Comp. Neurol. **194:** 555–570.
16. SWANSON, L.W. & P.E. SAWCHENKO. 1980. Paraventricular nucleus: a site for the integration of neuroendocrine and autonomic mechanisms. Neuroendocrinology **31:** 410–417.

17. MORRIS, J.F., D.B. CHAPMAN & H.W. SOKOL. 1987. Anatomy and function of the classic vasopressin secreting hypothalamus-neurohypophyseal system. *In* Vasopressin: Principles and Properties. D.M. Gash & G.I. Boer, Eds.: 1–89. Plenum. New York.
18. BUIJS, R.M., D.F. SWAAB, J. DOGTEROM & F.W. VAN LEEUWEN. 1978. Intra and extrahypothalamic vasopressin and oxytocin pathways in the rat. Cell Tiss. Res. **186:** 423–433.
19. NILAVER, G, E.A. ZIMMERMAN, J. WITKINS, *et al.* 1980. Magnocellular hypothalamic projection to the lower brain stem and spinal cord of the rat. Immunocytochemical evidence for predominance of the oxytocin-neurophysin system compared to the vasopressin-neurophysin system. Neuroendocrinology **30:** 150–158.
20. SOFRONIEW, M.V. & U. SCHRELL. 1981. Evidence for a direct projection from oxytocin and vasopressin neurons in the hypothalamic paraventricular nucleus to the medulla oblongata: immunohistochemical visualization of both the horseradish peroxidase transported and the peptide produced by the same neurons. Neurosci. Lett. **22:** 211–217.
21. SAWCHENKO, P.E. & L.W. SWANSON. 1982. Immunohistochemical identification of neurons in the paraventricular nucleus of the hypothalamus that project to the medulla or to the spinal cord in the rat. J. Comp.Neurol. **205:** 260–272.
22. PALKOVITS, M. 1984. Distribution of neuropeptides in the central nervous system: a review of biochemical mapping studies. Progr. Neurobiol. **23:** 115–189.
23. VAN GIERSBERGEN, P.L.M., M. PALKOVITS & W. DE JONG. 1992. Involvement of neurotransmitters in the nucleus tractus solitarii in cardiovascular regulation. Physiol. Rev. **72:** 789–824.
24. MIURA, M. & D.J. REIS. 1969. Termination and secondary projections of carotid sinus nerve in the cat brain stem. Am. J. Physiol. **217:** 142–153.
25. SAWCHENKO, P.E. & L.W. SWANSON. 1981. Central noradrenergic pathways for the integration of hypothalamic neuroendocrine and autonomic responses. Science **214:** 685–687.
26. PALKOVITS, M. 1988. Neuronal circuits in central baroreceptor mechanism. *In* Progress in Hypertention, Vol 1. H. Saito, H. Parvez, S. Parvez & T. Nagatsu, Eds.: 387–409. VSP. Utrecht.
27. MICHELINI, L.C. 1994. Vasopressin in the nucleus tractus solitarius: a modulator of baroreceptor reflex control of heart rate. Braz. J. Med. Biol. Res. **27:** 1017–1032.
28. WEINDL, A. & M. SOFRONIEW. 1985. Neuroanatomical pathways related to vasopressin. *In* Neurobiology of Vasopressin. D. Ganten & D. Pfaff, Eds.: 137–195. Springer-Verlag. Berlin.
29. DOGTEROM, J., F.G.M. SNIJDEWINT & R.M. BUIJS. 1978. The distribution of vasopressin and oxytocin in the rat brain. Neurosci. Lett. **9:** 341–346.
30. VAN LEEUWEN, F.W., E.M. VAN DER BEEK, J.J. VAN HEERIKHUIZE, *et al.* 1987. Quantitative light microscopic autoradiographic localization of binding sites labelled with [$^3$H] vasopressin antagonist d(CH$_2$)$_5$Tyr(Me)VP in the rat brain, pituitary and kidney. Neurosci. Lett. **80:** 121–126.
31. TRIBOLLET, E., C. BARBERIS, S. JARD, *et al.* 1988. Localization and pharmacological characterization of high affinity binding sites for vasopressin and oxytocin in the rat brain by light microscopic autoradiography. Brain Res. **442:** 105–118.
32. PHILLIP, P.A., J.M. ABRAHAMS, J. KELLY, *et al.* 1988. Localization of vasopressin binding sites in rat brain by *in vitro* autoradiography using a radioiodinated V$_1$ receptor antagonist. Neuroscience **27:** 749–761.
33. MICHELINI, L.C. & L.G.H. BONAGAMBA. 1988. Baroreceptor reflex modulation by vasopressin microinjected into the nucleus tractus solitarii of conscious rats. Hypertension **11**(Suppl. I): I.75–I.79.
34. DUFLOTH, D.L., M. MORRIS & L.C. MICHELINI. 1997. Modulation of exercise tachycardia by vasopressin in the nucleus tractus solitarii. Am. J. Physiol. **273** (Regul. Integr. Comp. Physiol. **42**): R1271–R1282.
35. CLAUSEN, J.P. 1977. Effect of physical training on cardiovascular adjustments to exercise in man. Physiol. Rev. **57:** 779–815.
36. SCHEUER, J. & C.M. TIPTON. 1977. Cardiovascular adaptations to physical training. Annu. Rev. Physiol. **39:** 221–251.

37. SMITH M.L., D.L. HUDSON, H.M. GRAITZER & P.B. RAVEN. 1989. Exercise training bradycardia: the role of autonomic balance. Med. Sci. Sports Exercise **21:** 40–44.
38. NEGRÃO, C.E., E.D. MOREIRA, P.C. BRUM, *et al.* 1992. Vagal and sympathetic control of heart rate during exercise by sedentary and exercise-trained rats. Braz. J. Med. Biol. Res. **25:** 1045–1052.
39. NEGRAO, C.E., E.D. MOREIRA, M.C.L.M. SANTOS, *et al.* 1992. Vagal function impairment after exercise training. J. Appl. Physiol. **72:** 1749-1753.
40. BRAGA, D.C., E. MORI, K.T. HIGA, *et al.* 2000. Central oxytocin modulates exercise-induced tachycardia. Am. J. Physiol. Regul. Integr. Comp. Physiol. **278:** R1474–R1482.
41. RICHARD P., F. MOOS & M.J. FREUND-MERCIER. 1991. Central effects of oxytocin. Physiol. Rev. **71:** 331–370.
42. KADEKARO, M., J.Y. SUMMY-LONG, S. FREEMAN, *et al.* 1992. Cerebral metabolic responses and vasopressin and oxytocin during progressive water deprivation in rats. Am. J. Physiol. Regul. Integr. Comp. Physiol. **262:** R310–R317.
43. LUDWIG, M., M.F. CALLAHAN, I. NEUMANN, *et al.* 1994. Systemic osmotic stimulation increases vasopressin and oxytocin release within the supraoptic nucleus. J. Neuroendocrinol. **6:** 369–373.
44. MORRIS, M. & N. ALEXANDER. 1989. Baroreceptor influences on oxytocin and vasopressin secretion. Hypertension **13:** 110–114.
45. MORRIS, M., A.B. LUCION, P. LI & M.F. CALLAHAN. 1995. Central oxytocin mediates stress-induced tachycardia. J. Neuroendocrinol. **7:** 455–459.
46. PETERSSON, M., T. LUNDEBERG & K. UVNAS-MOBERG. 1997. Oxytocin decreases blood pressure in male but not female spontaneously hypertensive rats. J. Auton. Nerv. Syst. **66:** 15–18.
47. PETERSSON, M., T. LUNDEBERG & K. UVNAS-MOBERG. 1999. Short-term increase and long-term decrease of blood pressure in response to oxytocin-potentiating effect of female steroid hormones. J. Cardiovasc. Pharmacol. **33:** 102–108.
48. VERBALIS, J.G., M.P. MANGIONE & E.M. STRICKER. 1991. Oxytocin produces natriuresis in rats at physiological plasma concentrations. Endocrinology **128:** 1317–1322.
49. CALLAHAN, M.F., C.R. THORE, D.K. SUNDBERG, *et al.* 1992. Excitotoxin paraventricular nucleus lesions: stress and endocrine reactivity and oxytocin mRNA levels. Brain Res. **597:** 8–15.
50. MAIER, T., W.J. DAI, T. CSIKOS, *et al.* 1998. Oxytocin pathways mediate the cardiovascular and behavioral responses to substance P in the rat brain. Hypertension **31:** 480–486.
51. BARBERIS, C. & E. TRIBOLLET. 1996. Vasopressin and oxytocin receptors in the central nervous system. Crit. Rev. Neurobiol. **10:** 119–154.
52. CHARPAK, S., W.E. ARMSTRONG, M. MUHLETHALER & J.J. DREIFUSS. 1984. Stimulatory action of oxytocin on neurones of the dorsal motor nucleus of the vagus nerve. Brain Res. **300:** 83–89.
53. DREIFUSS, J.J., M. RAGGENBASS, S. CHARPAK, *et al.* 1988. A role of central oxytocin in autonomic functions: its action in the motor nucleus of the vagus nerve. Brain Res. Bull. **20:** 765–770.
54. ROGERS, R.C. & G.E. HERMANN. 1985. Dorsal medullary oxytocin, vasopressin, oxytocin antagonist, and TRH effects on gastric acid secretion and heart rate. Peptides **6:** 1143–1148.
55. GUTKOWSKA, J., M. JANKOWSKI, S. MUKADDAM-DAHER & S.M. MCCANN. 2000. Oxytovin is a cardiovascular hormone. Braz. J. Med. Biol. Res. **33:** 625–633.
56. PETTY, M.A., R.E. LANG, T. UNGER T & D. GANTEN. 1985. The cardiovascular effects of oxytocin in conscious male rats. Eur. J. Pharmacol. **112:** 203–210.
57. RUSS, R.D. & B.R. WALKER. 1994. Oxytocin augments baroreflex bradycardia in conscious rats. Peptides **15:** 907–912.
58. BOOTH, F.W. & D.B. THOMASON. 1991. Molecular and cellular adaptation of muscle in response to exercise: perspectives of various models. Physiol. Rev. **71:** 541–585.
59. AMARAL, S.L., T.M.T. ZORN & L.C. MICHELINI. 2000. Exercise training normalizes wall-to-lumen ratio of the gracilis muscle arterioles and reduces pressure in spontaneously hypertensive rats. J. Hypertens. **18:** 1563–1572.

60. ROBINSON, B.F., S.E. EPSTEIN, G.D. BEISER & E. BRAUNWALD. 1966. Control of heart rate by the autonomic nervous system: studies in man on the interrelation between baroreceptor mechanisms and exercise. Circ. Res. **19:** 400–411.
61. GALLO, JR., L., B.C. MACIEL, J.A. MARIN-NETO & L.E.B. MARTINS. 1989. Sympathetic and para-sympathetic changes in heart rate control during dynamic exercise induced by endurance training in man. Braz. J. Med. Biol. Res. **22:** 631–643.
62. HIGA, K.T., E. MORI, M. MORRIS & L.C. MICHELINI. Baroreflex control of heart rate by oxytocin in the solitary-vagal complex. Am. J. Physiol. Regul. Integr. Comp. Physiol. In press.
63. MICHELINI, L.C., M.C. MARCELO, J.A. AMICO & M. MORRIS. 1999. Baroreflex regulation is altered in mice lacking oxytocin. Soc. Neurosci. Abstr. **25**(Pt. 1): 12.
64. FERRARIO, C.M., M.C. CHAPELL, E.A. TALLANT, *et al.* 1997. Counter-regulatory actions of angiotensin-(1–7). Hypertension **30:** 535–541.
65. SANTOS, R.A.S., M.J. CAMPAGNOLE-SANTOS, N.C.V. BARACHO, *et al.* 1994. Characterization of a new angiotensin antagonist selective for angiotensin-(1–7): evidence that the actions of angiotensin-(1–7) are mediated by specific angiotensin receptors. Brain Res. Bull. **35:** 293–398.
66. LÜSCHER, T.F. & R.K. DUBEY. 1995. Endothelium and platelet-derived vasoactive substances: role in the regulation of vascular tone and growth. *In* Hypertension: Pathophysiology, Diagnosis and Management. J.H. Laragh & B.M. Brenner, Eds.: 609–630. Raven Press. New York.
67. LASH, J.M. & G. BOHLEN. 1992. Functional adaptations of rat skeletal muscle arterioles to aerobic exercise training. J. Appl. Physiol. **72:** 2052–2062.
68. KREGEL, K.C.J., M. OVERTON, D.R. SEALS, *et al.* 1990. Cardiovascular responses to exercise in the rat: role of corticotropin-releasing factor. J. Appl. Physiol. **68:** 561–567.

# Exercise and Sensory Integration

## Role of the Nucleus Tractus Solitarius

JEFFREY T. POTTS

*Department of Physiology, Wayne State University School of Medicine,
540 East Canfield Avenue, Detroit, Michigan 48201, USA*

ABSTRACT: Since NTS neurons receive synaptic input from many sensory modalities, it is crucial to understand the neuronal mechanisms involved in synaptic processing. We have proposed that GABA-containing neurons in the NTS are the primary target for somatic afferent fibers activated by skeletal muscle contraction. In our model, local inhibition of baroreceptor signaling is necessary to counteract the increase in baroreceptor input such that NTS output is normalized and baroreflex sensitivity is maintained during exercise. This GABAergic mechanism, in conjunction with sympathoexcitation evoked by somatic afferents, preserves reflex sensitivity and resets the baroreflex, respectively. Unfortunately, there is insufficient data to date to support or refute the proposed role for GABA on baroreflex function during exercise. However, we feel that this model will be useful in formulating future experiments to explore these synaptic interactions.

KEYWORDS: Exercise; Nucleus tractus solitarius; Baroreceptor function; GABAergic neurons

## INTRODUCTION

Physical activity or exercise is perhaps the most profound challenge to circulatory homeostasis. It is well established that exercise is accompanied by sympathoexcitation.[1] Several neural mechanisms have been postulated to mediate the sympathoexcitatory response, including feedforward ("central command") and feedback (exercise pressor reflex, baroreceptor reflexes) mechanisms. These mechanisms provide the central nervous system (CNS) with critical inputs that establish the pattern of cardiovascular motor responses during exercise. A host of peripheral receptors (including the arterial and cardiopulmonary mechanoreceptors that normally inhibit sympathetic drive and skeletal muscle receptors that increase sympathetic drive) are also activated during exercise; their role in cardiovascular regulation has received a great deal of attention.[1–3] Specifically, the role of the arterial baroreflex has been challenged, owing to the prevailing sympathoexcitation during exercise.[4–7] Recent-

Address for correspondence: Jeffrey T. Potts, Ph.D., Department of Physiology, Wayne State University School of Medicine, 540 E. Canfield Ave., Detroit, MI 48201. Voice: 313-577-9295; fax: 313-577-5494.

jtpotts@med.wayne.edu

221

ly, however, it was reported that the human carotid baroreceptor reflex is reset and its overall sensitivity is retained during exercise.[8,9] The neural basis of this alteration in arterial baroreflex function is unknown.

This chapter will focus on the potential neural substrate(s) that mediate central resetting of the arterial baroreceptor reflex during exercise. In particular, the nucleus of the solitary tract (NTS), a primary sensory nucleus, will be examined with respect to its role in the neural processing of two discrete sensory inputs that are activated during exercise: arterial baroreceptors and somatosensory receptors. It is hypothesized that somatic and cardiovascular afferent inputs interact centrally in the NTS, where GABA neurons activated by somatic afferents inhibit baroreceptor signaling and thus contribute to sympathoexcitation during exercise. Data from anesthetized animals, as well as from an innovative *in situ* working heart–brain stem preparation (WHBP), will be presented and discussed in the context of how GABAergic neurons alter baroreceptor signaling in the NTS. Finally, we will speculate on the role of inhibition of baroreceptor signaling during exercise.

## THE NUCLEUS OF THE SOLITARY TRACT: ROLE AS A CENTRAL NEURAL SUBSTRATE DURING EXERCISE?

A number of regions along the neural axis have been implicated in shaping the cardiovascular responses evoked during exercise, including the NTS, the lateral reticular nucleus (LRN), the lateral tegmental field, the caudal and rostral ventrolateral medulla (VLM), the pons and midbrain periaqueductal gray (PAG), as well as the hypothalamus and motor cortex.[1,10–12] While all of these centers likely contribute to the autonomic responses evoked during exercise, the NTS is a particularly attractive brain stem site that may be involved in processing sensory inputs from somatic and cardiovascular receptors. The NTS is innervated by an array of cardiovascular afferents (arterial baro-/chemoreceptor afferents, cardiac vagal mechano/chemosensitive afferents, pulmonary mechanosensitive afferents)[13,14] and skeletal muscle receptors (mechano-/chemosensitive Aδ and C fiber afferents) that are activated during exercise.[2,3] Moreover, the NTS has extensive reciprocal connections with many other medullary and rostral brain structures involved in controlling autonomic outflow, including the pons, midbrain, thalamus, hypothalamus, and motor cortex.[13,15] Therefore, based on its anatomical location[13,14] and on the presence of a local network of excitatory and inhibitory interneurons[16,17] and neuroactive peptides,[18] the NTS is a likely candidate to process, integrate, and relay sensory signals to other brain sites involved in coordinating autonomic motor responses during exercise.

In the following sections we will discuss functional, anatomical, and electrophysiological evidence that supports the hypothesis that somatic and cardiovascular afferents interact centrally in the NTS. It should be noted that in addition to the NTS, there are other medullary and supramedullary regions that process somatosensory and cardiovascular inputs. However, this chapter will focus exclusively on the role of the NTS in this integration.

## INTERACTION BETWEEN THE ARTERIAL BARORECEPTOR AND SOMATOSENSORY RECEPTOR REFLEXES DURING EXERCISE

### *Functional Evidence*

The arterial baroreceptor reflex is the primary short-term controller of systemic blood pressure.[12,13] Several decades ago it was believed that the arterial baroreflex was inhibited during exercise.[5-7] However, recent studies in animals[19,20] and humans[8,9,20] have shown that the baroreflex is reset to the prevailing level of systemic pressure and continues to modulate heart rate and blood pressure during exercise with the same sensitivity (or gain) as at rest. Moreover, experiments that incorporated sinoaortic denervation in conscious exercising animals have provided additional evidence that baroreceptors play a role in patterning the cardiorespiratory responses during exercise.[6,19] These studies reported that in the chronic absence of baroreceptor input, blood pressure fell precipitously at the onset of exercise and failed to recover until exercise was terminated. This observation suggests that the pattern of cardiovascular adjustments evoked during exercise requires neural feedback from baroreceptor populations.

Over a century ago, Johansson[21] proposed that activation of a specific set of receptors in skeletal muscle contributed to the cardiovascular responses evoked during exercise (i.e., reflex increase in heart rate, arterial pressure, myocardial contractility). Since that time, many investigators have confirmed Johansson's hypothesis using a number of experimental models, including anesthetized and conscious animals, as well as human subjects.[22-29] It is now accepted that thinly myelinated A$\delta$ (predominantly mechanosensitive) and unmyelinated C fiber (predominantly chemosensitive) afferents or receptors that innervate skeletal muscle represent a major source of sensory input to spinal and supraspinal centers during exercise.[30-36] The majority of A$\delta$ and C fiber afferents synapse in dorsal horn laminae I–V at the cervical and lower lumbar/upper sacral levels of the spinal cord as well as in adjacent spinal segments.[37,38] These neurons synapse onto second-order neurons that project to supraspinal targets through a variety of ascending spinal pathways located in the lateral, ventrolateral, and dorsolateral quadrants of the spinal cord.[39-42] This neural feedback pathway, termed the exercise pressor reflex by McCloskey and Mitchell,[29] controls autonomic motor outflow, which alters cardiovascular activities (heart rate, cardiac output, regional blood flow, blood pressure).

Many central and efferent neural pathways, as well as effector organs, are common to both the arterial baroreflex and the exercise pressor reflex. Thus, it is likely that these two reflex pathways interact in some manner. Indeed, considerable efforts have been made to investigate the interaction between these two reflex pathways. Coote and Perez-Gonzalez[43] were the first to report that stimulation of the carotid sinus nerve inhibited the reflex responses evoked by group IV sensory afferents from skeletal muscle. This finding was later confirmed and extended by Abboud, Mark, and Thames.[44] These investigators reported that reflex renal vasoconstriction evoked by sciatic nerve stimulation was inhibited at high carotid sinus pressure and augmented at low carotid sinus pressure, suggesting that the interaction was dependent upon the level of sensory input from carotid baroreceptors. More recently, we have confirmed this notion.[45-47] Potts *et al.*[45,46] used a naturalistic paradigm to activate both carotid baroreceptors and skeletal muscle receptors and demonstrated that the site of interaction was localized to central autonomic circuits in the medulla. Potts and Mitchell[47] also tested the hypothesis that sensory input from skeletal muscle receptors was capable of modulating baroreflex function. In this study, we reported that neural input from mechanically sensitive skeletal muscle receptors rapidly reset the carotid baroreflex in a manner that was previously proposed for central command.[1,20] Together, these studies demonstrate that sensory input from skeletal muscle receptors interacts centrally with carotid baroreceptor input. Moreover, these studies provide direct evidence that neural input from skeletal muscle contributes to resetting of the carotid baroreflex, as proposed in previous studies.[8,9] However, the key medullary nuclei and the cellular mechanisms involved in this interaction remain areas of active research. In the following section, anatomical evidence will be presented showing that the NTS receives synaptic input from both arterial baroreceptors and somatosensory receptors.

### Neuroanatomical Evidence

Neuroanatomical studies have provided direct evidence that somatosensory afferents project to the NTS.[37,40–42] Degeneration techniques have demonstrated that projection neurons located in the ventrolateral quadrant of the spinal cord project to several medullary nuclei, including the NTS.[40] Transganglionic transport of horseradish peroxidase (HRP) indicated that HRP was transported from skeletal muscle to the dorsal horn of the spinal cord as well as to brain stem regions, including the NTS.[37] Moreover, when HRP was microinjected into the NTS, dorsal horn neurons in laminae I–VII of the lower lumbar and upper sacral spinal cord were retrogradely labeled.

Other strategies have also been employed to selectively trace sensory neurons from the spinal cord to the brain stem. For instance, the recent development of Fos-like immunohistochemistry has been successfully used to map polysynaptic neural pathways.[48,49] This technique is based on the observation that the cellular proto-oncogene c-fos encodes a nuclear phosphoprotein, Fos. Because activation of the c-fos gene and the subsequent expression of Fos protein in neurons parallel synaptic activity, detection of Fos protein has the potential to serve as a marker of polysynaptic pathways in the CNS. Several studies have taken advantage of this technique to map out the central neuronal pathways of the arterial baroreceptor reflex,[50–54] as well as to identify medullary regions that are activated during exercise.[55–57] Iwamoto et al. examined the pattern of Fos labeling in the brain following a bout of treadmill exercise in conscious rats.[55] They reported that many regions in the lower brain stem (NTS, LRN, caudal/rostral VLM), as well as in the midbrain PAG, the parabrachial nucleus, and the hypothalamus, expressed Fos protein. However, since these animals were conscious and performing volitional exercise, the primary source of neural input responsible for Fos expression could not be identified. To determine the Fos pattern evoked by somatosensory afferents, Li and colleagues[57] selectively activated somatic afferents by static muscle contraction in baroreceptor- denervated (sinoaortic denervation plus vagotomy) and anesthetized cats. They reported that Fos immunoreactivity was present in many of the same cardiovascular-related brain stem nuclei as reported by Iwamoto et al.[55] (including the NTS) despite concomitant synaptic input from peripheral baroreceptors and central locomotor centers. Thus, these

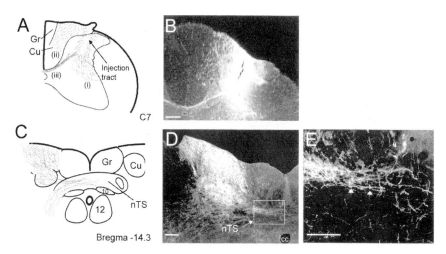

**FIGURE 1.** Example of neuronal labeling in the rat using the anterograde tracer biotin dextran amine (BDA). **(A)** Schematic of a cross-section of the cervical spinal cord (C7) showing the distribution of BDA-labeled fibers. **(B)** Intense BDA labeling in laminae I–V surrounding the injection tract. Distinctive clustering of positively labeled fibers was found: (i) to project to the ventrolateral quadrant of the spinal cord ipsilateral to the injection; (ii) in the dorsomedial aspect of the white matter corresponding to the cuneate nucleus; and (iii) in the contralateral dorsal horn via a well-defined fiber tract extending medially from laminae IV and crossing the midline at laminae X. **(C)** Schematic of a cross-section of the caudal medulla (Bregma −14.3 mm) showing the location of BDA-labeled fibers in the nucleus of the solitary tract (NTS) and the cuneate nucleus. **(D)** Dark-field image illustrating extensive labeling in the dorsal columns (cuneate nucleus only) and also in the dorsolateral, medial, and commissural subdivisions of the NTS. **(E)** High-power magnification (40×) of the medial and commissural subdivisions of the caudal NTS showing robust BDA-labeled fibers and terminal-like elements (↑). *Bar* represents 500 μm; cc, central canal; Cu, cuneate nucleus; Gr, gracile nucleus; NTS, nucleus tractus solitarius; 10, dorsal motor nucleus of the vagus; 12, hypoglossal nucleus.

findings provide somewhat more definitive evidence that selective stimulation of somatic afferents activate known medullary neural circuits that control central sympathetic outflow.

The topographical organization of cardiovascular inputs to the NTS is complex. Generally speaking, there is some organization of sensory innervation in the NTS; however, this is limited to gustatory inputs in the rostral NTS.[58] In contrast, there is considerably less organization within the caudal NTS, where the majority of cardiovascular inputs synapse.[59] In an attempt to characterize the innervation pattern of somatic afferents, we are using tract tracing techniques to map the central projection targets of putative somatosensory spinal neurons from the superficial dorsal horn to the NTS (i.e., second-order neurons that transmit Aδ and C fiber afferent inputs from skeletal muscle). In these experiments, the anterograde tracer biotinylated dextran amine (BDA) is microinjected into the cervical spinal cord (C6–C8) of rats, and samples of spinal cord and brain stem tissue are harvested 10–12 days later. Standard immunohistochemistry is then performed on frozen sections using 3-3′-diaminoben-

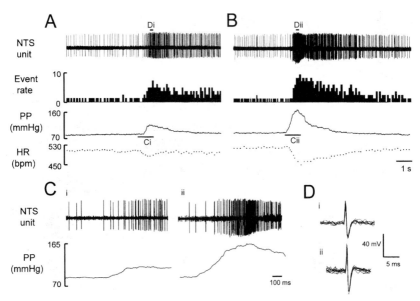

**FIGURE 2.** An example of the discharge pattern of a barosensitive NTS neuron in response to a physiological pressure stimulus in the working heart–brain stem preparation of the rat. (**A** and **B**) This spontaneously active neuron increased its discharge frequency proportionally with the rise in systemic pressure. This was accompanied by graded reflex reductions in heart rate. (**C**) The peak discharge pattern of this neuron occurred at peak pressure, and it appeared to be linearly encoded to the input pressure signal. (**D**) Ten superimposed sweeps of action potentials recorded at peak pressure. PP, perfusion pressure; HR, heart rate.

zidine and nickel intensification as the chromagen. An example from one of our experiments is illustrated in FIGURE 1. Spinal neurons that took up the tracer were localized throughout laminae I–V of the cervical spinal cord (see panels A and B). Positively labeled fibers were visible throughout the caudal-rostral extent of the medulla, including the NTS, LRN, VLM, and the spinal trigeminal tract. Within the caudal NTS, BDA-labeled fibers and terminal-like processes were localized to the medial, dorsomedial, dorsolateral, and commissural subdivisions. An example of the labeling pattern in the commissural subdivision of the NTS is shown in panels C–E in FIGURE 1. Terminal axons and synaptic boutons were visible in the dorsal third of the commissural NTS. These findings are in general agreement with earlier studies that reported that sensory fibers from the lower lumbar and upper sacral spinal cord projected to the caudal NTS.[37,40,41] In addition, our findings demonstrate that sensory neurons from the superficial dorsal horn in the cervical spinal cord of rats also project to regions of the caudal NTS that receive primary afferents from arterial baroreceptors.[14] Based on these findings, we propose that the caudal NTS is likely a neural substrate for the central interaction between somatic and cardiovascular afferent inputs. In the following section, the electrophysiological basis of this interaction will be discussed.

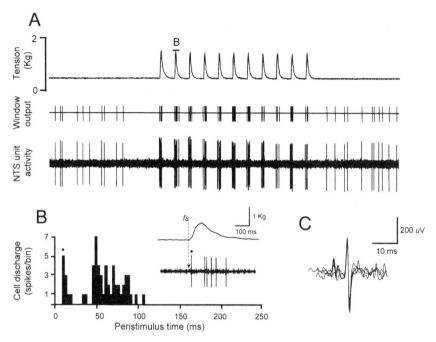

**FIGURE 3.** Example of the discharge pattern of an NTS neuron that was synaptically driven by somatosensory input recorded in the cat. **(A)** This somatosensitive neuron discharged vigorously in response to intermittent contraction of the hindlimb produced by ventral root stimulation. **(B)** Peristimulus time histogram showing the cumulative response of this neuron to 11 intermittent contractions (bin size = 200 ms). This cell displayed a short-latency (~65 ms) unimodal response that consisted of a train of 5–8 action potentials. The peak discharge frequency (~35 Hz) coincided with peak hindlimb tension development (see *inset*). **(C)** Five superimposed sweeps of action potentials recorded during a single hindlimb contraction. *fs*, onset of forelimb stimulation; •, stimulus artifact.

## *Electrophysiological Evidence*

Innervation of the NTS by primary baroreceptor afferent fibers has been well documented.[10–13,60–63] However, the encoding of blood pressure by target NTS neurons is not well understood. Barosensitive neurons, unlike baroreceptor afferent fibers, rarely possess pulse-rhythmic activity, although their activity may be cardiac-phase related.[60,61] Several different types of synaptic responses have been recorded from NTS neurons in response to electrical stimulation of baroreceptor and somatic afferents, or to changes in blood pressure and muscle tension.[60,61,64,65] An example of a characteristic discharge pattern of a barosensitive NTS neuron is shown in FIGURE 2. This neuron was spontaneously active, possessed a cardiac-related rhythm, and responded with an abrupt increase in its firing rate when systemic pressure was increased. The peak bursting rate of the neuron appeared to be related to the magnitude of the pressure stimulus. In addition to this type of response pattern, many other excitatory and inhibitory synaptic responses have been recorded from barosensitive NTS neurons.[60–65] Therefore, due to the diversity of spiking patterns, the heterogeneity of afferent inputs, and the difficulty in characterizing the medullary targets for NTS neurons, the precise role of this nucleus in sensory processing remains an area of considerable interest and active investigation.

Currently, we are attempting to characterize the local interaction between NTS neurons that receive synaptic input from somatic and cardiovascular receptors so that we may better understand how the NTS coordinates autonomic response patterns. Our approach is to selectively activate different sensory afferent populations supplying arterial baroreceptors and skeletal muscle receptors and to characterize the synaptic responses evoked by NTS neurons.[62] We have identified a unique population of NTS neurons that are synaptically activated by somatic afferents and that appear to be completely insensitive to inputs from arterial baroreceptors. These neurons were localized throughout the caudal NTS and did not appear to have any specific topographical organization. An example of the discharge pattern of one such neuron is illustrated in FIGURE 3. This neuron was spontaneously active and did not possess a cardiac-related rhythm. When the neuron was tested for barosensitivity, its firing pattern was not altered, suggesting that it did not receive synaptic input from arterial baroreceptors. However, when somatic afferents were stimulated by skeletal muscle contraction (ventral root stimulation of the triceps surae), this cell evoked a train of action potentials. A peristimulus-timed histogram revealed that this neuron evoked a unimodal discharge pattern that had a mean latency of 65 ms (see FIG. 3b). This observation is in general agreement with the short latency unimodal pattern reported by Toney and Mifflin[64] in a recent study examining the effect of somatosensory inputs on the firing patterns of NTS neurons. This NTS population represents 50% of the neurons that we have recorded to date; however, the "functional phenotype" for this population is as yet unknown. In the following section, we will present recent data that suggests that this NTS population consists of GABAergic neurons that are activated by contraction-sensitive somatic afferents.

## WORKING HEART–BRAIN STEM PREPARATION AS AN EXPERIMENTAL MODEL TO INVESTIGATE THE SYNAPTIC INTERACTIONS BETWEEN BARORECEPTOR AND SOMATIC AFFERENTS

In an attempt to facilitate experiments to determine the cellular basis for the interaction between somatic and cardiovascular afferents in the NTS, we have adopted the working heart–brain stem preparation (WHBP). A schematic illustration of this preparation is shown in FIGURE 4. The major advantages of this preparation include: (1) mechanical stability that facilitates electrophysiological recording techniques, such as whole-cell recording from functionally identified brain stem neurons; (2) easy access to the extracellular environment; (3) absence of anesthesia; and (4) preservation of a variety of reflex neural pathways such as baroreceptor, chemoreceptor, cardiac, cardiopulmonary, and gastrointestinal reflexes. The details describing this model can be found elsewhere.[66] Recently, we reported that activation of forelimb afferents evoked a coordinated pattern of cardiorespiratory responses in young rats (4–6 weeks) using the WHBP.[67] Because this is a reduced *in situ* preparation, somatic afferents were activated by electrically induced contraction of the forelimb. Forelimb contraction elicited robust cardiorespiratory responses that were eliminated by

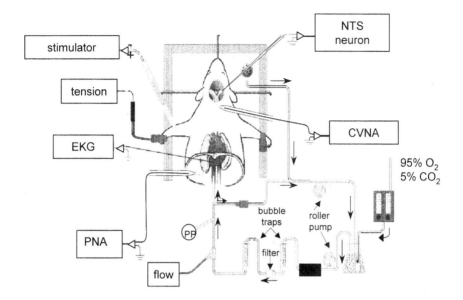

**FIGURE 4.** Schematic illustration of the working heart–brain stem preparation (WHBP) in the rat. Ringers solution is perfused from a reservoir by a roller pump. Before perfusing the preparation via the thoracic aorta the perfusate is heated and filtered, and air bubbles are removed. Perfusion rate (Flow) and pressure (PP) are recorded. Suction electrodes record phrenic (PNA) and cervical vagus (CVNA) nerve activities, and heart rate is derived from the electrocardiogram (EKG). Skeletal muscle afferents are activated by electrically evoked contractions of the forelimb; tension development is measured via a strain gauge. Arterial baroreceptors are activated by increases in perfusion pressure generated by the perfusion pump. Single-unit activity from NTS neurons is recorded extracellularly using glass microelectrodes.

denervating the forelimb or by neuromuscular blockade. These findings suggest that the cardiorespiratory responses were reflex in origin and were evoked by contraction-sensitive sensory fibers that innervated skeletal muscle in a reduced *in situ* preparation in the rat. Moreover, the pattern of cardiorespiratory responses evoked in this preparation was remarkably similar to the pattern produced in other animal models as well as in humans.[21–25]

We are currently using this preparation to investigate the potential role of GABAergic inhibition in the interaction between somatic and cardiovascular afferents. GABA (γ-aminobutyric acid) is the primary fast inhibitory neurotransmitter in the NTS.[18] Moreover, it has been shown that inhibitory signaling by GABA modulates baroreflex function.[16,17,68] However, the role of GABA in the central interaction between baroreceptor and somatic afferents is not known. We hypothesize that GABA neurons in the NTS are activated by somatic afferents and inhibit baroreceptor signaling. Activation of such an inhibitory mechanism is needed to counteract the elevation in afferent input from arterial baroreceptors during exercise in order to normalize NTS neuronal discharge and, thereby, baroreflex sensitivity. To test this hypothesis, we conducted a series of experiments using the WHBP in which we

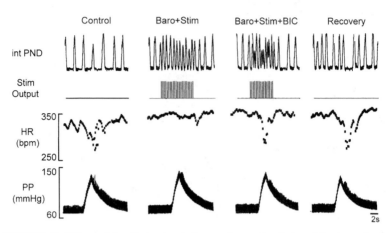

**FIGURE 5.** Effect of forelimb stimulation on baroreflex-induced bradycardia in the working heart–brain stem preparation. Forelimb stimulation attenuated the reflex bradycardia evoked by the arterial baroreceptor reflex (Baro + Stim). Bilateral microinjection of bicuculline blocked GABA$_A$ receptors in the NTS and restored the reflex bradycardia during forelimb stimulation (Baro + Stim + BIC). This finding suggests that forelimb afferents may attenuate baroreflex function by releasing GABA in the NTS that inhibits baroreceptor signaling. int PND, integrated phrenic nerve discharge; Stim output, output from stimulator used to contract the forelimb; HR, heart rate; PP, perfusion pressure.

reversible blocked GABA$_A$ receptors in the NTS with bicuculline methiodine.[69] An example from one of our experiments is shown in FIGURE 5. Prior to GABA$_A$ receptor blockade, the reflex bradycardia evoked by the arterial baroreflex was attenuated when skeletal muscle afferents were activated by contraction of the forelimb (Baro + Stim). However, when GABA$_A$ receptors in the NTS were blocked by bilateral microinjection of bicuculline methiodine, the reflex bradycardia was immediately restored (Baro + Stim + BIC). Based on these findings, we suggest that stimulation of somatic afferents activate GABA neurons, which, in turn, suppress the baroreceptor signaling in the NTS. It should be noted, however, that since a single input stimulus was used to activate the baroreflex system, it was not possible to determine whether the blunted bradycardia resulted from resetting of the baroreflex or whether reflex sensitivity was inhibited. Nonetheless, these data provide clear evidence that somatic afferents inhibit baroreceptor signaling in the NTS. In the following section, we will provide a hypothetical model of the central interaction between baroreceptor and somatosensory receptors and will discuss the potential role for GABAergic inhibition in the NTS during exercise.

## HYPOTHETICAL MODEL FOR THE CENTRAL INTERACTION BETWEEN BARORECEPTOR AND SOMATOSENSORY RECEPTOR AFFERENTS

Our overall goal is to determine the underlying mechanism(s) for baroreflex resetting during exercise. Current literature supports the concept that the arterial

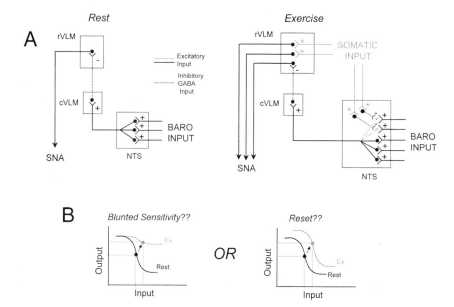

**FIGURE 6.** Hypothetical model illustrating potential synaptic interactions between somatic and baroreceptor afferents in the NTS. **(A)** *Left panel* outlines the medullary neural baroreflex pathway illustrating GABAergic inhibition of sympathetic premotor neurons in the rostal VLM. *Right panel* illustrates the effect of somatosensory afferents on neuronal activity in the NTS and rostral VLM. It is proposed that somatic afferents activate a GABAergic mechanism in the NTS to normalize NTS output and thus retain reflex sensitivity ("gain controller"). In addition, somatic afferents activate sympathetic premotor neurons in the rostral VLM that mediate sympathoexcitation ("set-point controller"). **(B)** Proposed outcome of the central interactions between somatic and baroreceptor afferents on arterial baroreflex function. See text for detailed discussion of model.

baroreceptor reflex is reset during exercise.[8,9,19,20] In addition, work from our own laboratory has shown: (1) afferent input from skeletal muscle resets the carotid baroreflex by increasing threshold pressure for reflex bradycardia and sympathoinhibition;[47] and (2) somatic afferents inhibit baroreceptor signaling in the NTS by activating GABAergic neurons.[69] Together, these results suggest that sensory input from skeletal muscle alters arterial baroreflex function. However, can baroreflex resetting be explained by activation of a GABAergic mechanism in the NTS?

Previous work by McWilliam and colleagues reported an apparent inhibition of the carotid baroreflex by somatic afferent input in decerebrate cats.[70,71] It was also suggested that somatic afferents inhibit barosensitive NTS neurons via a GABAergic mechanism.[72] In an attempt to assimilate these data with our findings, we have proposed a hypothetical model that highlights the potential synaptic interactions between somatic and baroreceptor afferents within the medulla (see Fig. 6). In this simplified model, sensory input from arterial baroreceptors tonically inhibits sympathetic premotor neurons in the rostral VLM via the well-established central neural baroreflex pathway.[10,13] The model predicts that at rest (left panel) sympathetic nerve activity (SNA) is inhibited when baroreceptor input is increased. During exercise, the baroreflex continues to operate as a negative feedback controller, however at heightened levels of baroreceptor input and sympathoexcitation. The elevation in baroreceptor input results from increases in arterial pulse pressure and the rate of rise of pressure (dP/dt), as well as the modest rise in mean arterial blood pressure that accompanies dynamic exercise.[20] This increase in afferent drive should activate NTS neurons and inhibit sympathetic outflow; however, instead, dynamic exercise is accompanied by marked sympathoexcitation. Therefore, baroreceptor signaling must be inhibited in order to counteract the elevation in afferent input. We speculate that this inhibition is produced by a GABAergic mechanism in the NTS and that baroreflex resetting is produced by two independent neural circuits activated by somatic afferents: one circuit controling the "set-point" of the reflex, and the other controling "reflex sensitivity." This schema is illustrated in FIGURE 6 (right panel). First, it has been previously shown that somatic afferents increase central sympathetic outflow by activating sympathetic premotor neurons in the rostral VLM.[73–75] Activation of this neural circuit evokes sympathoexcitation to establish the "dc level" about which the baroreflex will operate during exercise. We hypothesize that this neural circuit represents a virtual "set-point controller" for the reflex. Second, we have presented data that supports the concept that somatosensory afferents activate GABA neurons in the NTS.[69] We speculate that this GABAergic mechanism proportionally inhibits barosensitive NTS neurons to counteract augmented input from arterial baroreceptors. Conceptually, inhibiting baroreceptor signaling would normalize NTS output and thus maintain reflex sensitivity. We speculate that this neural circuit represents a virtual "gain controller" for the baroreflex. Together, activation of these two independent neural circuits renders the arterial baroreflex operational during exercise at a heightened level of centrally generated sympathetic activity.

This is our current working hypothesis. If this hypothesis proves to be correct, then activation of the set-point and gain controller circuits by somatic afferents represents a source of peripheral neural input to reset the baroreflex and retains its overall sensitivity. However, in addition to this mechanism, other sources of synaptic input may be involved in resetting the baroreflex during exercise (i.e., central command).

Future research endeavors should be designed to: (1) identify the synaptic interactions, neurochemical phenotype, and projection targets of functionally identified NTS neurons that are activated by baroreceptor and somatic receptor afferent input; (2) provide a better understanding of the neuroanatomical relationship between GABAergic neurons in the NTS and cardiovascular and somatic afferents; and (3) determine the relative degree of resetting that is attributed to inhibitory mechanisms in the NTS. Together, results from these experiments will help us to better understand the role of the NTS network in cardiovascular control during exercise and locomotion.

## ACKNOWLEDGMENTS

I would like to express my gratitude to Jere H. Mitchell, M.D., for his continued support and encouragement. I would also like to thank Julian F. R. Paton, Ph.D., for his insight and fruitful discussions in preparing this manuscript. This work was supported by the American Heart Association TX Affiliate (97G-101) and the National Institutes of Health (HL59167 and HL06296).

## REFERENCES

1. WALDROP, T.G., F.L. ELDRIDGE, G.A. IWAMOTO & J.H. MITCHELL. 1996. Central neural control of respiration and circulation during exercise. In Handbook of Physiology, Exercise: Regulation and Integration of Multiple Systems. L.B. Rowell & J.T. Shepherd, Eds.: 333–380. Oxford University Press. New York.
2. KAUFMAN, M.P. & H.V. FORSTER. 1996. Reflexes controlling circulatory, ventilatory and airway responses to exercise. In Handbook of Physiology, Section 12, Exercise: Regulation and Integration of Multiple Systems: 381–447. American Physiological Society. Bethesda, MD.
3. MITCHELL, J.H., M.P. KAUFMAN & G.A. IWAMOTO. 1983. The exercise pressor reflex: its cardiovascular effects, afferent mechanisms, and central pathways. Annu. Rev. Physiol. 45: 229–242.
4. BRISTOW, J.D., E.B. BROWN, D.J.C. CUNNINGHAM, et al. 1971. Effect of bicycling on the baroreflex regulation of pulse interval. Circ. Res. 38: 582–593.
5. MANCIA, G., J. IANNOS, G.G. JAMIESON, et al. 1978. Effect of isometric handgrip exercise on the carotid sinus baroreceptor reflex in man. Clin. Sci. Mol. Med. 54: 33–37.
6. MCRITICHIE, R.J., S.F. VATNER, D. BOETTCHER, et al. 1976. Role of arterial baroreceptors in mediating cardiovascular response to exercise. Am. J. Physiol. 230: 85–89.
7. STAESSEN, J., R. FIOCCHI, R. FAGARD, et al. 1987. Progressive attenuation of the carotid baroreflex control of blood pressure and heart rate during exercise. Am. Heart J. 114: 765–772.
8. POTTS, J.T., X. SHI & P.B. RAVEN. 1993. Carotid baroreflex responsiveness during dynamic exercise in humans. Am. J. Physiol. 265: H1928–H1938.
9. PAPELIER, Y., P. ESCOURROU, J.P. GAUTHIER & L.B. ROWELL. 1994. Carotid baroreflex control of blood pressure and heart rate in man during dynamic exercise. J. Appl. Physiol. 77: 502–506.
10. LOEWY, A.D. 1990. Central autonomic pathways. In Central Regulation of Autonomic Functions. A.D. Loewy & K.M. Spyer, Eds.: 88–103, Oxford University Press. New York.
11. KAO, F.F., S.S. MEI, A.M. BABICH & I.R. MOSS. 1977. Central organization of exercise input. In Central Interaction Between Respiratory and Cardiovascular Control Systems. H.P. Koepchen, S.M. Hilton & A. Trzebski, Eds.: 158–168. Springer-Verlag. New York.
12. JORDAN, D. 1995. CNS integration of cardiovascular regulation. In Cardiovascular Regulation. D. Jordan & J. Marshall, Eds.: 1–14. Portland Press. London.
13. SPYER, K.M. 1994. Central nervous mechanisms contributing to cardiovascular control. J. Physiol. (Lond.) 474(1): 1–19.
14. CIRIELLO, J., S.L. HOCHSTENBACH & S. RODER. 1994. Central projections of baroreceptor and chemoreceptor afferent fibers in the rat. In Nucleus of the Solitary Tract. I.R.A. Barraco, Ed.: 35–50. CRC Press. Boca Raton, FL.
15. TER HORST, G.J. & C. STREEFLAND. 1994. Ascending projections of the solitary tract nucleus. In Nucleus of the Solitary Tract. I.R.A. Barraco, Ed.: 35–50. CRC Press. Boca Raton, FL.
16. KAWAI, Y. & E. SENBA. 1996. Organization of excitatory and inhibitory local networks in the caudal nucleus of tractus solitarius of rats revealed in in vitro slice preparation. J. Comp. Neurol. 373: 309–321.
17. KAWAI, Y. & E. SENBA. 1999. Electrophysiological and morphological characterization of cytochemically defined neurons in the caudal nucleus tractus solitarius of the rat. Neuroscience 89: 1347–1355.
18. LAWRENCE A.J. & B. JARROTT. 1996. Neurochemical modulation of cardiovascular control in the nucleus tractus solitarius. Prog. Neurobiol. 48: 21–53.

19. MELCHER, A. & D.E. DONALD. 1981. Maintained ability of carotid baroreflex to regulate arterial pressure during exercise. Am. J. Physiol. 241: H838–H849.
20. ROWELL, L.B., D.S. O'LEARY & D.S. KELLOGG. 1996. Integration of cardiovascular control systems in dynamic exercise. In Handbook of Physiology, Section 12, Exercise: Regulation and Integration of Multiple Systems: 770–840. American Physiological Society. Bethesda, MD.
21. JOHANSSON, J.E. 1893. Uber die Ewinwirkung der Musdeltatigkeit auf die Atmun und die Hertzatigeit. Scand. Arch. Physiol. 5: 20–66.
22. ALAM, M. & F.H. SMIRK. 1937. Observation in man upon a blood pressure raising reflex arising from the voluntary muscles. J. Physiol. (Lond.) 89: 372–383.
23. COOTE, J.H., S.M. HILTON & J.F. PEREZ-GONZALEZ. 1971. The reflex nature of the pressor response to muscular exercise. J. Physiol. (Lond.) 214: 789–804.
24. DIEPSTRA, G., W. GONYEA & J.H. MITCHELL. 1980. Cardiovascular response to static exercise during selective autonomic blockade in the conscious cat. Circ. Res. 47: 530–535.
25. LIND, A.R. 1983. Cardiovascular adjustments to isometric contractions: static effort. In Handbook of Physiology, The Cardiovascular System III: 947–967. American Physiological Society. Bethesda, MD.
26. MARK, A.L., R.G. VICTOR, C. NERHED & B.G. WALLIN. 1985. Microneurographic studies of the mechanisms of sympathetic nerve responses to static exercise in humans. Circ. Res. 57: 461–469.
27. MATSUKAWA, K., P.T. WALL, L.B. WILSON & J.H. MITCHELL. 1994. Reflex stimulation of cardiac sympathetic nerve activity during static muscle contraction in cats. Am. J. Physiol. 267: H821–H827.
28. MATSUKAWA, K., P.T. WALL, L.B. WILSON & J.H. MITCHELL. 1992. Neurally mediated renal vasoconstriction during isometric muscle contraction in cats. Am. J. Physiol. 31: H833–H838.
29. McCLOSKEY, D.I. & J.H. MITCHELL. 1972. Reflex cardiovascular and respiratory response originating in exercising muscle. J. Physiol. (Lond.) 224: 173–186.
30. KAUFMAN, M.P., J.C. LONGHURST, K.J. RYBICKI, et al. 1983. Effects of static muscle contraction on impulse activity of groups III and IV afferents in cats. J. Appl. Physiol. 55: 105–112.
31. KAUFMAN, M.P., T.G. WALDROP, K.J. RYBICKI, et al. 1984. Effects of static and rhythmic twitch contractions on the discharge of group III and IV muscle afferents. Cardiovasc. Res. 18: 663–668.
32. KNIFFKI, K.D., S. MENSE & R.F. SCHMIDT. 1978. Responses of group IV afferent units from skeletal muscle to stretch, contraction, and chemical stimulation. Exp. Brain Res. 31: 511–522.
33. KNIFFKI, K.D., S. MENSE & R.F. SCHMIDT. 1981. Muscle receptors with fine afferent fibers which may evoke circulatory reflexes. Circ. Res. 48: I25–I31.
34. MENSE, S. & S. STAHNKE. 1983. Responses in muscle afferent fibers of slow conduction velocity to contractions and ischaemia in the cat. J. Physiol. (Lond.) 342: 383–397.
35. SATO, A. & R.F. SCHMIDT. 1973. Somatosympathetic reflexes: afferent fibers, central pathways, discharge characteristics. Physiol. Rev. 53: 916–947.
36. IWAMURA, Y., Y. UCHINO, S. OZAWA & N. KUDO. 1969. Excitatory and inhibitory components of somato-sympathetic reflex. Brain Res. 16: 351–358.
37. KALIA, M., S.S. MEI & F.F. KAO. 1981. Central projections from ergoreceptors (C fibers) in muscle involved in cardiopulmonary responses to static exercise. Circ. Res. 48: I48–I62.
38. LIGHT, A.R. & E.R. PERL. 1979. Re-examination of the dorsal root projection to the spinal dorsal horn including observations on the differential termination of coarse and fine fibers. J. Comp. Neurol. 186: 117–132.
39. KOZELKA, J.W. & R.D. WURSTER. 1985. Ascending spinal pathways for somato-autonomic reflexes in the anesthetized dog. J. Appl. Physiol. 58: 1832–1839.
40. MENETRY, D. & A. BASBAUM. 1987. Spinal and trigeminal projections to the nucleus of the solitary tract: a possible substrate for somatovisceral and viscerovisceral reflex activation. J. Comp. Neurol. 255: 439–450.

41. NYBERG, G. & A. BLOMQVIST. 1984. The central projection of muscle afferent fibers to the lower medulla and upper spinal cord: an anatomical study in the cat with transganglionic transport method. J. Comp. Neurol. **230:** 99–109.
42. ROSSI, G.F. & A. BRODAL. 1956. Spinal afferents to the trigeminal sensory nuclei and the nucleus of the solitary tract. J. Comp. Neurol. **16:** 321–332.
43. COOTE, J.H. & J.F. PEREZ-GONZALEZ. 1970. The response of some sympathetic neurons to volleys in various afferent nerves. J. Physiol. (Lond.) **208:** 261–278.
44. ABBOUD, F.M., A.L. MARK & M.D. THAMES. 1981. Modulation of the somatic reflex by carotid baroreceptors and by cardiopulmonary afferents in animals and humans. Circ. Res. **48**(6): 131–137.
45. POTTS, J.T., G.A. HAND, J. LI & J.H. MITCHELL. 1998. Central interaction between carotid baroreceptors and skeletal muscle receptors inhibits sympathoexcitation. J. Appl. Physiol. **84**(4): 1158–1165.
46. POTTS J.T. & J. LI. 1998. Interaction between carotid baroreflex and exercise pressor reflex depends on baroreceptor afferent input. Am. J. Physiol. **274:** H1841–H1847.
47. POTTS, J.T. & J.H. MITCHELL. 1998. Rapid resetting of carotid baroreceptor reflex by afferent input from skeletal muscle receptors. Am. J. Physiol. **275:** H2000–H2008.
48. MORGAN, J.I. & T. CURRAN. 1991. Stimulus-transcription coupling in the nervous system: involvement of the inducible proto-oncogene Fos and jun. Annu. Rev. Neurosci. **14:** 421–451.
49. DRAGUNOW, M. & R. FAULL. 1989. The use of *c-fos* as a metabolic marker in neuronal pathway tracing. J. Neurosci. Methods **29:** 261–265.
50. DEAN, C. & J.L. SEAGARD. 1995. Expression of *c-fos* protein in the nucleus tractus solitarius in response to physiological activation of carotid baroreceptors. Neuroscience **69**(1): 249–257.
51. DEAN, C. & J.L. SEAGARD. 1997. Mapping of carotid baroreceptor subtype projections to the nucleus tractus solitarius using *c-fos* immunohistochemistry. Brain Res. **758:** 201–208.
52. ERICKSON, J.T. & D.E. MILLHORN. 1991. Fos-like protein is induced in neurons of the medulla oblongata after stimulation of the carotid sinus nerve in awake and anesthetized rats. Brain Res. **567:** 11–24.
53. LI, Y-W. & R.A.L. DAMPNEY. 1992. Expression of *c-fos* protein in the medulla oblongata of conscious rabbits in response to baroreceptor activation. Neurosci. Lett. **144:** 70–74.
54. McKITRICK, T.L. KRUKOFFM & F.R. CALARESU. 1992. Expression of *c-fos* protein in the rat brain after electrical stimulation of the aortic depressor nerve. Brain Res. **599:** 215–222.
55. IWAMOTO, G.A., S.M. WAPPEL, G.M. FOX, *et al.* 1996. Identification of diencephalic and brain stem cardiorespiratory areas activated during exercise. Brain Res. **726:** 109–122.
56. LI, J., G.A. HAND, J.T. POTTS & J.H. MITCHELL. 1997. C-*fos* expression in the medulla induced by static muscle contraction in cats. Am. J. Physiol. **272:** H48–H56.
57. LI, J., J.T. POTTS & J.H. MITCHELL. 1998. Effect of barodenervation on *c-fos* expression in the medulla induced by static muscle contraction in cats. Am. J. Physiol. **274:** H901–H908.
58. BLESSING, W.H. 1997. Anatomy of the lower brainstem. *In* The Lower Brainstem and Bodily Homeostasis: 29–100. Oxford University Press. New York.
59. PATON, J.F.R. 1999. The Shapey-Schafer prize lecture. Nucleus tractus solitarii: integrating structures. Exp. Physiol. **84:** 815–833.
60. ROGERS, R.F., J.F.R. PATON & J.S. SCHWABER. 1993. NTS neuronal responses to arterial pressure and pressure changes in the rat. Am. J. Physiol. **265:** R1355–R1368.
61. ROGERS, R.F., W.C. ROSE & J.S. SCHWABER. 1996. Simultaneous encoding of carotid sinus pressure and dP/dt by NTS target neurons of myelinated baroreceptors. J. Neurophysiol. **76**(4): 2644–2660.
62. POTTS, J.T., J. LI & T.G. WALDROP. 1998. Extracellular recordings from nucleus tractus solitarii neurons: response to arterial baroreceptor and skeletal muscle receptor inputs. FASEB J. **12**(3): A353.

63. PATON, J.F.R. 1998. Pattern of cardiorespiratory afferent convergence to solitary tract neurons driven by pulmonary vagal C-fiber stimulation in the mouse. J. Neurophysiol. **79:** 2365–2373.
64. TONEY, G.M. & S.W. MIFFLIN. 2000. Sensory modalities conveyed in the hindlimb somatic afferent input to nucleus tractus solitarius. J. Appl. Physiol. **88:** 2062–2073.
65. HAYWARD, L.F. & R.B. FELDER. 1995. Cardiac rhythmicity among NTS neurons and its relationship to sympathetic outflow in rabbits. Am. J. Physiol. **269:** H923–H933.
66. PATON, J.F.R. 1996. A working heart-brainstem preparation of the mouse. J. Neurosci. Methods **65:** 63–68.
67. POTTS, J.T., K.M. SPYER & J.F.R. PATON. 2000. Somatosympathetic reflex in a working heart-brainstem preparation of the rat. Brain. Res. Bull. **53**(1): 59–67.
68. TSUKAMOTO, K. & A.F. SVED. 1993. Enhanced gamma-aminobutyric acid–mediated responses in nucleus tractus solitarius of hypertensive rats. Hypertension **22:** 819–825.
69. POTTS, J.T., J.F.R. PATON & J.H. MITCHELL. 2001. Spatial distribution of GABAergic interneurons and somatosensory afferents in the nucleus tractus solitarius: implications for arterial baroreceptor signalling. Submitted for publication.
70. MCWILLIAM, P.N. & T. YANG. 1991. Inhibition of cardiac vagal component of baroreflex by group III and IV afferents. Am. J. Physiol. **260:** H730–H734.
71. MCWILLIAM, P.N., T. YANG & L.X. CHEN. 1991. Changes in the baroreceptor reflex at the start of muscle contraction in the decerebrate cat. J. Physiol. (Lond.) **436:** 549–558.
72. MCMAHON, S.E., P.N. MCWILLIAMS, J. ROBERTSON & J.C. KAYE. 1992. Inhibition of carotid sinus baroreceptor neurons in the nucleus tractus solitarius of the anesthetized cat by electrical stimulatioin of hindlimb afferents (abstr.). J. Physiol. (Lond.) **452:** 224P.
73. BAUER, R.M., T.G. WALDROP, G.A. IWAMOTO & M.A. HOLZWARTH. 1992. Properties of ventrolateral medullary neurons that respond to muscle contraction. Brain Res. Bull. **28:** 167–178.
74. MORRISON, S.F. & D.J. REIS. 1989. Reticulospinal vasomotor neurons in the RVL mediate the somatosympathetic reflex. Am. J. Physiol. **256:** R1084–R1097.
75. RUGGERI, P., R. ERMIRIO, C. MOLINARI & F.R. CALARESU. 1995. Role of ventrolateral medulla in reflex cardiovascular responses to activation of skin and muscle nerves. Am. J. Physiol. **268:** R1464–R1471.

# Synaptic and Neurotransmitter Activation of Cardiac Vagal Neurons in the Nucleus Ambiguus

JIJIANG WANG,[a] MUSTAPHA IRNATEN,[a] ROBERT A. NEFF,[a]
PRIYA VENKATESAN,[a] CORY EVANS, [a] ARTHUR D. LOEWY,[b] THOMAS C.
METTENLEITER,[c] AND DAVID MENDELOWITZ[a]

[a]Department of Pharmacology, George Washington University,
Washington, District of Columbia 20037, USA

[b]Department of Anatomy and Neurobiology, Washington University School of Medicine,
St. Louis, Missouri 63110, USA

[c]Federal Research Center for Virus Diseases of Animals, Institute of Molecular Biology,
Friedrich-Loeffler Institutes, D-17498 Insel Riems, Germany

ABSTRACT: Cardiac vagal neurons play a critical role in the control of heart
rate and cardiac function. These neurons, which are primarily located in the
nucleus ambiguus (NA) and the dorsal motor nucleus of the vagus (DMNX),
dominate the neural control of heart rate under normal conditions. Cardiac vagal activity is diminished and unresponsive in many disease states, while restoration of parasympathetic activity to the heart lessens ischemia and
arrhythmias and decreases the risk of sudden death. Recent work has demonstrated that cardiac vagal neurons are intrinsically silent and therefore rely on
synaptic input to control their firing. To date, three major synaptic inputs to
cardiac vagal neurons have been identified. Stimulation of the nucleus tractus
solitarius evokes a glutamatergic pathway that activates both NMDA and non-
NMDA glutamatergic postsynaptic currents in cardiac vagal neurons. Acetylcholine excites cardiac vagal neurons via three mechanisms, activating a direct
ligand-gated postsynaptic nicotinic receptor, enhancing postsynaptic non-
NMDA currents, and presynaptically by facilitating transmitter release. This
enhancement by nicotine is dependent upon activation of pre- and postsynaptic
P-type voltage-gated calcium channels. Additionally, there is a GABAergic
innervation of cardiac vagal neurons. The transsynaptic pseudorabies virus
that expresses GFP (PRV-GFP) has been used to identify, for subsequent
electrophysiologic study, neurons that project to cardiac vagal neurons. Bartha
PRV-GFP-labeled neurons retain their normal electrophysiological properties,
and the labeled baroreflex pathways that control heart rate are unaltered by
the virus.

KEYWORDS: Parasympathetic; Heart rate; Cardiac; Medulla; PRV; GFP;
Virus; GABA; AMPA; Kainate; NMDA; Nicotine; Acetylcholine; Cholinergic

[d]Address for correspondence: David Mendelowitz, Department of Pharmacology, George
Washington University, 2300 Eye St. NW, Washington, D.C. 20037. Voice: 202-994-3466; fax:
202-994-2870.

dmendel@gwu.edu

## INTRODUCTION

Preganglionic parasympathetic cardiac neurons play a critical role in the control of heart rate and cardiac function. Previous work has unequivocally demonstrated that the normal low heart rate and respiratory sinus arrhythmia present in healthy animals and humans are determined primarily by the tonic firing and reflex control of parasympathetic cardiac neurons in the brain stem. These neurons, which are primarily located in the nucleus ambiguus (NA) and the dorsal motor nucleus (DMNX) of the vagus, dominate the neural control of heart rate under normal conditions and also influence the prognosis of many cardiovascular disorders, such as sudden cardiac death, ventricular fibrillation, and myocardial ischemia (FIG. 1).

Cardiac vagal activity is diminished and unresponsive in many disease states, and a delay in the inhibitory actions of this autonomic motor system following exercise

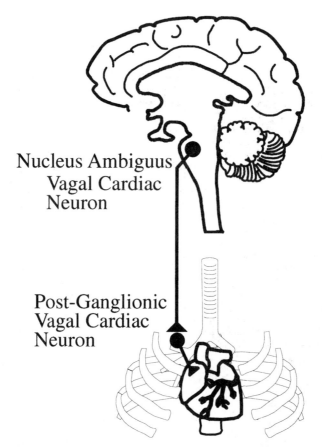

**FIGURE 1.** Preganglionic cardiac vagal neurons are located in the nucleus ambiguus as well as the dorsal motor nucleus of the vagus. The axons from preganglionic cardiac vagal neurons travel down the vagus nerve and synapse upon postganglionic cardiac vagal neurons in cardiac ganglia that are mostly in fat pads at the base of the heart.

is a powerful predictor of overall mortality.[1] Restoration of cardiac vagal activity prevents ischemia and reperfusion-induced arrhythmias and decreases risk of sudden death after myocardial infarction.[2] This and other work have suggested that increases in cardiac vagal activity could be an effective clinical target in heart diseases.

Recent work in the rat has demonstrated that cardiac vagal neurons in the NA do not possess pacemaker-like firing activities and are intrinsically silent.[3] The synaptic innervation of cardiac vagal neurons is therefore critical for the tonic and reflex evoked changes in cardiac vagal activity that control heart rate. Recent work will be reviewed that has shown that there are three major synaptic inputs to cardiac vagal neurons that activate glutamatergic, cholinergic, and GABAergic presynaptic and postsynaptic receptors. The neurons that project to cardiac vagal neurons can be identified and studied *in vitro* using a transsynaptic PRV virus that expresses GFP.

## GLUTAMATERGIC INPUTS TO CARDIAC VAGAL NEURONS

One of the more functionally important pathways innervating vagal cardiac neurons is from solitary tract nucleus (NTS) neurons. The NTS is the site of the first central synapse for visceral sensory neurons, including arterial baroreceptors.[4] NTS neurons project to "higher" brain nuclei, as well as other nuclei in the brain stem that are critical for efferent sympathetic and parasympathetic activity including the NA.[4] This work tested whether stimulation of the NTS would activate a monosynaptic pathway to cardiac vagal neurons in the NA. In addition, the postsynaptic receptors on cardiac vagal neurons that were activated by stimulation of this pathway were identified.

Individual cardiac vagal neurons were labeled by applying the fluorescent retrograde tracer, rhodamine, to the synaptic terminals of these neurons located in fat pads at the base of the heart. The animals were then sacrificed 2–3 days after the initial surgery and cardiac vagal neurons could be visually identified by the presence of the fluorescent rhodamine tracer in their cell bodies. Identified cardiac vagal neurons were imaged with differential interference contrast (DIC) optics, infrared illumination, and an infrared-sensitive CCD camera to gain better spatial resolution and to visually guide and position the patch pipette onto the surface of the identified neuron. The pipette was advanced until obtaining a giga-ohm seal between the pipette tip and the cell membrane of the identified neuron. Access to the intracellular compartment of the neuron was obtained by allowing nystatin to form pores in the cell membrane.

The brain slices were continuously perfused (2–3 mL/min) with a perfusate of the following composition: NaCl (125 mM), KCl (3 mM), $CaCl_2$ (2 mM), $NaHCO_3$ (26 mM), dextrose (5 mM), HEPES (5 mM), constantly bubbled with 95% $O_2$, 5% $CO_2$, and maintained at pH 7.4. Drugs used in this study were the NMDA antagonist, D-2-amino-5-phosphonovalerate (AP5, 50 μM final bath concentration); and the non-NMDA antagonists, 6-cyano-7-nitroquinoxaline-2,3-dione (CNQX, 50 μM final bath concentration) and (in one experiment) NBQX (50 μM final bath concentration). In addition, concanavalin A (Con A, 0.3 mg/mL) and cyclothiazide (Cyclo, 100 μM) were used to remove the desensitization of kainate and AMPA receptors, respectively. Drugs were applied to the neurons by addition into the perfusate. Picrotoxin (100 μM), strychnine (1 μM), and prazosin (10 μM) were added

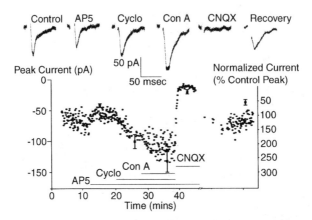

**FIGURE 2.** Stimulation of the NTS evokes rapidly activating and inactivating, and long-lasting, excitatory synaptic currents in cardiac vagal neurons. The selective NMDA receptor antagonist AP5 blocks the long-lasting component: *top, second trace*; and *bottom graph*. The non-NMDA currents are enhanced by both concanavalin A (Con A, 0.3 mg/mL; *top, third trace*; and *bottom graph*) and cyclothiazide (Cyclo, 100 µM; *top, fourth trace*; and *bottom graph*), which remove the desensitization of kainate and AMPA receptors, respectively. The non-NMDA antagonist CNQX (*top, fifth trace*; and *bottom graph*) blocks the AMPA and kainate synaptic currents.

to the bath perfusate to prevent GABAergic, glycine, and $\alpha_1$-adrenergic currents, respectively. Patch pipettes were filled with a solution consisting of K-Gluconate (130 mM), HEPES (10 mM), EGTA (10 mM), $CaCl_2$ (1 mM), $MgCl_2$ (1 mM), and nystatin (258 units/mL). The stimulating electrode was placed in the dorsomedial NTS, a location that receives a dense innervation from aortic baroreceptor fibers. Criteria that were used to limit the stimulation to a monosynaptic pathway from the NTS to vagal cardiac neurons in the NA included shortness of the latency with a constant latency for each cell and ability to follow paired synaptic activation at frequencies of 50–100 Hz.

Stimulation of the pathway from the NTS activated excitatory NMDA and non-NMDA receptor-mediated postsynaptic currents in vagal cardiac neurons in the NA (Fig. 2). The NMDA antagonist AP5 blocked the long-lasting component of the synaptic response. To identify the relative contribution of AMPA and kainate receptors, Cyclo and Con A, agents that remove the desensitization of AMPA and kainate receptors, respectively, were applied. Both Cyclo and Con A typically augmented the non-NMDA synaptic responses, indicating that most cardiac vagal neurons possess both AMPA and kainate receptors that are activated upon stimulation of the NTS. CNQX, a selective non-NMDA receptor blocker, abolished these synaptic responses.[5]

This monosynaptic projection from NTS to vagal cardiac neurons in the NA most likely plays an essential role in cardiovascular control. This pathway may constitute the essential excitatory link in the baroreflex pathway from NTS neurons that are excited (either directly or polysynaptically) by baroreceptors to cardioinhibitory cardiac vagal neurons.

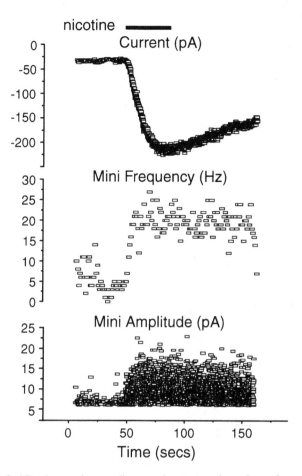

**FIGURE 3.** Nicotine excites cardiac vagal neurons via at least three mechanisms. Nicotine evokes an inward current (*top*) and augments non-NMDA minisynaptic currents by increasing their frequency (*middle*) and postsynaptic amplitude (*bottom*). α7 nicotinic blockers such as α-bungarotoxin can block the increase in mini frequency. The increase in frequency, amplitude, and inward current evoked by nicotine are also dependent on activation of voltage-gated calcium currents.

## CHOLINERGIC INPUTS TO CARDIAC VAGAL NEURONS

Acetylcholine excites cardiac vagal neurons via at least three sites of action.[6,7] Cardiac vagal neurons possess a postsynaptic nicotinic receptor that, when activated, evokes a depolarizing inward current that reverses at approximately −10 mV (FIG. 3). In addition, nicotine acts at different presynaptic and postsynaptic sites to facilitate glutamatergic neurotransmission. Presynaptic nicotinic receptors increase the frequency of transmitter release and can be blocked by αBgtx, indicating these presynaptic receptors likely contain the α7 subunit of the nicotinic receptor. In

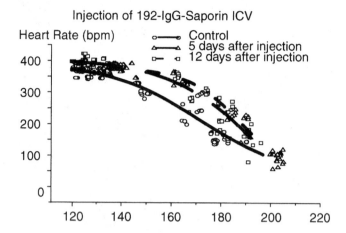

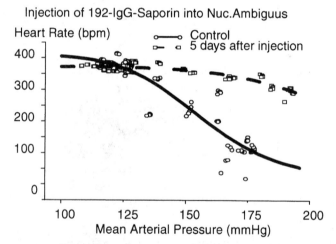

**FIGURE 4.** Infusions of phenylephrine for 4–8 seconds (1 mg/mL) evoked increases in blood pressure and reflex-mediated decreases in heart rate in chronically instrumented, unrestrained conscious rats. Intracerebral ventricular (ICV) injection of the selective cholinergic neuroimmunotoxin 192-IgG-Saporin had no effect on the baroreflex either 5 or 12 days after injection (*top*). Microinjection of 192-IgG-Saporin into the NA blunted the baroreflex at 5 days (*bottom*).

addition, nicotine augments postsynaptic non-NMDA currents via an αBgtx-insensitive receptor.

The mechanisms by which αBgtx-sensitive nAChRs increase the frequency of spontaneous release of transmitter onto cardiac vagal neurons depend on the activation of voltage-gated calcium channels. Although αBgtx-sensitive nAChRs have a high permeability to calcium, our recent work has shown that the calcium influx elicited from activation of the nicotinic channels is insufficient to cause spontaneous transmitter release.[8] Instead, spontaneous transmitter release seems to depend upon nicotine-evoked presynaptic depolarization and subsequent activation of presynaptic voltage-dependent calcium channels. The nicotine-evoked increase in presynaptic transmitter release can be blocked by broad calcium channel antagonists and specifically by antagonists of the P-type voltage-gated calcium channel.[8]

To investigate the role of cholinergic pathways to cardiac vagal neurons *in vivo*, we utilized an antineuronal immunotoxin that can ablate specific neuronal populations. The neuroimmunotoxin 192-IgG-Saporin is selectively taken up by cholinergic nerve terminals and transported back to cholinergic cell bodies, and then selectively destroys these cholinergic neurons that synapse at the microinjection site.[9]

Intracerebral ventricular injection of 192-IgG-Saporin does not produce any alteration of the baroreflex control of heart rate even after 12 days postinjection (FIG. 4). However, when microinjected into the NA, 192-IgG-Saporin blunted the baroreflex control of cardiac vagal activity in chronically instrumented, unrestrained animals (FIG. 4). The blunting of the baroreflex control of heart rate was first evident after three days and reached a steady-state inhibition by day 5. Respiratory sinus arrhythmia was also diminished. The blunting of the baroreflex and respiratory sinus arrhythmia with microinjection of 192-IgG-Saporin into the NA is supportive of the hypothesis proposed from the cellular work that cholinergic inputs to cardiac vagal neurons are excitatory and facilitate glutamatergic synaptic pathways that innervate cardiac neurons.

## GABAERGIC INPUTS TO CARDIAC VAGAL NEURONS

*In vivo* studies have strongly suggested that there is a tonically active GABAergic input to cardiac vagal neurons that plays an important role in the tonic and reflex control of heart rate. Blockade of $GABA_A$ receptors by microinjection of bicuculline into the NA produces a dose-dependent slowing of heart rate, which can be reversed by the $GABA_A$ receptor agonist, muscimol.[10] $GABA_A$ agonists microinjected in the NA prevent the reflex slowing of the heart in response to blood pressure increases evoked with phenylephrine.[10]

Recent work has shown that cardiac vagal neurons are constantly inhibited by spontaneous GABAergic synaptic input that can be blocked by bicuculline[11] (FIG. 5). Inhibiting action potential discharge blocks this spontaneous activity. This is in contrast to spontaneous excitatory synaptic inputs on cardiac vagal neurons that occur in the presence of TTX and thus do not depend on action potential generation.[6] Stimulation of the NTS monosynaptically evokes GABAergic postsynaptic currents in cardiac vagal neurons that can also be blocked by bicuculline.[11] The GABAergic pathway to cardiac vagal neurons may play an important role in the inhibition of cardiac neurons that occurs during inspiration.

## NEURONS THAT PROJECT TO CARDIAC VAGAL
## NEURONS IDENTIFIED BY PRV-GFP

The Bartha strain of pseudorabies virus (PRV), an attenuated swine alphaherpesvirus, can be used as a transsynaptic marker of neural circuits. Bartha PRV invades neuronal networks in the central nervous system through peripherally projecting

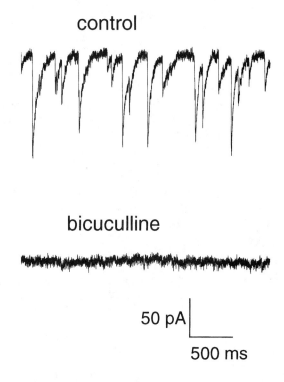

**FIGURE 5.** Cardiac vagal neurons demonstrate spontaneous inhibitory postsynaptic GABAergic currents (*top*). These synaptic inputs can be blocked by the $GABA_A$ antagonist bicuculline (*bottom*).

axons, replicates in these parent neurons, and then travels transsynaptically to continue labeling the second- and higher-order neurons in a time-dependent manner.[12] To visualize and record from neurons *in vitro* that determine the vagal motor outflow to the heart, we used a Bartha PRV mutant that expresses green fluorescent protein (GFP).[13,14] Neurons that project to cardiac vagal neurons include superior laryngeal, periambiguus, and NTS neurons.[14] Bartha PRV-GFP-labeled neurons retain their normal electrophysiological properties, and the baroreflex control of heart rate is unaltered by the virus[14] (FIG. 6).

This novel transsynaptic virus permits *in vitro* studies of identified neurons within functionally defined neuronal systems, including networks that mediate cardiovascular and respiratory function and interactions. It is anticipated that this virus can be used to identify other neurons that synapse upon cardiac vagal neurons, which can then be studied electrophysiologically. It is also likely that this virus can be utilized to introduce gene products other than GFP to deliberately alter the function of specific neurons in central nervous system pathways that control cardiorespiratory function.

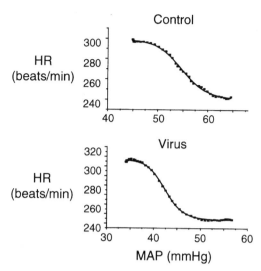

**FIGURE 6.** Infusions of phenylephrine for 2–4 s (1 mg/mL) evoked increases in mean arterial pressure (MAP, mmHg) and reflex-mediated decreases in heart rate (HR, beats/min) in 7- to 11-day-old rats. Labeling the cardiac vagal neurons and the neurons that project to them with the transsynaptic pseudorabies virus that expresses green fluorescent protein (PRV-GFP) did not alter the function of the labeled baroreflex pathway (control animal, *upper graph*; virus-labeled animal, *lower graph*). Initial heart rate, midpoint of the reflex, minimal heart rate, and gain of the reflex were not significantly different in virus-treated rats versus control rats. Baroreflex studies were conducted 3 days after injection of 0.5–20 μL of PRV-GFP virus [titer = $10^8$ plaque-forming units per milliliter (pfu/mL)] into the pericardial sac onto the fat pads at the base of the heart.

## SUMMARY

Recent work has shown that there are at least three major neurotransmitter and synaptic inputs to cardiac vagal neurons. Glutamate, released upon stimulation of the NTS, activates NMDA, AMPA, and kainate receptors in cardiac vagal neurons. It is likely that this pathway plays an important role in mediating the baroreflex-evoked and vagally mediated decrease in heart rate that occurs in response to increases in blood pressure. Stimulation of the NTS also activates a GABAergic pathway to cardiac vagal neurons. This pathway may be involved in generating respiratory sinus arrhythmia and, in particular, the inhibition of cardiac vagal neurons that occurs during inspiration. Nicotinic receptors are also likely involved in mediating respiratory sinus arrhythmia and likely act to excite cardiac vagal neurons during postinspiration. Acetylcholine released from respiratory neurons would activate postsynaptic nicotinic receptors and would directly excite cardiac vagal neurons. In addition, the release of acetylcholine would increase the frequency of glutamatergic synaptic inputs perhaps from the synaptic terminals of NTS neurons via activation of presynaptic α7-containing nicotinic receptors. This presynaptic action might be the mechanism responsible for the increased gain of the baroreflex during postinspiration. At least one source of cholinergic input to cardiac vagal neurons originates from superior laryngeal neurons colocalized in the NA. Advances using transsynaptic PRV that expresses GFP should help identify and characterize other neurons and pathways that determine cardiac vagal activity and the parasympathetic control of heart rate.

## REFERENCES

1. COLE, C.R. *et al.* 1999. Heart-rate recovery immediately after exercise as a predictor of mortality. N. Engl. J. Med. **341**(18): 1351–1357.
2. LAROVERE, M.T. *et al.* 1988. Baroreflex sensitivity, clinical correlates, and cardiovascular mortality among patients with a first myocardial infarction. Circulation **78**: 816–824.
3. MENDELOWITZ, D. 1996. Firing properties of identified parasympathetic cardiac neurons in the nucleus ambiguus. Am. J. Physiol. **271**: H2609–H2614.
4. LOEWY, A.D. & K.M. SPYER. 1990. Central Regulation of Autonomic Functions. Oxford University Press. London/New York.
5. NEFF, R.A., M. MIHALEVICH & D. MENDELOWITZ. 1998. Stimulation of NTS activates NMDA and non-NMDA receptors in rat cardiac vagal neurons in the nucleus ambiguus. Brain Res. **792**: 277–282.
6. NEFF, R.A. *et al.* 1998. Nicotine enhances presynaptic and postsynaptic glutamatergic neurotransmission to activate cardiac parasympathetic neurons. Circ. Res. **83**(12): 1241–1247.
7. MENDELOWITZ, D. 1998. Nicotine excites cardiac vagal neurons via three sites of action. Clin. Exp. Pharmacol. Physiol. **25**: 453–456.
8. WANG, J., M. IRNATEN & D. MENDELOWITZ. 2001. Agatoxin-IVA sensitive calcium channels mediate the presynaptic and postsynaptic nicotinic activation of cardiac vagal neurons in rats. J. Neurophysiol. **85**(1): 164–168.
9. HOLLEY, L.A. *et al.* 1994. Cortical cholinergic deafferentation following the intracortical infusion of 192 IgG-saporin: a quantitative histochemical study. Brain Res. **663**(2): 277–286.
10. DIMICCO, J.A. *et al.* 1979. GABA receptor control of parasympathetic outflow to heart: characterization and brain stem localization. Science **204**: 1106–1109.
11. WANG, J., M. IRNATEN & D. MENDELOWITZ. 2001. Characteristics of spontaneous and evoked GABAergic synaptic currents in cardiac vagal neurons in rats. Brain Res. **889**(1–2): 78–83.
12. JANSEN, A.S. *et al.* 1995. Central command neurons of the sympathetic nervous system: basis of the fight-or-flight response. Science **270**: 644–646.
13. JONS, A. & T.C. METTENLEITER. 1997. Green fluorescent protein expressed by recombinant pseudorabies virus as an *in vivo* marker for viral replication. J. Virol. Methods **66**(2): 283–292.
14. IRNATEN, M., R.A. NEFF, J. WANG *et al.* 2001. Activity of cardiorespiratory networks revealed by transsynaptic virus expressing GFP. J. Neurophysiol. **85**(1): 435–438.

# Excitatory Inputs to the RVLM in the Context of the Baroreceptor Reflex

ALAN F. SVED,[a] SATORU ITO,[b] CHRISTOPHER J. MADDEN,[a]
SEAN D. STOCKER,[a] AND YOSHIHARU YAJIMA[a]

[a]Department of Neuroscience, University of Pittsburgh,
Pittsburgh, Pennsylvania 15260, USA

[b]Second Department of Internal Medicine, Nihon University School of Medicine,
Tokyo, Japan

ABSTRACT: The central neural circuit mediating baroreceptor control of sympathetic vasomotor outflow involves an excitatory projection from arterial baroreceptors to nucleus tractus solitarius, an excitatory projection from nucleus tractus solitarius to the caudal ventrolateral medulla, an inhibitory projection from the caudal ventrolateral medulla to the rostral ventrolateral medulla (RVLM), and an excitatory projection from the RVLM to sympathetic preganglionic neurons in the spinal cord. For this circuit to be operational, the relevant neurons in the RVLM must be tonically active. Indeed, numerous studies have demonstrated that RVLM vasomotor neurons are tonically active; however, little is known regarding the nature of the tonic excitatory drive to these neurons. We present a model in which RVLM vasomotor neurons are tonically excited by inputs to the RVLM that can be blocked by the excitatory amino acid receptor antagonist, kynurenic acid, as well as an input from the caudal ventrolateral medulla that is not sensitive to kynurenic acid.

KEYWORDS: Rostral ventrolateral medulla; Caudal ventrolateral medulla; Caudal pressor area; Excitatory amino acids; Sarthran

## CENTRAL BARORECEPTOR PATHWAYS

Arterial baroreceptors influence the control of a variety of processes relevant to the control of the circulation, including autonomic regulation of the heart and vasculature,[1,2] renal function,[3] water drinking,[4] and the activity of vasopressin-secreting cells.[5] Of these, baroreceptor control of the heart and vasculature has received the most attention because of its prominence in the control of arterial blood pressure (AP). As AP increases, there is an increase in baroreceptor afferent input, which leads to a decrease in sympathetic nerve activity directed to the heart and blood vessels, accompanied by increased vagal parasympathetic cardiac activity; the converse responses are produced by decreases in AP.

Baroreceptor afferent nerves, arising from stretch-sensitive endings in the carotid sinus and aortic arch, project via the aortic depressor nerves and carotid sinus nerves

Address for correspondence: Dr. Alan F. Sved, Department of Neuroscience, University of Pittsburgh, 446 Crawford Hall, Pittsburgh, PA 15260. Voice: 412-624-6996; fax: 412-624-9198.
sved@bns.pitt.edu

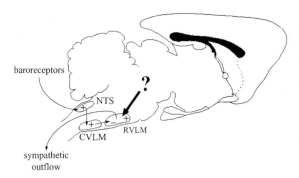

**FIGURE 1.** Schematic diagram of the neural circuitry underlying the baroreceptor reflex. Baroreceptor afferents terminate in NTS and provide an excitatory input onto these neurons. The central circuitry of the baroreflex involves an excitatory projection from NTS to the CVLM, an inhibitory projection from CVLM to the RVLM, and an excitatory projection from RVLM to preganglionic sympathetic neurons, thereby influencing sympathetic outflow. However, the excitatory input(s) onto RVLM neurons that drives the tonic activity of these neurons is presently unknown (*bold arrow*).

to the nucleus tractus solitarius (NTS) in the dorsomedial medulla.[6] Thus, the NTS contains the secondary sensory neurons involved in mediating baroreceptor reflexes. The neural pathways via which these secondary sensory neurons influence sympathetic and parasympathetic activity have been a focus of research, and now these pathways are well established. Baroreceptor-evoked changes in cardiac parasympathetic nerve activity appear to be mediated by a direct excitatory projection from second-order sensory neurons in the NTS to preganglionic parasympathetic neurons in the nucleus ambiguus.[7] In contrast, the central baroreceptor pathway controlling sympathetic vasomotor outflow is somewhat more complex, with an increase in baroreceptor afferent nerve activity causing the inverse change in sympathetic nerve activity. The chain of neurons includes a projection from the NTS to a region of the caudal ventrolateral medulla (CVLM). The CVLM provides a projection to neurons in the rostral ventrolateral medulla (RVLM) that then provide the descending influence upon sympathetic preganglionic neurons in the spinal cord.[8,9] Since functionally, an increase in AP and baroreceptor afferent nerve activity leads to inhibition of sympathetic vasomotor outflow, there must be an inhibitory link at some point in this pathway. This occurs at the level of the projection from the CVLM to RVLM.[10] Thus, it is now well accepted that the central circuitry involved in baroreceptor-mediated control of sympathetic outflow comprises an excitatory projection from NTS to CVLM, an inhibitory projection from CVLM to RVLM, and an excitatory projection from RVLM to preganglionic sympathetic vasomotor neurons (FIG. 1). Although additional interneurons may also be involved at any of these sites, inclusion of such neurons is not required to explain existing data and is not supported by the short latency of baroreceptor-evoked sympathoinhibition.

Despite the widespread acceptance of this model of central baroreceptor mechanisms, this model must necessarily be incomplete. Specifically, RVLM neurons must be tonically active, or neither inhibition nor disinhibition of these neurons would influence their activity. The nature of this excitatory drive of vasomotor neurons in the RVLM is the focus of this short review.

## EXCITATORY DRIVE OF RVLM VASOMOTOR NEURONS: PACEMAKER POTENTIALS?

RVLM vasomotor neurons, characterized as spinally projecting and barosensitive, are indeed tonically active.[11] This tonic activity of RVLM vasomotor neurons must depend upon either tonically active synaptic input to these neurons or their ability to generate spontaneous action potentials. Initial evidence that RVLM vasomotor neurons act as pacemaker cells and generate spontaneous action potentials came from studies by Guyenet and colleagues showing that, following injection of kynurenic acid (KYN) into the cisterna magna, RVLM vasomotor neurons displayed a constant discharge pattern[12] and that ramplike autodepolarizations were observed in spinally projecting RVLM neurons recorded intracellularly in an *in vitro* neonatal rat brain stem slice preparation.[13] However, dissociated spinally projecting RVLM neurons recorded *in vitro* did not display these pacemaker-like characteristics.[14] Although these conflicting observations have yet to be resolved, *in vivo* intracellular recordings of spinally projecting, barosensitive RVLM neurons provide no evidence for pacemaker activity in these neurons.[15] Rather, each action potential appears to be preceded by fast excitatory postsynaptic potentials. Thus, the tonic activity of RVLM vasomotor neurons is driven by a predominance of excitatory synaptic input to these cells.

## EXCITATORY DRIVE OF RVLM VASOMOTOR NEURONS: NEURONAL INPUTS?

Since tonically active inputs to the vasomotor neurons of the RVLM drive the baseline activity of these neurons, the source of this tonic excitatory input must arise from one or a combination of afferents to the RVLM. Neuroanatomical studies examining which brain regions project to the vasomotor area of the RVLM have documented a limited number of inputs to this area. In the rat, studies have demonstrated projections to the vasomotor area of the RVLM from CVLM, NTS, area postrema, raphe nuclei,[16] A5 neurons,[17] hypothalamic paraventricular nucleus (PVN),[18] central amygdaloid nucleus,[19] periaqueductal gray (PAG),[20] parabrachial nucleus,[21] and lateral hypothalamic area (LHA).[22] Unfortunately, only limited areas within the brain were investigated in these studies; thus, it is likely that areas providing input to the vasomotor region of the RVLM were overlooked. Surprisingly, no study to date has investigated the input to the vasomotor region of the RVLM from the entire brain in the rat. However, studies in the cat that have been more complete in this respect have demonstrated inputs to the vasomotor area of the RVLM from CVLM, NTS, Kolliker-Fuse nucleus (KF), PVN, LHA, medial vestibular nucleus,[23] and PAG.[24] Consistent with these observations, in the rat, projections to the nucleus paragigantocellularis lateralis, an area that encompasses the vasomotor area of the RVLM, have been demonstrated from the aforementioned areas as well as the medial prefrontal cortex (mPFC);[25] minor projections have been demonstrated from inferior colliculus, A5 area, locus coeruleus, gigantocellular nucleus, cochlear nucleus, and zona incerta.[25,26] Thus, major inputs to the vasomotor region of the RVLM in the rat likely consist of CVLM, NTS, KF, PVN, LHA, PAG, central amygdaloid nucleus, and mPFC. However, to the extent that the studies have been done, inhibition of not one of these regions leads to a marked decrease in AP. One possible reason for the failure to find afferent sources to the RVLM that drive tonic RVLM activity is readily apparent: it might be that two or more of these regions provide tonic excitatory input to RVLM vasomotor neurons and therefore a marked decrease in AP would only be observed following the inhibition of the correct combination of these regions. It is also possible that a region providing a portion of the excitatory drive to RVLM might be missed by this type of lesion approach if the region was functionally heterogeneous and provided tonic inhibition as well as excitation of the RVLM. Nonetheless, it should be possible to eliminate the tonic excitatory drive to RVLM vasomotor neurons and this manipulation should cause AP to decrease to the same extent as direct inhibition of the RVLM.

An alternative way of experimentally approaching the excitatory drive of RVLM vasomotor neurons focuses on the neurotransmitters used by inputs to RVLM rather than their anatomical origin. In this regard, the first class of neurotransmitters that comes to mind is the excitatory amino acid (EAA) transmitters, particularly L-glutamate, as EAA are the fast excitatory transmitters at the vast majority of excitatory brain synapses. However, studies conducted in the mid-1980s demonstrated that injection into the RVLM of KYN, an antagonist of ionotropic EAA receptors, had little effect on baseline blood pressure or the baroreceptor reflex in anesthetized rats;[27,28] similar results have recently been reported in conscious rats.[29] In contrast,

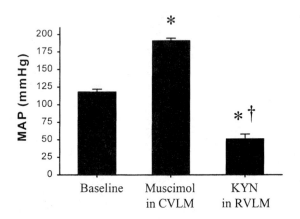

FIGURE 2. Mean arterial pressure (MAP) in chloralose-anesthetized rats at baseline conditions, 3 min after bilateral injection of muscimol (200 pmol) into the CVLM, and then 5 min after bilateral injection of kynurenic acid (KYN, 2.7 nmol) into the RVLM. Note that inhibition of CVLM increases MAP significantly above baseline values ($P < 0.05$); however, after blockade of excitatory amino acid transmission in RVLM, MAP decreased significantly below baseline levels ($P < 0.05$). Values are means ± SE ($n = 4$). *Significant difference from baseline MAP ($P < 0.05$). †Significant difference from MAP following muscimol into CVLM ($P < 0.05$). (Results were taken from Ref. 30.)

KYN injected into the RVLM does eliminate certain other evoked cardiovascular responses, such as the pressor response evoked by stimulation of the sciatic nerve.[28] The obvious conclusion from these studies is that ionotropic EAA receptors are not involved in the maintenance of baseline activity in RVLM vasomotor neurons and they are not essential for the baroreceptor reflex. While it is clear from these studies that KYN-sensitive receptors are not essential for the baroreceptor reflex, there are alternative explanations for the lack of a decrease in AP. For example, it is possible that injection of KYN into the RVLM not only removes a tonically active drive to RVLM vasomotor neurons, but simultaneously removes a tonically active inhibitory input that offsets the loss of the excitatory input. Indeed, our recent evidence supports this hypothesis.[30] Following inhibition of the CVLM, to eliminate the major inhibitory input to RVLM, inhibition of EAA receptors in RVLM decreased AP to levels significantly below the initial resting AP (FIG. 2).[30] This indicates that the CVLM contributed a non-EAA excitatory input to RVLM in addition to the inhibitory input. The observation that injection of KYN into the RVLM following inhibition of CVLM decreased AP to approximately the same level as direct inhibition of the RVLM suggests that a non-EAA input to the RVLM from the CVLM plus an EAA input to the RVLM account for much of the basal excitatory drive of RVLM vasomotor neurons.

## A TONICALLY ACTIVE EAA-MEDIATED INPUT TO RVLM

The experiment described above provides strong support for a tonically active EAA-mediated, KYN-sensitive input to RVLM contributing to the baseline drive of RVLM vasomotor neurons. Nonetheless, injection of KYN into the RVLM of anesthetized rats does not alter AP, presumably because it simultaneously removes an inhibitory input to the RVLM originating from the CVLM. Thus, KYN injected into the RVLM removes both an excitatory influence on vasomotor neurons and an equal inhibitory influence on these neurons.

At present, the source, or sources, of this tonically active EAA input to the RVLM is unclear. Based on reports by Weaver and colleagues that the pontine reticular formation might provide a tonically active EAA-mediated input to RVLM vasomotor neurons,[31–33] we tested whether, following CVLM inhibition, inhibition of the pontine reticular formation would markedly decrease AP. Indeed, that is what occurred.[34] However, it does not appear that the relevant region of the pontine reticular formation projects directly to the RVLM[25] (unpublished observations). Clearly, the nature of this input requires additional study.

## AN EXCITATORY INPUT TO THE RVLM FROM THE CVLM

The observation that KYN decreases AP to below-baseline levels only when the CVLM is inhibited suggests that the CVLM provides an excitatory input to RVLM vasomotor neurons that is not blocked by KYN. While the existence of this input was initially quite speculative, a recent report by Natarajan and Morrison[35] provides additional evidence for the existence of such a projection. Furthermore, their data indicate that the caudal pressor area (CPA) acts to increase sympathetic vasomotor outflow and AP via stimulation of this excitatory input from CVLM to RVLM since the pressor response that is evoked by stimulation or disinhibition of the CPA can be prevented by inhibition of the ipsilateral CVLM or blockade of EAA receptors with KYN injected into CVLM.[35] The CPA is a region in the caudal-most extent to the ventrolateral medulla, initially identified by the increased AP that occurred upon injection of glutamate into this region.[36] Pressor responses evoked from CPA are prevented by inhibition of the RVLM[36,37] and stimulation of the CPA excites RVLM vasomotor neurons,[38] indicating that the effects of the CPA on AP are mediated via the RVLM. Furthermore, the drive of vasomotor outflow from CPA appears to con-tribute to the tonic maintenance of AP since inhibition of the CPA results in a depressor response.[35,37] Curiously, injection of glycine into the CPA seems to reduce AP to a greater extent than GABA or GABA agonists; this might result from marked GABAergic drive to these neurons under basal conditions, a possibility further sup-ported by the recent observation that injection of a GABA receptor antagonist into the CPA produces a large increase in AP.[35] However, despite the evidence that the CPA tonically influences RVLM vasomotor neurons, neuroanatomical studies have failed to find a direct projection from CPA to RVLM.[16] Taken together, it appears that the CPA contributes significantly to the tonic maintenance of AP in anesthetized rats by driving an excitatory input from CVLM to RVLM rather than via a direct input to RVLM.

It is easy to incorporate the CPA into the model that we have previously suggested by including it as a primary drive to the sympathoexcitatory component of the CVLM (FIG. 3). Our previous data lead to the hypothesis that the excitatory input from CVLM to RVLM cannot be mediated by a KYN-sensitive input to RVLM,[30] and therefore the pressor response evoked by stimulation of the CPA should not be blocked by injection of KYN into the RVLM. Indeed, recent experiments demon-strate this to be the case.[39] Thus, the rat CVLM appears to be a heterogeneous region exerting both sympathoinhibitory and sympathoexcitatory influences on the RVLM. This CVLM sympathoexcitatory influence in rat may be analogous to the sympathoexcitatory input from the lateral tegmental field to the RVLM that has been described in cats.[40,41]

## OTHER TONIC EXCITATORY DRIVE OF RVLM VASOMOTOR NEURONS

Other neurotransmitter antagonists have been injected into the RVLM of anesthe-tized animals, and a few of these have been reported to lower AP.[42–48] The most prominent among these is the effect of the angiotensin antagonists, sarthran and sarile. Indeed, bilateral injection of sarthran or sarile into the RVLM of anesthetized rats or rabbits reduces AP and sympathetic nerve activity to a similar degree as direct inhibition of the RVLM.[44,47,48] Although these angiotensin analogs have been well characterized as angiotensin antagonists, the marked sympathoinhibition following injection of these drugs into the RVLM is not the result of blockade of AT1 recep-tors,[49,50] the predominant angiotensin receptor subtype in the RVLM. For example, selective AT1 receptor antagonists do not cause a decrease in AP when injected into

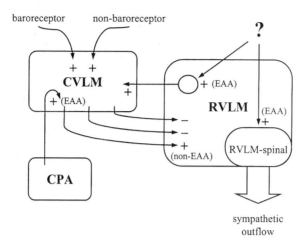

**FIGURE 3.** Schematic model of interactions between the CPA, CVLM, and RVLM. Excitatory amino acid inputs to the RVLM excite RVLM sympathoexcitatory neurons, as well as neurons that excite an inhibitory input mediated via the CVLM. The CPA provides a tonic excitatory input to CVLM neurons, which in turn excites RVLM neurons via a KYN-insensitive mechanism.

the RVLM[49–51] and sarthran injected into the RVLM still markedly decreases AP even when AT1 receptors in the RVLM are blocked.[49] Furthermore, the depressor action of sarthran can be prevented by coinjection of certain peptides that have no activity at AT1 receptors.[50] Nonetheless, sarthran and sarile do not nonspecifically inhibit RVLM neurons, as demonstrated by the observation that certain responses mediated by RVLM vasomotor neurons (e.g., somatic pressor response) remain following injection of these drugs[52] (unpublished observations). In addition, co-injection of certain angiotensin peptides can prevent the actions of sarile and sarthran, but do not affect the actions of direct inhibitory compounds such as muscimol.[50] The nature of this sarthran-sensitive receptor is unknown at present.

How does the observation that sarthran-like drugs injected into the RVLM eliminate tonic support of AP fit with the model of excitatory drive of RVLM vasomotor neurons presented in FIGURE 3? More specifically, how can sarthran-like drugs injected into the RVLM block both an excitatory non-EAA-mediated input from the CVLM and an EAA-mediated input arising from somewhere other than the CVLM? One possibility is that these excitatory inputs are funneled through the sarthran-sensitive drive to the RVLM vasomotor neurons. There are two observations that provide indirect support for that possibility. First, whereas the decrease in AP caused by sarthran injected into the RVLM is very rapid,[47] that produced by KYN in CVLM-inhibited rats is more gradual,[30] suggesting that KYN might be acting indirectly on RVLM vasomotor neurons by removing excitation of a local excitatory mechanism. Second, angiotensin-like peptides that reverse the effects of sarthran have no effect on AP when injected into the RVLM in otherwise untreated rats, but these peptides raise AP when injected into the RVLM of rats following injection of KYN into the RVLM plus inhibition of the CVLM.[53] These data are consistent with the hypothesis that normally the sarthran-sensitive receptor is fully activated and that, following injection of KYN into the RVLM of CVLM-inhibited rats, there is withdrawal of this activation, allowing exogenous agonist to act. Whatever the actual explanation, the marked decrease in AP produced by bilateral injection of sarthran or sarile into the RVLM suggests that tonically active inputs to RVLM vasomotor neurons are mediated through this sarthran-sensitive mechanism. Nonetheless, sarthran does not prevent the pressor response caused by electrical stimulation of the sciatic nerve[52] (unpublished observation), indicating that not all excitatory inputs to RVLM vasomotor neurons are mediated via a sarthran-sensitive mechanism. Interestingly, however, it appears that injection of sarile into the RVLM does block the pressor response evoked by stimulation of the CPA.[39]

## EXCITATORY DRIVE OF C1 VERSUS NON-C1 RVLM VASOMOTOR NEURONS

Barosensitive, spinally projecting RVLM neurons can be divided into two populations based on neurochemical phenotype: those containing the enzyme phenylethanolamine-$N$-methyltransferase (PNMT) and other enzymes involved in catecholamine biosynthesis, known as the C1 cell population, and those that are not catecholaminergic. An interesting issue that arises in the context of excitatory input to RVLM vasomotor neurons is that of potential differences between these two groups of neurons. In this regard, it is noteworthy that spinally projecting barosensitive C1 neurons have a lower firing rate than spinally projecting non-C1 neurons under baseline conditions *in vivo*.[54] This difference in basal firing rate would be consistent with the existence of differential inputs to these two neuronal populations, or differential responsiveness to these inputs. Indeed, the two populations may have different inputs. For example, angiotensin II (Ang II) has been reported to selectively excite C1 neurons in the RVLM in an *in vitro* slice preparation.[55] However, since this effect of Ang II is mediated by AT1 receptors, and selective blockade of AT1 receptors in the RVLM does not influence baseline AP,[49–51] it appears either that this mechanism is not tonically active *in vivo* or that selective decreases in the activity of C1 neurons do not decrease AP. Alpha-2 agonists are another example of an input that has been reported to selectively influence the C1 cell population,[56] and alpha-2 receptors are selectively expressed in spinally projecting C1 neurons within the RVLM.[57] In this regard, it is interesting to note that microinjection of clonidine into the RVLM, a treatment that produces a marked depressor response in control rats, did not change AP in rats in which the C1 neurons had been destroyed[58] by prior injection into the RVLM of a selective immunotoxin.[59] One caveat of this experiment, however, is that the clonidine-evoked depressor response could be mediated by actions on presynaptic catecholaminergic terminals within the RVLM, which would also be eliminated by treatment with the toxin. Nonetheless, these observations are consistent with the idea that the two populations of RVLM vasomotor neurons receive differential inputs. However, whether the tonic drive of these neuronal populations differs remains unclear and is in need of further investigation.

## ROLE OF TONIC EXCITATORY DRIVE OF RVLM
## IN THE BARORECEPTOR REFLEX

Given this emerging model of tonic excitatory drive of the RVLM, it is appropriate to consider how to incorporate baroreceptor inputs. Very simply, baroreceptor input appears to be one inhibitory input to RVLM vasomotor neurons that acts on the background of tonically active inputs plus the currently active phasic inputs. However, there is little direct data regarding the specific influence of these tonically active excitatory inputs to RVLM vasomotor neurons on baroreceptor reflex responses.

## REFERENCES

1. DORWARD, P.K. *et al.* 1985. The renal sympathetic baroreflex in the rabbit: arterial and cardiac baroreceptor influences, resetting, and effect of anesthesia. Circ. Res. **57**(4): 618–633.
2. DORWARD, P.K., L.B. BELL & C.D. RUDD. 1990. Cardiac afferents attenuate renal sympathetic baroreceptor reflexes during acute hypertension. Hypertension **16**(2): 131–139.
3. DIBONA, G.F. & U.C. KOPP. 1997. Neural control of renal function. Physiol. Rev. **77**(1): 75–197.
4. STOCKER, S.D., E. STRICKER & A.F. SVED. 2001. Acute hypertension inhibits thirst stimulated by angiotensin II, hyperosmolality, or hypovolemia in rats. Am. J. Physiol. Regul. Integr. Comp. Physiol. **280**: R214–R224.
5. RENAUD, L.P. & C.W. BOURQUE. 1991. Neurophysiology and neuropharmacology of hypothalamic magnocellular neurons secreting vasopressin and oxytocin. Prog. Neurobiol. **36**(2): 131–169.
6. CIRIELLO, J., S. HOCHSTENBACH & S. RODER. 1994. Central projections of baroreceptor and chemoreceptor afferent fibers in the rat. *In* Nucleus of the Solitary Tract: 35–50. CRC Press. Boca Raton, FL.
7. NEFF, R.A., M. MIHALEVICH & D. MENDELOWITZ. 1998. Stimulation of NTS activates NMDA and non-NMDA receptors in rat cardiac vagal neurons in the nucleus ambiguus. Brain Res. **792**(2): 277–282.
8. DAMPNEY, R.A. 1994. Functional organization of central pathways regulating the cardiovascular system. Physiol. Rev. **74**(2): 323–364.
9. SVED, A.F. 1999. Cardiovascular system. *In* Fundamental Neuroscience: 1051–1062. Academic Press. New York.
10. SVED, A.F., S. ITO & C.J. MADDEN. 2000. Baroreflex dependent and independent roles of the caudal ventrolateral medulla in cardiovascular regulation. Brain Res. Bull. **51**(2): 129–133.
11. GUYENET, P. 1990. Role of ventral medulla oblongata in blood pressure regulation. *In* Central Regulation of Autonomic Functions: 145–167. Oxford University Press. London/New York.
12. SUN, M.K., J.T. HACKETT & P.G. GUYENET. 1988. Sympathoexcitatory neurons of rostral ventrolateral medulla exhibit pacemaker properties in the presence of a glutamate-receptor antagonist. Brain Res. **438**(1–2): 23–40.
13. SUN, M.K. *et al.* 1988. Reticulospinal pacemaker neurons of the rat rostral ventrolateral medulla with putative sympathoexcitatory function: an intracellular study *in vitro*. Brain Res. **442**(2): 229–239.
14. LIPSKI, J. *et al.* 1998. Whole cell patch-clamp study of putative vasomotor neurons isolated from the rostral ventrolateral medulla. Am. J. Physiol. Regul. Integr. Comp. Physiol. **274**(4, pt. 2): R1099–R1110.
15. LIPSKI, J. *et al.* 1996. Properties of presympathetic neurones in the rostral ventrolateral medulla in the rat: an intracellular study *in vivo*. J. Physiol. (Lond.) **490**(3): 729–744.
16. ROSS, C.A., D.A. RUGGIERO & D.J. REIS. 1985. Projections from the nucleus tractus solitarii to the rostral ventrolateral medulla. J. Comp. Neurol. **242**(4): 511–534.

17. SUN, M.K. & P.G. GUYENET. 1986. Effect of clonidine and gamma-aminobutyric acid on the discharges of medullo-spinal sympathoexcitatory neurons in the rat. Brain Res. **368**(1): 1–17.
18. SHAFTON, A.D., A. RYAN & E. BADOER. 1998. Neurons in the hypothalamic paraventricular nucleus send collaterals to the spinal cord and to the rostral ventrolateral medulla in the rat. Brain Res. **801**(1–2): 239–243.
19. TAKAYAMA, K. & M. MIURA. 1991. Glutamate-immunoreactive neurons of the central amygdaloid nucleus projecting to the subretrofacial nucleus of SHR and WKY rats: a double-labeling study. Neurosci. Lett. **134**(1): 62–66.
20. CAMERON, A.A. et al. 1995. The efferent projections of the periaqueductal gray in the rat: a Phaseolus vulgaris–leucoagglutinin study: II. Descending projections. J. Comp. Neurol. **351**(4): 585–601.
21. KRUKOFF, T.L., K.H. HARRIS & J.H. JHAMANDAS. 1993. Efferent projections from the parabrachial nucleus demonstrated with the anterograde tracer Phaseolus vulgaris leucoagglutinin. Brain Res. Bull. **30**(1–2): 163–172.
22. ALLEN, G.V. & D.F. CECHETTO. 1992. Functional and anatomical organization of cardiovascular pressor and depressor sites in the lateral hypothalamic area: I. Descending projections. J. Comp. Neurol. **315**(3): 313–332.
23. DAMPNEY, R.A. et al. 1987. Afferent connections and spinal projections of the pressor region in the rostral ventrolateral medulla of the cat. J. Auton. Nerv. Syst. **20:** 73–86.
24. CARRIVE, P., R. BANDLER & R.A. DAMPNEY. 1988. Anatomical evidence that hypertension associated with the defence reaction in the cat is mediated by a direct projection from a restricted portion of the midbrain periaqueductal grey to the subretrofacial nucleus of the medulla. Brain Res. **460**(2): 339–345.
25. VAN BOCKSTAELE, E.J., V.A. PIERIBONE & G. ASTON-JONES. 1989. Diverse afferents converge on the nucleus paragigantocellularis in the rat ventrolateral medulla: retrograde and anterograde tracing studies. J. Comp. Neurol. **290**(4): 561–584.
26. ANDREZIK, J.A., V. CHAN-PALAY & S.L. PALAY. 1981. The nucleus paragigantocellularis lateralis in the rat: demonstration of afferents by the retrograde transport of horseradish peroxidase. Anat. Embryol. **161**(4): 373–390.
27. GUYENET, P.G., T.M. FILTZ & S.R. DONALDSON. 1987. Role of excitatory amino acids in rat vagal and sympathetic baroreflexes. Brain Res. **407**(2): 272–284.
28. KIELY, J.M. & F.J. GORDON. 1994. Role of rostral ventrolateral medulla in centrally mediated pressor responses. Am. J. Physiol. Heart Circ. Physiol. **267**(4, pt. 2): H1549–H1556.
29. ARAUJO, G.C., O.U. LOPES & R.R. CAMPOS. 1999. Importance of glycinergic and glutamatergic synapses within the rostral ventrolateral medulla for blood pressure regulation in conscious rats. Hypertension **34**(4, pt. 2): 752–755.
30. ITO, S. & A.F. SVED. 1997. Tonic glutamate-mediated control of rostral ventrolateral medulla and sympathetic vasomotor tone. Am. J. Physiol. Regul. Integr. Comp. Physiol. **273**(2, pt. 2): R487–R494.
31. HAYES, K. & L.C. WEAVER. 1992. Tonic sympathetic excitation and vasomotor control from pontine reticular neurons. Am. J. Physiol. Heart Circ. Physiol. **263**(5, pt. 2): H1567–H1575.
32. KRASSIOUKOV, A.V. & L.C. WEAVER. 1993. Connections between the pontine reticular formation and rostral ventrolateral medulla. Am. J. Physiol. Heart Circ. Physiol. **265**(4, pt. 2): H1386–H1392.
33. HAYES, K., F.R. CALARESU & L.C. WEAVER. 1994. Pontine reticular neurons provide tonic excitation to neurons in rostral ventrolateral medulla in rats. Am. J. Physiol. Regul. Integr. Comp. Physiol. **266**(1, pt. 2): R237–R244.
34. ITO, S. & A. SVED. 1996. Pontine reticular formation contributes to the tonic control of blood pressure. Neurosci. Abstr. **22:** 850.
35. NATARAJAN, M. & S.F. MORRISON. 2000. Sympathoexcitatory CVLM neurons mediate responses to caudal pressor area stimulation. Am. J. Physiol. Regul. Integr. Comp. Physiol. **279**(2): R364–R374.
36. GORDON, F.J. & L.A. MCCANN. 1988. Pressor responses evoked by microinjections of L-glutamate into the caudal ventrolateral medulla of the rat. Brain Res. **457**(2): 251–258.

37. POSSAS, O.S. *et al.* 1994. A fall in arterial blood pressure produced by inhibition of the caudalmost ventrolateral medulla: the caudal pressor area. J. Auton. Nerv. Syst. **49**(3): 235–245.
38. CAMPOS, R.R. & R.M. MCALLEN. 1999. Tonic drive to sympathetic premotor neurons of rostral ventrolateral medulla from caudal pressor area neurons. Am. J. Physiol. Regul. Integr. Comp. Physiol. **276**(4, pt. 2): R1209–R1213.
39. YAJIMA, Y. & A.F. SVED. 2001. Caudal pressor area response is not mediated by excitatory amino acids in rostral ventrolateral medulla. FASEB J.**15**(5): A804.
40. BARMAN, S.M. & G.L. GEBBER. 1987. Lateral tegmental field neurons of cat medulla: a source of basal activity of ventrolateral medullospinal sympathoexcitatory neurons. J. Neurophysiol. **57**(5): 1410–1424.
41. BARMAN, S.M., G.L. GEBBER & H.S. ORER. 2000. Medullary lateral tegmental field: an important source of basal sympathetic nerve discharge in the cat. Am. J. Physiol. Regul. Integr. Comp. Physiol. **278**(4): R995–R1004.
42. WILLETTE, R.N. *et al.* 1984. Cardiovascular control by cholinergic mechanisms in the rostral ventrolateral medulla. J. Pharmacol. Exp. Ther. **231**(2): 457–463.
43. ARNERIC, S.P. *et al.* 1990. Synthesis, release, and receptor binding of acetylcholine in the C1 area of the rostral ventrolateral medulla: contributions in regulating arterial pressure. Brain Res. **511**(1): 98–112.
44. SASAKI, S. & R.A. DAMPNEY. 1990. Tonic cardiovascular effects of angiotensin II in the ventrolateral medulla. Hypertension **15**(3): 274–283.
45. LEE, S.B., S.Y. KIM & K.W. SUNG. 1991. Cardiovascular regulation by cholinergic mechanisms in rostral ventrolateral medulla of spontaneously hypertensive rats. Eur. J. Pharmacol. **205**(2): 117–123.
46. PRIVITERA, P.J., H. THIBODEAUX & P. YATES. 1994. Rostral ventrolateral medulla as a site for the central hypertensive action of kinins. Hypertension **23**(1): 52–58.
47. ITO, S. & A.F. SVED. 1996. Blockade of angiotensin receptors in rat rostral ventrolateral medulla removes excitatory vasomotor tone. Am. J. Physiol. Regul. Integr. Comp. Physiol. **270**(6, pt. 2): R1317–R1323.
48. TAGAWA, T. *et al.* 1999. Sympathoinhibition after angiotensin receptor blockade in the rostral ventrolateral medulla is independent of glutamate and gamma-aminobutyric acid receptors. J. Auton. Nerv. Syst. **77**(1): 21–30.
49. HIROOKA, Y., P.D. POTTS & R.A. DAMPNEY. 1997. Role of angiotensin II receptor subtypes in mediating the sympathoexcitatory effects of exogenous and endogenous angiotensin peptides in the rostral ventrolateral medulla of the rabbit. Brain Res. **772**(1–2): 107–114.
50. ITO, S. & A. SVED. 2000. Pharmacological profile of the depressor response elicited by sarthran in the rat ventrolateral medulla. Am. J. Physiol. Heart Circ. Physiol. **279**: H2961–H2966.
51. AVERILL, D.B. *et al.* 1994. Losartan, nonpeptide angiotensin II–type 1 (AT1) receptor antagonist, attenuates pressor and sympathoexcitatory responses evoked by angiotensin II and L-glutamate in rostral ventrolateral medulla. Brain Res. **665**(2): 245–252.
52. HIROOKA, Y. & R.A. DAMPNEY. 1995. Endogenous angiotensin within the rostral ventrolateral medulla facilitates the somatosympathetic reflex. J. Hypertens. **13**(7): 747–754.
53. ITO, S. & A. SVED. 2000. Evidence that tonically active excitatory amino acid (EAA) input to rostral ventrolateral medulla (RVLM) supports blood pressure via a sarthran sensitive receptor. FASEB J. **14**(4): A623.
54. SCHREIHOFER, A.M. & P.G. GUYENET. 1997. Identification of C1 presympathetic neurons in rat rostral ventrolateral medulla by juxtacellular labeling *in vivo*. J. Comp. Neurol. **387**(4): 524–536.
55. LI, Y.W. & P.G. GUYENET. 1996. Angiotensin II decreases a resting K+ conductance in rat bulbospinal neurons of the C1 area. Circ. Res. **78**(2): 274–282.
56. STORNETTA, R.L. *et al.* 1995. Alpha-2 adrenergic receptors: immunohistochemical localization and role in mediating inhibition of adrenergic RVLM presympathetic neurons by catecholamines and clonidine. Ann. N.Y. Acad. Sci. **763**: 541–551.
57. GUYENET, P.G. *et al.* 1994. Alpha 2A–adrenergic receptors are present in lower brainstem catecholaminergic and serotonergic neurons innervating spinal cord. Brain Res. **638**(1–2): 285–294.

58. MADDEN, C.J. & A.F. SVED. 2001. The effects of destruction of C1 neurons on rostral
    ventrolateral medulla–evoked cardiovascular responses. FASEB J. **15**(4): A472.
59. MADDEN, C.J. *et al.* 1999. Lesions of the C1 catecholaminergic neurons of the ventro-
    lateral medulla in rats using anti-DbetaH-saporin. Am. J. Physiol. Regul. Integr.
    Comp. Physiol. **277**(4, pt. 2): R1063–R1075.

# Regulation of Sympathetic Tone and Arterial Pressure by the Rostral Ventrolateral Medulla after Depletion of C1 Cells in Rats

P. G. GUYENET, A. M. SCHREIHOFER, AND R. L. STORNETTA

*Department of Pharmacology, University of Virginia, Charlottesville, Virginia 22908-0735, USA*

ABSTRACT: This review describes experiments designed to determine the role of bulbospinal (BS) C1 cells in regulating the sympathetic outflow and blood pressure. This goal was achieved by analyzing the physiological consequences of destroying BS C1 cells. These cells were destroyed by suicide transport of an anti-dopamine-beta-hydroxylase antibody conjugated to saporin (anti-DβH-SAP). Two to 3 weeks after spinal cord injection (T2–T6), the toxin destroyed 75–85% of BS C1 and C3 cells along with >95% of BS noradrenergic neurons (A5, A6, A7). The toxin spared BS noncatecholaminergic cells. Under anesthesia, toxin-treated rats had a normal blood pressure and an apparently normal sympathetic nerve discharge (SNA, splanchnic), and intravenous clonidine caused a normal degree of sympathoinhibition. Inhibition of rostral ventrolateral medulla (RVLM) neurons by bilateral injection of muscimol caused the same hypotension and sympathoinhibition as in control rats. The baroreflex range was 41% attenuated by the toxin, but the $MAP_{50}$ was unchanged. Sympathoexcitatory responses to stimulation of peripheral chemoreceptors with cyanide or to electrical stimulation of RVLM were severely depressed (60% to 80%) in toxin-treated rats. Rats in which A5 neurons were selectively destroyed had no deficit in the parameters tested. Unit recordings of BS RVLM neurons indicated that the toxin destroyed most barosensitive C1 neurons, but spared noncatecholaminergic lightly myelinated BS cells. In summary, the integrity of C1 neurons is not essential for the generation of SNA and the maintenance of BP under resting conditions, perhaps because these functions are performed primarily by noncatecholaminergic BS neurons. However, the deficits caused by treatment with anti-DβH-SAP indicate that BS C1 neurons play a crucial role in several sympathoexcitatory responses mediated by the RVLM.

KEYWORDS: Saporin; Dopamine-beta-hydroxylase; Splanchnic nerve

## INTRODUCTION

The rostral ventrolateral medulla (RVLM) is critical for the regulation of arterial pressure and cardiac output.[1,2] This region contains bulbospinal (BS) neurons that provide a largely monosynaptic input to sympathetic preganglionic vasomotor neurons (SPGNs).[3–5] The discharge properties of many RVLM BS neurons suggest

Address for correspondence: Patrice Guyenet, Ph.D., University of Virginia Health System, P. O. Box 800735, 1300 Jefferson Park Avenue, Charlottesville, VA 22908-0735. Voice: 804-924-9974; fax: 804-982-3878.

pgg@virginia.edu

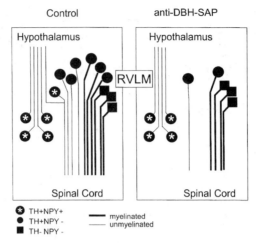

**FIGURE 1.** Effect of anti-DβH-saporin injection into the spinal cord on C1 and other RVLM bulbospinal barosensitive neurons. The RVLM contains bulbospinal neurons with a variety of phenotypes, including C1 cells and nonaminergic neurons. C1 cells are further subdivided into unmyelinated and lightly myelinated groups. Very few BS C1 cells express NPY mRNA, whereas all C1 cells with hypothalamic projection do so. This distinction provides a way to determine the proportion of bulbospinal C1 cells that are destroyed by the toxin. Anti-DβH-saporin selectively depleted bulbospinal C1 cells. The toxin spared C1 cells with projection elsewhere and it also spared the lightly myelinated barosensitive and bulbospinal cells of the RVLM. The toxin eliminated between 75% and 85% of bulbospinal C1 cells. It also destroyed bulbospinal noradrenergic neurons (A5, A6, and A7) not represented in the figure.

that they contribute a major excitatory drive to many types of SPGNs.[2,5,6] RVLM BS neurons are an obligatory synaptic relay for many sympathetic vasomotor reflexes, including the arterial baroreflex.[1,2,7] In particular, many BS RVLM neurons are profoundly inhibited by baroreceptor stimulation.[8,9] Their inhibition is thought to contribute greatly to the reduction in SPGN discharge rate during baroreceptor stimulation and thus to the overall sympathetic baroreflex.[1,2,7]

About two-thirds of RVLM BS express a catecholaminergic phenotype (C1 neurons) (FIG. 1). C1 neurons contain tyrosine-hydroxylase (TH), dopamine-β-hydroxylase (DβH), and phenylethanolamine-*N*-methyltransferase (PNMT) and are therefore assumed to release adrenaline and/or noradrenaline. Many C1 cells also contain peptides (e.g., enkephalins, neuropeptide Y) whose role in the spinal cord is largely undefined. BS C1 cells have either lightly myelinated or unmyelinated axons.[9] A large fraction of BS C1 neurons are inhibited by stimulation of arterial baroreceptors.[9–11] About one-third of RVLM BS neurons are not catecholaminergic (FIG. 1).[9–11] As of yet, a phenotypic marker for these non-C1 cells has not been identified. Many of the non-C1 cells are highly active at rest and very barosensitive.[9] They have lightly myelinated axons and could be a source (or the source) of supraspinal glutamatergic drive from RVLM to vasomotor SPGNs.[9,12,13] Whether glutamate is released by C1 cells is unknown.

The relative contributions of the C1 cells and the noncatecholaminergic RVLM neurons to the generation of sympathetic tone are not known because, until recently, neither cell type could be targeted for selective destruction. However, a newly introduced immunotoxin produced by conjugating the ribosomal inactivating protein saporin to an anti-dopamine-beta-hydroxylase antibody (anti-DβH-SAP) now provides the potential means to lesion C1 cells while sparing noncatecholaminergic neurons.[14,15]

The following review briefly describes the extent and selectivity of the lesions that can be achieved with spinal administration of anti-DβH-SAP. We also describe the autonomic deficits exhibited by rats with lesions of BS C1 neurons. The review summarizes data from three publications that should be consulted for experimental details.[16–18]

## SUICIDE TRANSPORT OF ANTI-DβH-SAP BY BULBOSPINAL CATECHOLAMINERGIC NEURONS

### *Quantitation and Anatomical Selectivity of Destruction*

The retrograde axonal transport of ribosome-inactivating proteins (RIP; e.g., ricin) has been used since the early 1980s as a tool to destroy neurons that project to the site of injection of the RIP (suicide retrograde transport).[19] The drawback of unconjugated toxins is that they are taken up nonselectively by nerve terminals and cannot be used to lesion specific chemical classes of neurons. Specificity can be built into the method by targeting the RIP to particular membrane receptors that transport the toxin to the intracellular space as they are internalized. For instance, the RIP saporin has been conjugated to an anti-dopamine-beta-hydroxylase antibody (anti-DβH-SAP).[14] Membrane-bound DβH is exteriorized during exocytosis and serves as a specific receptor for the internalization of anti-DβH-SAP into noradrenergic and adrenergic neurons. Once transported into the cell body, saporin blocks protein synthesis to cause the death and eventual elimination of the cell.[20]

We used this approach to produce selective lesions of bulbospinal catecholaminergic neurons. Several bilateral small injections of anti-DβH-SAP (total of 48 ng) were made into thoracic segments T2–T4 or T4–T6 in rats.[16–18] The effect of the toxin on C1 and other cells was examined 2 to 3 weeks later and quantified by one of two methods. In some cases,[16,18] we determined the effect of the toxin on the number of PNMT-immunoreactive (-ir) BS neurons labeled following injection of the retrogradely transported dye Fast Blue into the spinal cord. In others,[17] we determined the effect of the toxin on the number of PNMT-ir neurons lacking NPY mRNA. This second method was based on our prior finding that the vast majority of the C1 cells that project to the spinal cord (~90%) do not express NPY mRNA, whereas C1 cells with projections elsewhere express high levels of this mRNA (FIG. 1).[21] Both methods provided similar results: namely, an average destruction of between 75% and 85% of BS C1 neurons (FIG. 1). The toxin produced an equivalent reduction in the number of BS C3 cells and an even more massive reduction of BS noradrenergic neurons, including A5 neurons and those locus coeruleus neurons with projection to the spinal cord (>95%).[16] The toxin had no detectable effect on other types of BS neurons such as raphe serotonergic neurons and nonaminergic BS

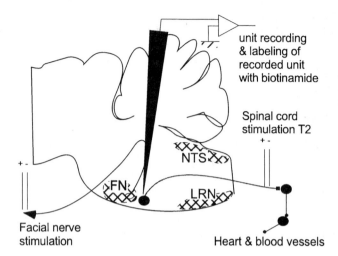

**FIGURE 2.** Method used to identify and label BS barosensitive neurons in the RVLM. The RVLM is identified by its location immediately posterior to the caudal end of the facial motor nucleus (FN). RVLM BS barosensitive neurons are recorded extracellularly and, once identified, are labeled with biotinamide using the method of Pinault.[33] Standard immuno-histochemical methods are then used to determine whether the biotinamide-labeled neurons contain TH or PNMT, that is, are C1 cells.

neurons within the RVLM.[16] C1 and other pontomedullary catecholaminergic neurons without spinal projection were also spared. Injections of the same amount of saporin conjugated to an anti-mouse IgG (control toxin) as opposed to the anti-DβH antibody had no effect on BS neurons, demonstrating that the uptake of saporin by bulbospinal neurons was a selective receptor-mediated process.[16] However, the anti-DβH-SAP conjugate and the control toxin both produced a persistent gliosis and some nonspecific neuronal loss at the spinal site of injection, suggesting that some saporin is taken up nonselectively by cell bodies at the site of injection.[16]

## SUICIDE TRANSPORT OF ANTI-DβH-SAP

### Effect on Electrophysiologically Identified RVLM Barosensitive BS Neurons

RVLM BS barosensitive neurons were recorded extracellularly and a subset of these cells were juxtacellularly labeled with biotinamide (FIG. 2). By testing whether the biotinamide-labeled neurons contained TH or PNMT, we were able to determine whether they were catecholaminergic.[17]

In intact rats or in animals treated with IgG-SAP (control rats), barosensitive BS neurons had axonal conduction velocities in the lightly myelinated and unmyelin-ated range.[9] All neurons with unmyelinated axons (conduction velocity < 1 m/s) were C1 cells. The remainder (conduction velocity from 1 to 7 m/s) were a mixture of C1 and noncatecholaminergic cells. Most barosensitive BS cells with axonal conduction velocity > 3 m/s were not C1 cells.[9] Out of 45 randomly sampled RVLM barosensitive neurons of all conduction velocities, 32 (71%) were found to be C1 cells in intact rats.

In rats treated with anti-DβH-SAP, BS neurons with low axonal conduction velocity (<1 m/s) and presumably unmyelinated axons were very rarely encountered, consistent with the loss of C1 neurons in histological material.[17] In these rats, the vast majority of surviving barosensitive BS neurons had conduction velocities above 3 m/s and thus were lightly myelinated.[17] In addition, the majority of these lightly myelinated neurons were not immunoreactive for TH or PNMT (11/13).[17]

In summary, anti-DβH-SAP produced a massive destruction of slowly conducting RVLM barosensitive neurons with the C1 phenotype. In contrast, the toxin spared many of the RVLM barosensitive neurons that are lightly myelinated, especially those that do not express TH or PNMT (FIG. 1). The electrophysiological properties of these surviving cells (discharge rate, sensitivity to baroreceptor activation) were comparable to those of neurons with the same conduction velocity found in intact rats.[17] Although massive, the destruction of bulbospinal barosensitive C1 cells was incomplete, in agreement with the histological data.[16,17] The selective resistance of the lightly myelinated cells to anti-DβH-SAP and the lack of demonstrable TH or PNMT in them both support the conclusion that they are not C1 cells.[9,17]

## IMMUNOLESION OF C1 AND OTHER BULBOSPINAL CATECHOLAMINERGIC CELL GROUPS WITH ANTI-DβH-SAP

### *Effects on Arterial Pressure, Resting Sympathetic Vasomotor Tone, Arterial Baroreflex, Bezold-Jarisch Reflex, and the Sympatholytic Effect of Clonidine*

Under anesthesia with halothane (1%) or chloralose, the mean arterial pressure (MAP) of rats treated with anti-DβH-SAP (lesioned rats) was the same as that of rats that had received injections of IgG-SAP or no spinal injection (control rats).[16–18] Apparently normal resting sympathetic nerve postganglionic activity (SNA) could be recorded from the greater splanchnic nerve of lesioned rats.[16–18]

In order to examine the baroreflex control of splanchnic SNA, MAP was raised with gradual aortic occlusion and lowered with i.v. sodium nitroprusside.[16] Plots of SNA (rectified and integrated) versus MAP were analyzed with a logistic function. Several parameters were quantified, such as the reflex midpoint ($MAP_{50}$), the percent SNA remaining at saturation of the reflex (lower plateau), the maximum SNA below baroreceptor threshold (upper plateau), and the gain of the reflex. Two series of experiments (experiment 1 reported in Ref. 16; experiment 2, unpublished data from Schreihofer and Guyenet) were performed in chloralose-anesthetized rats. These studies are summarized in FIGURE 3. In lesioned rats, the mid-operating point of the reflex ($MAP_{50}$) was unchanged by anti-DβH-SAP. However, the upper plateau expressed as a percent of resting SNA was decreased and the lower plateau was increased. These changes resulted in a consistent and significant decrease in the range of the reflex expressed as a percentage of baseline SNA (44% reduction in experiment 1; 38% in experiment 2). The gain of the reflex (% normalized SNA per mmHg at inflexion point of the logistic curve) was reduced in proportion to the over-

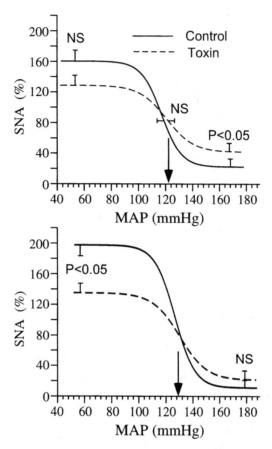

**FIGURE 3.** Effect of anti-DβH-saporin injection into the spinal cord on the sympathetic baroreflex. Two separate experiments are described, both performed in Sprague-Dawley rats under chloralose anesthesia. Experiment 1 **(top)** was made 1 hour after a crossover from halothane to chloralose anesthesia. Experiment 2 **(bottom)** was done 3 hours after the crossover. Each sigmoid curve represents the best fit of the relationship between splanchnic SNA (differential recording, 30–300 Hz, rectified and integrated) and mean arterial pressure for 5–8 rats. Control rats received IgG-SAP, a control toxin that does not lesion bulbospinal catecholaminergic neurons. Statistics evaluate the significance of the change in upper and lower plateaux and in $MAP_{50}$, the midpoint of the reflex.

all range (39%, experiment 1) by toxin treatment. These data appear consistent with the possibility that the toxin might have produced a slight reduction in the baro-sensitive component of splanchnic SNA at all levels of arterial pressure without causing much of a change in the degree of baroreceptor inhibition of this output. The maximum unnormalized range of the barosensitive component of splanchnic SNA (upper plateau minus lower plateau expressed in actual microvolts of the original signal) was slightly reduced by toxin treatment (29.8%, experiment 2), but the reduction failed to reach significance because of the inevitable scattering of the data.

In summary, the lesion of 75–85% of bulbospinal C1 cells along with >95% of the BS noradrenergic neurons has no effect on resting AP. The lesion produced relatively small changes in splanchnic nerve activity and in the sympathetic baroreflex consistent with a slight decrease in the barosensitive component of SNA at all levels of AP.

The sympathetic component of the Bezold-Jarisch reflex elicited by i.v. injection of a bolus of the 5-HT3 agonist phenylbiguanide (PBG) was unchanged (amplitude and duration) in lesioned animals.[16] The sympatholytic effect of clonidine administered iv was also unaffected by spinal treatment with anti-DβH-SAP.[17]

Thus, despite the large reduction in BS C1 neurons, the changes in AP, resting SNA, and cardiopulmonary reflexes were rather unremarkable. Could it be that sympathetic tone generation was taken over by a brain structure other than RVLM in animals with extensive lesions of BS C1 cells? To address this possibility, we determined the extent to which injection of the $GABA_A$ agonist muscimol decreases MAP and splanchnic SNA upon bilateral microinjection into RVLM.[17] These experiments demonstrated that the hypotension and the sympathoinhibition produced by muscimol were the same in toxin-treated animals (anti-DβH-SAP) as in controls (IgG-SAP).[17] Thus, RVLM remains the critical site for sympathetic tone generation and blood pressure maintenance after extensive lesion of BS catecholaminergic neurons including C1 and A5 cells.

## IMMUNOLESION OF C1 AND OTHER BULBOSPINAL CATECHOLAMINERGIC CELL GROUPS WITH ANTI-DβH-SAP

### *Effects on Sympathoexcitatory Responses*

The cardiovascular consequences of anti-DβH-SAP described so far were either absent or surprisingly small given the magnitude of the destruction of bulbospinal C1 cells and the importance classically assigned to these neurons in regulating sympathetic tone.[22] However, the c-Fos literature on C1 and other brain stem noradrenergic neurons suggests that these cells respond vigorously to stresses, be they somatic (hemorrhage, pain, prolonged hypotension) or psychological (fear, noise).[23,24] Might deficits in sympathetic response be more apparent when the brain stem sympathetic network is stimulated rather than in the resting state? To test this possibility, we analyzed the sympathetic response to brief stimulation of peripheral chemoreceptors with cyanide (i.v. bolus) or to direct electrical stimulation of the RVLM.[25]

The brief increase in splanchnic SNA caused by an i.v. bolus of cyanide was reduced by 80–100% in rats treated with anti-DβH-SAP, whereas this response persisted in rats treated with the control toxin (IgG-SAP).[16]

Intermittent electrical stimulation of the RVLM (single 0.5-ms pulses every 2 s) normally causes a large peak of evoked sympathetic activity in the splanchnic nerve. This evoked response was severely reduced (>65%) in rats treated with anti-DβH-SAP[17] (FIG. 4), but not in rats in which A5 neurons were lesioned with 6-OHDA and C1 cells were intact.[17] Finally, the rise in arterial pressure caused by repetitive stimulation of the RVLM (0.5 ms, 44 Hz, 10–60 µamps) was also significantly attenuated in rats treated with anti-DβH-SAP compared to control rats and to rats with selective

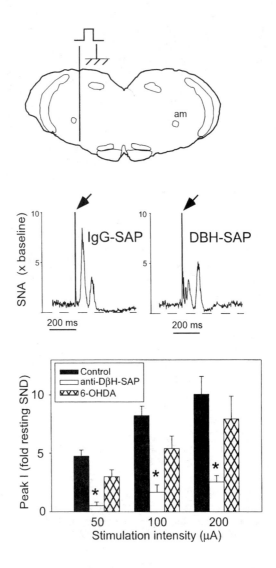

**FIGURE 4.** Effect of anti-DβH-saporin injection on the sympathetic response evoked by electrical stimulation of the RVLM. (**Top**) In halothane-anesthetized rats, the RVLM was stimulated with a monopolar electrode (0.5 Hz, 0.5 ms, 50–200 ms). (**Middle**) Example of evoked SNA response in a control rat (*left*) and in a rat treated with anti-DβH-SAP (*right*). Postganglionic SNA was recorded in the splanchnic nerve distal to the suprarenal ganglion (bipolar electrode, 30–300 Hz), amplified, and rectified. Peristimulus averaging of the evoked response (80 stimuli) was done, generating the patterns shown. Toxin treatment caused a dramatic reduction in peak I, the first and major peak of the evoked response. (**Bottom**) Group data showing the magnitude of the decrease in the amplitude of peak I caused by anti-DβH-saporin. The selective destruction of A5 neurons with 6-OHDA did not reproduce the effect of the combined lesion of C1 and A5 cells with anti-DβH-saporin. Significance evaluated by ANOVA (groups of 6–8 rats).

lesions of A5 neurons.[17] In brief, clear-cut sympathetic deficits could be uncovered in rats treated with anti-DβH-SAP when sympathoexcitatory rather than sympatho-inhibitory responses were examined. These effects were not mimicked by selectively lesioning A5 neurons.[17] Therefore, the deficits observed after administration of anti-DβH-SAP into the spinal cord are likely due primarily to the lesion of bulbospinal adrenergic neurons (C1 and, possibly, C3 neurons).

## INTERPRETATIONS AND CONCLUSIONS

### *Role of C1 and Other Bulbospinal Neurons in Generation of the Vasomotor Tone*

The deficits produced by lesioning C1 neurons (baroreflex range, peripheral chemoreflex, sympathoexcitatory responses to stimulation of the reticular formation) were always in the direction of a reduction in sympathoexcitation. These findings support the prevalent notion that C1 cells have a predominantly sympathoexcitatory function.[2,6,22] Until now, this notion rested on three lines of largely indirect evidence. First, C1 cells express c-Fos during stresses that elevate SNA and AP.[23,26–29] Second, many BS C1 cells are inhibited by baroreceptor stimulation.[9,30] Finally, BS C1 cells are located in the pressor area of the ventrolateral medulla and innervate SPGNs monosynaptically.[3,5,22] The present data provide a fourth and perhaps more direct evidence of a sympathoexcitatory function of C1 cells by showing that deficits in sympathoexcitatory responses result from lesioning these cells.

The more unusual finding of the present series of experiments is that a massive lesion of BS C1 and other catecholaminergic neurons had no effect on resting arterial pressure and little or no effect on sympathoinhibitory responses such as the baro-reflex, the Bezold-Jarisch reflex, or the sympatholytic effect of clonidine. In addition, the lesion appeared to have little effect on resting sympathetic tone, although the notorious difficulty in quantifying absolute levels of SNA across animals renders this statement tentative. The hypothesis that a structure distinct from RVLM had taken over after the lesion of C1 cells was clearly excluded because the ability of muscimol injections into RVLM to lower SNA and AP was unchanged by treatment with anti-DβH-SAP. Therefore, two explanations remain to account for the lack of effect of the toxin on many cardiovascular parameters. First, the destruction of even 75–85% of BS C1 cells may be efficiently compensated by adaptive changes (terminal sprouting from surviving C1 neurons and, perhaps, receptor supersensitivity at the preganglionic neuronal level). This possibility is compatible with observations made in other systems, most prominently the nigrostriatal dopaminergic pathway. In this case, dopaminergic cells must be reduced by more than 80% for symptomatic changes in extrapyramidal motor function to appear.[31,32] However, this explanation appears at odds with the large deficit in sympathoexcitatory responses triggered by stimulation of the RVLM or by activation of peripheral chemoreceptors.

Alternatively, although C1 neurons do have a sympathoexcitatory function, these cells may make a relatively small contribution to sympathetic tone generation and baroreflexes at rest. C1 cells may be recruited under specific stress conditions when SNA needs to be raised well beyond the resting state. This hypothesis requires that resting sympathetic tone be largely generated by noncatecholaminergic RVLM BS sympathoexcitatory neurons. In agreement with this notion, the RVLM contains tonically active barosensitive neurons that contain no TH or PNMT and are spared by treatment with anti-DβH-SAP.[9,17] In the absence of most C1 cells, these noncatecholaminergic RVLM neurons seem to have the ability to generate enough excitatory drive to SPGNs to maintain SNA and AP at a normal level.

In summary, injection of anti-DβH-SAP into the spinal cord results in the selective suicide transport of saporin by bulbospinal noradrenergic and adrenergic neurons. The cardiovascular deficits exhibited under anesthesia by rats treated with anti-DβH-SAP suggest that the integrity of adrenergic C1 neurons is not essential for sympathetic vasomotor tone generation under resting conditions. Instead, the lightly myelinated BS barosensitive RVLM neurons that are spared by treatment with anti-DβH-SAP may be sufficient to maintain a normal level of resting AP and SNA. However, the clear deficits observed during stimulation of the RVLM in rats treated with anti-DβH-SAP support the prevalent theory that C1 cells, when recruited, have a powerful sympathoexcitatory role.

## REFERENCES

1. DAMPNEY, R.A.L. 1994. The subretrofacial vasomotor nucleus: anatomical, chemical, and pharmacological properties and role in cardiovascular regulation. Prog. Neurobiol. **42:** 197–228.
2. GUYENET, P.G., N. KOSHIYA, D. HUANGFU et al. 1996. Role of medulla oblongata in generation of sympathetic and vagal outflows. In The Emotional Motor System: 127–144. Elsevier. Amsterdam/New York.
3. MILNER, T.A., S.F. MORRISON, C. ABATE & D.J. REIS. 1988. Phenylethanolamine-N-methyltransferase-containing terminals synapse directly on sympathetic preganglionic neurons in the rat. Brain Res. **448:** 205–222.
4. ZAGON, A. & A.D. SMITH. 1993. Monosynaptic projections from the rostral ventrolateral medulla-oblongata to identified sympathetic preganglionic neurons. Neuroscience **54:** 729–743.
5. JANSEN, A.S.P., X.V. NGUYEN, V. KARPITSKIY et al. 1995. Central command neurons of the sympathetic nervous system: basis of the fight-or-flight response. Science **270:** 644–646.
6. SUN, M.K. 1996. Pharmacology of reticulospinal vasomotor neurons in cardiovascular regulation. Pharmacol. Rev. **48:** 465–494.
7. SUN, M.K. 1995. Central neural organization and control of sympathetic nervous system in mammals. Prog. Neurobiol. **47:** 157–233.
8. BROWN, D.L. & P.G. GUYENET. 1985. Electrophysiological study of cardiovascular neurons in the rostral ventrolateral medulla in rats. Circ. Res. **56:** 359–369.
9. SCHREIHOFER, A.M. & P.G. GUYENET. 1997. Identification of C1 presympathetic neurons in rat rostral ventrolateral medulla by juxtacellular labeling "in vivo." J. Comp. Neurol. **387:** 524–536.
10. LIPSKI, J., R. KANJHAN, B. KRUSZEWSKA & M. SMITH. 1995. Barosensitive neurons in the rostral ventrolateral medulla of the rat in vivo: morphological properties and relationship to C1 adrenergic neurons. Neuroscience **69:** 601–618.
11. LIPSKI, J., R. KANJHAN, B. KRUSZEWSKA & W.F. RONG. 1996. Properties of presympathetic neurones in the rostral ventrolateral medulla in the rat: an intracellular study "in vivo." J. Physiol. (Lond.) **490:** 729–744.
12. DEUCHARS, S.A., S.F. MORRISON & M.P. GILBEY. 1995. Medullary-evoked EPSPs in neonatal rat sympathetic preganglionic neurones in vitro. J. Physiol. (Lond.) **487:** 453–463.
13. MORRISON, S.F., P. ERNSBERGER, T.A. MILNER et al. 1989. A glutamate mechanism in the intermediolateral nucleus mediates sympathoexcitatory responses to stimulation of the rostral ventrolateral medulla. Prog. Brain. Res. **81:** 159–169.

14. WRENN, C.C., M.J. PICKLO, D.A. LAPPI *et al.* 1996. Central noradrenergic lesioning using anti-DBH-saporin: anatomical findings. Brain Res. **740:** 175–184.
15. MADDEN, C., S. ITO, L. RINAMAN *et al.* 1999. Lesions of the C1 catecholaminergic neurons of the ventrolateral medulla in rats using anti-DBH-saporin. Am. J. Physiol. Regul. Integr. Comp. Physiol. **277:** R1063–R1075.
16. SCHREIHOFER, A.M. & P.G. GUYENET. 2000. Sympathetic reflexes in rats after depletion of bulbospinal catecholaminergic neurons with anti-DBH-saporin. Am. J. Physiol. Regul. Integr. Comp. Physiol. **279:** R729–R742.
17. SCHREIHOFER, A.M., R.L. STORNETTA & P.G. GUYENET. 2000. Regulation of sympathetic tone and arterial pressure by rostral ventrolateral medulla after depletion of C1 cells in rat. J. Physiol. (Lond.) **529:** 221–236.
18. SCHREIHOFER, A.M. & P.G. GUYENET. 2000. Role of presympathetic C1 neurons in the sympatholytic and hypotensive effects of clonidine in rats. Am. J. Physiol. Regul. Integr. Comp. Physiol. **279:** R1753–R1762.
19. WILEY, R.G., W.W. BLESSING & D.J. REIS. 1982. Suicide transport: destruction of neurons by retrograde transport of ricin, abrin, and modeccin. Science **216:** 889–890.
20. STIRPE, F. & L. BARBIERI. 1986. Ribosome-inactivating proteins up to date. FEBS Lett. **195:** 1–8.
21. STORNETTA, R.L., P.J. AKEY & P.G. GUYENET. 1999. Location and electrophysiological characterization of rostral medullary adrenergic neurons that contain neuropeptide Y mRNA in rat. J. Comp. Neurol. **415:** 482–500.
22. REIS, D.J., D.A. RUGGIERO & S.F. MORRISON. 1989. The C1 area of the rostral ventrolateral medulla oblongata: a critical brainstem region for control of resting and reflex integration of arterial pressure. Am. J. Hypertens. **2:** 363S–374S.
23. CHAN, R.K.W. & P.E. SAWCHENKO. 1994. Spatially and temporally differentiated patterns of c-Fos expression in the brainstem catecholaminergic cell groups induced by cardiovascular challenges in the rat. J. Comp. Neurol. **348:** 433–460.
24. CHAN, R.K.W. & P.E. SAWCHENKO. 1998. Organization and transmitter specificity of medullary neurons activated by sustained hypertension: implications for understanding baroreceptor reflex circuitry. J. Neurosci. **18:** 371–387.
25. GUYENET, P.G. & D.L. BROWN. 1986. Nucleus paragigantocellularis lateralis and lumbar sympathetic discharge in the rat. Am. J. Physiol. Integr. Comp. Physiol. **250:** R1081–R1094.
26. GIEROBA, Z.J., Y.H. YU & W.W. BLESSING. 1994. Vasoconstriction induced by inhalation of irritant vapour is associated with appearance of Fos protein in C1 catecholamine neurons in rabbit medulla oblongata. Brain Res. **636:** 157–161.
27. LI, Y.W. & R.A.L. DAMPNEY. 1994. Expression of Fos-like protein in the brain following sustained hypertension and hypotension in conscious rabbits. Neuroscience **61:** 613–634.
28. ERICKSON, J.T. & D.E. MILLHORN. 1994. Hypoxia and electrical stimulation of the carotid sinus nerve induce c-Fos-like immunoreactivity within catecholaminergic and serotonergic neurons of the rat brainstem. J. Comp. Neurol. **348:** 161–182.
29. STORNETTA, R.L., F.E. NORTON & P.G. GUYENET. 1993. Autonomic areas of rat brain exhibit increased Fos-like immunoreactivity during opiate withdrawal in rats. Brain Res. **624:** 19–28.
30. PILOWSKY, P., I.J. LLEWELLYN-SMITH, J. LIPSKI *et al.* 1994. Projections from inspiratory neurons of the ventral respiratory group to the subretrofacial nucleus of the cat. Brain Res. **633:** 63–71.
31. ZIGMOND, M.J. & E.M. STRICKER. 1984. Parkinson's disease: studies with an animal model. Life Sci. **35:** 5–18.
32. CHIUEH, C.C., R.S. BURNS, S.P. MARKEY *et al.* 1985. Primate model of parkinsonism: selective lesion of nigrostriatal neurons by 1-methyl-4-phenyl-1,2,3,6-tetrahydropyridine produces an extrapyramidal syndrome in rhesus monkeys. Life Sci. **36:** 213–218.
33. PINAULT, D. 1996. A novel single-cell staining procedure performed *in vivo* under electrophysiological control: morpho-functional features of juxtacellularly labeled thalamic cells and other central neurons with biocytin or neurobiotin. J. Neurosci. Methods **65:** 113–136.

# The Role of the Medullary Lateral Tegmental Field in the Generation and Baroreceptor Reflex Control of Sympathetic Nerve Discharge in the Cat

SUSAN M. BARMAN, HAKAN S. ORER, AND GERARD L. GEBBER

*Department of Pharmacology and Toxicology, Michigan State University, East Lansing, Michigan 48824, USA*

ABSTRACT: Data from experiments with single neuron recordings as well as central microinjections of *N*-methyl-D-aspartate (NMDA) and non-NMDA excitatory amino receptor antagonists that have led to a model of central sympathetic pathways that includes synaptic relays in the medullary lateral tegmental field (LTF) of the cat are summarized. Evidence is presented that (1) the LTF contains a population of tonically active sympathoexcitatory neurons that drive rostral ventrolateral medullary neurons, (2) blockade of non-NMDA receptors in the LTF significantly reduces basal levels of sympathetic nerve discharge (SND) and mean arterial pressure in baroreceptor-denervated cats, and (3) blockade of NMDA-mediated neurotransmission in the LTF prevents baroreceptor reflex control of SND. Thus, LTF neurons play an important role in the generation and baroreceptor reflex control of SND in the cat.

KEYWORDS: Cardiac-related rhythm; NMDA receptor antagonist; Non-NMDA receptor antagonist; Rostral ventrolateral medulla

## INTRODUCTION

Perhaps the most widely studied reflex pathway controlling sympathetic nerve discharge (SND) is that arising from arterial baroreceptors in the carotid sinus and aortic arch. Based largely on work in rats and rabbits, the most popular model[1,2] of the baroreceptor reflex is one in which afferent fibers terminate in the nucleus of the tractus solitarius (NTS), and neurons in this region project to and excite caudal ventrolateral medullary (CVLM) neurons. These CVLM neurons then project to and inhibit rostral ventrolateral medullary (RVLM) neurons with spinal axons that innervate the intermediolateral (IML) sympathetic nucleus in the thoracolumbar spinal cord. There is anatomical and electrophysiological evidence to support the existence of each element of this pathway.[2–5] Although it is generally agreed that RVLM-spinal neurons are a major source of excitatory drive to preganglionic sympathetic neurons in the IML,[6–8] there are conflicting views regarding the mechanisms respon-

Address for communication: Susan M. Barman, Department of Pharmacology and Toxicology, Michigan State University, East Lansing, MI 48824. Voice: 517-432-3154; fax: 517-353-8915.
barman@msu.edu

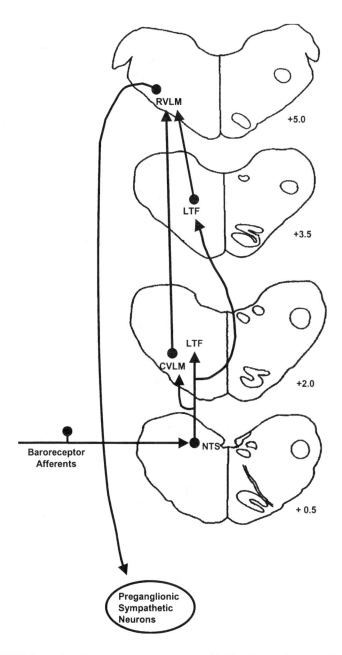

**FIGURE 1.** Model of central pathways responsible for the cardiac-related rhythm in sympathetic nerve discharge of the cat. +0.5–5.0 refers to distance in millimeters from the obex according to the stereotaxic atlas of Berman.[37] CVLM, caudal ventrolateral medulla; LTF, lateral tegmental field; NTS, nucleus of the tractus solitarius; RVLM, rostral ventro-lateral medulla.

sible for their basal discharges (see Ref. 9). Guyenet[7] has proposed that RVLM-spinal sympathoexcitatory (SE) neurons of the rat are inherently capable of generating their own activity and, thus, basal SND. In this model, baroreceptor inputs to RVLM neurons modulate their pacemaker activity. On the other hand, Lipski et al.[10] reported that the spontaneous activity of RVLM-spinal neurons in vivo can be attributed primarily, if not solely, to their synaptic inputs. In this case, baroreceptor reflex–mediated influences on RVLM neurons might arise, at least in part, from modulation of excitatory drive to the RVLM from other brain stem regions. Data summarized in this report support this view for the generation and baroreceptor reflex control of SND in the cat. In addition to the well-studied NTS→CVLM→RVLM pathway, the model of central pathways controlling SND shown in FIGURE 1 contains a synaptic relay in the medullary lateral tegmental field (LTF), which includes portions of nucleus reticularis parvocellularis and nucleus reticularis ventralis. Evidence will be presented showing that the LTF contains a population of tonically active SE neurons that drive RVLM-spinal neurons. Moreover, baroreceptor inputs to LTF neurons lead to their cardiac-related discharges as well as the cardiac-related rhythm in SND.

## INDICES OF BARORECEPTOR REFLEX CONTROL OF SND

One of the most commonly observed patterns of activity in sympathetic nerves is a cardiac-related rhythm (see Refs. 9 and 11). This rhythm has been identified in sympathetic nerves (preganglionic or postganglionic) of many species, including humans, and in the presence or absence of anesthesia. FIGURE 2A (top) shows oscillographic records of brachial arterial pressure (AP) and the naturally occurring discharges of the inferior cardiac postganglionic sympathetic nerve of a urethane-anesthetized, paralyzed, and artificially ventilated cat. By using a wide preamplifier bandpass (1–1000 Hz), the synchronized discharges of fibers comprising the nerve are viewed as slow waves (i.e., envelopes of spikes). Note that bursts of activity are locked in a 1:1 relationship to the cardiac cycle (i.e., a cardiac-related rhythm). As shown by the oscillographic records in FIGURE 2B (top), after baroreceptor denervation (bilateral section of the carotid sinus, aortic depressor, and vagus nerves), SND remains oscillatory, but bursts are no longer locked in a 1:1 relationship to the AP, and the intervals between consecutive slow waves become considerably more variable. The fact that oscillations persisted in SND after baroreceptor denervation was one of the first indications that the cardiac-related rhythm reflects baroreceptor-induced entrainment of a centrally generated irregular low-frequency ($\leq$6 Hz) oscillation in a 1:1 relationship to the AP.[12] It had previously been assumed that the cardiac-related pattern in SND was the simple consequence of the waxing and waning of central inhibition induced by pulse-synchronous baroreceptor afferent nerve activity.[13]

Although the cardiac-related rhythm is readily evident in the original recordings, autospectral analysis can be used to decompose SND into its frequency components. This becomes very useful in determining whether a particular intervention (e.g., baroreceptor denervation or microinjection of drugs into the brain stem) induces selective effects on SND. For the studies described in this report, autospectra of SND and AP were constructed by using a modified version[14] of the software of Cohen

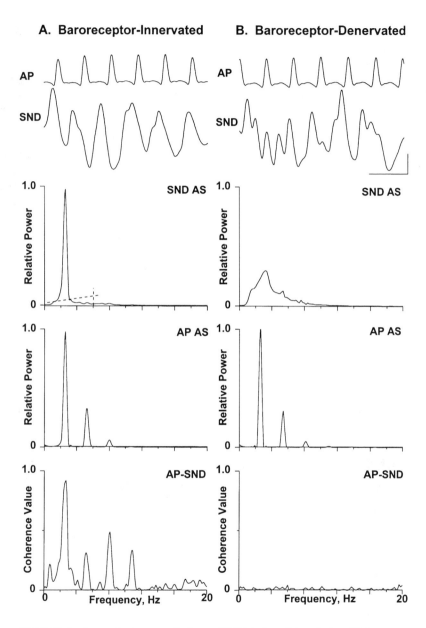

**FIGURE 2.** Sympathetic nerve discharge (SND) before **(A)** and after **(B)** baroreceptor denervation in a urethane-anesthetized cat. *Top*: Oscillographic records of brachial arterial pressure (AP) and inferior cardiac SND. Vertical calibration for SND is 30 μV; horizontal calibration is 0.5 s. *Bottom*: Traces are autospectra (AS) of SND and the AP and the corresponding coherence function. Spectra are based on 32 5-s windows; frequency resolution is 0.2 Hz per bin here and in subsequent figures. The autospectra of SND in (A) and (B) are displayed on the same power scale.

*et al.*[15] and Kocsis *et al.*[16] Fast Fourier Transform was performed on a minimum of
32 5-s windows of data blocks (5-ms sampling interval) with a frequency resolution
of 0.2 Hz/bin.

In the example shown in FIGURE 2A, when the baroreceptors were intact, most of
the power in the autospectrum of the discharges of the inferior cardiac nerve (SND
AS) was in a narrow band with a peak at the frequency of the heart beat (AP AS).
The power in the cardiac-related band of SND is one index of the baroreceptor
reflex. A macro written in Microsoft Excel version 7.0 was used to measure cardiac-
related power. Briefly, a line was fitted to connect the left and right limits of the
cardiac-related band of SND; cardiac-related power was calculated as the area above
the line. The 0- to 6-Hz total power was calculated by arithmetically summing the
values for the bins in this frequency range. The 0- to 6-Hz background power was
defined as 0- to 6-Hz total power minus cardiac-related power. Note that, after
baroreceptor denervation, most of the power in SND was distributed over a relatively
wide band, primarily at frequencies $\leq 6$ Hz (FIG. 2B).

In addition to the amount of cardiac-related power in SND, a second index of the
baroreceptor reflex is the strength of correlation of SND to the AP, which can be
quantified by using coherence analysis. The coherence value (scale: 0 to 1.0) is a
measure of the strength of linear correlation of two signals as a function of frequency.
As shown in FIGURE 2A, when the baroreceptors were intact, the AP-SND coherence
value at the frequency of the heartbeat was close to 1.0. In contrast, after baroreceptor denervation (FIG. 2B), the coherence value was reduced to a value not sig-

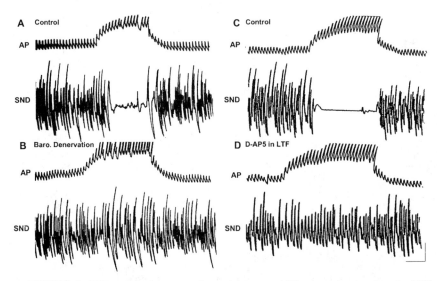

**FIGURE 3.** Effect of baroreceptor denervation or D-AP5 microinjection into the LTF
on the inhibition of SND during the pressor response produced by abrupt obstruction of the
abdominal aorta. Traces show brachial AP and inferior cardiac SND before (**A, C**) and after
(**B, D**) baroreceptor denervation or microinjection of D-AP5, respectively. Vertical calibration is 75 µV; horizontal calibration is 2 s.

nificantly different from 0.[17] Thus, the residual power in SND at the frequency of the heartbeat was not correlated (i.e., phase-locked) to the arterial pulse.

A third index of the baroreceptor reflex is the inhibition of SND accompanying an abrupt increase in mean arterial pressure (MAP) produced by inflating the balloon-tipped end of a Fogarty embolectomy catheter inserted into the abdominal aorta (aortic obstruction). In the example shown in FIGURE 3, SND was virtually completely suppressed before (A), but not changed after (B) baroreceptor denervation.

## LTF NEURONS WITH ACTIVITY CORRELATED TO SND

As demonstrated by using the techniques of single neuron spike–triggered averaging, arterial pulse–triggered analysis, and coherence analysis, the LTF contains neurons whose naturally occurring discharges are correlated to the cardiac-related rhythm in SND.[18–23] An example is shown in FIGURE 4. The arterial pulse–triggered average of SND and a histogram of LTF neuronal activity (FIG. 4B) showed that both

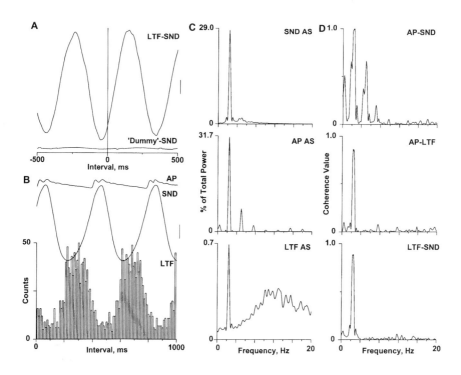

**FIGURE 4.** Identification of a medullary LTF neuron with activity correlated to the cardiac-related rhythm in SND. **(A)** Spike-triggered (*top*) and dummy-triggered (*bottom*) averages of SND (916 trials); bin width is 5 ms. **(B)** AP-triggered analysis (448 trials); bin width is 5 ms for averages of AP and SND, and 10 ms for histogram of LTF neuronal activity. **(C)** Autospectra of SND, AP, and LTF neuronal activity. **(D)** Coherence functions relating pairs of these signals. Vertical calibration is 20 μV in (A) and 40 μV in (B).

signals contained a cardiac-related component. The spike-triggered average (FIG. 4A) showed that this LTF neuron was most apt to fire 155 ms before the peak of the cardiac-related slow wave in inferior cardiac SND. The deflections in this average were of much greater amplitude than those in the corresponding "dummy" average of SND that was constructed by using a random pulse train having the same mean frequency as the LTF neuronal spike train. Frequency-domain analysis confirmed the results of time-domain analysis. Both the autospectra of SND and LTF neuronal activity (FIG. 4C) had a sharp peak at the frequency of the heartbeat; the peak in the LTF-SND coherence function (FIG. 4D) at the same frequency indicated that the cardiac-related discharges of these two signals were strongly correlated (coherence value of 0.89). As expected, LTF neuronal activity also was strongly correlated to the AP.

Two observations suggest that LTF neurons are contained in the efferent network responsible for the cardiac-related rhythm in SND. First, their activity remains locked in time to the peak of the cardiac-related slow wave in SND during changes in heart rate that shift the phase relations between the arterial pulse (a reflection of baroreceptor afferent nerve activity) and SND.[18] Second, their discharges are correlated to the irregular low-frequency oscillations in SND that replace the cardiac-related rhythm during baroreceptor unloading.[21]

LTF neurons with activity correlated to the cardiac-related rhythm in SND can be classified into two groups on the basis of their responses to baroreceptor reflex activation produced by aortic obstruction. The firing rates of neurons in the first group decrease in parallel to SND during baroreceptor reflex activation; thus, they are classified as putative SE neurons.[18,21–23] LTF-SE neurons fire significantly earlier than RVLM neurons during the inferior cardiac sympathetic nerve slow wave (as determined with spike-triggered averaging),[18,19,21] and antidromic mapping showed that their axons project to and appear to terminate in the RVLM.[19] Taken together, these data led to the proposal that these LTF neurons are a source of excitatory drive to RVLM-spinal neurons.[19,21] The second group of LTF neurons with cardiac-related activity are referred to as putative sympathoinhibitory (SI) neurons because their firing rates increase during the inhibition of SND produced by baroreceptor reflex activation.[20–23] The axons of these LTF neurons appear to terminate in the vicinity of raphespinal SI neurons.[20] However, LTF-SE and LTF-SI neurons cannot be distinguished on the basis of anatomical location, basal firing rates, or firing times relative to the peak of the inferior cardiac sympathetic nerve slow wave.[21]

## ROLE OF THE LTF IN BARORECEPTOR REFLEX CONTROL OF SND

The identification of LTF neurons with cardiac-related activity, by itself, does not indicate that these neurons play a role in baroreceptor reflex control of SND. We therefore designed a series of experiments to test the hypothesis that the LTF is an important synaptic relay in the baroreceptor reflex pathway.[24] These experiments made use of the fact that N-methyl-D-aspartate (NMDA) and non-NMDA receptors have been localized on neurons within caudal brain stem regions of the cat involved in control of cardiovascular function, including the LTF.[25] We determined the effects of blockade of excitatory amino acid (EAA) receptors in the LTF on the three indices of baroreceptor reflex function: amount of cardiac-related power in SND, strength of linear correlation (coherence value) of SND to the AP at the frequency of the heartbeat, and inhibition of SND during increased MAP produced by abrupt obstruction of the abdominal aorta.

The competitive NMDA receptor antagonist, D(−)-2-amino-5-phosphono-pentanoic acid (D-AP5), or the competitive non-NMDA receptor antagonist, 1,2,3,4-tetrahydro-6-nitro-2,3-dioxobenzo-[*f*]quinoxaline-7-sulfonamide (NBQX), was microinjected bilaterally into the LTF. Microinjections (300 pmol D-AP5 or 100 pmol NBQX in 100 nL saline) were made bilaterally in tracks located 2 and 3 mm rostral to the obex, 2.8–3 mm lateral to the midline, at depths of 3 and 4.5 mm from the dorsal surface. Multiple injections were made because neurons with activity correlated to SND are distributed over several millimeters within the LTF, extending from near the level of the obex to ~4 mm rostral to the obex, ~2–3 mm lateral to the midline, and ~2.5–4.7 mm below the dorsal medullary surface (see fig. 3 of Ref. 21). Because cardiac-related power in SND is dependent on the level of MAP, extreme care was taken to keep MAP the same before and after drug injection in these experiments.

The experimental protocol was as follows. An 80-s control data sample was collected after the micropipette was positioned at the first site to be injected. A complete set of injections was then made on the left and right sides of the medulla. Test 80-s data blocks were collected within 1–2 min after the injections, 10–15 min later, and then at 15- to 30-min intervals for up to 2 h to allow for recovery. Changes in SND were noted during or soon after completing the injection; however, the data

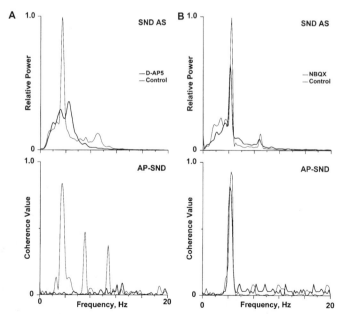

**FIGURE 5.** Effects of bilateral microinjection of D-AP5 **(A)** or NBQX **(B)** into the LTF of baroreceptor-innervated cats. Traces are overlapped AS of SND (*top*) and coherence functions relating SND to the AP (*bottom*) before (*thin line*) and 10–15 min after (*thick line*) microinjection.

block collected 10–15 min after the microinjection was used to quantify the effects of D-AP5 or NBQX on SND and the baroreceptor reflex. By this time, the maximum changes in SND had occurred and SND had reached a steady-state level. The time courses of action of NBQX and D-AP5 were similar to those reported by others when cardiovascular or respiratory changes were monitored after the microinjection of these drugs into the brain.[26–28]

The data in FIGURE 5A show the results from an experiment in which D-AP5 was microinjected bilaterally into the LTF. The autospectra of SND before and after microinjection of D-AP5 are displayed on the same power scale. The control auto-spectrum of SND (FIG. 5A, top, thin line) shows a prominent sharp peak at the frequency of the heartbeat, and the coherence value relating SND to the AP at this frequency was 0.84 (FIG. 5A, bottom, thin line). Within 15 min after bilateral micro-injection of D-AP5 into the LTF (FIG. 5A, thick lines), the cardiac-related rhythm in SND was eliminated as evidenced by an AP-SND coherence value near 0 at the frequency of the heartbeat. These changes were accompanied by an increase (141% of control) in 0- to 6-Hz background power in SND. Although not shown, SND recovered within 2 h.

FIGURE 6A summarizes the effects produced by bilateral microinjection of D-AP5 into the LTF of 7 cats. D-AP5 essentially abolished the cardiac-related rhythm in SND as indicated by the marked decrease in cardiac-related power and the low coherence value relating SND to the AP at the frequency of the heartbeat. These changes occurred despite the fact that MAP was held constant in these experiments in order to avoid changes in cardiac-related power in SND that might have occurred as the result of a change in the level of baroreceptor afferent nerve activity. The decrease in cardiac-related power in SND was accompanied by a significant increase in 0- to 6-Hz background power; however, 0- to 6-Hz total power was not significantly changed.

Bilateral microinjection of D-AP5 into the LTF also prevented the inhibition of SND during aortic obstruction. In the example shown in FIGURE 3, SND was inhibited before (C), but not after (D) the microinjection of D-AP5. Thus, the composite effects of the blockade of NMDA receptors in the LTF mimicked those accompanying baroreceptor denervation. Within 2 h after completing the injections of D-AP5, all of the indices of baroreceptor reflex control of SND returned to near control levels.

The data in FIGURE 5B show the results from an experiment in which NBQX was microinjected bilaterally into the LTF. In this case, the cardiac-related power in SND was decreased to 60% of control, and the AP-SND coherence value at the frequency of the heartbeat was slightly reduced from 0.93 to 0.78 at 10 min after bilateral micro-injection of NBQX. These changes were associated with a reduction in both 0- to 6-Hz background (82% of control) and 0- to 6-Hz total power (76% of control) in SND. Although not shown, power in SND returned to control values within 50 min after the injection of NBQX into the LTF.

FIGURE 6B summarizes the effects produced by bilateral microinjection of NBQX into the LTF of 11 cats. NBQX significantly and reversibly decreased cardiac-related power in SND. However, the magnitude of the change was significantly less than that produced by microinjection of D-AP5 into the LTF. In contrast to the effects of D-AP5, microinjection of NBQX significantly decreased 0- to 6-Hz total power and did not significantly change 0- to 6-Hz background power in SND. Moreover, although blockade of non-NMDA receptors in the LTF significantly decreased the AP-SND

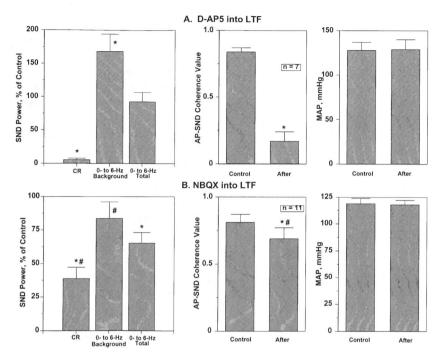

**FIGURE 6.** Summary of effects of bilateral microinjection of D-AP5 (**A**) and NBQX (**B**) into the LTF of baroreceptor-innervated cats. *Left*: Changes in cardiac-related (CR) power, 0- to 6-Hz background power, and 0- to 6-Hz total power in SND. *Middle*: Changes in the AP-SND coherence value at the frequency of the heartbeat. *Right*: Mean arterial pressure (MAP) was maintained constant in these experiments. *n*, Number of experiments; *, statistically different than control ($p \leq 0.05$; paired *t* test); #, statistically different than corresponding value for the effects of D-AP5 microinjected into the LTF ($p \leq 0.05$; unpaired *t* test).

coherence value at the frequency of the heartbeat, this value remained rather high, and microinjection of NBQX into the LTF failed to prevent the inhibition of SND during aortic obstruction (not shown). Thus, the effects of blockade of non-NMDA receptors in the LTF did not mimic the effects of baroreceptor denervation.

As discussed in the original publication,[24] the effects on SND produced by microinjection of EAA receptor antagonists into the LTF cannot be explained by spread of the injectate to the NTS or CVLM, regions identified as obligatory relays in the baroreceptor reflex pathway.[1-5,29-31] First, the reductions in SND cardiac-related power and AP-SND coherence value at the frequency of the heartbeat after microinjection of D-AP5 into the LTF were significantly greater than those produced by microinjection of D-AP5 into either the NTS or CVLM. Second, the inhibition of SND during abrupt aortic obstruction was blocked by microinjection of D-AP5 into the LTF, but not into the NTS or CVLM. Third, NBQX microinjection into the LTF decreased cardiac-related power in SND, whereas cardiac-related power was increased when NBQX was injected into the CVLM. Further evidence that the EAA receptor antagonists acted within the LTF to produce the observed changes in SND is that microinjection of D-AP5 or NBQX at sites in a track located 1.2–1.8 mm medial to the LTF (in the paramedian reticular formation) did not affect SND.[24,32]

There are at least two ways to explain how blockade of EAA receptors in the LTF could reversibly reduce or abolish cardiac-related power in SND. First, if EAA neurotransmission in this region is involved in the entrainment of irregular low-frequency oscillations in SND to pulse-synchronous baroreceptor afferent nerve activity, microinjection of the appropriate EAA receptor antagonist should convert the cardiac-related rhythm to irregular 0- to 6-Hz oscillations and thus disrupt the 1:1 locking of bursts of SND to the AP. This is indeed what occurred when D-AP5 was microinjected bilaterally into the LTF; that is, cardiac-related power in SND was significantly reduced and 0- to 6-Hz background power was significantly increased. D-AP5 also prevented the reflex-induced inhibition of SND that occurs during the pressor response produced by abrupt aortic obstruction. This observation also supports the view that NMDA receptor-mediated synaptic transmission in the LTF plays a pivotal role in the baroreceptor reflex pathway controlling SND. The effects of D-AP5 microinjection into the LTF are consistent with the possibility that baro-receptor-induced activation of LTF-SI neurons[20–23] is mediated by EAAs acting through NMDA receptors.

A second way in which cardiac-related power in SND could be decreased by blockade of EAA receptors in the LTF is by reducing the activity of LTF-SE neurons. Because these neurons are thought to be a source of excitatory drive to RVLM-spinal neurons,[19,21] reducing their activity would decrease SND. However, residual SND would still be cardiac-related provided that the mechanism for entrainment of SND to the AP was not affected. This scenario is consistent with the effects produced by microinjection of the non-NMDA receptor antagonist, NBQX, into the LTF. Thus, in contrast to the effects of D-AP5, NBQX appears to have lowered the level of excitatory output from the LTF without upsetting the baroreceptor reflex. This possibility prompted a second series of experiments in which the effects of EAA receptor blockade in the LTF were studied in baroreceptor-denervated cats.[32]

## ROLE OF THE LTF IN THE GENERATION OF BASAL SND

If activation of non-NMDA receptors in the LTF is involved in setting the level of excitatory drive to sympathetic nerves, as suggested by the data described above, bilateral microinjection NBQX into the LTF of baroreceptor-denervated cats should decrease SND and MAP. Moreover, if NMDA receptors in the LTF are predominantly involved in mediating baroreceptor influences on SND, bilateral microinjection of D-AP5 into the LTF should have little, if any, effect on SND or MAP in baroreceptor-denervated cats. To test these predictions, we quantified the effects of blockade of non-NMDA or NMDA receptors in the LTF on 0- to 6-Hz and total (0- to 20-Hz) power in SND as well as MAP of baroreceptor-denervated cats.[32]

FIGURE 7A shows the effects produced by microinjection of NBQX bilaterally into the LTF of a baroreceptor-denervated cat. The control autospectrum of SND (FIG. 7A, thin line) showed a dispersed band of power, primarily at frequencies ≤ 6 Hz. Although not shown, coherence analysis indicated that the baroreceptor denervation was complete (AP-SND coherence value at the frequency of the heartbeat was not

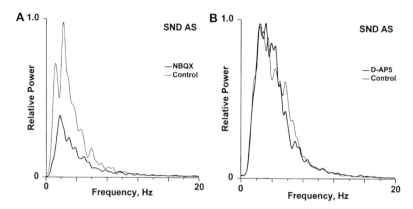

**FIGURE 7.** Effects of bilateral microinjection of NBQX (**A**) or D-AP5 (**B**) into the LTF of baroreceptor-denervated cats. Traces are overlapped AS of SND before (*thin line*) and 10 min after (*thick line*) microinjection.

significantly different from 0). The 0- to 6-Hz power and total power in SND were decreased to 41% and 45% of control, respectively, at 10 min after blockade of non-NMDA receptors in LTF (FIG. 7A, thick line). The reduction in SND was accompanied by a fall in MAP from 110 to 63 mmHg. As summarized in FIGURE 8A, 0- to 6-Hz power and total power in SND as well as MAP were significantly decreased at 10–15 min after bilateral microinjection of NBQX into the LTF of 7 baroreceptor-denervated cats. SND and MAP returned to control levels within 1 h after completing the microinjections of NBQX into the LTF.

D-AP5 was microinjected bilaterally into the LTF of 8 baroreceptor-denervated cats. As shown by the example in FIGURE 7B and summarized in FIGURE 8B, neither SND nor MAP was significantly changed by blockade of NMDA receptors in the LTF of baroreceptor-denervated cats.

These experiments are the first to show that non-NMDA (but not NMDA) receptor-mediated activation of medullary LTF neurons plays a key role in setting the resting level of SND and MAP in baroreceptor-denervated cats. The source of this EAA-mediated excitatory drive to LTF neurons remains to be determined.

As described in the original publication,[32] microinjection of either NBQX or D-AP5 into the RVLM significantly decreased SND and MAP; in fact, the changes produced by microinjection of NBQX into the RVLM and LTF were similar. Thus, the possibility should be considered that the decreases in SND and MAP after micro-injection of NBQX into the LTF resulted from spread of the injectate to the RVLM. Several arguments are presented in the original report to counter this possibility, leading to the conclusion that NBQX acted within the LTF to reduce SND and MAP.

The decreases in SND and MAP produced by microinjection of NBQX into the LTF may be due, at least in part, to removal of synaptic drive (i.e., disfacilitation) from this region to RVLM-spinal SE neurons. As described above, data are available to support the view that LTF-SE neurons are a source of excitatory drive to RVLM neurons.[18,21] When considered in conjunction with these earlier studies, the marked decrease in SND produced by microinjection of NBQX into the LTF supports the

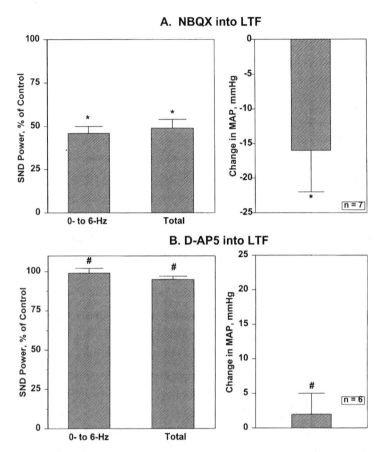

**FIGURE 8.** Summary of effects of bilateral microinjection of NBQX (**A**) and D-AP5 (**B**) into the LTF of baroreceptor-denervated cats. *Left*: Changes in 0- to 6-Hz power, and total power (0- to 20-Hz) in SND. *Right*: Changes in MAP. *n*, Number of experiments; *, statistically different than control ($p \leq 0.05$; paired *t* test); #, statistically different than corresponding value for the effects of D-AP5 microinjected into the LTF ($p \leq 0.05$; unpaired *t* test).

view that excitatory drive from the LTF is an important source of the discharges of RVLM-spinal SE neurons.

The decreases in SND and MAP produced by NBQX microinjection into the LTF and RVLM were comparable, but this does not necessarily mean that these two regions are of equal importance in setting the basal level of SND. First, because we did not determine dose-response relationships for EAA receptor antagonists, we do not know if the dose of NBQX used produced different degrees of blockade of non-NMDA receptors in the LTF and RVLM. Second, because microinjection of either NBQX or D-AP5 into the RVLM significantly reduced SND, combined blockade of non-NMDA and NMDA receptors in the RVLM may have lowered SND to a greater extent than blockade of EAA neurotransmission in the LTF. Third, we do not know the extent to which neurotransmitters other than EAAs or intrinsic pacemaker properties determine the level of activity of LTF and RVLM neurons and, therefore, the level of SND. Indeed, blockade of EAA receptors in either the LTF or the RVLM did not reduce inferior cardiac SND to the level (<10% of control) seen after complete cervical spinal cord transection.[33,34] This implies that other brain stem regions or mechanisms other than EAA-mediated activation of LTF and RVLM neurons contribute to basal SND. Fourth, we might have actually underestimated the effects on SND and MAP produced by blockade of non-NMDA receptors on LTF-SE neurons. It is possible that the decrease in SND due to inactivation of these neurons with NBQX was partially masked by a simultaneous blockade of EAA receptors on LTF-SI neurons that would have increased SND.[20,21] Thus, the data available do not allow us to compare the relative degrees to which the LTF and RVLM determine the resting level of SND and MAP.

## CLOSING REMARKS

As reviewed in reference 35, in the 1930s the dorsolateral medullary reticular formation (including the portion of the LTF studied here) was viewed as a critical brain region involved in cardiovascular control. SND and MAP were increased by electrical simulation and decreased after electrolytic lesion of the LTF. With the advent of modern neuroanatomical tract-tracing techniques, the focus of attention switched to the RVLM, a region that provides direct input to the IML.[36] By the early 1980s, many laboratories reported that chemical stimulation of the RVLM produced marked increases in SND and MAP, and chemical inactivation of the RVLM reduced MAP to levels seen in spinal animals.[6–8] Because the axons of RVLM-SE neurons traverse the LTF en route to the spinal cord, changes in MAP and SND induced by electrical stimulation or ablation of the LTF have been attributed to activation or destruction of the projections of RVLM neurons.[8] The data summarized in this report challenge this view and support the model of central neural control of SND shown in FIGURE 1. Most importantly, the effects produced by microinjection of EAA receptor antagonists into the LTF demonstrate that neurons in this region contribute to the generation and baroreceptor reflex control of SND of the cat.

Is the LTF in the cat an anatomically displaced, but functional equivalent of the CVLM in the rat? This is not likely to be the case. Whereas the LTF in the cat and CVLM in the rat have obligatory roles in mediating baroreceptor reflex–induced changes in SND, the mechanisms by which this happens is quite different. In the rat, CVLM neurons that receive baroreceptor input project to and inhibit (via GABA release) RVLM-spinal SE neurons.[1,3,5] In contrast, baroreceptor-induced inhibition of LTF-SE neurons is presumed to disfacilitate RVLM-spinal SE neurons of the cat.

Hopefully, the studies summarized here will stimulate new interest in the role of the LTF in the control of SND and MAP. Whereas important novel information concerning central sympathetic control mechanisms has been provided by these studies, the results also lead to new questions such as "What is the source of EAA-mediated excitatory drive to LTF neurons?" and "Are LTF neurons a source of the EAA receptor-mediated synaptic drive to RVLM-spinal SE neurons?"

## ACKNOWLEDGMENTS

These studies were supported by Grant No. HL-33266 from the National Heart, Lung, and Blood Institutes.

## REFERENCES

1. BLESSING, W.W. 1997. The Lower Brainstem and Bodily Homeostasis. Oxford University Press. London/New York.
2. SVED, A.F. & F.J. GORDON. 1994. Amino acids as central neurotransmitters in the baroreceptor reflex pathway. News Physiol. Sci. **9:** 243–246.
3. AGARWAL, S.K., A.J. GELSEMA & F.R. CALARESU. 1990. Inhibition of rostral VLM by baroreceptor activation is relayed through caudal VLM. Am. J. Physiol. Regul. Integr. Comp. Physiol. **258:** R1271–R1278.
4. AICHER, S.A., O.S. KURUCZ, D.J. REIS & T.A. MILNER. 1995. Nucleus of the tractus solitarius efferent terminals synapse on neurons in the caudal ventrolateral medulla that project to the rostral ventrolateral medulla. Brain Res. **693:** 51–63.
5. JESKE, I., S.F. MORRISON, S.L. CRAVO & D.J. REIS. 1993. Identification of baroreceptor reflex interneurons in the caudal ventrolateral medulla. Am. J. Physiol. Regul. Integr. Comp. Physiol. **264:** R169–R178.
6. DAMPNEY, R.A.L. 1994. Functional organization of central pathways regulating the cardiovascular system. Physiol. Rev. **74:** 323–364.
7. GUYENET, P.G. 1990. Role of the ventral medulla oblongata in blood pressure regulation. *In* Central Regulation of Autonomic Functions: 145–167. Oxford University Press. London/New York.
8. ROSS, C.A., D.A. RUGGIERO, D.H. PARK *et al.* 1984. Tonic vasomotor control by the rostral ventrolateral medulla: effects of electrical and chemical stimulation of the area containing C1 adrenaline neurons on arterial pressure, heart rate, and plasma catecholamines and vasopressin. J. Neurosci. **4:** 474–494.
9. BARMAN, S.M. & G.L. GEBBER. 2000. "Rapid" rhythmic discharges of sympathetic nerves: sources, mechanisms of generation, and physiological relevance. J. Biol. Rhythms. In press.
10. LIPSKI, J., R. KANJHAN, B. KRUSZEWSKA & W. RONG. 1996. Properties of presympathetic neurons in the rostral ventrolateral medulla in the rat: an intracellular study *in vivo*. J. Physiol. (Lond.) **490:** 729–744.
11. MALPAS, S.C. 1997. The rhythmicity of sympathetic nerve activity. Prog. Neurobiol. **56:** 65–96.
12. TAYLOR, D.G. & G.L. GEBBER. 1975. Baroreceptor mechanisms controlling sympathetic nervous rhythms of central origin. Am. J. Physiol. **228:** 1002–1013.
13. ADRIAN, E.D., G.W. BRONK & G. PHILLIPS. 1932. Discharges in mammalian sympathetic nerves. J. Physiol. (Lond.) **74:** 133–155.
14. GEBBER, G.L., S. ZHONG, S.M. BARMAN *et al.* 1994. Differential relationships among the 10-Hz rhythmic discharges of sympathetic nerves with different targets. Am. J. Physiol. Regul. Integr. Comp. Physiol. **267:** R387–R399.
15. COHEN, M.I., W.R. SEE, C.N. CHRISTAKOS & A.L. SICA. 1987. High-frequency and medium-frequency components of different inspiratory nerve discharges and their modification by various inputs. Brain Res. **417:** 148–152.
16. KOCSIS, B., G.L. GEBBER, S.M. BARMAN & M.J. KENNEY. 1990. Relationships between activity of sympathetic nerve pairs: phase and coherence. Am. J. Physiol. Regul. Integr. Comp. Physiol. **259:** R549–R560.
17. BENIGNUS, V.A. 1970. Correction to "estimation of the coherence spectrum and its confidence interval using the Fast Fourier Transform". IEEE Trans. Audio Electroacoust. **AU-18:** 320.
18. BARMAN, S.M. & G.L. GEBBER. 1983. Sequence of activation of ventrolateral and dorsal medullary sympathetic neurons. Am. J. Physiol. Regul. Integr. Comp. Physiol. **245:** R438–R447.

19. BARMAN, S.M. & G.L. GEBBER. 1987. Lateral tegmental field neurons of cat medulla: a source of basal activity of ventrolateral medullospinal sympathoexcitatory neurons. J. Neurophysiol. **57:** 1410–1424.

20. BARMAN, S.M. & G.L. GEBBER. 1989. Lateral tegmental field neurons of cat medulla: a source of basal activity of raphespinal sympathoinhibitory neurons. J. Neurophysiol. **61:** 1011–1024.

21. GEBBER, G.L. & S.M. BARMAN. 1985. Lateral tegmental field neurons of cat medulla: a potential source of basal sympathetic nerve discharge. J. Neurophysiol. **54:** 1498–1512.

22. VAYSSETTES-COURCHAY, C., F. BOUYSSET, M. LAUBIE & T.J. VERBEUREN. 1997. Central integration of the Bezold-Jarisch reflex in the cat. Brain Res. **744:** 272–278.

23. VAYSSETTES-COURCHAY, C., F. BOUYSSET, T.J. VERBEUREN & M. LAUBIE. 1993. Role of the lateral tegmental field in central sympathoinhibitory effects of 8-hydroxy-2-(di-*n*-propylamino)tetralin in the cat. Eur. J. Pharmacol. **236:** 121–130.

24. ORER, H.S., S.M. BARMAN, G.L. GEBBER & S.M. SYKES. 1999. Medullary lateral tegmental field: an important synaptic relay in the baroreceptor reflex pathway of the cat. Am. J. Physiol. Regul. Integr. Comp. Physiol. **277:** R1462–R1475.

25. AMBALAVANAR, R., C.L. LUDLOW, R.J. WENTHOLD *et al.* 1998. Glutamate receptor subunits in the nucleus of the tractus solitarius and other regions of the medulla in the cat. J. Comp. Neurol. **402:** 75–92.

26. JUNG, R., E.N. BRUCE & P.G. KATONA. 1991. Cardiorespiratory responses to glutamatergic antagonists in the caudal ventrolateral medulla of rats. Brain Res. **564:** 286–295.

27. SOLTIS, R.P., J.C. COOK, A.E. GREGG & B.J. SANDERS. 1997. Interaction of GABA and excitatory amino acids in the basolateral amygdala: role in cardiovascular regulation. J. Neurosci. **17:** 367–374.

28. SOMOGYI, P., J.B. MINSON, D. MORILAK *et al.* 1988. Evidence for an excitatory amino acid pathway in the brainstem and for its involvement in cardiovascular control. Brain Res. **496:** 401–407.

29. CRAVO, S.L., S.F. MORRISON & D.J. REIS. 1991. Differentiation of two cardiovascular regions within caudal ventrolateral medulla. Am. J. Physiol. Regul. Integr. Comp. Physiol. **261:** R985–R994.

30. GORDON, F.J. 1987. Aortic baroreceptor reflexes are mediated by NMDA receptors in caudal ventrolateral medulla. Am. J. Physiol. Regul. Integr. Comp. Physiol. **252:** R628–R633.

31. OHTA, H. & W.T. TALMAN. 1994. Both NMDA and non-NMDA receptors in the NTS participate in the baroreceptor reflex in rats. Am. J. Physiol. Regul. Integr. Comp. Physiol. **267:** R1065–R1070.

32. BARMAN, S.M., G.L. GEBBER & H.S. ORER. 2000. Medullary lateral tegmental field: an important source of basal sympathetic nerve discharge in the cat. Am. J. Physiol. Regul. Integr. Comp. Physiol. **278:** R995–R1004.

33. ZHONG, S., Z-S. HUANG, G.L. GEBBER & S.M. BARMAN. 1993. Role of the brain stem in generating the 2- to 6-Hz oscillation in sympathetic nerve discharge. Am. J. Physiol. Regul. Integr. Comp. Physiol. **265:** R1026–R1035.

34. ZHONG, S., M.J. KENNEY & G.L. GEBBER. 1991. High power, low frequency components of cardiac, renal, splenic, and vertebral sympathetic nerve activities are uniformly reduced by spinal cord transection. Brain Res. **556:** 130–134.

35. BARMAN, S.M. 1990. Brainstem control of cardiovascular function. *In* Brainstem Mechanisms of Behavior: 353–381. Wiley. New York.

36. ZAGON, A. & A.D. SMITH. 1993. Monosynaptic projections from the rostral ventrolateral medulla oblongata to identified sympathetic preganglionic neurons. Neuroscience **54:** 729–743.

37. BERMAN, A.L. 1968. The Brain Stem of the Cat: A Cytoarchitectonic Atlas with Stereotaxic Coordinates. University of Wisconsin Press. Madison, WI.

# Differential Regulation of Sympathetic Outflows to Vasoconstrictor and Thermoregulatory Effectors

SHAUN F. MORRISON

*Department of Physiology, Northwestern University Medical School, Chicago, Illinois 60611, USA*

ABSTRACT: The medullary premotor neurons determining the sympathetic outflow regulating cardiac function and vasoconstriction are located in the rostral ventrolateral medulla (RVLM). The present study sought evidence for differential characteristics and baroreceptor reflex sensitivities between the sympathetic nerve activity (SNA) controlling brown adipose tissue (BAT) metabolism and thermogenesis and cardiovascular SNA such as that controlling mesenteric vasoconstriction via the splanchnic (SPL) nerve. The tonic discharge of sympathetic nerves is determined by the inputs to functionally specific sympathetic preganglionic neurons from supraspinal populations of premotor neurons. Under normothermic conditions, BAT SNA was nearly silent, while SPL SNA exhibited sustained, large-amplitude bursts. Disinhibition of neurons in the rostral raphe pallidus (RPa), a potential site of sympathetic premotor neurons controlling BAT SNA, or icv injection of prostaglandin $E_2$, a pyrogenic stimulus, elicited a dramatic increase in BAT SNA. SPL SNA was strongly influenced by the baroreceptor reflex as indicated by a high coherence to the arterial pressure, while activated BAT SNA exhibited no correlation with the arterial pressure. Since these characteristics and reflex responses in sympathetic outflow have been shown to arise from the ongoing or altered discharge of sympathetic premotor neurons, the marked differences between SPL SNA and BAT SNA provide strong evidence supporting the hypothesis that vasoconstriction and thermogenesis (metabolism) are controlled by distinct populations of sympathetic premotor neurons, the former in the RVLM and strongly baroreceptor-modulated and the latter potentially in the RPa exhibiting little influence of baroreceptor reflex activation.

KEYWORDS: Baroreceptor reflex; Brown adipose tissue; Frequency domain; GABA inhibition; Hypothermia; Raphe pallidus; Rostral ventrolateral medulla; Sympathetic nerve activity; Thermogenesis; Vasoconstriction

## INTRODUCTION

Although nearly every tissue in the body, with perhaps the exception of skeletal muscle fibers, receives a sympathetic innervation, the characteristics of the sympathetic outflows to the blood vessels and heart have been most extensively studied.

Address for correspondence: Shaun F. Morrison, Department of Physiology (M211), Northwestern University Medical School, 303 E. Chicago Avenue, Chicago, IL 60611. Voice: 312-503-5024; fax: 312-503-5101.

s-morrison2@northwestern.edu

Many years of systematic and maintained experimental effort have also provided detailed anatomical and electrophysiological information on the central nervous system networks controlling the sympathetic nerve activity (SNA) to the cardiovascular system. Thus, while our understanding of the central neural basis for the generation of basal cardiovascular sympathetic tone and for the reflex regulation of SNA to the blood vessels and heart is quite comprehensive, we know comparatively little about the central substrates underlying the regulation of noncardiovascular tissues.

One of the groups of noncardiovascular tissues whose central regulatory circuits are becoming of increasing interest is that involved in energy homeostasis and thermoregulation. As obesity reaches epidemic proportions in our society, an understanding of the central control of energy metabolism and thermogenesis will become increasingly important in the discovery of novel approaches to reducing adiposity.[1] Although brown adipose tissue (BAT) is not common in humans after infancy, it is the principal, sympathetically regulated, energy-metabolizing tissue in the rat and serves as a model effector system in the rat for experiments to delineate central pathways involved in the generation and control of the sympathetic outflows influencing energy metabolism and thermoregulation.

As with most tissues, the sympathetic nerves to BAT contain axons whose discharge regulates the activity of a particular tissue cell type, in this case, the capacity of the brown adipocytes to convert the energy stored in fatty acids to heat production, as well as axons that innervate the blood vessels within the tissue to maintain a blood flow that is appropriate for the level of tissue activity.[2] To increase our understanding of the functional organization of the central networks controlling the sympathetic outflows to energy metabolism/thermoregulatory effectors and how they might differ from the extensively studied sympathetic circuits controlling cardiovascular tissues, the present experiments contrast the responses to cardiovascular and thermoregulatory stimuli in BAT SNA with those in splanchnic (SPL) SNA, a visceral vasoconstrictor efferent nerve.

A critical aspect in delineating the supraspinal pathways controlling a functionally specific sympathetic discharge is the identification and characterization of the sympathetic premotor neurons for the particular function. While the medullary premotor neurons determining the sympathetic outflow regulating cardiac function and vasoconstriction have been extensively studied in the rostral ventrolateral medulla (RVLM),[3–6] the localization and identification of the sympathetic premotor innervation of BAT sympathetic preganglionic neurons have not been accomplished. Recently, indirect evidence has been provided for a role for raphe neurons in the premotor regulation of BAT SNA and BAT thermogenesis. Cold exposure has been shown to produce a dramatic increase in Fos immunoreactivity that is selectively concentrated in the rostral raphe pallidus (RPa) and to a lesser degree in the raphe obscurus.[7,8] Additionally, the RPa contains neurons with projections to sympathetic preganglionic neurons,[9–11] including those that control BAT function.[12] Also consistent with the existence of BAT sympathetic premotor neurons in RPa is the finding that activation of RPa neurons evoked a selective and maximal increase in BAT SNA that was independent of neurons in the RVLM.[13] In the present study, the differential sensitivities of SNA to the baroreceptor reflex and to intracerebroventricular (icv) prostaglandin $E_2$ (PGE$_2$) were used to suggest that the sympathetic premotor neurons determining BAT SNA have different functional characteristics from those mediating cardiovascular functions such as visceral vasoconstriction via SPL SNA.

## METHODS

Sprague-Dawley rats (300–450 g) were anesthetized intravenously with urethane (0.8 g/kg) and chloralose (80 mg/kg) after induction with 3% isoflurane in 100% $O_2$ and cannulation of a femoral artery, a femoral vein, and the trachea for monitoring arterial pressure, injecting drugs, and artificial ventilation, respectively. Animals were positioned prone in a stereotaxic frame (incisor bar: −4.0 mm) with a spinal clamp on the T10 vertebra, paralyzed with D-tubocurarine (0.3 mg initial dose, 0.1 mg/h supplements), and artificially ventilated with 100% $O_2$ (50 cycles per minute; tidal volume: 3 mL). Small adjustments in minute ventilation were made as necessary to maintain end-tidal $CO_2$ between 3.5% and 4.5%. Throughout most of the experiment, colonic temperature was maintained at 37.5°C with a heat lamp and a heating plate beneath the animal. To provide a natural stimulus for the activation of the sympathetic nerve discharge to BAT, body temperature was lowered by removing the heat sources and, in some cases, placing dry ice in contact with the metal heating plate beneath the animal. This caused temperature to fall from 37.5°C to between 34°C and 35°C within 10 minutes, at which time the heat sources were turned on and body temperature returned to 37.5°C.

Postganglionic SNA to BAT was recorded from the central cut end of a small nerve bundle dissected from the ventral surface of the right interscapular BAT after dividing the fat pad along the midline and reflecting it laterally. Using a dorsal approach, postganglionic SNA was recorded from the central cut end of the left SPL nerve as it exited from the suprarenal ganglion. Both SNAs were filtered from 1 to 300 Hz amplified with a Cyberamp 380 (Axon Instruments) and digitized (22 kHz) and recorded (Neurodata) on VCR tape along with the arterial pressure.

A microinjection pipette (tip outside diameter: 20 μm) was positioned stereotaxically in the RPa after a partial occipital craniotomy. Relative to lambda, the coordinates for the RPa were anterior-posterior, −3.5 mm; medio-lateral, 0.0 mm; and dorso-ventral, −9.4 mm below the dural surface. At the end of each experiment, the micropipette was withdrawn vertically, refilled with a 1% solution of fast green dye, and repositioned at the microinjection site, and dye was electrophoretically deposited (15 μA anodal direct current for 15 minutes). Following perfusion and histologic processing, the locations of the microinjection sites in the RPa were plotted on camera lucida drawings of sections through the rostral medulla.[14] For icv injection of $PGE_2$, a stainless-steel tube, 0.5 mm inside diameter, was positioned in the left lateral ventricle (coordinates relative to bregma: anterior-posterior, −1.2 mm; medio-lateral, 1.5 mm; and dorso-ventral, −3.4 mm below the dural surface) and connected via polyethylene tubing to a 10-μL syringe containing $PGE_2$ (1 μg/1 μL).

Following digitization at 1 kHz, signals were analyzed with software written in the ASYST programming environment. The BAT and SPL SNA amplitudes were derived from autospectral analysis. For each experimental condition, average autospectra of the SNA were obtained by dividing 20.5-second data records into nine 4.1-second segments with a 50% overlap. The value of the autospectra at each frequency was computed as the mean value of the powers at that frequency in the individual autospectra of these nine segments. The amplitudes of the sympathetic nerve activities were taken as the root-mean-square value of the total power in the 1–10 Hz band of the averaged autospectra. Ordinary and partial coherences among nerve activities

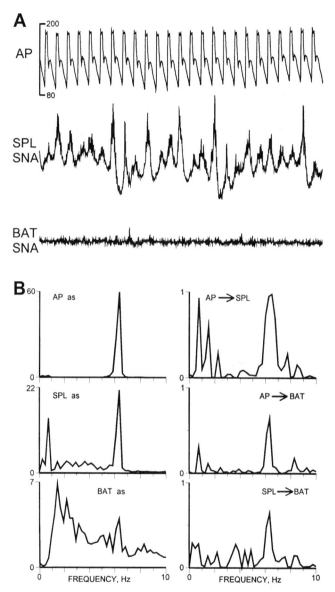

**FIGURE 1.** Brown adipose and splanchnic sympathetic efferent responses to acute hypothermia. **(A)** Brown adipose tissue sympathetic nerve activity (BAT SNA) at normothermia (37.5°C), tonic splanchnic sympathetic nerve activity (SPL SNA), and arterial pressure (AP). **(B)** Autospectra (as; ordinate is % of total power) of AP, SPL SNA, and BAT SNA under normothermic conditions; note the prominent peaks at the heart rate frequency, and ordinary coherences (ordinate is coherence) between AP and BAT SNA (AP > BAT), between AP and SPL SNA (AP > SPL), and between SPL and BAT SNAs (SPL > BAT); note the common baroreceptor-mediated modulation of SPL and BAT SNAs under these conditions. (*Figure 1 continued on following page.*)

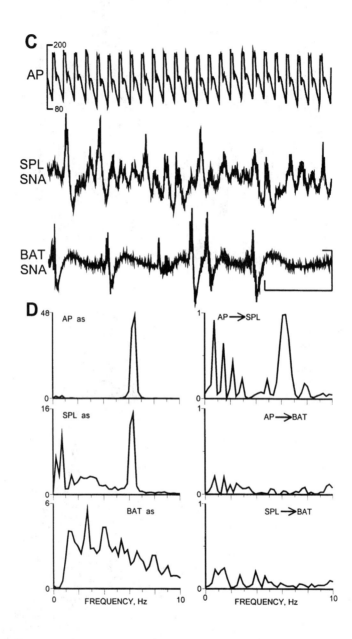

**FIGURE 1 — *Continued.* (C)** Large-amplitude bursts in BAT SNA, with little change in the amplitude of SPL SNA during hypothermia (34.6°C). **(D)** Autospectra (as; ordinate is % of total power) of AP, SPL SNA, and BAT SNA during hypothermia. Under these conditions, there are no frequencies at which AP or SPL SNA exhibits a high level of coherence with BAT SNA, although the high AP > SPL coherence at the heart rate is maintained. (Adapted from reference 13.)

were computed according to published algorithms.[15,16] Statistical significance was assessed with the Student's $t$ test, with $p < 0.05$.

## RESULTS

In the absence of conditions that stimulate energy metabolism in BAT, that is, at normothermia maintained by external heating sources in urethane/chloralose-anesthetized rats, the sympathetic discharge to BAT is characterized by low amplitude bursts (FIG. 1A). In most animals, these bursts were correlated with the cardiac cycle, yielding AP to BAT SNA coherence values (FIG. 1B) greater than 0.6. Simultaneously recorded, SPL SNA, a measure of visceral vasoconstrictor sympathetic outflow, was characterized by large-amplitude bursts (FIG. 1A) synchronized to the cardiac cycle as indicated by the large peak in the SPL autospectrum at the cardiac frequency (FIG. 1B). These bursts were strongly correlated with the arterial pulse, usually yielding AP to SPL SNA coherence values (FIG. 1B) greater than 0.9. These data are consistent with the presence of a low level of baroreceptor reflex–modulated, vasoconstrictor sympathetic outflow in BAT SNA at rest and a markedly higher level in SPL SNA under the same control conditions. The sympathetic premotor neurons in the RVLM whose discharge is modulated by the baroreceptor reflex and which are responsible for maintaining basal cardiovascular sympathetic tone[3,6,13] are the likely source of the excitation to the sympathetic preganglionic neurons comprising the vasoconstrictor components of both BAT SNA and SPL SNA.

Removal of the heating sources and chilling of the heating plate beneath the rat produced a reduction in core temperature and a hypothermic stimulation of cutaneous receptors that reflexively stimulated BAT SNA and BAT thermogenesis (FIG. 1C). Activated BAT SNA was characterized by large-amplitude bursts that were similar in character to those in SPL SNA, but were never synchronized to the cardiac cycle. This was indicated by the absence of a peak in the BAT SNA autospectrum at the cardiac frequency and by AP to BAT SNA coherence values at the cardiac frequency that were less than 0.3 (FIG. 1D). Acute hypothermic stimulation of BAT thermogenesis resulted in a mean increase in BAT SNA of more than 400% of control. In contrast, acute hypothermia induced a mean increase in SPL SNA of less than 25% in these same animals and did not alter the predominant cardiac-related pattern of burst discharge in SPL SNA (FIG. 1C), which remained highly coherent to the arterial pulse (FIG. 1D). Since the principal sources of sympathoexcitation arise from supraspinal premotor neurons, the induction of a large increase in BAT SNA in the form of bursts that were not synchronized to the cardiac cycle, in conjunction with a very modest increase in SPL SNA, provides strong support for the hypothesis that increases in BAT thermogenesis are mediated by a different population of sympathetic premotor neurons than those that regulate vasoconstriction. Indeed, at least a portion of the increase in overall SPL SNA was likely to have been the result of hypothermia-stimulated activation of axons that innervate BAT depots within the SPL distribution,[13] such as those surrounding the adrenal gland and the kidney.

Activation of a potential sympathetic premotor neuron population innervating BAT sympathetic preganglionic neurons controlling BAT thermogenesis should produce a marked increase in BAT SNA and BAT temperature. If sympathetic premotor neurons for BAT SNA are distinct and spatially separate from those regulating SPL

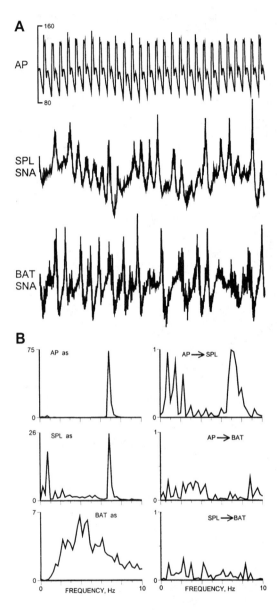

**FIGURE 2.** Maximal responses in brown adipose and splanchnic sympathetic outflows following disinhibition of neurons in the rostral raphe pallidus. **(A)** Brown adipose tissue sympathetic nerve activity (BAT SNA) and tonic splanchnic sympathetic nerve activity (SPL SNA) following microinjection of bicuculline into raphe pallidus. **(B)** Autospectra (as; ordinate is % of total power) of and coherences (ordinate is coherence) among AP, BAT SNA, and SPL SNA following disinhibition of raphe pallidus neurons. Note the high level of power in BAT SNA and the absence of high coherence between AP or SPL and BAT (*lower traces*). (Adapted from reference 13.)

visceral vasoconstriction, such stimulation may produce little change in SPL SNA amplitude. To determine if neurons in RPa, a site containing neurons that project to the spinal sympathetic intermediolateral nucleus,[9-11] would meet this criterion, changes in BAT SNA and SPL SNA were observed following disinhibition of RPa neurons with local microinjection of bicuculline. As shown in FIGURE 2A, micro-injection of bicuculline (60 nL, 1 mM) into RPa resulted in a dramatic and sustained increase in BAT SNA (compare with control in FIG. 1A), with only a minor elevation in the level of SPL SNA (compare with control in FIG. 1A). At the peak of the bicuculline-evoked response, the mean increase in BAT SNA was greater than 1500% of control, while that in SPL SNA was less than 35% of control SPL SNA. As in the response to acute hypothermia, the bursts in BAT SNA following dis-inhibition of RPa neurons were not coherent with the arterial pressure (FIG. 2B). The mean AP to BAT SNA coherence at the cardiac frequency was less than 0.2, although there was no bicuculline-induced change in the strong cardiac modulation of SPL SNA, resulting in a mean AP to SPL SNA coherence at the cardiac frequency greater than 0.9. These results are consistent with the hypothesis that RPa contains sympa-thetic premotor neurons for BAT SNA and that these are different from those in the RVLM regulating SPL vasoconstriction. Interestingly, the very low level of BAT SNA at normothermia and the large increases in BAT SNA evoked by blockade of $GABA_A$ receptors in RPa suggest that physiologically stimulated increases in BAT SNA and BAT thermogenesis arise from reduced activity of a potent, tonically active GABAergic inhibition of BAT sympathetic premotor neurons in RPa.

A physiological stimulus that can induce large increases in BAT SNA comparable to those resulting from disinhibition of RPa neurons is the icv application of the pyrogenic stimulus, $PGE_2$. This prostaglandin plays a role in the activation of hypo-thalamic neurons and efferent pathways involved in the autonomic component of the acute-phase reaction to inflammatory stimuli that results in an increase in body tem-perature,[17-20] at least partly through an increase in BAT thermogenesis.[21] As shown in FIGURE 3, icv $PGE_2$ produced a marked increase in the amplitude and frequency of bursts in BAT SNA. The absence of a peak in the autospectrum of BAT SNA at the heart rate (FIG. 3B) indicates that the central networks responsible for generating the elevated level of BAT SNA due to icv $PGE_2$ are not modulated by baroreceptor reflex inputs. These results indicate that the activity in the networks generating BAT SNA is relatively insensitive to activation of the baroreceptor reflex, a major acute modulator of cardiovascular SNA whose effects are one of the hallmarks used to identify sympathetic premotor neurons in the RVLM.[3,6,22]

## DISCUSSION

The level and bursting characteristics of basal SNA to cardiovascular targets are directly attributable to the discharge of their sympathetic premotor neurons in the RVLM.[3,6,23] Similarly, the reduction in vasoconstrictor and cardiac SNA that occurs following baroreceptor reflex stimulation is mediated through an inhibition of the sympathetic premotor neurons in RVLM that govern the level of sympathetic dis-charge to these tissues.[3,6] From these fundamental properties of the central sympa-thetic network derived from studies on vasoconstrictor SNA, the marked differences between BAT SNA and SPL SNA in their basal discharge characteristics and in their

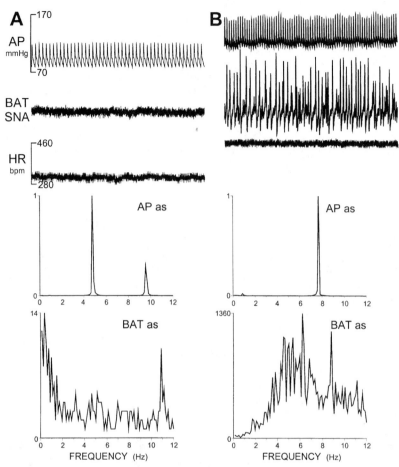

**FIGURE 3.** Increases in arterial pressure (AP), heart rate (HR), and sympathetic out-flow to brown adipose tissue (BAT) evoked by intracerebroventricular prostaglandin $E_2$ (PGE$_2$). **(A)** AP, BAT sympathetic nerve activity (SNA), and HR under control, normo-thermic conditions. Autospectra of AP (AP as) and BAT SNA (BAT as) under control con-ditions. Ordinate of the AP autospectrum is normalized to maximum power. **(B)** AP, BAT SNA, and HR and autospectra of AP (AP as) and BAT SNA (BAT as) during the peak of the response to icv PGE$_2$. Note the absence of a peak in the autospectrum of BAT SNA at the cardiac frequency.

frequency components indicative of baroreceptor reflex modulation lead to the con-clusion that distinct populations of sympathetic premotor neurons control the sym-pathetic discharge to these functionally disparate tissues. These differences include (a) the amplitudes of the basal discharge under normothermic conditions, (b) the selective activation of BAT SNA by hypothermia, by disinhibition of RPa neurons, and by PGE$_2$, and (c) the frequency characteristics of activated BAT SNA versus SPL SNA, including the prominent, heart rate–related peak in the autospectrum of

SPL SNA, but not BAT SNA, indicative of baroreceptor reflex modulation. Together, these results are consistent with the hypothesis that the sympathetic outflow determining the level of energy metabolism in BAT and of BAT thermogenesis is controlled by a different population of premotor neurons than that determining the mesenteric vasoconstrictor sympathetic outflow via the SPL nerve. The absence of any spectral indication of a significant baroreceptor reflex modulation of activated BAT SNA, coupled with the demonstration that increases in arterial pressure inhibit SPL SNA, but not BAT SNA,[8] suggests that the sympathetic network generating BAT SNA is not influenced by the level of arterial pressure and that baroreceptor reflex regulation may be selectively targeted to those sympathetic outflows, primarily cardiovascular, with premotor neurons in the RVLM. In this regard, the cardiac modulation of basal BAT SNA seen under normothermic conditions is consistent with the existence of a small population of vasoconstrictor fibers[2] in the sympathetic nerves to BAT whose activity is controlled by baroreceptor-modulated, sympathetic premotor neurons in the RVLM. As the ganglion cell axons innervating adipocytes become active in response to hypothermia, icv administration of $PGE_2$, or disinhibition of RPa neurons, their much larger number and the absence of a baroreceptor regulation of the discharge of their premotor neurons result in a nearly immediate loss of any correlation between the AP and activated BAT SNA. This was true during the large increases in BAT SNA following disinhibition of RPa neurons as well as during the more modest activations of BAT SNA in response to icv $PGE_2$ and to hypothermia. Activation of the sympathetic input to adipocytes may also induce nitric oxide production as a mechanism of matching BAT blood flow to metabolism and thermogenesis.[24]

The finding that disinhibition of neurons in the region of the rostral RPa produced a potentially maximal increase in BAT SNA with only a minimal rise in SPL SNA suggests that RPa contains neurons that are differentially involved in the regulation of BAT thermogenesis versus visceral vasoconstrictor tone. Additional evidence leads to the speculation that RPa is a site of BAT sympathetic premotor neurons. Anatomically, neurons in RPa project to the spinal intermediolateral cell column containing sympathetic preganglionic neurons.[9–12] In studies involving inactivation of sympathetic premotor neurons in the RVLM, disinhibition of RPa neurons was still capable of producing a robust increase in BAT SNA.[13] The size of the BAT SNA response to blockade of $GABA_A$ receptors in RPa indicates that the neurons in RPa that influence BAT SNA are normally under a strong tonic GABAergic inhibition and suggests that reductions in the level of this inhibitory input may be the basis for physiologically evoked increases in BAT SNA and thermogenesis.[8] In this regard, the similarity between the characteristics of the bursts in BAT SNA evoked by disinhibition of RPa and by icv administration of $PGE_2$ is consistent with the hypothesis that disinhibition of RPa neurons mediates the $PGE_2$-evoked increase in BAT SNA and BAT thermogenesis.

Two overlapping mechanisms have been proposed for the fundamental medullary substrate allowing differential and selective control of the sympathetic outflows to different cardiovascular tissues (i.e., different vascular beds and the heart). Frequency domain analysis of the discharge from multiple sympathetic nerves has led Gebber to suggest the existence of a distinct brain stem generator module (oscillator) for each cardiovascular sympathetic efferent nerve.[23] The dynamic coupling of these oscillators would underlie the patterning of sympathetic outflows to the different

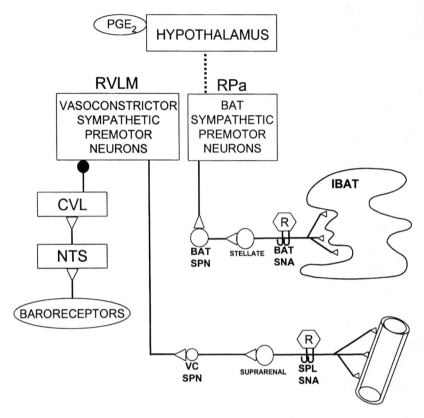

**FIGURE 4.** Schematic illustration of the hypothesized sympathetic premotor neuronal regulation of brown adipose tissue (BAT) thermogenesis and splanchnic (SPL) vasoconstriction (VC) by the raphe pallidus (RPa) and the rostral ventrolateral medulla (RVLM), respectively. The principal site of ganglion cells (stellate ganglion) innervating the interscapular BAT (IBAT) is shown, as is the suprarenal ganglion that contributes much of the postganglionic component of SPL sympathetic nerve activity (SNA). Nerve recording sites (R) are also illustrated. Functionally distinct and spatially separate populations of sympathetic premotor neurons determine the discharge of VC and BAT sympathetic preganglionic neurons (SPN). The baroreceptor reflex selectively influences the discharge of cardiovascular sympathetic premotor neurons in the RVLM via activation of neurons in the nucleus of the tractus solitarius (NTS) that activate inhibitory neurons in the caudal ventrolateral medulla (CVLM). PGE$_2$ may increase BAT SNA via hypothalamic efferents that result in a disinhibition of BAT sympathoexcitatory neurons in RPa. Not shown are (1) the minor VC component of BAT SNA that is controlled by sympathetic premotor neurons in the RVLM and (2) the minor BAT component of SPL SNA that is controlled by premotor neurons in the RPa.

cardiovascular tissues necessary to support behavior and homeostatic reflexes. Based on differential sympathetic nerve responses to microstimulation of different regions of the RVLM, McAllen has proposed that functionally specific, but spatially overlapping populations of RVLM sympathetic premotor neurons account for the ability to selectively regulate individual cardiovascular sympathetic efferents.[25]

These concepts can be merged if premotor neurons are incorporated in the generator modules. The results of the present study provide support for an extension of these hypotheses to include anatomically separate populations of sympathetic premotor neurons (and their attendant oscillator circuits) as a basis for the differential control of cardiovascular and noncardiovascular sympathetic outflows.

The data in the present study support a model for differential control of functionally distinct sympathetic outflows that is based on functionally distinct populations of sympathetic premotor neurons.[4,13,23,25] FIGURE 4 summarizes this model for differential control of BAT thermogenesis and vasoconstrictor tone, with the incorporation of the hypothesized location of BAT premotor neurons in RPa. The schematic diagram illustrates (a) the differential sympathetic premotor regulation of vasoconstrictor outputs and of thermogenic (metabolic) outflows, (b) the restriction of the influence of the baroreceptor reflex to the former, and (c) the potential pathway via the hypothalamus by which $PGE_2$ produces selective increases in BAT SNA and body temperature. Several components of the sympathetic regulation of overall cardiovascular function, including cardiac rate, cardiac contractility, vasoconstriction, and adrenal medullary catecholamine secretion, are controlled by premotor neurons in the RVLM[3–6,25,26] whose activity is strongly modulated by the baroreceptor reflex. Although speculative, it seems likely that a similarly diverse constellation of sympathetic outputs influencing metabolism and thermoregulation will be under the control of sympathetic premotor neurons in the RPa region and that the discharge of these premotor neurons will not be influenced by baroreceptor reflex activation.

## ACKNOWLEDGMENTS

This work was supported by NIDDK Grant No. DK-20378. I thank James B. Young for support of these investigations and insightful discussions of these data.

## REFERENCES

1. DULLOO, A.G. & S. SAMEC. 2000. Uncoupling proteins: do they have a role in body weight regulation? News Physiol. Sci. **15:** 313–318.
2. CANNON, B., J. NEDERGAARD, J.M. LUNDBERG et al. 1986. "Neuropeptide tyrosine" (NPY) is co-stored with noradrenaline in vascular, but not in parenchymal sympathetic nerves of brown adipose tissue. Exp. Cell Res. **164:** 546–550.
3. GUYENET, P.G. 1990. Role of the ventral medulla oblongata in blood pressure regulation. In Central Regulation of Autonomic Functions, pp. 145–167. Oxford University Press. London/New York.
4. MCALLEN, R.M. & C.N. MAY. 1994. Differential drives from rostral ventrolateral medullary neurons to three identified sympathetic outflows Am. J. Physiol. **267:** R935–R944.
5. CAMPOS, R.R. & R.M. MCALLEN. 1997. Cardiac sympathetic premotor neurons. Am. J. Physiol. **272:** R615–R620.
6. MORRISON, S.F., T.A. MILNER & D.J. REIS. 1988. Reticulospinal vasomotor neurons of the rat rostral ventrolateral medulla: relationship to sympathetic nerve activity and the C1 adrenergic cell group. J. Neurosci. **8:** 1286–1301.
7. BONAZ, B. & Y. TACHE. 1994. Induction of Fos immunoreactivity in the rat brain after cold-restraint induced gastric lesions and fecal excretion. Brain Res. **652:** 56–64.

8. MORRISON, S.F., A.F. SVED & A.M. PASSERIN. 1999. GABA-mediated inhibition of raphe pallidus neurons regulates sympathetic outflow to brown adipose tissue. Am. J. Physiol. **276:** R290–R297.

9. LOEWY, A.D. 1981. Raphe pallidus and raphe obscurus projections to the intermediolateral cell column in the rat. Brain Res. **222:** 129–133.

10. STRACK, A.M., W.B. SAWYER, J.H. HUGHES et al. 1989. A general pattern of CNS innervation of the sympathetic outflow demonstrated by transneuronal pseudorabies viral infections. Brain Res. **491:** 156–162.

11. BACON, S.J., A. ZAGON & A.D. SMITH. 1990. Electron microscopic evidence of a monosynaptic pathway between cells in the caudal raphe nuclei and sympathetic preganglionic neurons in the rat spinal cord. Exp. Brain Res. **79:** 589–602.

12. BAMSHAD, M., C.K. SONG & T.J. BARTNESS. 1999. CNS origins of the sympathetic nervous system outflow to brown adipose tissue. Am. J. Physiol. **276:** R1569–R1578.

13. MORRISON, S.F. 1999. RVLM and raphe differentially regulate sympathetic outflows to splanchnic and brown adipose tissue. Am. J. Physiol. **276:** R962–R973.

14. PAXINOS, G. & C. WATSON. 1986. The Rat Brain in Stereotaxic Coordinates. Second edition. Academic Press. London/New York/Sydney.

15. BENDAT, J.S. & A.G. PIERSOL. 1986. Random Data, Analysis, and Measurement Procedures. Second edition. Wiley. New York.

16. GEBBER, G.L., S. ZHONG, S.M. BARMAN et al. 1994. Differential relationships among the 10-Hz rhythmic discharges of sympathetic nerves with different targets. Am. J. Physiol. **267:** R387–R399.

17. MILTON, A.S. 1998. Prostaglandins and fever. Prog. Brain Res. **115:** 129–139.

18. SAPER, C.B. 1998. Neurobiological basis of fever. Ann. N.Y. Acad. Sci. **856:** 90–94.

19. ELMQUIST, J.K., T.E. SCAMMELL, C.D. JACOBSON & C.B. SAPER. 1996. Distribution of Fos-like immunoreactivity in the rat brain following intravenous lipopolysaccharide administration. J. Comp. Neurol. **371:** 85–103.

20. COCEANI, F. & E.S. AKARSU. 1998. Prostaglandin $E_2$ in the pathogenesis of fever: an update. Ann. N.Y. Acad. Sci. **856:** 76–82.

21. FYDA, D.M., K.E. COOPER & W.L. VEALE 1991. Contribution of brown adipose tissue to central PGE1-evoked hyperthermia in rats. Am. J. Physiol. **260:** R59–R66.

22. BROWN, D.L. & P.G. GUYENET. 1985. Electrophysiological study of cardiovascular neurons in the rostral ventrolateral medulla in rats. Circ. Res. **56:** 359–369.

23. GEBBER, G.L., S. ZHONG & S.M. BARMAN. 1995. Synchronization of cardiac-related discharges of sympathetic nerves with inputs from widely separated spinal segments. Am. J. Physiol. **268:** R1472–R1483.

24. NISOLI, E., C. TONELLO, L. BRISCINI & M.O. CARRUBA. 1997. Inducible nitric oxide synthase in rat brown adipocytes: implications for blood flow to brown adipose tissue. Endocrinology **138:** 676–682.

25. MCALLEN, R.M., C.N. MAY & R.R. CAMPOS. 1997. The supply of vasomotor drive to individual classes of sympathetic neuron. Clin. Exp. Hypertens. **19:** 607–618.

26. MCALLEN, R.M. 1986. Action and specificity of ventral medullary vasopressor neurones in the cat. Neuroscience **18:** 51–59.

# Evidence for Central Organization of Cardiovascular Rhythms

NICOLA MONTANO, ALBERTO PORTA, AND ALBERTO MALLIANI

*Centro Ricerche Cardiovascolari, CNR, Dipartimento di Scienze Precliniche LITA di Vialba, Medicina Interna II, Ospedale "L. Sacco," Università degli Studi di Milano, Milano, Italy*

ABSTRACT: Spectral analysis of heart rate and arterial pressure variabilities is a powerful noninvasive tool that is increasingly used to infer alterations of cardiovascular autonomic regulation in a variety of physiological and pathophysiological conditions such as hypertension, myocardial infarction, and congestive heart failure. A most important methodological issue to properly interpret the results obtained by the spectral analysis of cardiovascular variability signals is represented by the attribution of neurophysiological correlates to these spectral components. In this regard, recent application of spectral techniques to the evaluation of the oscillatory properties of sympathetic efferent activity in animals as well as in humans offers a new approach to a better understanding of the relationship between cardiovascular oscillations and autonomic regulation. The data so far collected seem to suggest the presence of a centrally organized neural code, characterized by excitatory and inhibitory neural mechanisms subserving the genesis and the regulation of cardiovascular oscillations concerning the major variables of autonomic regulation.

KEYWORDS: Heart rate variability; Sympathetic activity; Spectral analysis; Baroreflex mechanisms

The neural regulation of circulatory function is mainly effected through the interplay of the sympathetic and vagal outflows, which are tonically and phasically modulated by means of the interaction of at least three major factors: (1) central integration, (2) peripheral inhibitory reflex mechanisms with negative feedback characteristics, and (3) peripheral excitatory reflex mechanisms with positive feedback characteristics.

Although there are situations, such as diving reflex, in which sympathetic and vagal drive may change in the same direction, in most physiological conditions, the activation of one outflow is accompanied by the inhibition of the other.[1–3] This is true for reflexes arising predominantly not only from the arterial baroreceptive areas, but also from the heart.

This interaction can be explored by assessing cardiovascular rhythmicity with an appropriate methodology. Application of spectral analysis to beat-to-beat cardiovascular variability has emerged as a powerful tool to study the dynamic interaction of sympathetic and vagal regulatory mechanisms.[1–3] The possibility of quantifying the

Address for correspondence: Nicola Montano, Centro Ricerche Cardiovascolari, CNR, DiSP LITA di Vialba, Università degli Studi di Milano, Ospedale "L. Sacco," Via G. B. Grassi 74, 20157 Milano, Italy. Voice: +39-02-38210535; fax: +39-02-38210533.
nicola.montano@unimi.it

small spontaneous beat-by-beat oscillations in cardiovascular variables such as RR interval and arterial pressure aroused a growing interest in view of the hypothesis that these rhythmical oscillations could provide some insight into the neural cardiovascular regulation. The oscillatory pattern that characterizes the spectral profile of heart rate and arterial pressure short-term variability consists of two major components, at low (LF, 0.04–0.15 Hz) and high (HF, synchronous with respiratory rate) frequency, respectively.[1,2]

The current status of research directed to understanding the origins and neurophysiological basis for the LF and HF components of RR interval variability will be reviewed here.

## CARDIOVASCULAR OSCILLATIONS AND THE
## AUTONOMIC NERVOUS SYSTEM

The respiration-related HF component is by general agreement attributed mainly to vagal mechanisms.[1,4,5] This conclusion was based on the disappearance of this component after vagotomy performed in experiments on decerebrate cats[6] or after muscarinic receptor blockade in conscious dogs[4] and humans.[7] Moreover, it has also been demonstrated that the mechanical effects of respiration may be involved in the modulation of this component.[8]

On the contrary, different hypotheses have been debated regarding LF oscillation of RR variability. At first, both vagal and sympathetic outflows were considered to determine oscillations in this part of the spectrum, together with the hypothetical participation of other regulatory mechanisms such as the renin-angiotensin system.[4] A different interpretation has been later advanced, proposing that the LF oscillation in RR interval is related to sympathetic modulation as a result of two factors: (1) a baroreflex response to the 0.1-Hz Mayer waves in arterial pressure (the LF blood pressure oscillations)[9] and (2) the consequence of baroreflex buffering of the HF blood pressure oscillations resulting in a resonant LF oscillation—due to the delay in the sympathetic control loop of baroreflex mechanisms.[10] It has also been suggested that the 0.1-Hz oscillation of RR interval and blood pressure variability may also rely upon the central rhythmic organization of neural activity integrating peripheral negative- and positive-feedback reflex mechanisms in the context of a physiological closed-loop model.[1]

Therefore, it is important to assess directly the rhythmic content of the activity of neural pathways involved in the control of cardiovascular function to evaluate the presence of coherent oscillatory patterns linking sympathetic outflows and cardiovascular target functions.

## LF AND HF OSCILLATIONS IN SYMPATHETIC
## SUPRASPINAL STRUCTURES

In a study[11] performed on decerebrate, artificially ventilated cats, we observed the presence of the two main rhythms, LF and HF, in the variability of the discharge of cardiac sympathetic efferent fibers. Both these oscillatory components were highly coherent with the similar spectral components detectable in the variability of RR interval and systolic arterial pressure (SAP) and underwent parallel changes during hemodynamic maneuvers. Namely, increases in sympathetic efferent discharge, induced by decreases in arterial pressure, were associated with simultaneous increases in the LF component of sympathetic discharge, RR, and SAP variability. Concurrently, the HF component was decreased in all the spectra. Opposite changes in spectral components were induced by increases in arterial pressure. This study[11] furnished the first evidence of a reciprocal relation between LF and HF oscillations in the sympathetic neural outflow.

We addressed the issue of whether the LF and HF rhythms originate centrally in a subsequent study.[12] Arterial pressure and the discharge of medullary neurons, localized in areas involved in the regulation of sympathetic activity, were recorded in anesthetized, vagotomized, sinoaortic denervated cats. Both LF and HF components were detected in the discharge variability of single neurons and were coherent with blood pressure oscillations. While the observation of an HF oscillation was not unexpected, as it is known that brain stem sympathetic-related neurons receive inputs from the central respiratory rhythm generator, the finding of an LF oscillation in single neuron discharge variability suggests that this rhythm is generated at a central level. Moreover, in some cases, an LF component was present in the neuron discharge variability while absent in the spectral profile of blood pressure variability, further reinforcing the view that LF is not necessarily dependent upon the functional integrity of baroreceptive mechanisms.

## LF AND HF OSCILLATIONS IN SYMPATHETIC SPINAL STRUCTURES

The most convincing finding in favor of the wide distribution of these oscillations was the detection of LF and HF components in the sympathetic nerve discharge, RR interval, and SAP variabilities of cats after high cervical spinal section and bilateral vagotomy.[13]

It is known that neural regulation of cardiovascular function is integrated not only at supraspinal level, but also at spinal level, thereby including sympatho-sympathetic reflexes.[14,15] In fact, spinal structures provide a tonic sympathetic discharge compatible with resting blood pressure within a physiological range.[16,17] Moreover, Fernandez de Molina and Perl[18] in cats and Kaminsky *et al.*[19] in dogs reported that experimental animals with cervical spinal section could exhibit oscillations of the sympathetic efferent discharge in phase with Mayer's waves (corresponding to the LF spectral component). Accordingly, when heart rate and arterial pressure variabilities were studied in tetraplegic patients,[20,21] it was found that about half of them had LF oscillations in both RR interval and arterial pressure variability.

To address the issue of a widespread neural genesis for the LF oscillations, we evaluated the spectral content of cardiac efferent sympathetic discharge and RR interval variability in decerebrate vagotomized cats before and after spinal section at the C1 level.[22] Both LF and HF components were detected in sympathetic discharge, RR interval, and systolic arterial pressure before spinal section. The two components were still present in sympathetic nerve activity and cardiovascular variabilities after C1 spinal section. It was interesting to observe[22] that, in these conditions, a moderate rise in arterial pressure, obtained with aortic constriction, induced a marked increase in sympathetic efferent activity, through a positive-feedback sympatho-sympathetic excitatory spinal reflex. During this reflex sympathetic excitation, both LF and HF components of sympathetic discharge variability were increased in their absolute values. Interestingly, LF and HF components when expressed in normalized units (nu) were unchanged during sympathetic excitation.

Thus, the reciprocal changes that most often characterize the responsiveness of LF nu and HF nu seem to depend upon a supraspinal integration as they were present in decerebrate animals,[10] but undetectable during a spinal reflex. Dorsal root section from C6 to T8 vertebral segments abolished the reflex sympathetic excitation. In short, it appears that spinal mechanisms contribute to the genesis of LF oscillations.

The presence of the HF component in RR and SAP variabilities of spinal animals is explained by the positive-pressure artificial ventilation that is capable of markedly affecting hemodynamic conditions. However, the mechanical stimulus related to ventilation was also likely to activate somatic and visceral afferents projecting to the spinal cord and thereby spinal reflex mechanisms contributing to the presence of HF component in sympathetic discharge.[23] Indeed, after dorsal root section, coherence between ventilation and sympathetic spectral components was no longer present. On the other hand, $HF_{RR}$ and $HF_{SAP}$ oscillations have been observed in heart-transplanted patients,[8] that is, in a situation in which cardiac vagal innervation is not present.

Moreover, it is important to point out that the detection of an $LF_{RR}$ in the absence of cardiac vagal innervation strengthens the view that this rhythm can, at least in some circumstances, derive solely from sympathetic modulation.

## BAROREFLEX MECHANISMS AND LF OSCILLATION OF HEART RATE VARIABILITY

While it is quite probable that baroreflex mechanisms might modulate LF amplitude, it is unlikely that LF genesis can be attributed exclusively to these mechanisms. From a neurophysiological point of view, an increase in the output of a neural oscillator can be induced by increasing a rhythmic input to it or by reducing some tonic inhibitory activity restraining its intrinsic rhythmicity. An increased input from baroreceptors was clearly obtained by Sleight et al.[9] with their mechanical stimulation, obtained by neck chamber, but a limitation of this model was, indeed, that it transformed a closed-loop system into an open input-output relation.

Tachycardia accompanying standing or hypotension is attributed in part to the sympathetic excitation that occurs as a release phenomenon caused by a reduction of baroreceptor nerve activity. The reduction of the rhythmic input to the nervous centers would be accompanied by a relative increase in LF component.

Conversely, in conditions such as mental stress or physical exercise, during which there is a simultaneous presence of tachycardia and hypertension, the baroreceptor firing should increase. However, the LF component is increased as well in these circumstances. In addition, there are conditions such as experimental myocardial ischemia during which an LF increase can occur in the absence of arterial pressure changes.[24,25] Incidentally, in resting conscious dogs, an LF component is usually present in arterial pressure variability, but usually absent in RR variability, in spite of the high baroreflex gain. Also, the baroreflex gain is known to be decreased during standing, mental stress, and exercise,[26,27] conditions all characterized by an increased sympathetic activity. All the above elements support the hypothesis that the LF rhythm seems to be intrinsic in sympathetic excitation, independently of its genesis.

A further demonstration ruling out the mandatory role of baroreceptor mechanisms was obtained by a study[28] performed on two patients with severe congestive heart failure (CHF) who underwent the implantation of a left ventricular assist device (LVAD). This device, used as a bridge to cardiac transplantation in intractable heart failure, obtains oxygenated blood from the native left ventricle and sends it to the arterial circulation. Thus, these patients represented a unique model in which native heart rate variability was completely uncorrelated to blood pressure variability (determined by the artificial pump frequency and stroke). The two CHF subjects did not show an LF oscillation in RR variability, which was restored after LVAD implantation.[28] Hence, the presence of an LF oscillation in RR interval independent of any oscillation in blood pressure suggests that this rhythm is a fundamental property of the central autonomic outflow. On the other hand, the above observation does not preclude an important role of the baroreflex in modulating this rhythm since the baroreflex circuitry can oscillate quite efficiently in the LF range.[9]

## OSCILLATORY PATTERN OF MUSCLE
## SYMPATHETIC NERVE ACTIVITY

The advent, in recent years, of direct intraneural microneurographic recordings of efferent sympathetic nerve traffic to both muscle blood vessels (MSNA) and skin blood vessels (SSNA) has allowed us to address this issue also in human beings.[29,30]

Previous studies in human healthy volunteers reported the presence of both LF and HF oscillations in the spectral profile of MSNA.[31,32] However, these studies did not investigate the correlation between the neural and cardiovascular oscillatory patterns.

In our first study,[33] we intended to determine the effects of sympathetic excitation (inducing graded hypotension) and of sympathetic inhibition (inducing graded hypertension) on the traditional indices (bursts and amplitude) and on spectral components of MSNA. During sympathetic activation induced by nitroprusside administration, we observed an increase of the LF oscillation in the variability of MSNA, RR, and arterial pressure. Conversely, sympathetic inhibition and vagal activation induced by phenylephrine administration were characterized by a predominance of the HF components in all variability signals.

The simultaneous evaluation of spectral measures of MSNA and RR interval variability allowed us to directly address the issue of which spectral measure of RR interval variability may better reflect changes in autonomic state. Our results showed that the use of LF nu and HF nu or the LF/HF ratio provides the strongest correlation with attendant changes in MSNA (assessed by amplitude or by normalized power of spectral components rather than bursts/min). The synchronous changes in the LF and HF of both MSNA and RR interval variabilities during different levels of sympathetic drive are suggestive of common central mechanisms governing both sympathetic and parasympathetic cardiovascular modulation.

Similar results were obtained in a subsequent study[34] in which a gravitational (i.e., a tilt maneuver) rather than a pharmacological stimulus was used to increase sympathetic activity.

These data, confirming those previously obtained in cats,[10] suggest that the two main oscillatory rhythms are, respectively, markers of excitation (LF) and inhibition (HF) and that, in healthy subjects, these rhythms are modulated in a reciprocal manner. Indeed, changes in the central excitatory-inhibitory balance might induce reciprocal changes not only in average impulse activity of central vagal and sympathetic motor neurons, but also in the balance between LF and HF rhythms that can be observed in peripheral target organs.[35]

In this sense, a recent study[36] in which we evaluated the effects of low and high doses of atropine on MSNA and cardiovascular variabilities appears particularly relevant. In humans, low-dose atropine is known to decrease heart rate and to increase respiratory sinus arrhythmia because of an increase in parasympathetic activity. Vice versa, high doses of atropine are parasympatholytic, markedly increasing heart rate and decreasing heart rate variability. Whether the vagotonic effect of low-dose atropine is due to a peripheral effect on the sinoatrial node or to a central neural mechanism is not clear. On the other hand, it is unknown whether a similar vagotonic effect is also exerted by high-dose atropine since any central effect would be masked by muscarinic blockade at the sinoatrial node. We addressed this question by assessing the effects of the vagotonic (low dose) or vagolitic (high dose) actions of atropine on the spectral components of MSNA variability.

We observed[36] that low-dose atropine was associated with an increase in the HF and a decrease in the LF oscillation of both RR interval and MSNA variability without changes in arterial blood pressure. High-dose atropine induced a similar increase in the HF and decrease in the LF of MSNA variability. Thus, the study of oscillatory characteristics of cardiovascular signals reveals a central vagotonic effect able to modulate the sympathetic nerve traffic to peripheral blood vessels.

## SUMMARY

In numerous circumstances, the increase in sympathetic activity seems to be associated with a simultaneous enhancement of its LF rhythm and, conversely, with a decrease of its HF component. The reciprocal organization seems to be a fundamental characteristic of central autonomic cardiovascular control.

The relative distribution of power between these two oscillatory frequencies is tightly linked to changes in the strength of the signal, so one oscillatory frequency is a marker of excitation (LF) and the other is a marker of inhibition (HF). A state of excitation would be accompanied by an increased sympathetic activity with its rhythmic characteristics, conveying at the periphery the predominance of the LF component; conversely, the contribution of vagal activity to the LF component would be minimal because vagal activity would be simultaneously inhibited.

On the other hand, a state of inhibition, such as that occurring during reflexes mediated by vagal afferents, would be accompanied by an increased vagal activity conveying at the periphery the increase in HF component.

In physiological conditions, LF and HF oscillations, both likely to have a central and peripheral mixed origin, would reflect, in their normalized values or as LF/HF ratio, the state of the central balance between excitation and inhibition coupled with the pattern of sympathovagal balance. We hypothesize that, if this is true, a similar behavior of the oscillatory pattern should be detectable also in the variability of discharge of vagal fibers. In preliminary ongoing experiments (unpublished) in which we recorded cardiovascular vagal activity in decerebrate rats, we observed an increase in LF nu and a decrease in HF nu of vagal discharge variability during a hypotensive maneuver despite the reduction in the average vagal activity, while the increase in vagal outflow induced by a hypertensive maneuver was accompanied by a decrease in LF nu and an increase in HF nu. Thus, the detection of the two rhythms from one autonomic neural output may represent a window on the central organization of the neural mechanisms subserving cardiovascular oscillations.

## REFERENCES

1. MALLIANI, A., M. PAGANI, F. LOMBARDI *et al.* 1991. Cardiovascular neural regulation explored in the frequency domain. Res. Adv. Ser. Circ. **184:** 482–492.
2. MALLIANI, A. 1999. The pattern of sympathovagal balance explored in the frequency domain. News Physiol. Sci. **14:** 111–117.
3. MALLIANI, A., M. PAGANI, N. MONTANO *et al.* 1998. Sympathovagal balance: a reappraisal. Circulation **98:** 2640–2644.
4. AKSELROD, S., D. GORDON, F.A. HUBEL *et al.* 1981. Power spectrum analysis of heart rate fluctuations: a quantitative probe of beat to beat cardiovascular control. Science **213:** 220–222.
5. TASK FORCE OF THE EUROPEAN SOCIETY OF CARDIOLOGY AND THE NORTH AMERICAN SOCIETY OF PACING AND ELECTROPHYSIOLOGY. 1996. Heart rate variability: standards and measurement, physiological interpretation, and clinical use. Circulation **93:** 1043–1065.
6. CHESS, G.F., R.M.K. TAM & F.R. CALARESU. 1975. Influence of cardiac neural inputs on rhythmic variations of heart period in the cat. Am. J. Physiol. **228:** 775–780.
7. SELMAN, A., A. MCDONALD, R. KITNEY *et al.* 1982. The interaction between heart rate and respiration: part I—experimental studies in man. Automedica **4:** 131–139.
8. BERNARDI, L., B. BIANCHINI, G. SPADACINI *et al.* 1995. Demonstrable cardiac reinnervation after human heart transplantation by carotid baroreflex modulation of RR interval. Circulation **92:** 2895–2903.
9. SLEIGHT, P., M.T. LA ROVERE, A. MORTARA *et al.* 1995. Physiology and pathophysiology of heart rate and blood pressure variability in humans: is power spectral analysis largely an index of baroreflex gain? Clin. Sci. **88:** 103–109.
10. DE BOER, W., J.M. KAREMAKER & J. STRACKEE. 1987. Hemodynamic fluctuations and baroreflex sensitivity in humans: a beat-to-beat model. Am. J. Physiol. (Heart Circ. Physiol.) **253:** 680–689.
11. MONTANO, N., F. LOMBARDI, T. GNECCHI RUSCONE *et al.* 1992. Spectral analysis of sympathetic discharge, R-R interval, and systolic arterial pressure in decerebrate cats. J. Auton. Nerv. Syst. **40:** 21–32.
12. MONTANO, N., T. GNECCHI RUSCONE, A. PORTA *et al.* 1996. Presence of vasomotor and respiratory rhythms in the discharge of single medullary neurons involved in the regulation of cardiovascular system. J. Auton. Nerv. Syst. **57:** 116–122.
13. MONTANO, N., T. GNECCHI RUSCONE, A. PORTA *et al.* 1996 (August 25–29). Occurrence in the discharge of the isolated sympathetic spinal outflow of a rhythmicity in phase with vasomotor activity. XVIIIth Congress of the European Society of Cardiology (Birmingham, U.K.): no. P1035.
14. MALLIANI, A., F. LOMBARDI, M. PAGANI *et al.* 1975. Spinal cardiovascular reflexes. Brain Res. **87:** 239–246.
15. COOTE, J.H. 1988. The organization of cardiovascular neurons in the spinal cord. Rev. Physiol. Biochem. Pharmacol. **110:** 147–157.

16. SHERRINGTON, C.S. 1906. The Integrative Action of the Nervous System. Yale University Press. New Haven, CT.
17. BEACHAM, W.S. & E.R. PERL. 1964. Background and reflex discharge of sympathetic preganglionic neurons in the spinal cat. J. Physiol. **172:** 400–416.
18. FERNANDEZ DE MOLINA, A. & E.R. PERL. 1965. Sympathetic activity and the systemic circulation in the spinal cat. J. Physiol. (Lond.) **181:** 82–102.
19. KAMINSKI, R.J., G.A. MEYER & D.L. WINTER. 1970. Sympathetic unit activity associated with Mayer waves in the spinal dog. Am. J. Physiol. **219:** 1768–1771.
20. GUZZETTI, S., C. COGLIATI, C. BROGGI et al. 1994. Influences of neural mechanisms on heart period and arterial pressure variabilities in quadriplegic patients. Am. J. Physiol. **266:** H1112–H1120.
21. KOH, J., T.E. BROWN, L.A. BEIGHTOL et al. 1994. Human autonomic rhythms: vagal cardiac mechanisms in tetraplegic subjects. J. Physiol. (Lond.) **474:** 483–495.
22. MONTANO, N., C. COGLIATI, V.J. DIAS DA SILVA et al. 2000. Effects of spinal section and of a positive feedback excitatory reflex on sympathetic and heart rate variability. Hypertension **36:** 1029–1034.
23. SICA, A.L., B.W. HUNDLEY, D.A. RUGGIERO et al. 1997. Emergence of lung-inflation-related sympathetic nerve activity in spinal cord transected neonatal swine. Brain Res. **767:** 380–383.
24. BERNARDI, L., F. KELLER, M. SANDERS et al. 1989. Respiratory sinus arrhythmia in the denervated human heart. J. Appl. Physiol. **67:** 1447–1455.
25. RIMOLDI, O., S. PIERINI, A. FERRARI et al. 1990. Analysis of short-term oscillations of R-R and arterial pressure in conscious dogs. Am. J. Physiol. **258:** H967–H976.
26. PAGANI, M., V.K. SOMERS, R. FURLAN et al. 1988. Changes in autonomic regulation induced by physical training in mild hypertension. Hypertension **12:** 600–610.
27. IELLAMO, F., P. PIZZINELLI, M. MASSARO et al. 1999. Muscle metaboreflex contribution to sinus node regulation during static exercise: insights from spectral analysis of heart rate variability. Circulation **100:** 27–32.
28. COOLEY, R.L., N. MONTANO, C. COGLIATI et al. 1998. Evidence for a central origin of the low-frequency oscillation in RR interval variability. Circulation **98:** 556–561.
29. WALLIN, G. 1983. Intraneural recording and autonomic function in man. In Autonomic Failure, pp. 36–51. Oxford University Press. London/New York.
30. MARK, A.L., R.G. VICTOR, C. NERHED et al. 1985. Microneurographic studies of the mechanisms of sympathetic nerve responses to static exercise in humans. Circ. Res. **57:** 461–469.
31. ECKBERG, D.L., C. NERHED & B.C. WALLIN. 1985. Respiratory modulation of muscle sympathetic and vagal cardiac outflow in man. J. Physiol. (Lond.) **365:** 181–196.
32. SAUL, J.P., R.F. REA, D.L. ECKBERG et al. 1990. Heart rate and muscle sympathetic nerve variability during reflex changes of autonomic activity. Am. J. Physiol. **258:** H713–H721.
33. PAGANI, M., N. MONTANO, A. PORTA et al. 1997. Relationship between spectral components of cardiovascular variabilities and direct measures of muscle sympathetic nerve activity in humans. Circulation **95:** 1441–1448.
34. FURLAN, R., A. PORTA, F. COSTA et al. 2000. Oscillatory patterns in sympathetic neural discharge and cardiovascular variables during orthostatic stimulus. Circulation **101:** 886–892.
35. MALLIANI, A. 2000. Principles of Cardiovascular Neural Regulation in Health and Disease. Kluwer. Boston/Dordrecht/London.
36. MONTANO, N., C. COGLIATI, A. PORTA et al. 1998. Central vagotonic effects of atropine modulate spectral oscillations of sympathetic nerve activity. Circulation **98:** 1394–1399.

# Heterogeneous Receptor Distribution in Autonomic Neurons

SUE A. AICHER

*Oregon Health Sciences University, Neurological Sciences Institute,*
*Beaverton, Oregon 97006, USA*

ABSTRACT: The central nervous system components for baroreflex regulation of sympathetic outflow include specific sets of neurons in the brain and spinal cord. Critical nuclei containing sympathetic baroreceptive neurons are the nuclei of the solitary tract, regions of the caudal and rostral ventrolateral medulla, and the intermediolateral cell column in the spinal cord. While many other brain regions project to these nuclei, cells in these areas appear to form the minimal required pathway for baroreflex control of sympathetic outflow. Synaptic connections have been identified between cells in these nuclei that are consistent with a serial relay from baroreceptor afferents through the brain stem and to sympathetic preganglionic neurons in the spinal cord. In recent years, we have examined the distribution of receptor proteins in these neurons, with a focus on receptors that are most likely to modulate the activity of these cells. In three studies examining the distribution of different receptors on distinct neurons, each study found some type of heterogeneity in the distribution of each receptor within a particular type of neuron. This heterogeneity was seen with regard to the distribution of receptor protein within the dendritic tree of individual neurons, as well as between pre- and postsynaptic sites on the same cell. This heterogeneous distribution of receptors suggests that receptors undergo dendritic targeting within autonomic neurons. This receptor trafficking may be regulated by heterogeneous afferent input to autonomic neurons and could be changed under conditions where afferent activity is significantly altered.

KEYWORDS: Blood pressure; Cardiovascular; Electron microscopy; Ultrastructure; Opioid receptors; Glutamate receptors; Nucleus tractus solitarius; Intermediolateral cell column; Rostral ventrolateral medulla

## INTRODUCTION

The neurons that mediate the sympathoinhibitory effects of baroreceptor activation are located in at least three distinct regions of the medulla oblongata: (1) the nuclei of the solitary tract, which receive baroreceptive sensitive primary afferents; (2) the caudal ventrolateral medulla (CVL), which contains barosensitive GABAergic interneurons that project to the rostral ventrolateral medulla (RVL); and (3) the RVL, which contains adrenergic and nonadrenergic neurons that are sympatho-

Address for correspondence: Sue A. Aicher, Ph.D., Oregon Health Sciences University, Neurological Sciences Institute, 505 NW 185th Avenue, Beaverton, OR 97006. Voice: 503-418-2550; fax: 503-418-2501.
aichers@ohsu.edu

excitatory and project to sympathetic preganglionic neurons in the intermediolateral cell column (IML) of the spinal cord.[1–5] The net effect of activation of this reflex pathway following stretch of the baroreceptors in the periphery is a reduction in sympathetic outflow from the central nervous system, which leads to a fall in systemic blood pressure if the baroreceptor activation is of sufficient duration.

The anatomy and physiology of this baroreflex system have been extensively documented. The neurons that mediate baroreceptor reflex sympathoinhibition are regulated by a number of neurotransmitters, as well as exogenously applied chemicals, including glutamate and opioids.[6–8] However, little is known about the cellular distribution of receptor proteins in these cells. In several recent studies, we have examined the pre- and postsynaptic distribution of important receptor proteins in relation to neurons that are likely to mediate baroreceptive sympathoinhibition. All of these studies used dual immunogold and immunoperoxidase labeling to identify the following: (1) a particular cell group of interest and (2) a specific receptor protein.[9–12] This tissue was then examined by electron microscopy to determine the subcellular distribution of the receptor in relation to the cells of interest.

## NMDA RECEPTORS ARE LOCATED IN SOME DENDRITIC TARGETS OF ADRENERGIC TERMINALS IN THE SPINAL CORD

In the first study, we tested the hypothesis that NMDA receptors are located at sites that are postsynaptic to RVL terminals in the IML.[9] To identify RVL projections to the thoracic spinal cord, we used an antibody to phenylethanolamine-$N$-methyl-transferase (PNMT), the synthetic enzyme for epinephrine, which labels adrenergic terminals. The C1 adrenergic cells are a major sympathoexcitatory cell group in the medulla and they provide the adrenergic input to the thoracic spinal cord.[3,4] Therefore, PNMT-labeled terminals in the IML mainly arise from the RVL. To identify NMDA receptors, we used an antibody against the R1 subunit of the NMDA receptor since this subunit is required for functional channels to form.[13]

As part of the analysis, the spinal cord was sectioned in the horizontal plane for half of the animals and in the coronal plane for the other half of the animals. The basis for this approach was to test the hypothesis that the degree of receptor detection in the targets of axon terminals would differ if the cells were sectioned along the plane of the primary dendritic branches or across them (FIG. 1). It has been postulated that some preganglionic neurons, at least in the cat, are oriented primarily in the horizontal plane.[14] Therefore, we would hypothesize that the postsynaptic receptor would more likely be detected in horizontal spinal cord sections (FIG. 1). We found that, indeed, more of the dendritic targets of PNMT-containing axon terminals in the IML contained NMDA R1 receptor subunit if the spinal cord was sectioned horizontally than if it was sectioned coronally (FIG. 2).[9] Also, the dendrites were larger in the horizontally sectioned spinal cords (FIG. 2). Since the same population of axon terminals was being examined and labeling conditions were identical, this difference suggests two things: (a) the dendrites of sympathetic preganglionic neurons in the rat spinal cord that are contacted by PNMT terminals extend further in the horizontal plane than in the coronal plane of the spinal cord; and (b) because a greater area of the dendrites are viewed in the horizontal plane, we were more likely to detect the receptor in these dendrites. These results further suggest that there is selective tar-

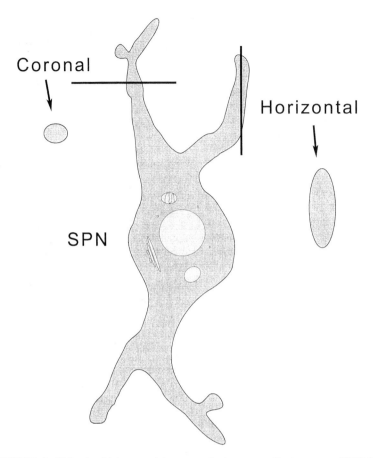

**FIGURE 1.** If the dendritic tree of the sympathetic preganglionic neuron (SPN) is oriented primarily in the horizontal plane of the spinal cord, coronal sections of spinal cord would often sample dendrites of these cells perpendicularly to their plane of orientation, while horizontal sections would sample more often along the long axis of dendrites. The experimental results found that, indeed, dendrites receiving PNMT afferents were larger in horizontal spinal cord sections than coronal spinal cord sections (see text and FIG. 2).

geting of NMDA receptors within the dendrites that are contacted by PNMT-containing terminals in the spinal cord. If receptors were randomly distributed within these cells and/or were very closely associated with PNMT terminals, the plane of section analyzed should not have been a factor. These results were our first indication that we can detect dendritic trafficking of receptors within specific groups of autonomic neurons.

The major assumption of these studies is that dendrite size at the electron microscopic level is related to the distance of the dendrite out on the dendritic tree (FIG. 3) or to the amount of branching seen in the cell. Using this type of analysis, we can

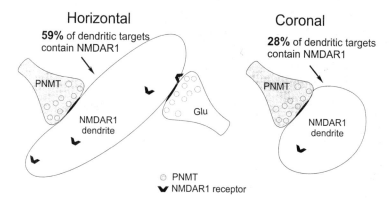

**FIGURE 2.** The likelihood of finding NMDA R1 receptor protein in dendritic targets of PNMT terminals was greater for spinal cords cut horizontally (59%) than for those cut coronally (28%), suggesting that these receptors are more closely associated with other excitatory afferents to these cells (possibly glutamatergic) and that these dendrites are more preferentially oriented in the horizontal plane of the spinal cord.

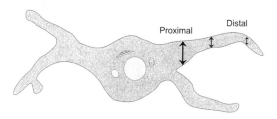

**FIGURE 3.** These experiments assume that the cross-sectional diameter of dendrites closer to the somata (proximal) is greater than the diameter of dendrites further away from the somata (distal).

determine if other receptors are differentially distributed within the dendrites of autonomic neurons and/or their afferents.

## OPIOID RECEPTORS ARE DIFFERENTIALLY DISTRIBUTED WITHIN RVL SYMPATHOEXCITATORY NEURONS

In another study, we examined the distribution of the μ-opioid receptor protein (MOR1) in C1 adrenergic neurons in the RVL. Both endogenous and exogenous opioids are known to regulate blood pressure and sympathetic outflow,[15,16] and the RVL sympathoexcitatory neurons are a major autonomic target of these ligands.[17,18] This study again used an antibody against PNMT to detect adrenergic neurons in the RVL and an antibody directed against the cloned μ-opioid receptor, MOR1. We found MOR1 in the dendrites of C1 adrenergic neurons in the RVL, but it was preferentially

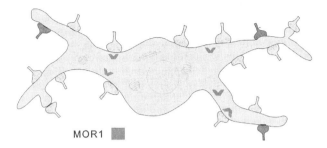

MOR1 ■

**FIGURE 4.** Schematic summary of two studies showing that postsynaptic MOR1 is found in larger dendrites of RVL neurons, while presynaptic MOR1 profiles contact more distal dendrites.

detected in larger dendrites.[11] We also found MOR1 in axons and axon terminals contacting adrenergic dendrites. Interestingly, the profiles containing presynaptic MOR1 were preferentially apposed to smaller PNMT-containing dendrites that did not contain postsynaptic MOR1.[11] These results indicate that there is a targeting of MOR1 within adrenergic neurons, as well as within specific afferents that contact these neurons (FIG. 4). It is possible that postsynaptic MOR1 is associated with select sets of afferents that target proximal portions of C1 neurons, such as afferents from the CVL,[19] and that presynaptic MOR1 is associated with afferents that target more distal C1 dendrites, such as afferents from the NTS.[19] While the source of these MOR1 afferents remains to be determined, these results clearly show that there is selective targeting of the same receptor to distinct pre- and postsynaptic sites within a population of chemically homogeneous neurons.

In a second experiment to address whether there is actually heterogeneous receptor distribution within individual baroreceptive neurons, we used a method to label single neurons that were functionally characterized[20] and then examined the receptor distribution within these neurons using immunogold-labeling methods. The cell labeling was conducted in collaboration with Drs. Patrice Guyenet and Ann Schreihofer at the University of Virginia and the ultrastructural analyses were conducted in collaboration with Dr. Teresa Milner at the Weill Medical College of Cornell University. In these studies, we were able to demonstrate that, within individual neurons, some dendrites contained MOR1 labeling, while others did not.[12] Also, there was a trend for the receptor-containing dendrites to be larger than dendrites that received MOR1-labeled afferents. This pattern of distribution was similar to what we had seen with large populations of C1 adrenergic neurons in the RVL. Therefore, a heterogeneous receptor distribution could be demonstrated in individual neurons with known baroreceptive function.

In a previous study, we noted that there was a topographic organization to the projections from two other brain stem autonomic regions, the NTS and the CVL, onto C1 adrenergic RVL neurons.[19] CVL afferents are more likely to contact the somata and proximal dendrites of C1 RVL neurons, while NTS afferents are more likely to contact distal dendrites of C1 cells. We hypothesize then that these two types of afferents may be differentially regulated by ligands of the μ-opioid receptor.

## SUMMARY

The studies described have shown that receptor protein is distributed in a heterogeneous manner within C1 neurons, their afferents, and their dendritic targets in the spinal cord. It is likely that a similar heterogeneity exists for presynaptic receptor modulation of other afferents to these and other baroreceptive neurons. Our data support the notion that receptor trafficking is regulated within these neurons, but the mechanisms for this regulation are not known. It remains to be determined if this receptor trafficking is coupled to selective afferent innervation of autonomic neurons and whether changes in afferent activity may lead to alterations in postsynaptic receptor distribution.

## ACKNOWLEDGMENTS

This work was supported by an Established Investigator Award from the American Heart Association and by NIH Grant No. HL56301. I thank Aarti Patel, Sarita Sharma, James Kraus, and Alla Goldberg for technical assistance. I would also like to thank Ida Llewellyn-Smith, whose comments on previous studies inspired the comparison of horizontal and coronal spinal cord sections. The experiments described were conducted while I was at the Weill Medical College of Cornell University.

## REFERENCES

1. CHALMERS, J. & P. PILOWSKY. 1991. Brainstem and bulbospinal neurotransmitter systems in the control of blood pressure. J. Hypertens. 9: 675–694.
2. SPYER, K.M. 1994. Central nervous mechanisms contributing to cardiovascular control. J. Physiol. (Lond.) 474: 1–19.
3. REIS, D.J., S. MORRISON & D.A. RUGGIERO. 1988. The C1 area of the brain stem in tonic and reflex control of blood pressure. Hypertension 11: I8–I13.
4. RUGGIERO, D.A., S.L. CRAVO, E. GOLANOV et al. 1994. Adrenergic and non-adrenergic spinal projections of a cardiovascular-active pressor area of medulla oblongata: quantitative topographic analysis. Brain Res. 663: 107–120.
5. AICHER, S.A., T.A. MILNER, V.M. PICKEL & D.J. REIS. 2000. Anatomical substrates for baroreflex sympathoinhibition. Brain Res. Bull. 51: 107–110.
6. SUN, M.K. 1996. Pharmacology of reticulospinal vasomotor neurons in cardiovascular regulation. Pharmacol. Rev. 48: 465–494.
7. MATSUMURA, K., I. ABE, M. TOMINAGA et al. 1992. Differential modulation by μ- and δ-opioids on baroreceptor reflex in conscious rabbits. Hypertension 19: 648–652.
8. MORRISON, S.F., J. CALLAWAY, T.A. MILNER & D.J. REIS. 1991. Rostral ventrolateral medulla: a source of the glutamatergic innervation of the sympathetic intermediolateral nucleus. Brain Res. 562: 126–135.
9. AICHER, S.A., B-I. HAHN & T.A. MILNER. 2000. N-Methyl-D-aspartate-type glutamate receptors are found in post-synaptic targets of adrenergic terminals in the thoracic spinal cord. Brain Res. 856: 1–11.
10. AICHER, S.A., A. GOLDBERG, S. SHARMA & V.M. PICKEL. 2000. μ-Opioid receptors are present in vagal afferents and their dendritic targets in the medial nucleus tractus solitarius. J. Comp. Neurol. 422: 181–190.
11. AICHER, S.A., J.A. KRAUS, S. SHARMA et al. 2001. Selective distribution of μ-opioid receptors in C1 adrenergic neurons and their afferents. J. Comp. Neurol. 433: 23–33.

12. AICHER, S.A., A.M. SCHREIHOFER, J.A. KRAUS et al. 2001. μ-Opioid receptors are present in functionally identified sympathoexcitatory neurons in the rat rostral ventrolateral medulla. J. Comp. Neurol. **433:** 34–47.
13. HOLLMANN, M. & S. HEINEMANN. 1994. Cloned glutamate receptors. Annu. Rev. Neurosci. **17:** 31–108.
14. MORGAN, C.W., W.C. DE GROAT, L.A. FELKINS & S-J. ZHANG. 1993. Intracellular injection of neurobiotin or horseradish peroxidase reveals separate types of preganglionic neurons in the sacral parasympathetic nucleus of the cat. J. Comp. Neurol. **331:** 161–182.
15. HASSEN, A.H., G. FEUERSTEIN & A.I. FADEN. 1982. μ receptors and opioid cardiovascular effects in the NTS of rat. Peptides **3:** 1031–1037.
16. WILLETTE, R.N., A.J. KRIEGER & H.N. SAPRU. 1982. Blood pressure and splanchnic nerve activity are reduced by a vagally mediated opioid action. J. Cardiovasc. Pharmacol. **4:** 1006–1011.
17. HAYAR, A. & P.G. GUYENET. 1998. Pre- and postsynaptic inhibitory actions of methionine-enkephalin on identified bulbospinal neurons of the rat RVL. J. Neurophysiol. **80:** 2003–2014.
18. BARABAN, S.C., R.L. STORNETTA & P.G. GUYENET. 1995. Effects of morphine and morphine withdrawal on adrenergic neurons of the rat rostral ventrolateral medulla. Brain Res. **676:** 245–257.
19. AICHER, S.A., R.H. SARAVAY, S.L. CRAVO et al. 1996. Monosynaptic projections from the nucleus tractus solitarii to C1 adrenergic neurons in the rostral ventrolateral medulla: comparison with input from the caudal ventrolateral medulla. J. Comp. Neurol. **373:** 62–75.
20. SCHREIHOFER, A.M. & P.G. GUYENET. 1997. Identification of C1 presympathetic neurons in rat rostral ventrolateral medulla by juxtacellular labeling in vivo. J. Comp. Neurol. **387:** 524–536.

# Integrative Sympathetic Baroreflex Regulation of Arterial Pressure

KENJI SUNAGAWA,[a,b] TAKAYUKI SATO,[c] AND TORU KAWADA[b]

[b]The National Cardiovascular Center Research Institute, Osaka 5658565, Japan

[c]Department of Physiology II, Kochi Medical School, Nankoku, Kochi, Japan

ABSTRACT: The baroreflex system is the most important negative feedback control system functioning physiologically to attenuate the effects of rapid perturbation in arterial pressure. However, the complexity of the system resulting from the closed-feedback loop, nonlinearity, and system memory makes detailed quantitative characterization of the baroreflex system difficult. To overcome such limitations, we proposed a framework to decompose the baroreflex loop into two major arcs, that is, the mechanoneural arc and neuromechanical arc. Steady state analysis indicated that such decomposition allowed us to analytically determine the operating point by equilibrating two respective function curves. Dynamic analysis suggested that the mechanoneural arc accelerated the slow mechanical response of the neuromechanical arc. The acceleration mechanism in the mechanoneural arc optimized arterial pressure regulation in achieving both stability and quickness. Establishment of such an integrative framework allowed the development of an artificial feedback control system able to regulate sympathetic vasomotor tone.

KEYWORDS: Baroreflex; Transfer function; Bionic baroreflex system

## INTRODUCTION

The baroreflex system is the most important negative feedback control system functioning physiologically to attenuate the effects of rapid perturbation in arterial pressure. For instance, the change in arterial pressure induced by a postural change is sensed by arterial baroreceptors located within the walls of the aortic arch and the internal carotid arteries. This fall in pressure is neurally encoded and relayed via afferent pathways to a brain stem vasomotor center, and it then immediately causes an appropriate degree of compensatory vasoconstriction through the activation of efferent sympathetic pathways. Without such compensation, even the simple act of standing would cause a significant fall in arterial pressure and potentially the loss of consciousness. Furthermore, it is well known that many cardiovascular diseases involve baroreflex dysfunction. Therefore, it is important clinically as well as physiologically to understand the characteristics of the baroreflex system. However, the complexity of the system resulting from the closed-feedback loop, nonlinearity, and system memory makes detailed quantitative analyses difficult. To overcome such

[a]Address for correspondence: Kenji Sunagawa, The National Cardiovascular Center Research Institute, 5-7-1 Fujishirodai, Suita, Osaka 5658565, Japan. Voice: +81-6-6833-5012, ext. 2509; fax: +81-6-6872-7485.

sunagawa@ri.ncvc.go.jp

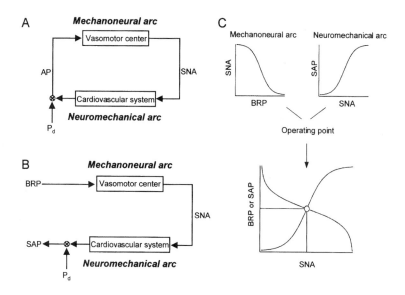

**FIGURE 1.** Sympathetic arterial baroreflex system in closed-loop (**A**) and open-loop (**B**) conditions. Pd indicates external disturbance to arterial pressure (AP). In open-loop condition, the relationship between baroreceptor pressure (BRP) and sympathetic nerve activity (SNA) and that between SNA and systemic arterial pressure (SAP) can be measured quantitatively. When the two curves characterizing the two relationships are plotted on an equilibrium diagram, the intersection of the two curves is the operating point of AP and SNA under closed-loop conditions of the feedback system (**C**). (Reproduced from reference 1 with permission of the authors and publisher.)

limitations, we recently developed a framework to decompose the baroreflex loop into two major arcs, that is, the mechanoneural arc and neuromechanical arc.[1,2] Decomposition of the total arc into the major arcs provided a platform to determine analytically the operating point[1] and to predict numerically the dynamic behavior[2] of the baroreflex system. Establishment of such a conceptual platform allowed the development of an artificial feedback control system able automatically to regulate sympathetic vasomotor tone.[3]

## ANALYTICAL FRAMEWORK FOR UNDERSTANDING STEADY STATE SYMPATHETIC BAROREFLEX CONTROL OF ARTERIAL PRESSURE

Earlier studies have revealed the baroreceptor-mediated control of sympathetic nerve activity[4] and the sympathetic control of heart rate and cardiovascular mechanics.[5,6] However, an analytical approach for identifying an operating point of the arterial baroreflex has not been developed. Such an approach is needed for an integrative understanding of the mechanism by which the arterial pressure at the operating point is determined under the closed-loop condition of the feedback system. To overcome such limitations, we developed a framework to decompose the baroreflex loop into two major arcs, that is, the mechanoneural arc and neuromechanical arc.[1]

FIGURE 1A is a simplified diagram representing the characteristics of the sympathetic arterial baroreflex system. Disturbance in arterial pressure is immediately sensed by arterial baroreceptors. The vasomotor center responsively modifies its command over sympathetic vasomotor nerve activity (SNA). Sympathetic nerve activity governs heart rate and the mechanical properties of the heart and vessels, which themselves exert direct influence over systemic arterial pressure (SAP). This circulatory nature of the baroreflex feedback system makes it difficult to characterize analytically the system behavior. To overcome this problem, we opened the feedback loop and divided the system into a controlling element and controlled element (FIG. 1B). We denoted the controlling element as a mechanoneural arc and the controlled element as the neuromechanical arc. In the mechanoneural arc, the input is pressure-sensed by the arterial baroreceptors and the output is sympathetic nerve activity. In the neuromechanical arc, the input is sympathetic nerve activity and the output is arterial pressure. They are positively correlated as shown in the top right panel of FIGURE 1C. Because the variables characterizing the functions of the two arcs are common, we superimposed the two curves and analytically identified the operating point, that is, the point defined by the arterial pressure and sympathetic nerve activity under the closed-loop conditions of the feedback system, as an intersection between them on an equilibrium diagram (FIG. 1C). We examined the validity of this framework in animal experiments.

In anesthetized, vagotomized rats, we characterized the mechanoneural arc and neuromechanical arc under open-loop conditions and predicted the closed-loop equilibrium (operating-point) pressure. Shown in FIGURE 2A is a representative example of original tracings of carotid sinus pressure, sympathetic nerve activity, and arterial pressure. The responses of sympathetic nerve activity and arterial pressure to a given level of carotid sinus pressure were remarkably consistent and reproducible throughout the one-hour recording protocol. The fact that arterial pressure appears to be a mirror image of carotid sinus pressure indicates that the arterial baroreflex is a negative feedback system. FIGURES 2B and 2C display the relationship between carotid sinus pressure and sympathetic nerve activity and that between sympathetic nerve activity and arterial pressure of the example. Both curves characterizing the mechanoneural and neuromechanical arcs were sigmoidal and could be well described by the four-parameter logistic equation models. We obtained the equilibrium operating-point pressures by superimposing two function curves (FIG. 2D). Predicted operating-point pressures by this framework were then compared against the equilibrium pressures under the closed-loop condition. The predicted pressures highly correlated with the measured pressures ($y = 0.99x + 1.1$, $r = 0.99$, SEE = 2.4 mmHg).

This analytical framework provides unique views of the integrative characteristics of steady state baroreflex responses. In particular, its ability to separate the set-point pressure from the operating-point pressure should be emphasized. According to the feedback control theory, sympathetic nerve activity would be totally deactivated should arterial pressure equal the set-point pressure. In the engineering term, this is called the reference signal. As can be seen in FIGURE 2B, sympathetic nerve activity becomes very low at the arterial pressure of 160 mmHg, indicating that the set-

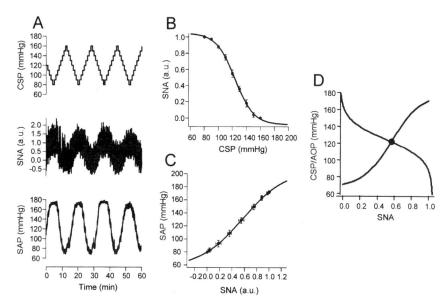

**FIGURE 2.** Original tracings of carotid sinus pressure (CSP), sympathetic nerve activity (SNA), and systemic arterial pressure (SAP) in baseline state (**A**), and graphs showing the relationship between CSP and SNA (**B**) and between SNA and SAP (**C**). Values in B and C: mean ± SD. (Reproduced from reference 1 with permission of the authors and publisher.)

point pressure is about 160 mmHg. However, the operating-point pressure is about 120 mmHg, which is much lower than the set-point pressure. The difference between the set-point pressure and operating-point pressure is determined by the total feedback loop gain. This is to say that the gain of the baroreflex loop is not high enough to match the operating-point pressure to the set-point pressure. Since the total loop gain is the product of the slopes of two curves, the gain changes with the operating pressure, as does the capacity of attenuating pressure disturbances.

This framework could explain a mechanism of the determination of the operating point of the sympathetic baroreflex system under steady state conditions. However, in the feedback system, dynamic characteristics determine system stability and quickness. Hence, we evaluated the dynamic characteristics of both the mechano-neural arc and neuromechanical arc.

## DYNAMIC CHARACTERISTICS OF THE BAROREFLEX SYSTEM AND ITS PHYSIOLOGICAL ROLE

In the negative feedback system, closed-loop behavior is determined not only by the total loop gain, but also by its dynamic characteristics. The dynamic system characteristics govern the stability of the system and the quickness of its responses. Because the output of the baroreflex system depends not only on the instantaneous input, but also on the history of the input change,[7,8] we cannot thoroughly characterize the system properties unless we analyze its dynamic properties. In the baroreflex regulation of systemic arterial pressure, the regulatory signal passes quickly through the mechanoneural arc, whereas changes in pressure resulting from the effector response through the neuromechanical arc occur rather slowly because the change in systemic arterial pressure involves multiple mechanical responses at the efferent nerve–effector junction. These responses comprise vascular resistance,[4] vascular unstressed volume,[5] heart rate, and ventricular contractility. Because quick and stable control of systemic arterial pressure is crucial, we hypothesized that the mechanoneural arc compensates for the slow mechanical responses of the neuro-mechanical arc, thereby improving the quality of SAP regulation.

In anesthetized, vagotomized rabbits, we isolated the carotid sinuses bilaterally. To evaluate the dynamic characteristics of the baroreflex system, according to a Gaussian white-noise technique,[9] we altered intrasinus pressure randomly and rapidly. We then estimated the transfer function from carotid sinus pressure to sympathetic nerve activity characterizing the mechanoneural arc and that from sympathetic nerve activity to arterial pressure characterizing the neuromechanical arc.[2] The transfer function is a well-established measure used to represent the frequency-dependent characteristics and thereby the dynamic characteristics of the system. The transfer function from input $x$ to output $y$ was estimated with a fast Fourier transform algorithm (FFT). We obtained ensembled autospectrum of $x$ and the cross-spectrum between the two through the FFT. Taking the ratio of the cross-spectrum to the auto-spectrum yields the transfer function. It represents the input-output relation of a given system over the frequencies of interest.

The left panel of FIGURE 3 shows the average transfer function of the mechano-neural arc. The modulus of the mechanoneural arc transfer function was fairly constant below 0.1 Hz. It increased above that frequency up to 1 Hz. The gain increased

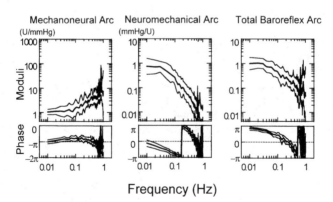

Frequency (Hz)

**FIGURE 3.** Average transfer functions of mechanoneural arc (**left**), neuromechanical arc (**middle**), and total baroreflex arc (**right**) from 12 rabbits. The *bold line* and two *thin lines* indicate mean and SD. *Top*: Modulus of transfer function indicating gain from input to output. Gain increases with frequencies in the mechanoneural arc (left). Gain decreases with frequencies in the neuromechanical and total baroreflex arcs (middle and right). *Bottom*: Phase shift from input to output. Phase of mechanoneural arc and that of total arc are predominantly out of phase, indicating the properties of a negative feedback system. (Reproduced from reference 2 with permission of the authors and publisher.)

with frequencies, indicating the derivative nature of the mechanoneural arc. The estimated slope of the modulus curve between 0.1 and 1 Hz was 6.1 ± 0.06 dB/octave. The phase of the mechanoneural arc was nearly out of phase over a wide frequency range. The features of the transfer function resemble a first-order high-pass filter with a lag time. The middle panel of FIGURE 3 shows the transfer function of the neuromechanical arc. The modulus of the transfer function was fairly constant below 0.07 Hz and decreased at >0.07 Hz. The estimated slope of the modulus curve between 0.1 and 1 Hz was −11 ± 1.48 dB/octave. The phase was in phase in the low-frequency range and increasingly delayed in the high-frequency range. The phase was out of phase at 0.2 Hz. The observed characteristics of the transfer function approximated a second-order low-pass filter with a lag time. The right panel of FIGURE 3 shows the transfer function of the total baroreflex loop. The modulus at the lowest frequency, which approximates the steady state baroreflex gain, was 1.04 ± 0.68. The modulus of the transfer function was reasonably constant below 0.05 Hz and decreased above 0.05 Hz. The slope of the modulus curve between 0.1 and 1 Hz was −6.01 ± 0.9 dB/octave, approximating the first-order low-pass filter. Although the modulus contours of the total baroreflex loop and the neuromechanical arc transfer functions approximate low-pass filter characteristics, the slope of the former was significantly less than that of the latter in the high-frequency range. This is because the high-pass filter characteristics of the mechanoneural arc significantly compensated for the steep negative slope of the neuromechanical arc transfer function. The mechanoneural arc quickened the response of the systemic arterial pressure.

    Increasing the gain of the baroreflex in the high-frequency range certainly accelerates the response in systemic arterial pressure under open-loop conditions. Under closed-loop conditions, however, too much acceleration could result in

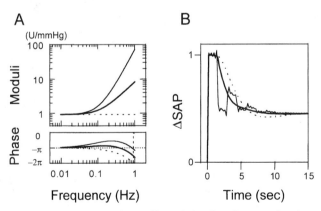

**FIGURE 4.** Simulation study of the effect of the changing transfer characteristics of the mechanoneural arc on the closed-loop response to a step pressure perturbation. Elimination of the high-pass filter characteristics significantly slowed the response to a step change in arterial pressure (*dotted line* in A and B). Doubling the order of high-pass filter characteristics (*thin line* in A and B) quickened response time to a step pressure change but resulted in oscillation of arterial pressure, indicating instability of the system. (Reproduced from reference 2 with permission of the authors and publisher).

instability in pressure regulation. Therefore, to examine the physiological implication of the acceleration of the mechanoneural arc, we simulated the closed-loop
arterial pressure regulation to an exogenous step pressure perturbation while altering
the dynamic characteristics of the mechanoneural arc. FIGURE 4 shows the effect of
changes in acceleration on the pressure response to the step exogenous perturbation.
The corner frequency of the transfer function of the mechanoneural arc was unchanged. We changed the slope from 0 to 12 dB/octave. The native system (bold line
in FIG. 4A) with characteristics of a first-order high-pass filter gave a steady state
pressure response that was approximately one-half the amplitude of pressure perturbation (bold line in FIG. 4B). The time required to reach 50% of the steady state
response was $2.71 \pm 0.64$ s. When we eliminated the high-pass filter characteristics
from the mechanoneural arc (dotted line in FIG. 4A), the response time was significantly prolonged by 50% ($4.1 \pm 1.52$ s) (dotted line in FIG. 4B). When we doubled
the slope of the modulus of the transfer function (thin line in FIG. 4A), the pressure
response became oscillatory, indicating the instability of the system (thin line in
FIG. 4B). Thus, the native characteristics of the mechanoneural arc were fairly
optimal in achieving quickness and stability in regulating arterial blood pressure.

## A BIONIC BAROREFLEX SYSTEM

The success of the detailed characterization of the baroreflex system led us to develop an intelligent neural prosthesis that restores the normal baroreflex function in
patients with central baroreflex failure.[3] Patients with neurological disorders such as
Shy-Drager syndrome,[10] baroreceptor deafferentiation,[11] and traumatic spinal cord
injuries[12] present central baroreflex failure and a severely impaired quality of life as
a consequence. In such patients, peripheral sympathetic neurons have the potential
to release norepinephrine in response to direct electrical stimuli. Unfortunately,
although various interventions such as salt loading, cardiac pacing, and adrenergic
agonists have been used to treat orthostatic hypotension, most patients nevertheless
remain bedridden for an extensive period. To rescue those patients, we attempted
functional replacement of the vasomotor center with a bionic baroreflex system in a
rat model of central baroreflex failure
A simplified diagram representing the characteristics of the native baroreflex
system is provided in FIGURE 5A. In the native baroreflex system, change in arterial
pressure (SAP) induced by external disturbance in pressure (Pd) is sensed by arterial
baroreceptors. The change in pressure initiates a reflex change in vasomotor sympathetic outflow and is accordingly buffered. The primary reflex center is located in the
brain stem. In the bionic baroreflex system (FIG. 5B), a micromanometer functions
as the baroreceptor, a computer as the vasomotor center, and an electrical stimulator
as the preganglionic sympathetic neuron. On the basis of measured changes in
arterial pressure, the artificial vasomotor center executes real-time operations that
determine the frequency of the electrical stimulation necessary for compensatory
adjustment of arterial pressure to the desired level and then commands an electrical
stimulator to deliver a stimulus of the same frequency to a sympathetic vasomotor
nerve. To enable the bionic baroreflex system to mimic the functioning of the native
baroreflex system, it is necessary to quantitatively identify the operating rule that
underlies native baroreflex function and to implant it into the bionic baroreflex sys-

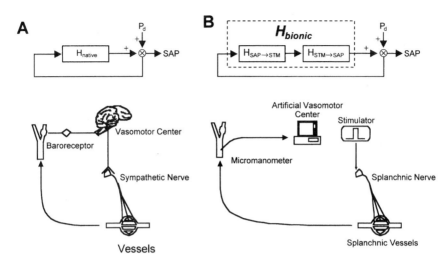

**FIGURE 5.** Block diagrams of native **(A)** and bionic **(B)** baroreflex systems. In the native baroreflex system, change in arterial pressure (SAP) induced by external disturbance in pressure (Pd) is sensed by arterial baroreceptors. The change in pressure initiates a reflex change in vasomotor sympathetic outflow and is thereby buffered. The primary reflex center is located in the brain stem. In the bionic baroreflex system, a catheter-tipped micromanometer functions as the baroreceptor, a computer as the vasomotor center, and an electrical simulator (STM) as the preganglionic sympathetic neuron. $H_{NATIVE}$ denotes the open-loop transfer function of the native baroreflex system. $H_{SAP-STM}$ and $H_{STM-SAP}$ are open-loop transfer functions from SAP to STM and from STM to SAP, respectively. Overall open-loop transfer function of bionic baroreflex system is given by $H_{SAP-STM} \times H_{STM-SAP}$. (Reproduced from reference 3 with permission of the authors and publisher.)

tem. Thus, we first analyzed under open-loop conditions the input-output relation characterizing native baroreflex function ($H_{NATIVE}$) by using a white-noise identification method.[9] We then identified the open-loop transfer function ($H_{STM-SAP}$) from electrical stimulation to systemic arterial pressure. Finally, we determined the open-loop transfer function required for the artificial vasomotor center of the bionic baroreflex system, that is, $H_{SAP-STM}$, by a simple process of division, namely, $H_{NATIVE}/H_{STM-SAP}$. The transfer function $H_{SAP-STM}$ represents the operating rule characterizing quantitatively the dynamics of how the artificial vasomotor center should operate in its stimulation of the sympathetic vasomotor nerve to mimic the native baroreflex. We chose celiac ganglia as the site of sympathetic efferent stimulation.

The significance of our investigation is most readily demonstrated by the representative example shown in FIGURE 6A, where we evaluated the performance of the bionic baroreflex system in response to rapid progressive hypotension secondary to sudden sympathetic withdrawal in an anesthetized, vagotomized rat. Sensing the rapid fall in systemic arterial pressure, the bionic baroreflex system automatically computed stimulation frequency and appropriately stimulated the sympathetic nerve to prevent systemic arterial pressure from falling >25% in 10 s. FIGURE 6B summarizes the results obtained for 16 rats, demonstrating the effectiveness of bionic

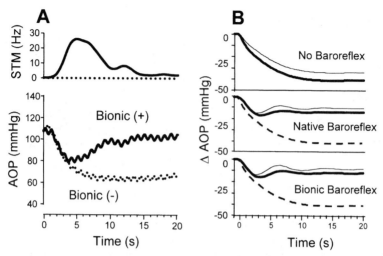

**FIGURE 6.** Efficacy of bionic baroreflex system during rapid progressive hypotension induced by sudden sympathetic withdrawal. Sympathetic withdrawal was evoked by increasing carotid sinus pressure to ~160 mmHg. **(A)** Representative example of on-line real-time operation of bionic baroreflex system. While sensing changes in arterial pressure (AOP), the bionic baroreflex system automatically computed the frequency of stimulation (STM) of the greater splanchnic nerve and drove a stimulator. When the bionic baroreflex system was inactive, AOP fell rapidly and severely. **(B)** Time courses of changes in AOP. Data are expressed by mean (*solid line* ± SD [*broken lines*]) for 16 rats. For comparison, mean data during no baroreflex are also shown by *dotted lines*. When no baroreflex system was active, AOP fell monotonically and reached a minimum in 10 s. On the other hand, when native baroreflex was active, AOP reached a nadir in 5 s and then increased to a plateau. A similar time course of AOP change by the native baroreflex system was well reproduced by the bionic baroreflex system. (Modified from reference 3 with permission of the authors and publisher.)

baroreflex system performance in buffering systemic arterial pressure fall in response to sympathetic withdrawal. With normal operation of the native baroreflex prevented and without bionic compensation (no baroreflex), arterial pressure fell by $49 \pm 8$ mmHg in 10 s in response to sympathetic withdrawal. However, with the bionic baroreflex system placed on-line with real-time execution (bionic baroreflex), the arterial pressure fall was suppressed by $22 \pm 6$ mmHg at the nadir and by $16 \pm 5$ mmHg at the plateau. These effects were statistically indistinguishable from those of the native baroreflex system. The bionic baroreflex system indeed reproduced the native baroreflex in a model of central baroreflex failure.

## LIMITATIONS

There are some limitations in the presented studies. Because we bilaterally cut the vagal nerves in all studies, the effect of the vagal system was not included. Although the baroreflex modulation of systemic arterial pressure is likely to be predominantly regulated through the sympathetic nervous system, the dynamic as well as static properties of the baroreflex system might be different when vagally mediated effects on the heart rate are present. Further examination concerning the vagal contribution remains to be investigated. Anesthetic agents used in the present study could also affect the baroreflex properties. Further examination concerning how the anesthesia affects the baroreflex should be performed in the conscious condition. Therefore, our results should be interpreted carefully.

## CONCLUSIONS

The baroreflex system is the most important negative feedback control system functioning physiologically to attenuate the effects of rapid perturbation in arterial pressure. However, the complexity of the system resulting from the closed-feedback loop, nonlinearity, and system memory makes detailed quantitative characterization difficult. To overcome such limitations, we proposed a framework to decompose the baroreflex loop into two major arcs, that is, the mechanoneural arc and neuro-mechanical arc. Decomposition of the total arc into the major arcs provided a platform to determine the operating point and numerically predict the dynamic behavior of the baroreflex system analytically. Establishment of such an integrative framework led us to develop an artificial feedback control system able automatically to regulate sympathetic vasomotor tone, that is, a bionic baroreflex system.

## REFERENCES

1. SATO, T., T. KAWADA, M. INAGAKI *et al.* 1999. New analytic framework for understanding sympathetic baroreflex control of arterial pressure. Am. J. Physiol. **276:** H2251–H2261.
2. IKEDA, Y., T. KAWADA, M. SUGIMACHI *et al.* 1996. Neural arc of baroreflex optimizes dynamic pressure regulation in achieving both stability and quickness. Am. J. Physiol. **271:** H882–H890.
3. SATO, T., T. KAWADA, T. SHISHIDO *et al.* 2000. Novel therapeutic strategy against central baroreflex failure: a bionic baroreflex system. Circulation **100:** 299–304.
4. DIBONA, G.F., S.Y. JONES & V.L. BROOKS. 1995. ANG II receptor blockade and arterial baroreflex regulation of renal nerve activity in cardiac failure. Am. J. Physiol. **269:** R1189–R1196.
5. CARNEIRO, J.J. & D.E. DONALD. 1977. Blood reservoir function of dog spleen, liver, and intestine. Am. J. Physiol. **232:** H67–H72.
6. SHOUKAS, A.A. & K. SAGAWA. 1973. Control of total systemic vascular capacity by the carotid sinus baroreceptor reflex. Circ. Res. **33:** 22–33.
7. KUBOTA, T., J. ALEXANDER, JR., R. ITAYA *et al.* 1992. Dynamic effects of carotid sinus baroreflex on ventriculoarterial coupling studied in anesthetized dogs. Circ. Res. **70:** 1044–1053.
8. SUGIMACHI, M., T. IMAIZUMI, K. SUNAGAWA *et al.* 1990. A new method to identify dynamic transduction properties of aortic baroreceptors. Am. J. Physiol. **258:** H887–H895.
9. MARMARELIS, P.Z. & V.Z. MARMARELIS. 1978. Analysis of Physiological Systems: The White-Noise Approach. Plenum. New York.
10. SHY, M. & G.A. DRAGER. 1960. A neurological syndrome associated with orthostatic hypotension: a clinico-pathologic study. Arch. Neurol. **3:** 511–527.
11. LEE, H.T., J. BROUN & W.E. FEE, JR. 1997. Baroreflex dysfunction after nasopharyngectomy and bilateral carotid isolation. Arch. Otolaryngol. Head Neck Surg. **123:** 434–437.
12. MATTHEWS, J.M., G.D. WHEELER, R.S. BURNHAM *et al.* 1997. The effects of surface anesthesia on the autonomic dysreflexia response during functional electrical stimulation. Spinal Cord **35:** 647–651.

# Central Baroreflex Resetting as a Means of Increasing and Decreasing Sympathetic Outflow and Arterial Pressure

STEPHEN E. DiCARLO[a] AND VERNON S. BISHOP[b]

[a]Wayne State University School of Medicine, Detroit, Michigan 48201, USA

[b]The University of Texas Health Science Center at San Antonio, San Antonio, Texas 78339-3900, USA

ABSTRACT: The arterial baroreflex has two important functions. First, the arterial baroreflex is a negative feedback reflex that regulates arterial pressure around a preset value called a set or operating point. Second, the arterial baroreflex also establishes the prevailing systemic arterial pressure when the operating point is reset. That is, modulating the response of barosensitive neurons in the central nervous system (CNS) establishes the operating point or prevailing systemic arterial pressure. Therefore, the operating point of the arterial baroreflex is not fixed, but is variable over a wide range of pressures and is determined by a variety of inputs from the peripheral and central nervous systems. At the onset of dynamic exercise, heart rate (HR) and sympathetic nerve activity (SNA) increase abruptly and dramatically. The initial increase in HR and SNA is mediated by central command. Central command operates by resetting the operating point of the arterial baroreflex to a higher pressure. In this situation, the operating point of the arterial baroreflex is above the prevailing arterial pressure, which elicits a blood pressure error. This error is corrected by activating SNA and inhibiting parasympathetic nerve activity, which increases cardiac output and peripheral resistance and, consequently, arterial pressure. After exercise, loss of central command and enhanced activity of the cardiopulmonary reflex resets the operating point of the arterial baroreflex to a lower pressure. In this situation, the operating point of the arterial baroreflex is below the prevailing arterial pressure, which elicits a blood pressure error. This error is corrected by inhibiting SNA, which decreases peripheral resistance and consequently arterial pressure. In these situations, central resetting of the arterial baroreflex is a means of increasing and decreasing sympathetic outflow and arterial pressure.

KEYWORDS: Autonomic nervous system; Exercise; Post-exercise hypotension; Hypotension

The autonomic and cardiovascular responses to both isometric and dynamic exercise have been studied for many years.[1,2] Although it is well established that there are striking differences in the hemodynamics and autonomic responses to these two

Address for correspondence: Stephen E. DiCarlo, Ph.D., Department of Physiology, 6213 Scott Hall, 540 E. Canfield Avenue, Detroit, Michigan 48201–1928. Voice: 313-577-1557; fax: 313-577-5494.

sdicarlo@med.wayne.edu

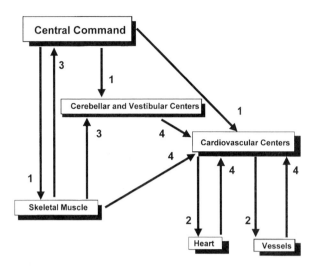

**FIGURE 1.** Model of the proposed mechanisms responsible for the initiation and integration of the autonomic response during whole-body dynamic exercise. At the onset of exercise, central command sends a motor program to the cerebellar and vestibular centers and simultaneously activates skeletal muscle to produce movement and cardiovascular centers to increase heart rate and arterial pressure (1). The cardiovascular centers, acting via the autonomic nervous system, increases heart rate and arterial pressure (2). The quality and intensity of movement is sent back to central command and the cerebellar and vestibular systems so that adjustments in the motor program can be made (3) (i.e., the movement matches the program). Signals from the heart (cardiopulmonary receptors), blood vessels (arterial baroreceptors), muscles (muscle metaboreceptors), and cerebellar and vestibular systems modify the cardiovascular responses (4) so that the intensity of muscle movement is matched by cardiovascular responses. (From DiCarlo and Bishop.[48] Reprinted by permission.)

forms of muscle activation, authors often draw conclusions concerning autonomic control during dynamic exercise from data obtained from both forms of exercise.[2] This is inappropriate since it has led to generalizations that do not pertain to whole-body dynamic exercise. Therefore, this discussion will focus on the autonomic mechanisms involved with whole-body dynamic exercise in man, dog, rabbit, and rat.

FIGURE 1 presents a model of the proposed mechanisms responsible for the initiation and integration of the autonomic response during whole-body dynamic exercise. At the onset of exercise, central command sends a motor program to the cerebellar and vestibular centers and simultaneously activates skeletal muscle to produce movement and cardiovascular centers to increase heart rate (HR) and arterial pressure (1). The cardiovascular centers, acting via the autonomic nervous system, increases HR and arterial pressure (2). The quality and intensity of movement is sent back to central command and the cerebellar and vestibular systems so that adjustments in the motor program can be made (3) (i.e., the movement matches the program). Signals from the heart (cardiopulmonary receptors), blood vessels (arterial baroreceptors), muscles (muscle metaboreceptors), and cerebellar and vestibular system modify the cardiovascular responses (4) so that the intensity of muscle movement is matched by cardiovascular responses.

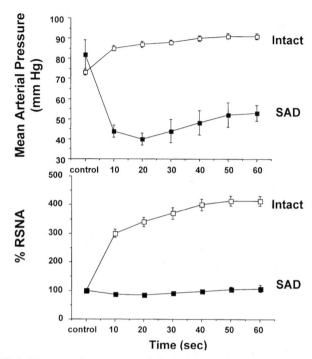

**FIGURE 2.** Mean arterial pressure and renal sympathetic nerve activity (RSNA) before and during the first 60 seconds of dynamic exercise in intact and SAD rabbits. SAD converted the sympathoexcitatory responses to inhibitory responses at the onset of exercise. These results suggest that central command operates through the arterial baroreflex. SAD = sinoaortic-denervated. (Modified by permission from DiCarlo and Bishop.[5])

Central command is the concept of a feed-forward parallel, simultaneous activation of neuronal circuits that control cardiovascular and motor function. However, the anatomic description of central command is not well defined. Specifically, direct action of higher centers (signals originating from the brain rostral to the circulatory control areas in the medulla) descend or "irradiate" onto the motor centers to initiate movement and simultaneously onto the cardiovascular centers to regulate sympathetic and parasympathetic activity to the heart and blood vessels.[1,3,4] In this context, cardiovascular function is increased simultaneously with the onset of activity. Furthermore, central command continues to mediate the autonomic responses during exercise via its role in muscle recruitment.

Central command may be operating through the arterial baroreflex.[5] This conclusion is based on experimental evidence documenting that the pressor response at the onset of exercise is attenuated in sinoaortic-denervated (SAD) dogs.[6,7] Furthermore in the absence of functional arterial baroreceptors, the onset of exercise is characterized by reductions in arterial pressure, HR, and sympathetic nerve activity (SNA) in SAD rabbits.[5,8] For example, FIGURE 2 presents arterial pressure and SNA before and during the first 60 seconds of dynamic exercise in intact and SAD rabbits. SAD converted the sympatho-excitatory responses to inhibitory responses at the onset of exercise. These results suggest that central command operates through the arterial baroreflex. If central command operated independently of the arterial baroreflex, one would expect an exaggerated increase in arterial pressure and SNA at the onset of exercise in SAD rabbits. Instead arterial pressure and SNA fell markedly at the onset of dynamic exercise and did not recover to control levels during the period of exercise, indicating that functional arterial baroreflexes are required for the sympatho-excitatory response at the onset of exercise.[5]

Ludbrook and Potocnik[9] also reported that arterial baroreflexes are required during spontaneous motor activity in rabbits. The normal small increases in arterial pressure and HR associated with spontaneous motor activity (postural changes, exploration, grooming, eating) changed to sharp decreases of these variables after SAD. Sharp decreases in arterial pressure occurring with behavioral activity after SAD have been reported in the rabbit,[10] dog,[11] and cat.[12] These results suggest that the arterial baroreflex facilitates rapid increases in arterial pressure and HR in response to a variety of forms of everyday activity.[9] These results in the rabbit are consistent with earlier results in the dog. For example, Walgenbach and Donald[13] recorded arterial pressure during graded exercise in SAD dogs. At the onset of exercise, arterial pressure fell and did not recover to pre-exercise levels in SAD dogs.

The studies cited above document that functional arterial baroreceptors are required for the sympatho-excitatory responses at the onset of exercise. However, these results present an apparent paradox. The arterial baroreflex functions as a short-term, negative feedback regulator of arterial pressure. An increased arterial pressure elicits an arterial baroreflex-mediated bradycardia and sympatho-inhibition that compensates for the elevation in pressure. Conversely, a decreased arterial pressure elicits an arterial baroreflex-mediated tachycardia and sympatho-excitation that compensates for the decrease in pressure. It is apparent, however, that there are situations when both arterial pressure and HR increase simultaneously (i.e., dynamic exercise).[14,15] This apparent paradox (simultaneous increase in HR and arterial pressure) may be explained by a resetting of the operating point (pressure sought by the reflex) of the arterial baroreflex to a higher pressure.[5,14,16–20] That is, the operating point of the baroreflex is shifted to a higher pressure so that the reflex now operates (considers "normal") around the new higher pressure.

What evidence exists that demonstrates that central command mediates the sympatho-excitatory response at the onset of exercise by shifting the operating point of the arterial baroreflex towards higher pressures? We tested the hypothesis that the operating point of the arterial baroreflex is shifted toward higher pressures at the onset of exercise and that the magnitude of the exercise pressor response and the increase in SNA is determined by the extent of the shift of the operating point.[5] A delay in the exercise pressor response would increase SNA, whereas an increase in the rate of development of the exercise pressor response would attenuate the increase in SNA. The approach involved recording renal sympathetic nerve activity (RSNA), arterial pressure, and HR before and during 60 seconds of treadmill running under control conditions (when arterial pressure was allowed to increase normally) and when the exercise pressor response was attenuated by an intravenous infusion of nitroglycerin (NTG). When the exercise response was attenuated by intravenous infusions of NTG, RSNA significantly increased above the control run, presumably to

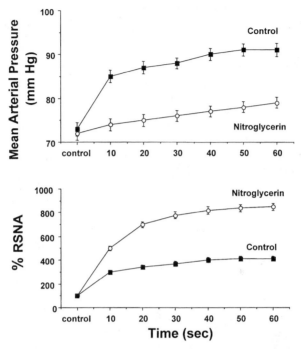

**FIGURE 3.** Relationship between mean arterial pressure and renal sympathetic nerve activity (RSNA) vs. time during the onset of exercise. Control curve represents normal response. Nitroglycerin curve illustrates response when initial rate and magnitude of increase in blood pressure were delayed with intravenous infusions of nitroglycerin. When the blood pressure response was attenuated by intravenous infusions of nitroglycerin, RSNA significantly increased above the control run, presumably to raise MAP to some preset value. (From DiCarlo and Bishop.[5] Reprinted by permission.)

raise blood pressure to some preset value (FIG. 3). These data suggest that the baroreflex is reset upward during exercise, thus contributing to the cardiovascular adjustments required to match the metabolic requirements.

Additional support for arterial baroreflex resetting is provided in an interesting set of experiments by Walgenbach and Donald.[13] These investigators surgically denervated the aortic baroreceptors, then fixed carotid sinus pressure at the pre-exercise level. Preventing the carotid baroreceptors from responding to the stress of exercise by vascular isolation and exposure to a static pressure resulted in an immediate decrease in arterial pressure at the onset of exercise. However, hypertension developed during exercise which was maintained throughout the 5-min recovery period. The authors concluded that the carotid baroreflex acts to offset the decrease in arterial pressure at the start of exercise. Furthermore, these results are consistent with the concept that during exercise the operating point of the baroreflex is shifted to a higher pressure and thus permits the arterial pressure to increase with exercise. Similarly, Ludbrook and Graham[8] have shown that at the onset of exercise in the rabbit, despite

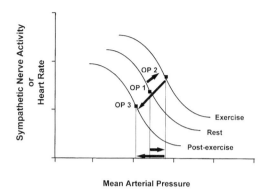

**FIGURE 4.** Proposed model illustrating arterial baroreflex resetting during and after exercise. The arterial baroreflex is a negative feedback reflex that regulates arterial pressure around a preset value called the operating point (OP 1). The arterial baroreflex also establishes the prevailing arterial pressure when the operating point is reset. At the onset of exercise, central command resets the operating point to a higher pressure (OP 2). This upward resetting mediates the simultaneous increase in arterial pressure and sympathetic nerve activity. After exercise, loss of central command may result in a downward resetting of the operating point (OP3) to a pressure below the resting operating point (OP 1). This downward resetting mediates the simultaneous decrease in arterial pressure and sympathetic nerve activity.

an increase in mean arterial pressure (MAP; 22 mmHg), the tonic depressor effects of the baroreceptors were suppressed rather than enhanced. The investigators concluded that the operating point of the reflex rose faster than did the arterial pressure. These data are consistent with the hypothesis that at the onset of exercise, central command resets the operating point of the arterial baroreflex and mediates the simultaneous increase in arterial pressure and SNA (FIG. 4).

Arterial baroreflex resetting may occur centrally at the nucleus tractus solitarius (NTS) by modulating the response of barosensitive neurons.[5,21–25] Central command may reduce the sensitivity of NTS neurons (FIG. 5A) and thus reduce the responses to arterial baroreceptor input (FIG. 5B). Once the sensitivity is reduced, there is a reduced NTS activity for any given arterial baroreceptor input (FIG. 5B). The reduced NTS activity may reset the operating point of the arterial baroreflex to a higher pressure (FIG. 5C).

These results document that the arterial baroreflex has two important functions. First, the arterial baroreflex is a negative feedback reflex that regulates arterial pressure around a preset value called a set or operating point. Second, the arterial baroreflex also establishes the prevailing systemic arterial pressure when the operating point is reset.[26] That is, modulating the response of barosensitive neurons in the CNS establishes the operating point or prevailing systemic arterial pressure.[5,21] Therefore, the operating point of the arterial baroreflex is not fixed, but is variable over a wide range of pressures and is determined by a variety of inputs from the peripheral and central nervous systems.[26]

Resetting of the operating point of the arterial baroreflex to a lower pressure may be responsible for the post-exercise reduction in sympathetic outflow and arterial

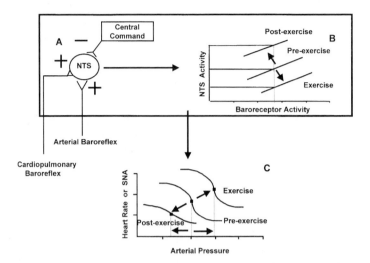

**FIGURE 5.** Schematic representation suggesting that the operating point of the arterial baroreflex can be shifted to higher or lower pressures. Arterial baroreflex resetting may occur centrally at the nucleus tractus solitarius (NTS) by modulating the response of barosensitive neurons. Central command may reduce the sensitivity of NTS neurons (**A**). Once the sensitivity is reduced, there is a reduced NTS activity for any given arterial baroreceptor input (**B**). The reduced NTS activity may reset the operating point of the arterial baroreflex to a higher pressure (**C**). After exercise, the operating point of the arterial baroreflex is shifted to a lower pressure. Sensitization of barosensitive neurons may be mediated by a post-exercise facilitation of inhibitory cardiopulmonary reflexes. Once sensitized, there is an increased NTS activity for any given arterial baroreceptor input (**B**). Enhanced NTS activity resets the operating point of the arterial baroreflex to a lower pressure (**C**). Downward resetting of the arterial baroreflex would account for the hypotension, sympathoinhibition and absence of reflex tachycardia that occurs following a single bout of dynamic exercise. (Modified with permission from Bishop and Mifflin.[21])

pressure (FIG. 4). The best model available to test this hypothesis may be the spontaneous hypertensive rat (SHR), because the SHR has exaggerated post-exercise responses.[23,27–34] For example, FIGURE 6 presents mean arterial pressure before, during, and after exercise (panel A) and lumbar sympathetic nerve activity (LSNA) before and after exercise (panel B) in the SHR. After exercise both mean arterial pressure and LSNA were reduced below the pre-exercise level.[32] Similarly, after exercise, HR and cardiac sympathetic tonus were reduced below the pre-exercise level.[27] These results suggest that the operating point of the arterial baroreflex may have been lowered after exercise since a reduction in arterial pressure should elicit an arterial baroreflex-mediated increase in HR and SNA. If this hypothesis is correct, then removal of the arterial baroreflex should prevent the hypotension and sympatho-inhibition that occurs following acute exercise. To address this question, post-exercise autonomic responses were measured in sinoaortic-denervated (SAD) and intact hypertensive rats. FIGURE 7 presents arterial pressure and cardiac sympathetic tonus before (no-exercise) and after exercise (post-exercise) in intact and SAD hypertensive rats. After exercise, both arterial pressure and cardiac sympathetic tonus

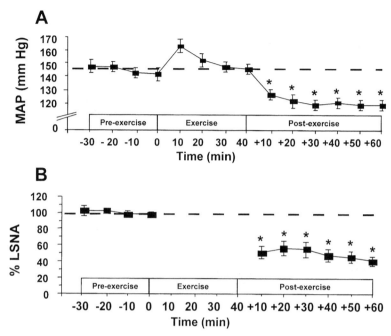

**FIGURE 6.** Mean arterial pressure (MAP) before, during, and after exercise (**A**) and lumbar sympathetic nerve activity (LSNA) before and after exercise (**B**) in the SHR. After exercise both MAP and LSNA were reduced below the pre-exercise level. These results suggest that the arterial baroreflex may have been altered after exercise since a reduction in arterial pressure should elicit an arterial baroreflex-mediated increase in SNA. (From Kulics et al.[32] Reprinted by permission.)

were reduced below pre-exercise levels in intact rats. However, SAD prevented post-exercise reductions in arterial pressure and cardiac sympathetic tonus. These results demonstrate that the arterial baroreflex is required for post-exercise reductions in arterial pressure and cardiac sympathetic tonus in the SHR.

Recent evidence supports the concept that a single bout of dynamic exercise shifts the operating point of the arterial baroreflex to a lower pressure.[23,28,35–37] Halliwill and colleagues[36] reported significant reductions in baseline muscle sympathetic nerve activity (MSNA) which was associated with a downward shift of the SNA-arterial pressure relationship after a single bout of dynamic exercise. Similarly, Hara and Floras[37] reported that the arterial baroreflex control of MSNA was preserved after treadmill exercise at 70% of HR reserve in normotensive men, but was shifted to a lower operating point (reset).

In addition to the importance of arterial baroreceptor afferent activity in resetting the operating point of the arterial baroreflex, other sensory afferents may also contribute. In some instances, certain afferent input may act to enhance the upward resetting, while in other cases, afferent input may cause a resetting of the operating point to lower pressures.[24,25,31,38–40] Indeed, in rabbits, daily exercise increases the inhibitory influence of cardiopulmonary afferents on heart rate, blood pressure, and

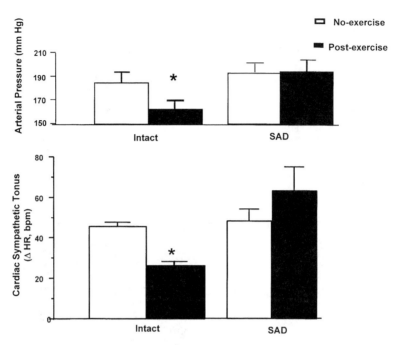

**FIGURE 7.** Arterial pressure and cardiac sympathetic tonus before (no-exercise) and after exercise (post-exercise) in intact and sinoaortic-denervated (SAD) hypertensive rats. After exercise, arterial pressure and cardiac sympathetic tonus were reduced below pre-exercise levels in intact rats. However, SAD prevented post-exercise reductions in arterial pressure and cardiac sympathetic tonus. These results demonstrate that the arterial baroreflex is required for post-exercise reductions in arterial pressure and cardiac sympathetic tonus in SHR. (Modified with permission from Chandler and DiCarlo.[23])

sympathetic outflow.[41,42] Furthermore, daily exercise blunted the upward resetting of the operating point of the arterial baroreflex during exercise by enhancing the cardiopulmonary baroreflex. Blockade of cardiac afferents restored the upward resetting of the operating point to that observed prior to daily exercise.[43]

Similarly, the cardiopulmonary reflex may contribute to post-exercise resetting of the arterial baroreflex. Several studies have demonstrated that a single bout of dynamic exercise enhances the inhibitory influence of the cardiopulmonary reflex on the sympathetic nervous system. For example, mild exercise (30 minutes of upright exercise on a cycle ergometer at 50% of $VO_2$ max) induced a sustained (3 hours) post-exercise reduction in systolic ($-9 \pm 2$ mmHg) and diastolic ($-4 \pm 2$ mmHg) blood pressure in individuals with hypertension.[44] The authors concluded that an exercise-induced reduction in blood pressure was primarily the result of cardiopulmonary baroreflex inhibition of peripheral vascular resistance.[35] Similarly, the effect of blocking cardiac afferent receptors on the post-exercise-induced reduction in arterial pressure was examined in the SHR. In this study, cardiac afferent blockade prevented post-exercise hypotension. With cardiac afferents intact, post-exercise mean arterial pressure (MAP) decreased ($-29 \pm 5$ mmHg) below the pre-exercise level. Blockade of the cardiac efferents did not affect the post-exercise hypotensive response ($-26 \pm$ 4 mmHg). However, combined cardiac efferent and afferent blockade attenuated the post-exercise fall in MAP ($-7 \pm 4$ mmHg).[31] In addition, Bennett and colleagues[45] examined forearm vascular resistance response to lower body subatmospheric pressure (LBSP) before and after exercise. LBSP unloads (reduces the stimulation of) the cardiopulmonary baroreceptors by causing venous pooling. The investigators reported a greater increase in forearm vascular resistance during LBSP after exercise, suggesting that cardiopulmonary receptors exert a greater inhibitory influence on the vasculature after exercise. Finally, in conscious SAD dogs, Daskalopoulos and colleagues[46] demonstrated that the cardiopulmonary baroreflex is responsible for decreasing systemic vascular resistance after exercise. These data suggest that the inhibitory influence of cardiac afferents on the circulation may be enhanced after exercise.

These studies are consistent with the following model (Fig. 4). At the onset of exercise, central command resets the operating point of the arterial baroreflex to a higher pressure. This resetting mediates the simultaneous increase in arterial pressure and sympathetic nerve activity. After exercise, loss of central command and enhanced activity of the cardiopulmonary reflex results in a downward resetting of the operating point of the arterial baroreflex below the original operating point. This resetting mediates the simultaneous post-exercise decrease in arterial pressure and SNA.

To test this hypothesis, we examined the relationship between arterial pressure and HR before and after a single bout of dynamic exercise in SHR.[28] After exercise both arterial pressure and HR were reduced below pre-exercise levels. Furthermore, the range, the pressure at the midpoint of the pressure range, the HR at the midpoint of the HR range, the minimum and maximum HR, and the gain of the arterial baroreflex control of HR were reduced after exercise (Fig. 8). These data suggest that post-

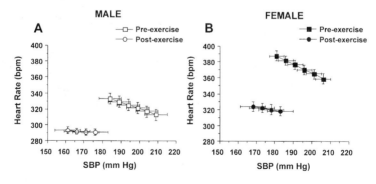

**FIGURE 8.** Group means for the arterial baroreflex regulation of heart rate in a pre-exercise and post-exercise period for male (**A**) and female (**B**) SHR. Absolute data were plotted as group means to determine the relationship between systolic blood pressure and heart rate. After a single bout of dynamic exercise, the arterial baroreflex function curve was shifted downwards and to the left, and this shift was accompanied by a reduction in the range, maximum, and gain in both male and female SHR. (Modified with permission from Chandler et al.[28])

exercise reductions in arterial pressure are mediated by both a reduction in gain and a resetting of the operating point of the arterial baroreflex to a lower pressure.

Arterial baroreceptor resetting may occur centrally at the nucleus tractus solitarius (NTS) as a result of sensitization of barosensitive neurons (FIG. 5A).[28] Sensitization of barosensitive neurons could be mediated by a post-exercise facilitation of inhibitory cardiopulmonary reflexes, since cardiac afferent blockade attenuated the hypotensive effect of a single bout of dynamic exercise,[31] and other investigators have shown that the influence of inhibitory cardiac afferents on the circulation may be enhanced after exercise.[44,45] Alternatively, muscle afferents may sensitize NTS neurons since Shyu and colleagues[39] have shown post-stimulatory hypotension after sciatic nerve stimulation and muscle afferents synapse in the NTS.[40] Once sensitized, there is an increased NTS activity for any given arterial baroreceptor input (FIG. 5B). The enhanced NTS activity resets the operating point of the arterial baroreflex to a lower pressure (FIG. 5B). Resetting of the arterial baroreflex would account for the hypotension, sympathoinhibition and absence of reflex tachycardia that occurs following a single bout of dynamic exercise (FIG. 7).

## SUMMARY

At the onset of dynamic exercise, HR and SNA increase abruptly and dramatically. The initial increase in HR is due to withdrawal of tonic parasympathetic activity mediated by the feedforward influence of central command. Similarly, the initial increase in SNA is mediated by central command. Furthermore, central command continues to mediate the autonomic responses during exercise via its role in muscle recruitment. Central command appears to operate by resetting the operating point of the arterial baroreflex to a higher pressure. In this situation, the operating point of the arterial baroreflex is above the prevailing arterial pressure, which elicits a blood pressure error. This error is corrected by activating SNA and inhibiting parasympathetic activity, which increases cardiac output and peripheral resistance and consequently arterial pressure. The arterial baroreflex also monitors and corrects any change in arterial pressure induced by increases in body temperature (cutaneous vasodilation) or other stressors. After exercise loss of central command and enhanced activity of the cardiopulmonary reflex resets the operating point of the arterial baroreflex to a lower pressure. In this situation, the operating point of the arterial baroreflex is below the prevailing arterial pressure, which elicits a blood pressure error. This error is corrected by inhibiting SNA and activating parasympathetic activity, which decreases peripheral resistance and consequently arterial pressure. In these situations, central resetting of the arterial baroreflex is a means of increasing or decreasing sympathetic outflow and arterial pressure.[47,48]

## REFERENCES

1. KROGH, A. & J. LINDHARD. 1913. The regulation of respiration and circulation during the initial stages of muscular work. J. Physiol. (London) 51: 59–90.
2. MITCHELL, J.H. & P.B. RAVEN. 1994. Cardiovascular response and adaptation to exercise. In Physical Activity, Fitness, and Health: International Proceedings and Con-

sensus Statement. C. Couchard, R. Shepherd & T. Stephens, Eds. Human Kinetics Publishers. Champaign, IL

3. ROWELL, L.B. 1980. What signals govern the cardiovascular responses to exercise? Med. Sci. Sports Exerc. **12:** 307–315.

4. WALDROP, T.G., F.L. ELDRIDGE, G.A. IWAMOTO & J.H. MITCHELL. 1996. Central neural control of respiration and circulaiton during exercise. *In* Exercise: Regulation and Integration of Multiple Systems. L.B. Rowell & J.T. Shepherd, Eds. American Physiological Society. Bethesda, MD.

5. DICARLO, S.E. & V.S. BISHOP. 1992. Onset of exercise shifts operating point of arterial baroreflex to higher pressures. Am. J. Physiol. Heart Circ. Physiol. **262:** H303–307.

6. KRASNEY, J.A., M.G. LEVITZKY & R.C. KOEHLER. 1974. Sinoaortic contribution to the adjustment of systemic resistance in exercising dogs. J. Appl. Physiol. **36:** 679–685.

7. ARDELL, J.L., A.M. SCHER & L.B. ROWELL. 1980. Effects of baroreceptor denervation on the cardiovascular response to dynamic exercise. *In* Arterial Baroreceptors and Hypertension. Peter Sleight, Ed. Oxford University Press. Oxford, UK

8. LUDBROOK, J. & W.F. GRAHAM. 1985. Circulatory responses to onset of exercise: role of arterial and cardiac baroreflexes. Am. J. Physiol. Heart Circ. Physiol. **248:** H457–H467.

9. LUDBROOK, J. & S.J. POTOCNIK. 1986. Circulatory changes during spontaneous motor activity: role of arterial baroreflexes. Am. J. Physiol. Heart Circ. Physiol. **250:** H426–H433.

10. ALEXANDER, N. & M. DECUIR. 1966. Low arterial pressure in awake rabbits without carotid sinus and aortic nerves. Proc. Soc. Exp. Biol. Med. **121:** 766–769.

11. COWLEY, A.W., JR., J.F. LIARD & A.C. GUYTON. 1973. Role of baroreceptor reflex in daily control of arterial blood pressure and other variables in dogs. Circ. Res. **32:** 564–576.

12. BACCELLI, G., R. ALBERTINI, A. DEL BO, *et al.* 1981. Role of sinoaortic reflexes in hemodynamic patterns of natural defense behaviors in the cat. Am. J. Physiol. **240:** H421–H429.

13. WALGENBACH, S.C. & D.E. DONALD. 1983. Inhibition by carotid baroreflex of exercise-induced increases in arterial pressure. Circ. Res. **52:** 253–262.

14. POTTS, J.T., X.R. SHI & P.B. RAVEN. 1993. Carotid baroreflex responsiveness during dynamic exercise in humans. Am. J. Physiol. Heart Circ. Physiol. **265:** H1928–H1938.

15. ROWELL, L.B., D.S. O'LEARY & D.L. KELLOGG, JR. 1996. Integration of the cardiovascular control systems in dynamic exercise. *In* Handbook of Physiology. Exercise: Regulation and Integration of Multiple Systems. L.B. Rowell & J.T. Shepherd, Eds. American Physiological Society. Bethesda, MD.

16. MELCHER, A. & D.E. DONALD. 1981. Maintained ability of carotid baroreflex to regulate arterial pressure during exercise. Am. J. Physiol. Heart Circ. Physiol. **241:** H838–H849.

17. O'LEARY, D.S. 1996. Heart rate control during exercise by baroreceptors and skeletal muscle afferents. Med. Sci. Sports Exerc. **28:** 210–217.

18. O'LEARY, D.S. & D.P. SEAMANS. 1993. Effect of exercise on autonomic mechanisms of baroreflex control of heart rate. J. Appl. Physiol. **75:** 2251–2257.

19. ROWELL, L.B. & D.S. O'LEARY. 1990. Reflex control of the circulation during exercise: chemoreflexes and mechanoreflexes. J. Appl. Physiol. **69:** 407–418.

20. PAPELIER, Y., P. ESCOURROU, J.P. GAUTHIER & L.B. ROWELL. 1994. Carotid baroreflex control of blood pressure and heart rate in men during dynamic exercise. J. Appl. Physiol. **77:** 502–506.

21. BISHOP, V.S. & S.W. MIFFLIN. 1992. Central neural mechanism in the cardiovascular response to exercise. *In* Central Neural Mechanisms of Cardiovascular Regulation. J. Ciriello & G. Kunos, Eds. Springer Verlag/Birkhauser. Berlin.

22. BISHOP, V.S. 1994. Carotid baroreflex control of blood pressure and heart rate in men during dynamic exercise [editorial]. J. Appl. Physiol. **77:** 491–492.

23. CHANDLER, M.P. & S.E. DICARLO. 1997. Sinoaortic denervation prevents postexercise reductions in arterial pressure and cardiac sympathetic tonus. Am. J. Physiol. Heart Circ. Physiol. **273:** H2734–H2745.

24. POTTS, J.T., G.A. HAND, J. LI & J.H. MITCHELL. 1998. Central interaction between carotid baroreceptors and skeletal muscle receptors inhibits sympathoexcitation. J. Appl. Physiol. **84:** 1158–1165.
25. POTTS, J.T. & J. LI. 1998. Interaction between carotid baroreflex and exercise pressor reflex depends on baroreceptor afferent input. Am. J. Physiol. Heart Circ. Physiol. **274:** H1841–H1847.
26. SAGAWA, K. 1983. Baroreflex control of the systemic arterial pressure and vascular bed. *In* Handbook of Physiology. The Cardiovascular System. Peripheral Circulation and Organ Blood Flow. J.T. Shepherd and F.M. Abboud, Eds. American Physiological Society. Bethesda, MD.
27. CHANDLER, M.P. & S.E. DICARLO. 1998. Acute exercise and gender alter cardiac autonomic tonus differently in hypertensive and normotensive rats. Am. J. Physiol. Reg. Integ. Comp. Physiol. **274:** R510–R516.
28. CHANDLER, M.P., D.W. RODENBAUGH & S.E. DICARLO. 1998. Arterial baroreflex resetting mediates postexercise reductions in arterial pressure and heart rate. Am. J. Physiol. Heart Circ.Physiol. **275:** H1627–H1634.
29. CHEN, Y., M.P. CHANDLER & S.E. DICARLO. 1995. Acute exercise attenuates cardiac autonomic regulation in hypertensive rats. Hypertension **26:** 676–683.
30. CHEN, Y., M.P. CHANDLER & S.E. DICARLO. 1997. Daily exercise and gender influence postexercise cardiac autonomic responses in hypertensive rats. Am. J. Physiol. Heart Circ. Physiol. **272:** H1412–H1418.
31. COLLINS, H.L. & S.E. DICARLO. 1993. Attenuation of postexertional hypotension by cardiac afferent blockade. Am. J. Physiol. Heart Circ. Physiol. **265:** H1179–H1183.
32. KULICS, J.M., H.L. COLLINS & S.E. DICARLO. 1999. Postexercise hypotension is mediated by reductions in sympathetic nerve activity. Am. J. Physiol. Heart Circ. Physiol. **276:** H27–H32.
33. OVERTON, J.M., M.J. JOYNER & C.M. TIPTON. 1988. Reductions in blood pressure after acute exercise by hypertensive rats. J. Appl. Physiol. **64:** 748–752.
34. DICARLO, S.E., H.L. COLLINS, M.G. HOWARD, *et al.* 1994. Postexertional hypotension: a brief review. Sports Med. Training Rehab. **5:** 17–27.
35. CLÉROUX, J., A. KOUAMÉ, A. NADEAU, *et al.* 1992. Baroreflex regulation of forearm vascular resistance after exercise in hypertensive and normotensive humans. Am. J. Physiol. Heart Circ. Physiol. **263:** H1523–H1531.
36. HALLIWILL, J.R., J.A. TAYLOR & D.L. ECKBERG. 1996. Impaired sympathetic vascular regulation in humans after acute dynamic exercise. J.Physiol. **495:** 279–288.
37. HARA, K. & J.S. FLORAS. 1992. Effects of naloxone on hemodynamics and sympathetic activity after exercise. J. Appl. Physiol. **73:** 2028–2035.
38. DICARLO, S.E. & V.S. BISHOP. 1988. Exercise training attenuates baroreflex regulation of nerve activity in rabbits. Am. J. Physiol. Heart Circ. Physiol. **255:** H974–H979.
39. SHYU, B.C., S.A. ANDERSSON & P. THOREN. 1984. Circulatory depression following low frequency stimulation of the sciatic nerve in anesthetized rats. Acta Physiol. Scand. **121:** 97–102.
40. TONEY, G.M. & S.W. MIFFLIN. 1994. Time-dependent inhibition of hindlimb somatic afferent inputs to nucleus tractus solitarius. J. Neurophysiol. **72:** 63–71.
41. DICARLO, S.E. & V.S. BISHOP. 1990. Regional vascular resistance during exercise: role of cardiac afferents and exercise training. Am. J. Physiol. **258:** H842–H847.
42. DICARLO, S.E. & V.S. BISHOP. 1990. Exercise training augments cardiac afferents inhibition of baroreflex function in conscious rabbits. Am. J. Physiol. Heart Circ. Physiol. **258:** H212–H220.
43. DICARLO, S.E., L.K. STAHL & V.S. BISHOP. 1997. Daily exercise attenuates the sympathetic nerve response to exercise by enhancing cardiac afferents. Am. J. Physiol. Heart Circ. Physiol. **273:** H1606–H1610.
44. CLÉROUX, J., N. KOUAMÉ, A. NADEAU, *et al.* 1992. Aftereffects of exercise on regional and systemic hemodynamics in hypertension. Hypertension **19:** 183–191.
45. BENNETT, T., R.G. WILCOX & I.A. MACDONALD. 1984. Post-exercise reduction of blood pressure in hypertensive men is not due to acute impairment of baroreflex function. Clin. Sci. **67:** 97–103.

46. DASKALOPOULOS, D.A., J.T. SHEPHERD & S.C. WALGENBACH. 1984. Cardiopulmonary reflexes and blood pressure in exercising sinoaortic-denervated dogs. J. Appl. Physiol. **57:** 1417–1421.
47. BISHOP, V.S. & S.E. DICARLO. 1994. Role of vagal afferents in cardiovascular control. *In* Vagal Control of the Heart: Experimental Basis and Clinical Implications. M.N. Levy & P.J. Schwartz, Eds. Futura Publishing Co. Mount Kisco, NY.
48. DICARLO, S.E. & V.S. BISHOP. 1999. Exercise and the autonomic nervous system. *In* Handbook of Clinical Neurology: The Autonomic Nervous System. Part 1. Normal Functions. O. Appenzeller, Ed. Elsevier. New York.

# Effects of Exercise Training on Baroreflex Control of the Cardiovascular System

EDUARDO MOACYR KRIEGER,[a] GUSTAVO JOSÉ JUSTO DA SILVA,[a] AND CARLOS EDUARDO NEGRÃO[b]

[a]Unit of Hypertension, Heart Institute (InCor), Medical School, University of São Paulo, São Paulo, Brazil

[b]Unit of Cardiovascular Rehabilitation and Exercise Physiology, Heart Institute (InCor), Medical School, and Laboratory of Exercise Physiology, School of Physical Education and Sports, University of São Paulo, São Paulo, Brazil

ABSTRACT: Dynamic exercise training has been recommended as an antihypertensive therapy and as a way to modify the effects of many cardiovascular risk factors (Arakawa, 1993; Arroll and Beaglehole, 1992; Kelly and McClellan, 1994: see references 1–3 in the paper). However, the mechanisms underlying the blood-pressure lowering effect of chronic exercise are still poorly understood. It has been suggested that a decrease in sympathetic tone is one of the major effects elicited by chronic exercise on the cardiovascular system. The importance of the sympathetic component is confirmed in this review, since it was found that in spontaneously hypertensive rats (SHR) a marked decrease in sympathetic activity occurred after exercise training. Moreover, our findings suggest that this effect is mediated by improving the depressed baroreceptor function, which is, in part, responsible for the attenuation of the baroreflex sensitivity observed in the sedentary SHR (Krieger et al., 1998, 1999; see references 4 and 5 in the paper).

KEYWORDS: Baroreceptor reflex; Exercise training; Sympathetic nerve activity; Hypertension; Spontaneously hypertensive rat (SHR)

## 1. EFFECTS OF EXERCISE TRAINING ON SYMPATHETIC NERVE ACTIVITY

### 1.1. Normotensive Rats

One of the most striking effects of exercise training on the cardiovascular system is the presence of resting bradycardia. Depending on the mode, intensity, and duration of exercise training, and also on the animal species studied, the mechanisms responsible for the bradycardic effect vary according to the relative importance of three major factors: the increase in vagal tone, the decrease in sympathetic tone, and the altered sensitivity of the cardiac pacemaker cells to neurotransmitters (for references, see Negrão et al.[6]).

Address for correspondence: Eduardo Moacyr Krieger, M.D., Ph.D., Unidade de Hipertensão, InCor-Instituto do Coração da Faculdade de Medicina da Universidade de São Paulo, Av. Dr. Enéas de Carvalho Aguiar, 44, São Paulo, Brazil, 05403-000. Voice: 55 11 30695048/5391; fax: 55 11 30695048.

edkrieger@incor.usp.br

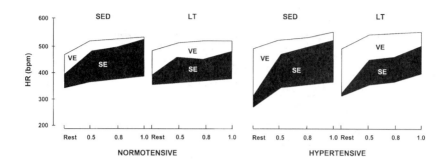

**FIGURE 1.** Contribution of vagal (VE) and sympathetic (SE) effects on the heart rate at rest and during exercise (0.5, 0.8, and 1.0 mph on 15% grade) in sedentary (SED) and exercise-trained (LT) normotensive rats, and in sedentary (SED) and exercise-trained (LT) SHR. The differences in heart rate before and after administration of methylatropine and propranolol were used to calculate vagal and sympathetic effects, respectively. Note that the decrease in tachycardic responses in normotensives and SHR after exercise training was caused by a partial withdrawal of vagal activity and a smaller increase in sympathetic activity. (Adapted from Negrão *et al.*[7] and Gava *et al.*[12] Reproduced by permission.)

In a study of normotensive rats subjected to chronic dynamic exercise training on a treadmill, we observed that one of the major determinants of resting bradycardia was a reduction in the pacemaker activity accompanied by an unexpected decrease in sensitivity of the bradycardic response to vagal stimulation and methacholine administration,[6] and an actual decrease in parasympathetic tone. However, a decrease in sympathetic tone was also demonstrated when a pharmacological blockade with methylatropine and propranolol was performed in exercise-trained rats.[7] Moreover, the significant attenuation of tachycardia during an acute bout of dynamic exercise in exercise-trained rats was attributed to a slight withdrawal of parasympathetic activity, as well as to a smaller increase in sympathetic activity. These results show that exercise training, in fact, reduces sympathetic nerve activity (FIG. 1). Is the reduction of sympathetic activity observed in exercise-trained rats restricted to the heart? Does it extend to other territories that could influence the regulation of total peripheral resistance? Using a multifiber preparation to record renal sympathetic nerve activity, we found in normotensive rats that a 13-week period of exercise training significantly decreased resting renal sympathetic nerve activity[8] (FIG. 2). Direct evidence that the activity of the peripheral sympathetic nerves is attenuated by exercise training has been obtained in different species, including cats[9] and humans.[10] If the decrease in renal sympathetic nerve activity is representative of a general reduction in sympathetic tone to all the areas, it is surprising that exercise training does not decrease blood pressure in normotensive rats. It is possible that local mechanisms (endothelial, myogenic, metabolic, etc.) may counteract the lower neurogenic tone, thus maintaining the peripheral resistance and the blood pressure at normal levels.[11]

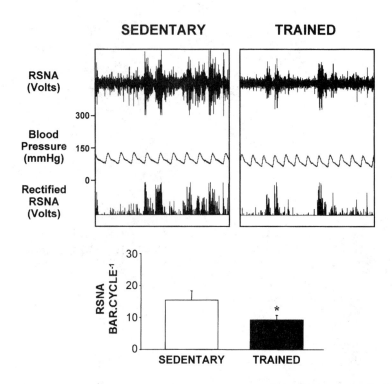

**FIGURE 2.** (**Upper panel**) Renal sympathetic nerve activity (RSNA), pulsatile blood pressure, and rectified RSNA in a sedentary rat and an exercise-trained rat. (**Lower panel**) Averaged RSNA expressed in bars/cycle in sedentary and exercise-trained normotensive rats. Note the decrease in RSNA produced by exercise training. * = Significant difference when compared to sedentary, $p \leq .05$. (Adapted from Negrão et al.[8] Reproduced by permission.)

### 1.2. Spontaneously Hypertensive Rats

In spontaneously hypertensive rats (SHR), we have also observed that exercise training decreases resting heart rate mainly due to a decrease in cardiac sympathetic tone. Indeed, low-intensity exercise training performed at 50% of the maximal oxygen uptake ($VO_2$ max), but not high-intensity training (85% of $VO_2$ max), reduces sympathetic tone (FIG. 3) without altering vagal tone or intrinsic heart rate.[12] The fact that the sympathetic tone was increased in sedentary SHR and that the low-intensity exercise training actually reduced sympathetic tone to a level similar to that of normotensive sedentary rats are important aspects. Therefore, exercise training normalizes the increased sympathetic tone existing in sedentary SHR. This attenuation of sympathetic tone to the heart seems to be the major mechanism responsible for the reduction of arterial hypertension in exercise-trained SHR,[13] since reductions in heart rate and cardiac output completely account for the reduction of blood pressure. Similar to the results observed in normotensive rats, exercise training also attenuated the sympathetic excitation and tachycardia produced by progressive dynamic exercise in SHR (FIG. 1).

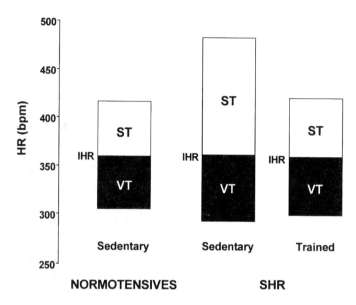

**FIGURE 3.** Sympathetic (ST) and vagal (VT) tone in sedentary normotensive rats and in sedentary and exercise-trained SHR. Intrinsic heart rate (IHR) was calculated after double blockade by methacholine and propranolol; ST is the difference between heart rate measured after methacholine and the IHR; VT is the difference between heart rate measured after propranolol and the IHR. Note that exercise training normalized the increased ST in SHR, bringing the ST to a level similar to that observed in normotensive rats. (Adapted from Negrão *et al.*[6] and Gava *et al.*[12] Reproduced by permission.)

## 2. INFLUENCE OF EXERCISE TRAINING ON BAROREFLEX CONTROL OF CARDIOVASCULAR SYSTEM

### 2.1. Normotensive Rats

It is well known that arterial and cardiopulmonary baroreflexes and the chemoreflex contribute significantly to the reflex control of circulation. We therefore thought that regular exercise could provoke a partial decrease in sympathetic activity by enhancing the gain-sensitivity of the baroreflexes. To test this hypothesis, we studied the effect of a 13-week period of dynamic exercise training on the baroreflex control of heart rate in normotensive rats. The sensitivity of arterial baroreflex control of heart rate was analyzed by producing transient increases and decreases in arterial pressure by i.v. injections of phenylephrine and sodium nitroprusside, respectively. The magnitude of baroreflex bradycardia was significantly less in exercise-trained rats compared with sedentary rats (FIG. 4A). In contrast, the magnitude of baroreflex tachycardia was significantly greater in exercise-trained rats (FIG. 4B). These data indicate that exercise training affects baroreflex bradycardia and tachycardia in opposite directions. We have also observed that the decreased baroreflex bradycardia in exercise-trained rats was accompanied by decreased bradycardic responses to

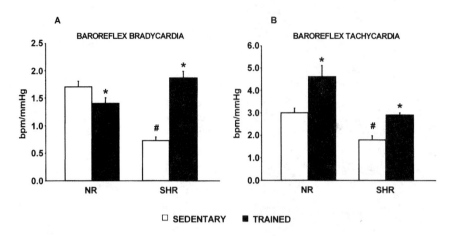

**FIGURE 4.** Baroreflex sensitivity for (**A**) bradycardia and (**B**) tachycardia, analyzed by $\Delta$ heart rate /$\Delta$ mean arterial pressure indexes in sedentary and exercise-trained normotensive rats (NR) and in sedentary and exercise-trained SHR. Note that exercise training decreased bradycardic sensitivity and increased tachycardic sensitivity in normotensive rats. In SHR, exercise training improved both bradycardia and tachycardia sensitivities, which were markedly depressed in the sedentary condition. * = Significant difference when compared to sedentary, $p \leq .05$. # = Significant difference when compared to sedentary normotensive rats, $p \leq .05$. (Adapted from Kelly and McClellan[4] and Brum et al.[21] Reproduced by permission.)

electrical stimulation of the peripheral end of the cut vagus nerve and methacholine administration.[7] Therefore, the attenuated reflex bradycardia was caused at least in part by decreased responsiveness of the efferent pathway of the reflex. Conversely, the increased baroreflex tachycardia in exercise-trained rats could be explained by an increase in baroreflex sensitivity, as will be discussed later in this chapter.

The effect of exercise training on baroreflex sensitivity in humans is controversial.[14–17] The variable results in human and animal studies may be attributed to different methodological approaches and differences between species. Increases in baroreflex sensitivity in exercise-trained human subjects have been demonstrated using a sigmoidal logistic function to characterize the baroreflex.[15,16] In contrast, the attenuation in baroreflex sensitivity has been described by means of baroreflex bradycardia index[7] or by regression analysis, fitting changes in mean arterial pressure to corresponding heart rate.[7] Data from our laboratory have shown that baroreflex sensitivity obtained by the sigmoidal logistic function in rats is similar to the baroreflex tachycardia index, but is approximately twofold greater than the baroreflex bradycardia index.[18] Our results demonstrate that exercise training changes the baroreflex tachycardia and baroreflex bradycardia in opposite directions. Therefore, baroreflex sensitivity calculated from the sigmoidal logistic function may mainly reflect the changes in baroreflex tachycardia. The changes in baroreflex bradycardia may not be readily observed using the logistic function analysis. Kingwell et al. found that the sensitivity of baroreflex control of heart rate was not altered by exercise training in normotensive humans under control conditions.[17] However, these investigators did observe a decreased baroreflex sensitivity after exercise training when the cardiac sympathetic response was blocked by propranolol, suggesting a decrease in the sensitivity of parasympathetic-mediated baroreflex bradycardia.[17]

When the baroreflex control of renal sympathetic nerve activity was studied in conscious exercise-trained normotensive rats, a decreased resting renal sympathetic nerve activity was confirmed, but the baroreflex sensitivity was actually attenuated.[8] DiCarlo and Bishop[19] also observed a decreased sensitivity of the arterial baroreflex control of renal sympathetic nerve activity in exercise-trained rabbits, which they attributed to an enhanced inhibition by the cardiopulmonary reflex.

## 2.2. Spontaneously Hypertensive Rats

In SHR, in which baroreflex control of heart rate is greatly attenuated, the effect of exercise training was remarkable, bringing the baroreflex sensitivity close to the normal values.[20] Indeed, the baroreflex bradycardia in SHR, which represented only 35% of the values exhibited by the normotensive rats, was markedly improved after exercise training up to 82% of the value seen in normotensive rats (FIG. 4A and 4B). The baroreflex sensitivity of the tachycardic responses in SHR, which during the control condition was only 32% of that seen in normotensive rats, increased up to 83% of normal after exercise training. Therefore, exercise training almost completely reversed the depressed baroreflex sensitivity observed in sedentary SHR. Preliminary experiments have indicated that the impaired baroreflex control of renal sympathetic nerve activity in SHR also improves after exercise training.[21]

Baroreflex sensitivity is markedly depressed in SHR.[22] The improvement in baroreflex control of both heart rate and peripheral sympathetic activity (renal sympathetic nerve activity) in SHR by low-intensity exercise training is expected to enhance the buffering capacity of the baroreflex, thus reducing blood pressure variability and sympathetic influences on the cardiovascular system. Similarly, an increased arterial baroreflex sensitivity after exercise training has been observed in hypertensive human subjects.[23,24]

## 3. INFLUENCE OF EXERCISE TRAINING ON BARORECEPTOR GAIN-SENSITIVITY

Since the attenuated baroreflex sensitivity in sedentary SHR is partially due to impaired afferent baroreceptor sensitivity,[25] we considered the possibility that low-intensity exercise training may restore baroreflex sensitivity in SHR by increasing the sensitivity of baroreceptor afferents to changes in arterial pressure. Arterial pressure and the activity of the aortic depressor nerve (aortic baroreceptor multifiber preparation) were measured in sedentary and exercise-trained normotensive rats and sedentary and exercise-trained SHR.[26]

The magnitude of the changes in aortic baroreceptor activity induced by changes in systolic arterial pressure increased significantly in exercise-trained normotensive rats ($2.09 \pm 0.1$ vs. $1.44 \pm 0.1\%$/mmHg) and exercise-trained SHR ($0.92 \pm 0.1$ vs. $0.71 \pm 0.1\%$/mmHg) compared with their respective sedentary control groups.[26] Likewise, maximum aortic baroreceptor gain-sensitivity was significantly higher in exercise-trained normotensive rats ($2.25 \pm 0.19$ vs. $1.77 \pm 0.03\%$/mmHg) and exer-

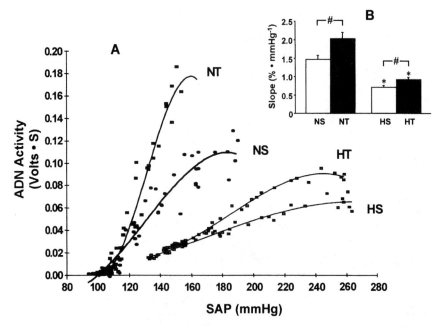

**FIGURE 5. (Panel A)** Comparison of aortic depressor nerve (ADN) activity–systolic arterial pressure (SAP) relationship in sedentary (NS) and exercise-trained (NT) normotensive rats and sedentary (HS) and exercise-trained (HT) SHR. **(Panel B)** The average values of the slope sensitivity of both groups. Note that exercise training improved aortic baroreceptor gain-sensitivity in both normotensive and spontaneously hypertensive rats. However, baroreceptor gain-sensitivity in SHR was restored only partially back to the level observed in sedentary normotensive rats by the exercise training. * = Significant difference when compared to NS, $p \le .05$. # = Significant difference between sedentary rats and exercise-trained rats, $p \le .05$. (Adapted from Brum et al.[26] Reproduced by permission.).

cise-trained SHR ($1.07 \pm 0.04$ vs. $0.82 \pm 0.05\%$/mmHg) compared with their respective sedentary control groups (FIG. 5).

These data represent the first demonstration that dynamic exercise training increases the gain-sensitivity of the afferent limb of the aortic baroreflex in normotensive rats as well as in SHR. In normotensive rats, exercise training increased baroreceptor gain-sensitivity by 38%. In SHR, training increased gain-sensitivity significantly, but only partly back to the level observed in sedentary normotensive rats (FIG. 5). The improvement of afferent aortic baroreceptor gain-sensitivity in SHR partially explains the recovery of baroreflex sensitivity after exercise training.

Since exercise training enhanced baroreceptor function, it was somewhat surprising that only baroreflex-mediated tachycardia was increased, while baroreflex-mediated bradycardia was actually decreased. This paradox can be explained by the decreases in bradycardic responses to efferent vagal nerve stimulation and methacholine administration that were observed after exercise training.[7] The impaired efferent function may exceed the increase in baroreceptor sensitivity, resulting in decreased baroreflex-mediated bradycardia.

According to the mechanoelastic concept, in the presence of increased vascular compliance, the same pulse pressure can result in increased baroreceptor activation.[27] Since exercise training increases intrinsic aortic compliance in rats[28] and arterial compliance in humans,[29,30] we postulate that the improvement in aortic baroreceptor gain-sensitivity may be due to an increase in aortic compliance. The failure of exercise training to increase arterial compliance in SHR[31] suggests that this mechanism may not explain the training-induced increase in baroreceptor sensitivity in SHR. Endothelial changes following exercise training is another attractive hypothesis that may explain the training-induced increase in aortic baroreceptor gain-sensitivity. Both the magnitude and frequency of shear stress on endothelial cells during exercise increase the release of endothelial factors[29] that may lead to increased baroreceptor activity. In fact, Yen *et al.*[32] reported that exercise training increases the vasodilatory response to acetylcholine in SHR. The increase in aortic baroreceptor gain-sensitivity can also be explained by a reduction of sympathetic nerve activity. Exercise training reduces muscle sympathetic nerve activity[10] and norepinephrine spillover[33] in humans, and reduces renal sympathetic nerve activity in rats.[8] Inhibition of sympathetic nerve activity could modify the distensibility of the carotid sinus area,[34-36] and consequently increase afferent baroreceptor discharge in SHR. Alternatively, it is possible that the blood withdrawal or infusion used to generate the baroreceptor function curve may have altered cardiopulmonary receptor activity and affected the aortic baroreceptor gain-sensitivity via interaction between reflex influences. However, this does not seem to be the case. During hypotension/deactivation of cardiopulmonary receptors, and hence, increase in sympathetic nerve activity, no differences in the aortic baroreceptor pressure threshold were found between sedentary and exercise-trained rats.[26] The marked increase in gain-sensitivity of afferent baroreceptors after exercise training, in both normotensive and hypertensive rats, was most evident at higher levels of arterial pressure.

## 4. CONCLUDING REMARKS

Our analysis of the antihypertensive benefits of exercise training in SHR provides the following conclusions:

(1) The antihypertensive effect is produced by low-intensity, but not high-intensity exercise training;

(2) The reduction in blood pressure is the result of decreases in heart rate and cardiac output rather than decreases in total peripheral resistance;

(3) Exercise training attenuates the influence of the sympathetic nervous system on the heart of SHR;

(4) An improvement of the depressed baroreceptor function and baroreflex sensitivity appears to contribute importantly to the benefits elicited by exercise training.

Finally, more studies are needed to clarify the relative contributions of the changes in function of afferent, central, and efferent neural pathways and the sensitivity of the target organs to the overall decrease in sympathetic activity and arterial pressure observed after exercise training, and the reasons for the failure of sympathetic inhibition to decrease peripheral vascular resistance.

## ACKNOWLEDGMENTS

The financial support for the studies on the cardiovascular effects of exercise training was provided by grants from FAPESP (Fundação de Amparo a Pesquisa do Estado de São Paulo) and Fundação E.J. Zerbini.

## REFERENCES

1. ARAKAWA, K. 1993. Antihypertensive mechanism of exercise. J. Hypertens. **11:** 223–229.
2. ARROLL, B. & R. BEAGLEHOLE. 1992. Does physical activity lower blood pressure: a critical review of the clinical trials. J. Clin. Epidemiol. **45**(5): 439–447.
3. KELLEY, G. & P. MCCLELLAN. 1994. Antihypertensive effects of aerobic exercise: a brief meta-analytic review of randomized controlled trials. Am. J. Hypertens. **7:** 115–119.
4. KRIEGER, E.M., P.C. BRUM & C.E. NEGRÃO. 1998. Role of arterial baroreceptor function on cardiovascular adjustments to acute and chronic dynamic exercise. Biol. Res. **31:** 273–279.
5. KRIEGER, E.M., P.C. BRUM & C.E. NEGRÃO. 1999. Influence of exercise training on neurogenic control of blood pressure in spontaneously hypertensive rats. Hypertension **34**(Pt. 2): 720–723.
6. NEGRÃO, C.E., E.D. MOREIRA M.C.L.M. SANTOS, et al. 1992. Vagal function impairment after exercise training. J. Appl. Physiol. **72**(5): 1749–1753.
7. NEGRÃO, C.E., E.D. MOREIRA, P.C. BRUM, et al. 1992. Vagal and sympathetic control of heart rate during exercise by sedentary and exercise-trained rats. Braz. J. Med. Biol. Res. **25:** 1045–1052.
8. NEGRÃO, C.E., M.C. IRIGOYEN, E.D. MOREIRA, et al. 1993. Effect of exercise training on RSNA, baroreflex control, and blood pressure responsiveness. Am. J. Physiol. **265**(34): R365–R370.
9. NINOMIYA, I., K. MATSUKAWA & N. NISHIURA. 1988. Central and baroreflex control of sympathetic nerve activity to the heart and kidney in a daily life of the cat. Clin. Exp. Hypertens. **10**(Suppl. 1): 19–31.
10. GRASSI, G., G. SERAVALLE, D.A. CALHOUN & G. MANCIA. 1994. Physical training and baroreceptor control of sympathetic nerve activity in humans. Hypertension **23:** 294–301.
11. BRODY, M.J., K.M. BARRON, K. BERECEK, et al. 1983. Neurogenic mechanisms of experimental hypertension. *In* Hypertension, J. Genest, O. Kuchel, P. Hamet, and M. Cantin, Eds.: 117–139. McGraw-Hill. New York.
12. GAVA, N.S., A.S. VÉRAS-SILVA, C.E. NEGRÃO & E.M. KRIEGER. 1995. Low-intensity exercise training attenuates cardiac β-adrenergic tone during exercise in spontaneously hypertensive rats. Hypertension **26**(6): 1129–1133.
13. VÉRAS-SILVA, A.S., K.C. MATTOS, N. GAVA, et al. 1997. Low-intensity exercise training decreases cardiac output and hypertension in spontaneously hypertensive rats. Am. J. Physiol. **42:** H 2627–H 2631.
14. BARNEY, J.A., T.J. EBERT, L. GROBAN, et al. 1988. Carotid baroreflex responsiveness in high-fit and sedentary young men. J. Appl. Physiol. **65**(5): 2190–2194.
15. MCDONALD, P.M., A.J. SANFILIPPO & G.K. SAVARD. 1993. Baroreflex function and cardiac structure with moderate endurance training in normotensive men. J. Appl. Physiol. **4**(5): 2469–2477.
16. TATRO, D.L., G.A. DUDLEY & V.A. CONVERTINO. 1992. Carotid-cardiac baroreflex response and LBNP tolerance following resistance training. Med. Sci. Sports Exercise **24**(7): 789–796.
17. KINGWELL, B.A., A.M. DART, G.L. JENNINGS & P.I. KORNER. 1992. Exercise training reduces the sympathetic component of the blood pressure-heart rate baroreflex in man. Clin. Sci. **82:** 357–362.

18. FARAH, V.M., E.D. MOREIRA, M.D. PIRES, *et al.* 1999. Comparison of three methods for the determination of baroreflex sensitivity in conscious rats. Braz. J. Med. Biol. Res. **32:** 361–369.
19. DICARLO, S.E. & V.S. BISHOP. 1990. Exercise training enhances cardiac afferent inhibition of baroreflex function. Am. J. Physiol. **258**(1, Pt. 2): H212–H220.
20. SILVA, G.J.J., P.C. BRUM, C.E. NEGRÃO & E.M. KRIEGER. 1997. Acute and chronic effects of exercise on baroreflexes in spontaneously hypertensive rats. Hypertension **30**(Pt. 2): 714–719.
21. BRUM. P.C., F. IDA, E.D. MOREIRA, *et al.* 1998. Exercise training increases the baroreflex control of renal sympathetic nerve activity in spontaneously hypertensive rats (Abstr.). J. Hypertens. **16**(Suppl. 2): S 251.
22. IDA, F., E.D. MOREIRA, V.L.L. OLIVEIRA & E.M. KRIEGER. 1992. The magnitude of rapid resetting of the baroreceptors is attenuated in spontaneously hypertensive rats. Gen. Hypertens. **218:** 65–67.
23. SOMERS, V.K., J. CONWAY, J. JOHNSTON & P. SLEIGHT. 1991. Effects of endurance training on baroreflex sensitivity and blood pressure in borderline hypertension. Lancet **8**(337): 1363–1368.
24. PAGANI, M., V. SOMERS, R. FURLAN, *et al.* 1988. Changes in autonomic regulation induced by physical training in mild hypertension. Hypertension **12:** 600–610.
25. ANDRESEN, M.C. & M. YANG. 1989. Arterial baroreceptor resetting: contributions of chronic and acute processes. Clin. Exp. Pharmacol. Physiol. **15:** 19–30.
26. BRUM, P.C., G.J.J. SILVA, E.D. MOREIRA, *et al.* 2000. Exercise training increases baroreceptor gain-sensitivity in normal and hypertensive rats. Hypertension **36:** 1018–1022.
27. KIRCHHEIM, H.R. 1976. Systemic arterial baroreceptor reflexes. Physiol. Rev. **56:** 100–176.
28. KINGWELL, B.A., P.J. ARNOLD, G.L. JENNINGS & A.M. DART. 1997. Spontaneous running increases aortic compliance in Wistar-Kyoto rats. Cardiovasc. Res. **35:** 132–137.
29. CAMERON, J.D. & A.M. DART. 1994. Exercise training increases total systemic arterial compliance in humans. Am. J. Physiol. **266**(35): H693–H701.
30. KINGWELL, B.A., J.D. CAMERON, K.J. GILLIES, *et al.* 1995. Arterial compliance may influence baroreflex function in athletes and hypertensives. Am. J. Physiol. **268**(37): H411–H418.
31. KINGWELL, B.A., P.J. ARNOLD, G.L. JENNINGS & A.M. DART. 1998. The effects of voluntary running on cardiac mass and aortic compliance in Wistar-Kyoto and spontaneously hypertensive rats. J. Hypertens. **16:** 181–185.
32. YEN, M.H., J.H. YANG, J.R. SHEU, *et al.* 1995. Chronic exercise enhances endothelium-mediated dilation in spontaneously hypertensive rats. Life Sci. **57**(24): 2205–2213.
33. MEREDITH, I.T., P. FRIBERG & G.L. JENNINGS. 1991. Exercise training lowers resting renal but not cardiac sympathetic activity in man. Hypertension **18:** 575–582.
34. BAGSHAW, R.J. & L.H. PETERSON. 1972. Sympathetic control of the mechanical properties of the canine carotid sinus. Am. J. Physiol. **222**(6): 1462–1468.
35. BOLTER, C.P. & J.R. LEDSOME. 1976. Effect of cervical sympathetic nerve stimulation on canine carotid sinus reflex. Am. J. Physiol. **230**(4): 1026–1030.
36. SEAGARD, J.L., F.A. HOPP & J.P. KAMPINE. 1987. Effect of sympathetic sensitization of baroreceptors on renal nerve activity. Am. J. Physiol. **252**(21): R328–R335.

# CNS Effects of Ovarian Hormones and Metabolites on Neural Control of Circulation

CHERYL M. HEESCH AND C. MICHAEL FOLEY

*Department of Biomedical Sciences and Dalton Cardiovascular Research Center, University of Missouri, Columbia, Missouri 65211, USA*

ABSTRACT: Pregnant women often experience orthostatic hypotension, and pregnancy is associated with increased susceptibility to hemorrhagic hypotension. Experiments evaluating arterial baroreflex control of efferent sympathetic nerve activity in virgin and term-pregnant rats revealed that arterial baroreflex sympathoexcitation is attenuated, while sympathoinhibitory responses are well-maintained or potentiated. Following a hypotensive challenge, pregnant animals exhibit attenuated Fos expression in the rostral ventrolateral medulla (RVLM), suggesting that unloading of arterial baroreceptors results in less excitation of presympathetic neurons in the brain stem. Other experiments, in which afferent baroreceptor discharge was recorded, suggest that this was not due to differences in afferent baoreceptor function. GABAergic mechanisms are responsible for tonic inhibition of sympathoexcitatory neurons in the RVLM and the major metabolite of progesterone, $3\alpha$-OH-dihydroprogesterone ($3\alpha$-OH-DHP), which is elevated in pregnancy, is the most potent endogenous positive modulator of CNS $GABA_A$ receptor function. Additional experiments revealed that acutely administered $3\alpha$-OH-DHP, either intravenously or directly into the RVLM, mimicked the effects of pregnancy on baroreflex control of efferent sympathetic nerve activity and potentiated pressure sensitivity of spinally projecting RVLM neurons. Preliminary experiments using semiquantitative RT-PCR, evaluated the relative expression of three subunits ($\alpha_{1-3}$) of the $GABA_A$ receptor, and suggest that chronic exposure to elevated levels of ovarian hormones can result to changes in $GABA_A$ receptor subunit composition. It is likely that changes in control of sympathetic outflow in pregnancy are related to complex interactions between genomic and nongenomic actions of ovarian hormones and metabolites.

KEYWORDS: Arterial baroreflex; Pregnancy; Female; Progesterone; Allopregnanolone; $3\alpha$-OH-dihydroprogesterone; Neurosteroids; Rostral ventrolateral medulla

## EFFECTS OF PREGNANCY ON ARTERIAL BAROREFLEX FUNCTION

Normal pregnancy is characterized by an increase in plasma and blood volume, heart rate, and cardiac output (approximately 40%). Arterial blood pressure is actu-

Address for correspondence: Dr. Cheryl M. Heesch, University of Missouri Dalton Cardiovascular Research Center, Research Park, Columbia, MO 65211-3300. Voice: 513-882-2359; fax: 513-884-4232.

heeschc@missouri.edu

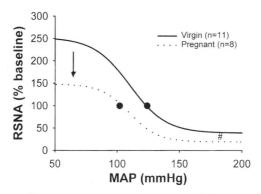

**FIGURE 1.** Mean RSNA baroreflex curves for virgin female and term-pregnant rats. Baseline MAP (*closed circles*) was lower in pregnant rats, and the ability to increase NA above baseline values was attenuated, as seen by a decrease in NA range and maximum NA (*arrow*). Minimum NA was less in pregnant compared with virgin rats (#). (Adapted from Masilamani and Heesch.[5] Reproduced with permission from The American Physiological Society.)

ally decreased, due to a substantial decrease in total peripheral resistance.[1,2] However, estimates of basal sympathetic outflow suggest that sympathetic nerve activity is either unchanged[3] or slightly increased.[4,5] Pregnant women have an increased incidence of orthostatic hypotension, and pregnant animals show increased sensitivity to the hypotensive effects of hemorrhage.[6,7] Experiments performed in anesthetized rabbits by Humphreys and Joels demonstrated that baroreflex control of mean arterial pressure[8] was altered by pregnancy. Carotid sinus baroreflex depressor responses were equivalent, but pressor responses were attenuated in pregnant compared to nonpregnant animals. Subsequent studies revealed that this was due to attenuated increases in vascular resistance in nonuterine circulatory beds,[9] rather than to attenuated changes in cardiac output[10] during baroreceptor unloading (low carotid sinus pressure) in pregnant animals. Although these data suggest that autonomic neural mechanisms may be involved, interpretation of the results is complicated by the fact that vascular responsiveness to circulating and neurally released vasoconstrictors is decreased in pregnancy.[11–13]

Experiments were performed in our laboratory, in which arterial baroreflex control of efferent renal sympathetic nerve activity (RSNA) was directly assessed in both anesthetized[14] and awake[5] virgin and term-pregnant Sprague-Dawley rats. Briefly, arterial blood pressure was increased and decreased from baseline values by graded intravenous infusions of phenylephrine and nitroprusside, and reflex changes in RSNA were recorded. The data were fit to a nonlinear logistic curve[15] that related RSNA (% baseline) to mean arterial pressure (MAP). Curve coefficients provided information related to nerve-activity range, maximum nerve activity, minimum nerve activity, and MAP at the curve midpoint. Slopes were calculated and served as an index of baroreflex sensitivity. FIGURE 1 shows mean baroreflex curves from chronically instrumented conscious virgin and term-pregnant rats. Baseline MAP was significantly lower in pregnant ($102 + 2.4$ mmHg) compared to virgin ($124 \pm 3.4$

mmHg) rats. Baroreflex sympathoinhibition in response to a hypertensive challenge was well maintained or even potentiated, while baroreflex sympathoexcitatory responses during a hypotensive challenge were attenuated by pregnancy. Similar experiments were performed in separate groups of virgin and pregnant rats, except that afferent baroreceptor discharge was recorded in the aortic depressor nerve. Consistent with the lower arterial pressure, the baroreceptor function curve midpoint was lower in term-pregnant rats (virgin = $140 \pm 2.7$; pregnant = $124 \pm 3.6$ mmHg). However, the shape of the afferent baroreceptor discharge curves was similar between virgin and term-pregnant animals.[16] Therefore, it seemed likely that a central nervous system (CNS) mechanism contributed to the attenuated sympathoexcitatory effects of pregnancy.

## EFFECTS OF PREGNANCY ON FOS
## EXPRESSION IN BRAIN STEM

Activation of peripheral arterial baroreceptors ultimately results in inhibition of tonically active sympathoexcitatory neurons in the rostral ventrolateral medulla (RVLM). The brain stem pathway that mediates this response is as follows. Baroreceptor afferent discharge results in excitation of secondary neurons predominantly in the ipsilateral nucleus tractus solitarius (NTS) in the medulla oblongata. Projections from the NTS to the caudal ventrolateral medulla (CVLM) excite neurons in this region, which then send an inhibitory GABAergic projection to the RVLM. Since RVLM neurons provide a tonic excitatory input to preganglionic sympathetic neurons in the intermediolateral cell column of the spinal cord, inhibition of efferent sympathetic nerve activity results.[17] In addition to baroreflex-mediated GABAergic inhibition of the RVLM, neurons in this area are also tonically inhibited by GABAergic inputs independent of afferent baroreceptor input.[18,19]

Using c-fos immunocytochemistry as a method for evaluating neuronal activation, several laboratories have consistently reported that hypotension results in increased Fos expression in specific brain stem regions associated with arterial baroreflexes.[20–23] Therefore, experiments were performed to determine if, following a hypotensive challenge, differences existed in Fos expression between virgin and term-pregnant rats. Rats chronically instrumented with arterial and venous catheters received either isotonic saline vehicle or hydralazine, which lowered arterial blood pressure to levels predicted to completely unload arterial baroreceptors. Similar to reports of others, [21–23] hypotension resulted in significant increases in total Fos expression in both the NTS and the CVLM. Because baroreceptor activation is decreased with decreased arterial pressure, the stimulus for increased Fos expression in the NTS and CVLM is currently unclear. Future experiments evaluating phenotype of the subpopulations of neurons expressing Fos following hypotension should provide insight. Of interest to our study, the increases in total Fos in the NTS and CVLM were similar in virgin and pregnant rats, and therefore those particular neuronal populations are unlikely to contribute to the differences in control of sympathetic outflow that have been observed. In contrast, although total Fos expression in the RVLM was increased in both virgin and term-pregnant rats, the increase was significantly less in the pregnant animals (FIG. 2). Interestingly, since there was no dif-

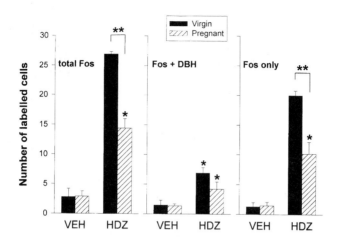

**FIGURE 2.** (**Left**) Total numbers of Fos-positive nuclei, (**middle**) numbers of Fos-positive cells also labeled for dopamine beta hydroxylase (DBH), and (**right**) numbers of Fos-positive cells not labeled for DBH in rostral ventrolateral medulla of virgin female or pregnant rats after vehicle (VEH) or hydralazine (HDZ). HDZ resulted in significant increases in Fos expression in all cases. Pregnant rats exhibited an attenuated increase in Fos following HDZ treatment (left), which was due to less of an increase in noncatecholamine synthesizing cells (C). *$P < 0.05$ compared with corresponding VEH-treated group; **$P < 0.05$ compared with HDZ-treated virgin females. (From Curtis *et al.*[24] Reproduced with permission from The American Physiological Society.)

ference in Fos expression in neurons containing the catecholamine synthetic enzyme, dopamine beta hydroxylase, it appears that a population of noncatecholaminergic neurons within the RVLM accounts for the difference between virgin and pregnant animals.[24]

Ovarian hormones and their metabolites are elevated in pregnancy and are likely candidates for mediating alterations in control of sympathetic outflow during pregnancy. Since gamma aminobutyric acid (GABA) is the primary inhibitory transmitter in the central baroreflex pathway, we considered that increased GABAergic influences in the RVLM might contribute to attenuated baroreflex sympathoexcitation, potentiated baroreflex sympathoinhibition, and attenuated Fos expression in the RVLM following a hypotensive challenge in term-pregnant animals. Of particular interest in this regard is the primary metabolite of progesterone, 3α-hydroxy-dihydroprogesterone (3α-OH-DHP), which has been shown to positively modulate CNS GABA$_A$ receptor function.[25,26]

## NEUROSTEROID MODULATION OF GABA$_A$ RECEPTORS

Throughout the CNS, the transmitter GABA mediates fast inhibitory responses by activation of GABA$_A$ receptors, which are ligand-gated chloride channels located in the plasma membrane.[27] GABA$_A$ receptors have several distinct allosteric modulatory sites, and certain endogenous ligands, termed neurosteroids, have been shown to bind to a unique site on the $GABA_A$ receptor complex and potentiate chloride conductance.[26,28] The neurosteroid 3α-OH-DHP, which is the major metabolite of progesterone, is the most potent endogenous positive modulator of CNS $GABA_A$ receptor function.[25,26] Both plasma and CNS levels of 3α-OH-DHP are elevated in pregnancy to levels that have been shown to potentiate GABA-mediated neuronal inhibition.[29,30]

Regional specificity has been demonstrated for neurosteroid modulation of $GABA_A$ ligand binding and function within the CNS;[31–33] however, the brain stem had not been closely studied. Therefore we examined the effects of the neurosteroid, 3α-OH-DHP, and its inactive isomer, 3β-OH-dyhydoprogesterone (3β-OH-DHP), on [$^3$H]flunitrazepam binding to $GABA_A$ receptors in medullary nuclei from female rats in the estrus stage of the estrous cycle.[34] This benzodiazapine ligand provides high resolution for autoradiographic analysis, and, in other systems, modulation of [$^3$H]flunitrazepam binding by neurosteroids has been used as an indicator of allosteric interactions with the $GABA_A$ receptor.[35,36] We found that *in vitro* exposure to 3α-OH-DHP, but not 3β-OH-DHP, resulted in potentiation of $GABA_A$ ligand binding in the NTS ($165 \pm 23.5\%$ control), CVLM ($173 \pm 18.3\%$ control), and RVLM ($176 \pm 6.1\%$ control). Thus, major medullary nuclei in the arterial baroreflex pathway are susceptible to positive modulation by the neuroactive metabolite of progesterone.

## EFFECTS OF PROGESTERONE METABOLITES ON ARTERIAL BAROREFLEX

Since the action of 3α-OH-DHP to positively modulate $GABA_A$ receptor function is a rapid membrane effect, we postulated that if 3α-OH-DHP was involved in modulating control of sympathetic outflow, exogenous administration of this progesterone metabolite should have acute effects on arterial baroreflex function. Arterial baroreflex control of efferent sympathetic nerve activity was assessed in virgin female rats (estrus stage of cycle) before, 15, and 30 min after intravenous administration of 3α-OH-DHP (160 μg/kg bolus + 1.6 μg/kg/min infusion).[37] Independent of changes in baseline arterial pressure, the baroreflex curve shifted to a lower operating pressure range within 15 min and sympathoexcitatory responses were attenuated by 30 min (FIG. 3). In contrast, administration of the same dose of inactive 3β-OH isomers of DHP had no effect on arterial baroreflex control of efferent sympathetic nerve activity (FIG. 4). Although 3α-OH-DHP is highly lipid soluble and therefore would have access to the CNS when administered intravenously, we considered the possibility that effects on peripheral baroreceptors might contribute to the baroreflex responses in these experiments. In a separate group of rats, a similar protocol was performed, except that afferent baroreceptor discharge was recorded in the aortic depressor nerve. The baroreceptor function curves were similar before, 15 min, and 30 min after intravenous 3α-OH-DHP, and baseline MAP was unchanged.[16] Thus, it appears that 3α-OH-DHP does not affect afferent baroreceptor discharge.

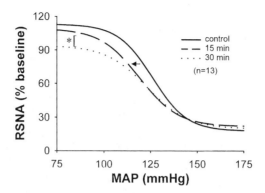

**FIGURE 3.** Mean RSNA baroreflex curves for virgin female rats before (control), 15 min after, and 30 min after intravenous administration of 3α-OH-DHP. Baseline MAP was not different among the three conditions (Control = 103 ± 4.6; 15 min = 103 ± 6.0; 30 min = 94 ± 12). However, within 15 min of 3α-OH-DHP administration, the arterial pressure at curve midpoint was decreased (*arrow*) and within 30 min maximum RSNA was decreased (*). $P < .05$. (From Heesch and Rogers.[37] Reproduced with permission from Blackwell Science Ltd.)

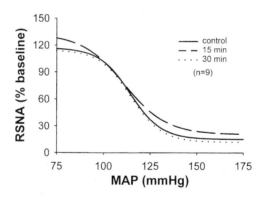

**FIGURE 4.** Mean RSNA baroreflex curves for virgin female rats before (control), 15 min after, and 30 min after intravenous administration of 3β-OH-DHP isomers. 3β-OH-DHP had no effect on baseline MAP or baroreflex control of sympathetic nerve activity. (From Heesch and Rogers.[37] Reproduced with permission from Blackwell Science Ltd.)

These results are consistent with a stereospecific, possibly nongenomic, action of 3α-OH-DHP on arterial baroreflex function, likely through an action in the CNS. Since potentiation of GABAergic influences in the RVLM would be consistent with the preceding observations, additional experiments were performed in separate groups of animals in which arterial baroreflex control of RSNA was tested before, 3 min, or 15 min after either 3α-OH-DHP or 3β-OH-DHP was microinjected into the RVLM (100 nL, 2 µM). By 15 min, 3α-OH-DHP, but not 3β-OH-DHP, microinjected into the RVLM resulted in attenuated baroreflex sympathoexcitatory responses,[38] similar to the effects observed 30 min following intravenous administration (FIGS. 3 and 4).

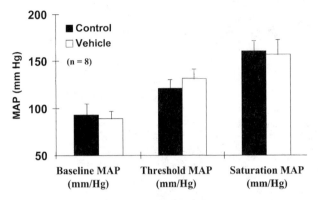

**FIGURE 5.** Effect of vehicle on RVLM neurons. Administration of vehicle (40% β-cyclodextrin) had no effect on baseline MAP, threshold pressure, or saturation pressure of RVLM neurons. *Bars* are values ± standard error of the mean. A paired *t*-test was used to compare control and vehicle responses. (From Laiprasert *et al.*[40] Reproduced with permission from The American Physiological Society.)

## 3α-OH-DHP POTENTIATES SYMPATHOINHIBITION IN THE RVLM

The purpose of the next study was to determine if circulating 3α-OH-DHP, in concentrations similar to those found in pregnancy (20–30 ng/μL),[26,30] acutely altered the arterial pressure sensitivity of spinally projecting neurons in the RVLM to endogenously released GABA. Urethane-anesthetized virgin female rats were prepared for extracellular recording of single-unit activity in the RVLM. Spinally projecting neurons were identified by advancing the recording electrode in the region of the RVLM while electrically stimulating the dorsolateral funiculus of the spinal cord, a region that contains descending axonal projections from the RVLM to spinal preganglionic sympathetic neurons in the intermediolateral cell column (IML).[39] Spontaneously firing neurons that were both antidromically activated by spinal-cord stimulation and greatly inhibited by elevations in arterial pressure were presumed to be presympathetic cardiovascular neurons of the RVLM[17] and were included in this study. Threshold pressure for inhibition of the neuron and saturation pressure where maximum inhibition occurred were determined during a gradual increase in MAP. Threshold and saturation pressure for a unit were determined before and 10 min following an intravenous bolus injection of either vehicle (44 μL, 40% β-cyclodextrin) or 3α-OH-DHP (44 μL, 1.12 μg/kg). FIGURE 5 shows that the vehicle had no effect on baseline MAP, or threshold and saturation pressures of RVLM neurons. In contrast, 10 min following intravenous administration of the neuroactive metabolite of progesterone, 3α-OH-DHP, both threshold and saturation pressures of RVLM neurons were decreased (FIG. 6). Since arterial baroreflex inhibition of RVLM neurons during an increase in MAP is mediated by GABA,[17] these results are consistent with the suggestion that circulating 3α-OH-DHP results in an increased sensitivity of RVLM neurons to endogenously released GABA.[40] This is supported by the observation that the sympathoinhibitory response to RVLM microinjection of the GABA$_A$

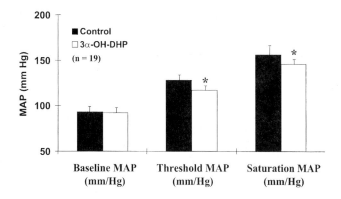

**FIGURE 6.** Effect of 3α-OH-DHP on RVLM neurons. 3α-OH-DHP had no effect on baseline MAP. However, threshold and saturation pressures of RVLM neurons were decreased 10 min following intravenous administration of 3α-OH-DHP. *Bars* are values ± standard error of the mean. A paired $t$-test was used to compare control and 3α-OH-DHP responses. (From Laiprasert *et al.*[40] Reproduced with permission from The American Physiological Society.)

agonist, isoguvacine (2 mmol, 20 nL) was potentiated by prior (2–3 min) microinjection of 3α-OH-DHP (2mmol, 30 nL) into the RVLM.[37]

## EFFECTS OF PREGNANCY ON GABA$_A$ RECEPTOR α-SUBUNITS IN THE RVLM

The ovarian hormones estrogen and progesterone are elevated in pregnancy. In rats, plasma levels of progesterone and its metabolites increase early, while estrogen levels progressively increase throughout pregnancy.[30,41] Since the effects of pregnancy on arterial baroreflex function are not well developed until late pregnancy[42] (Heesch, unpublished observation), we considered that prior exposure to estrogen in pregnancy might be important for the effects of 3α-OH-DHP to become fully evident. Estrogen has been proposed to augment GABAergic transmission within the CNS by multiple mechanisms,[43] including preferential synthesis of specific GABA$_A$ receptor subunits that confer maximum sensitivity to the neuroactive metabolite of progesterone. Compared to $\alpha_2$ subunit-containing GABA$_A$ receptors, GABA$_A$ receptors containing $\alpha_1$ subunits show increased sensitivity to positive modulation by 3α-OH-DHP.[44,45] Fenelon and Herbison[45] reported increased expression of GABA$_A$ $\alpha_1$ subunit mRNA in hypothalamic magnocellular oxytocin neurons in late pregnancy before parturition. In addition, the ratio of $\alpha_1$ relative to $\alpha_2$ GABA$_A$ receptor subunits in these neurons decreased prior to parturition and was associated with decreased positive modulation of GABA$_A$ receptor function by 3α-OH-DHP.[46]

Preliminary experiments were performed to evaluate, by semiquantitative reverse transcriptase-polymerase chain reaction (RT-PCR), the relative expression of three different GABA$_A$ receptor α subunits in the RVLM. mRNA was isolated [Dynabeads oligo (dT)$_{25}$] from homogenized tissue punches of the RVLM of female virgin and term-pregnant rats.[47] First strand cDNA synthesis was performed using reverse transcriptase (RT). Following RT, the cDNA was analyzed by PCR using primers for $GABA_A$ $\alpha_{1-3}$ subunits, glyceraldehyde phosphate dehydrogenase (GAPDH), tyrosine hydroxylase (TH), and phenylethanolamine-N-methyltransferase (PNMT).[48–50] A portion of the isolated mRNA from each punch was not treated with RT and used to check for contamination by genomic DNA (RT–). The PCR products were electrophorised, the gels were photographed and scanned, and the mass of each band was quantified by densitometry and compared with a quantitative DNA low molecular-weight ladder. All RVLM punches included in the study had detectable GAPDH, TH, and PMNT message signals and no detectable genomic DNA contamination (lack of a signal in the RT– reaction) (FIG. 7A). $GABA_A$ $\alpha_1$, $\alpha_2$, and to a lesser extent, $\alpha_3$ subunits were present in the RVLM (FIG. 7B). The average ratio of the mass of the PCR reactions for $\alpha_1:\alpha_2$ subunits tended to be reduced in pregnant compared to virgin rats (FIG. 7C). These data suggest that late pregnancy in rats may be associated with a change in the relative expression of $GABA_A$ $\alpha$ subunits. However, these preliminary results are not consistent with the hypothesis that pregnancy results in a relative increase in $\alpha_1$ subunit expression, an effect that could confer increased sensitivity to positive modulation of $GABA_A$ receptors by the neuroactive metabolite of progesterone, 3$\alpha$-OH-DHP. Future experiments using competitive RT-PCR, examining additional $GABA_A$ receptor subunits, and examining additional regions of the brain stem and forebrain will reveal more regarding possible effects of pregnancy and ovarian hormones on $GABA_A$ receptors.

## CONCLUSIONS

The studies described herein demonstrate that term pregnancy is characterized by attenuated arterial baroreflex sympathoexcitatory responses and potentiated sympathoinhibitory responses. Experiments using *c-fos* immunocytochemistry as a marker for neuronal activation, revealed that a hypotensive stimulus resulted in less activation of RVLM neurons in pregnant compared to virgin animals. Although baroreflex responses were evaluated in these experiments, it should be noted that the differences between pregnant and virgin animals were most evident at low arterial pressures, where arterial baroreceptor input would be expected to be minimal or nonexistent. Thus, if attenuated sympathoexcitation in pregnant animals is due to increased inhibitory influences within the CNS, the inhibitory effects are probably largely independent of arterial baroreceptors. Tonic inhibitory GABAergic inputs, separate from arterial baroreflexes, have been demonstrated in the RVLM.[18,19]

The major metabolite of progesterone, which is elevated in pregnancy, is the most potent endogenous positive modulator of CNS $GABA_A$ receptors.[25,26] Several lines of evidence from these studies indicate that acutely administered 3$\alpha$-OH-DHP, either intravenous or directly into the RVLM, potentiates sympathoinhibition resulting from endogenously released or exogenously administered GABA. These findings are consistent with a rapid nongenomic membrane effect of the neuroactive metabolite of progesterone on $GABA_A$ receptor function within the RVLM. Although the acute effects of 3$\alpha$-OH-DHP are qualitatively similar to the effects of pregnancy on control of sympathetic nerve activity, it is highly likely that other mechanisms also contribute. Estrogen, progesterone, neuroactive progesterone metabolites, and a host

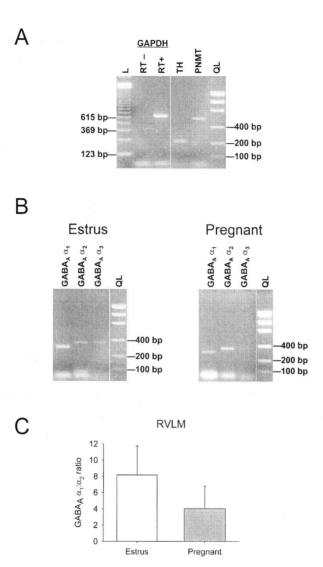

**FIGURE 7.** (**Panel A**) PCR detection of mRNA of GAPDH (625 bp), TH (220 bp), PNMT (548 bp) in the RVLM of an estrus rat. First strand cDNA synthesis reaction was performed in the presence (+) or absence (−) of RT. (**Panel B**) PCR detection of γ-aminobutyric acid$_A$ (GABA$_A$) $\alpha_{1-3}$ subunit mRNA in RVLM from an estrus and term-pregnant (day 21) rat. (**Panel C**) Comparison of GABA$_A$ $\alpha$1: $\alpha$2 ratio in estrus ($n = 3$) and term-pregnant ($n = 3$) rats. Values are mean ± SE. PCR products were electrophoresed on a 2% agarose gel and visualized with ethidium bromide staining. (ABBREVIATIONS: bp = base pairs; L = DNA ladder, 123-bp step molecular weight marker; QL = quantitative DNA ladder, 235 total ng of low DNA mass ladder.)

of other endocrine mediators are chronically elevated during pregnancy. Therefore, it is probable that a combination of genomic and nongenomic effects interact to produce the observed alterations in sympathetic outflow. Preliminary experiments suggest that term pregnancy might be associated with a change in $GABA_A$ receptor subunit expression. However, additional experiments are necessary to determine the exact nature of these changes, the mechanisms involved, and the functional consequences. In conclusion, the growing realization that ovarian hormones and metabolites have significant effects on CNS control of the sympathetic nervous system has important implications for evaluating gender differences and development of cardiovascular diseases that involve the sympathetic nervous system.

## REFERENCES

1. LINDHEIMER, M.D. & A.I. KATZ. 1992. Renal physiology and disease in pregnancy. *In* The Kidney: Physiology and Pathophysiology, D.W. Seldin and G. Giebisch, Eds.: 3371–3432. Raven Press. New York.
2. DE SWIET, M. 1991. The cardiovascular system. *In* Clinical Physiology in Obstetrics, G. Chamberlain, Ed.: 3–38. Blackwell Scientific Publincations. Oxford.
3. BARRON, W.M., S.K. MUJAIS, M. ZINAMAN, *et al.* 1986. Plasma catecholamine responses to physiologic stimuli in normal human pregnancy. Am. J. Obstet. Gynecol. **154:** 80–84.
4. LUBE, W.F. 1984. Hypertension in pregnancy. Drugs **28:** 170–188.
5. MASILAMANI, S.M.E. & C.M. HEESCH. 1997. Effects of pregnancy and progesterone metabolites on baroreflex control of sympathetic outflow and heart rate in conscious rats. Am. J. Physiol. Regul. Integrative Comp. Physiol. **272:** R924–R934.
6. BROOKS, V.L. & L.C. KEIL. 1994. Hemorrhage decreases arterial pressure sooner in pregnant compared with nonpregnant dogs: role of baroreflex. Am. J. Physiol. Heart Circ. Physiol. **266:** H1610–H1619.
7. BROOKS, V.L., C.M. KANE & L.S. WELCH. 1999. Regional conductance changes during hemorrhage in pregnant and nonpregnant conscious rabbits Am. J. Physiol. Regul. Integrative Comp. Physiol. **277:** R675–R681.
8. HUMPHREYS, P.W. & N. JOELS. 1974. The carotid sinus baroreceptor reflex in the pregnant rabbit. J. Physiol. **239:** 89–102.
9. HUMPHREYS, P.W. & N. JOELS. 1982. Reflex response of the rabbit hind-limb muscle vascular bed to baroreceptor stimulation and its modification by pregnancy. J. Physiol. **330:** 461–473.
10. HUMPHREYS, P.W. & N. JOELS. 1977. Changes in cardiac output and total peripheral resistance during the carotid sinus baroreceptor reflex in the pregnant rabbit. J. Physiol. **272:** 45–55.
11. FERRIS, T.F. 1983. The pathophysiology of toxaemia and hypertension during pregnancy. Drugs **25:** 198–205.
12. DAVIDGE, S. & M. MCLAUGHLIN. 1994. Endogenous modulation of the blunted adrenergic response in resistance-sized mesenteric areries from the pregnant rat. Am. J. Obstet. Gynecol. **167:** 1691–1698.
13. HINES, T. & K.W. BARRON. 1992. Effect of sinoaortic denervation on pressor responses in pregnant rats. Am. J. Physiol. Regul. Integrative Comp. Physiol. **262:** R1100–R1105.
14. CRANDALL, M.E. & C.M. HEESCH. 1990. Baroreflex control of sympathetic outflow in pregnant rats: effects of captopril. Am. J. Physiol. Regul. Integrative Comp. Physiol. **258:** R1417–R1423.
15. KENT, B.B., J.W. DRANE, B. BLUMENSTEIN & J.W. MANNING. 1972. A mathematical model to assess changes in the baroreceptor reflex. Cardiology **5F:** 295–310.
16. HEESCH, C.M., J.D. LAIPRASERT & R. HAMLIN. 2000. Effects of pregnancy and pregesterone metabolite on afferent baroreceptor discharge [Abstr.]. FASEB J. **14:** A68–A68.

17. GUYENET, P.C. 1990. Role of the ventral medulla oblongata in blood pressure regulation. *In* Central Regulation of Autonomic Function, A.D. Loewry and K.M. Spyer, Eds.: 145–167. Oxford Univ. Press. New York.
18. DAMPNEY, R.A.L. & S. SASAKI. 1991. Tonic control of subretrofacial vasomotor neurons in the rostral ventrolateral medulla. Clin. Exp. Pharmacol. Physiol. **18:** 97–100.
19. CRAVO, S.L., S.F. MORRISON & D.J. REIS. 1991. Differentiation of two cardiovascular regions within caudal ventrolateral medulla. Am. J. Physiol. Regul. Integrative Comp. Physiol. **261:** R985–R994.
20. BADOER, E., M.J. MCKINLEY, B.J. OLDFIELD & R.M. MCALLEN. 1993. A comparison of hypotensive and non-hypotensive hemorrhage on Fos expression in spinally projecting neurons of the paraventricular nucleus and rostral ventrolateral medulla. Brain Res. **610:** 216–223.
21. CHAN, R.K.W. & P.E. SAWCHENKO. 1994. Spatially and temporally differentiated patterns of *c-fos* expression in brainstem catecholaminergic cell groups induced by cardiovascular challenges in the rat. J. Comp. Neurol. **348:** 433–460.
22. GRAHAM, J.C., G.E. HOFFMAN & A.F. SVED. 1995. c-Fos expressions in brainstem in response to hypotension and hypertension in conscious rats. J. Auton. Nerv. Syst. **55:** 92–104.
23. LI, Y.W. & R.A.L. DAMPNEY. 1994. Expression of Fos-like protein in brain following sustained hypertension and hypotension in conscious rabbits. Neuroscience **61:** 613–634.
24. CURTIS, K.S., J.T. CUNNINGHAM & C.M. HEESCH. 1999. Fos expression in brain stem nuclei of pregnant rats after hydralazine-induced hypotension. Am. J. Physiol. Regul. Integrative Comp. Physiol. **277:** R532–R540.
25. ORCHINIK, M. & B. MCEWEN. 1993. Novel and classical actions of neuroactive steroids. Neurotransmissions **9:** 1–6.
26. PAUL, S.M. & R.H. PURDY. 1992. Neuroactive steroids. FASEB J. **6:** 2311–2322.
27. MACDONALD, R.L. & R.W. OLSEN. 1994. $GABA_A$ receptors channels. Annu. Rev. Neurosci. **17:** 569–602.
28. COSTA, E. 1998. From $GABA_A$ receptor diversity emerges a unified vision of GABAergic inhibition. Annu. Rev. Pharmacol. Toxicol. **38:** 321–350.
29. MAJEWSKA, M.D. 1992. Neurosteroids: endogenous bimodal modulators of the GABA receptor. Mechanism of action and physiological significance. Prog. Neurobiol. **38:** 379–395.
30. CONCAS, A., P. FOLLESA, M.L. BARBACCIA, *et al.* 2000. Physiolgoical modulation of $GABA_A$ receptor plasticity by progesterone metabolites. Eur. J. Pharmacol. **375:** 225–235.
31. NGUYEN, Q., D.W. SAPP, P.C. VAN NESS & R.W. OLSEN. 1995. Modulation of $GABA_A$ receptor binding in human brain by neuroactive steroids: species and brain regional differences. Synapse **19:** 77–87.
32. LAN, N.C., K.W. GEE, M.B. BOLGER & J.S. CHEN. 1991. Differential responses of expressed recombinant human $GABA_A$ receptors to neurosteroids. J. Neurochem. **57(5):** 1818–1821.
33. SCHMID, G., R. SALA, G. BONANNO & M. RAITERI. 1998. Neurosteroids may differentially affect the function of two native $GABA_A$ receptor subtypes in the rat brain. Naunyn-Schmiedebergs Arch. Pharmacol. **357:** 401–407.
34. GARRETT, K.M., K.W. BARRON, R. BRISCOE & C.M. HEESCH. 1997. Neurosteroid modulation of [$^3$H]flunitrazepam binding in the medulla: an autoradiographic study. Brain Res. **768:** 301–309.
35. FRIEDMAN, L., T.T. GIBBS & D.H. FARB. 1993. γ-Aminobutyric acid$_A$ receptor regulation: chronic treatment with pregnanolone uncouples allosteric interactions between steroid and benzodiazepine sites. Mol. Pharmacol. **44:** 191–197.
36. MAJEWSKA, M.D., N.L. HARRISON, R.D. SCHWARTZ, *et al.* 1981. Steroid hormone metabolites are barbiturate-like modulators of the GABA receptor. Science **232:** 1004–1007.
37. HEESCH, C.M. & R.C. ROGERS. 1995. Effects of pregnancy and progesterone metabolites on regulation of sympatheic outflow. Clin. Exp. Pharmacol. Physiol. **22:** 136–142.

38. HEESCH, C.M., J.D. LAIPRASERT, R.C. ROGERS & S. GHOSH. 1997. Effects of 3α-hydroxy dihydroprogesterone (3α-OH-DHP) in the rostral ventrolateral medulla (RVLM) of female rats [Abstr.]. Soc. Neurosci. Abstr. **23:** 153.
39. ROSS, C.A., D.A. RUGGIERO, T.H. JOH, *et al.* 1984. Rostral ventrolateral medulla: selective projections to the thoracic autonomic cell column from the region containing C1 adrenaline neurons. J. Comp. Neurol. **228:** 168–185.
40. LAIPRASERT, J.D., R.C. ROGERS & C.M. HEESCH. 1998. Neurosteroid modulation of arterial baroreflex-sensitive neurons in rat rostral ventrolateral medulla. Am. J. Physiol. Regul. Integrative Comp. Physiol. **274:** R903–R911.
41. GARLAND, H.O., J.C. ATHERTON, C. BAYLIS, *et al.* 1987. Hormone profiles for progesterone, oestradiol, prolactin, plasma renin activity, aldosterone and corticosterone during pregnancy and pseudopregnancy in two strains of rat: correlation with renal studies. J. Endocrinol. **113:** 435–444.
42. QUESNELL, R.R. & V.L. BROOKS. 1997. Alterations in the baroreflex occur late in pregnancy in conscious rabbits. Am. J. Obstet. Gynecol. **176:** 692–694.
43. HERBISON, A.E. 1997. Estrogen regulation of GABA transmission in rat preoptic area. Brain Res. Bull. **44:** 321–326.
44. SHINGAI, R., M.L. SUTHERLAND & E.A. BARNARD. 1991. Effects of subunit subtypes of the cloned GABA$_A$ receptor on the response to a neurosteroid. Eur. J. Pharmacol. **206:** 77–80.
45. FENELON, V.S. & A.E. HERBISON. 1996. Plasticity in GABA$_A$ receptor subunit mRNA expression by hypothalamic magnocellular neurons in the adult rat. J. Neurosci. **16:** 4872–4880.
46. BRUSSAARD, A.B., K.S. KITS, R.E. BAKER, *et al.* 1997. Plasticity in fast synaptic inhibition of adult oxytocin neurons caused by switch in GABA$_A$ receptor subunit expression. Neuron **19:** 1103–1114.
47. FOLEY, C.M., J.J. STANTON, E.M. PRICE, *et al.* 2000. GABA$_A$ receptor α1, α2, and α3 subunit expression in discrete cardiovascularly related brainstem regions in nonpregnant and pregnant rats [Abstr.]. FASEB J. **14:** A68–A68.
48. COMER, A.M., S. YIP & J. LIPSKI. 1997. Detection of weakly expressed genes in the rostral ventrolateral medulla of the rat using micropunch and reverse transcription-polymerase chain reaction techniques. Clin. Exp. Pharmacol. Physiol. **24:** 755–759.
49. CRISWELL, H.E., T.J. MCCOWN, S.S. MOY, *et al.* 1997. Action of zolpidem on responses to GABA in relation to mRNAs for GABA$_A$ receptor alpha subunits within single cells: evidence for multiple functional GABA$_A$ isoreceptors on individual neurons. Neuropharmacology **36:** 1641–1652.
50. LEMOULLEC, J.M., S. JOUQUEY, P. CORVOL & F. PINET. 1997. A sensitive reverse transcriptase polymerase chain reaction assay for measuring the effects of dehydration and gestation on rat amounts of vasopressin and ocytocin mRNAs. Mol. Cell. Endocrinol. **128:** 151–159.

# Central Angiotensin and Baroreceptor Control of Circulation

GEOFFREY A. HEAD AND DMITRY N. MAYOROV

*Neuropharmacology Laboratory, Baker Medical Research Institute,
St. Kilda Road Central, Melbourne, 8008, Australia*

888888

# Central Angiotensin and Baroreceptor Control of Circulation

GEOFFREY A. HEAD AND DMITRY N. MAYOROV

*Neuropharmacology Laboratory, Baker Medical Research Institute,
St. Kilda Road Central, Melbourne, 8008, Australia*

ABSTRACT: Angiotensin (Ang) receptors are located in many important central nuclei involved in the regulation of the cardiovascular system. While most interest has focused on forebrain circumventricular actions, areas of the brainstem such as the nucleus of the solitary tract and the ventrolateral medulla contain high concentrations of $AT_1$ receptors. The present review encompasses the physiological role of Ang II in the hindbrain, particularly in relation to its influence on baroreflex control mechanisms. In rabbits there are sympatho-excitatory $AT_1$ receptors in the rostral ventrolateral medulla (RVLM), accessible to Ang II from the cerebrospinal fluid. Activation of these receptors acutely increases renal sympathetic nerve activity (RSNA) and RSNA baroreflex responses. However, blockade of endogenous Ang receptors in the brainstem also shows sympathoexcitation, suggesting there is greater endogenous activity of a sympathoinhibitory Ang II action. Microinjections of angiotensin antagonists into the RVLM showed relatively little tonic activity of endogenous Ang II influencing sympathetic activity in conscious rabbits. However, Ang II receptors in the RVLM mediate sympathetic responses to airjet stress in conscious rabbits. Similarly with respect to heart rate baroreflexes, there appears to be little tonic effect of angiotensin in the brainstem in normal conscious animals. Chronic infusion of Ang II for two weeks into the fourth ventricle of conscious rabbits inhibits the cardiac baroreflex while infusion of losartan increases the gain of the reflex. These actions suggest that Ang II in the brainstem modulates sympathetic responses depending on specific afferent and synaptic inputs in both the short term but importantly also in the long term, thus forming an important mechanism for increasing the range of adaptive response patterns.

KEYWORDS: Ang II; $AT_1$ receptors; Losartan; Renal sympathetic activity; Baroreflexes; Chemoreflexes; Rostral ventrolateral medulla; Blood pressure; Rabbits

## INTRODUCTION

Much evidence exists to suggest that within the central nervous system (CNS), there is a renin-angiotensin system comprising angiotensinogen as the substrate and synthetic enzymes that produce the various forms of angiotensin (Ang).[1–3] But it has been the discovery of the localization of Ang II receptors in important nuclei throughout the brain of many different species that has been the key to understanding

Address for correspondence: Dr. Geoffrey A. Head, Baker Medical Research Institute, P.O. Box 6492, St. Kilda Road Central, Melbourne, 8008, Australia. Voice: 61 3 9522 4333; fax: 61 3 9521 1362.
Geoff.Head@baker.edu.au

361

the potential function of this Ang system.[4–7] Perhaps the most well studied of these is body fluid homeostasis and the regulation of the cardiovascular system. There are high concentrations of Ang receptors in regions that regulate thirst, body fluid, and blood pressure such as the subfornical organ, organum vasculosum laminae terminalis, and the area postrema.[2,8,9] These regions do not have a blood–brain barrier and can respond to circulating levels of Ang II, thus providing an important link from the kidney to the brain.[10,11] Other regions in the brainstem such as the nucleus tractus solitarii (NTS), the rostral ventrolateral medulla (RVLM), the caudal ventrolateral medulla (CVLM), and the intermediolateral column of the spinal cord are also rich in Ang receptors and are key integrative sites involved in central cardiovascular regulation but possess a blood–brain barrier that normally prevents any direct contact from circulating Ang. Presumably, these receptors are activated by an endogenous Ang system involving either Ang II or Ang III as neurotransmitters or neuromodulators. Thus, it would appear that Ang not only plays an important role in the regulation of the cardiovascular system within the kidney and vasculature but also within in the CNS.[2,12]

For the last decade it has been possible to discriminate Ang II receptor subtypes using nonpeptide Ang II receptor antagonists.[13,14] These highly selective Ang II receptor ligands such as losartan and PD123177 have provided evidence for the existence of two Ang II receptor subtypes, termed $AT_1$ and $AT_2$.[13] $AT_1$ receptors, of which there are two isoforms,[15] have been found in the highest concentrations in rostral forebrain areas such as the circumventricular organs and hypothalamus while the less prevalent $AT_2$ receptors are found in higher concentrations in areas such as the cerebellum and thalamus.[16,17] However, despite several decades of study, we are not really clear on how Ang in different regions of the brain participates in the physiological regulation of the cardiovascular system. Perhaps more importantly, it is not clear how central Ang II contributes to pathophysiological conditions such as hypertension or heart failure. It would be an oversimplification to suggest that there is one brain Ang system, and care must be taken to separate anatomically distinct but related regions of the brain. Of particular interest have been the brainstem nuclei involved in the generation of sympathetic vasomotor tone and integration of baroreceptor afferent information. Baroreflexes are critical in the short-term regulation of arterial pressure[18–20] and are vital to reduce the impact of fluctuations by altering sympathetic vasomotor activity or heart rate and cardiac output.[21] The present brief review discusses the role of central Ang in modulating cardiovascular reflex mechanisms. Since most reviews and experimental studies have concentrated on the forebrain regions, the particular focus of this paper will be to highlight the cardiovascular actions of Ang within the brainstem.

## CARDIOVASCULAR EFFECTS OF INTRAVENTRICULAR ANGIOTENSIN

Many studies have shown that stimulation of central Ang II receptors in various species results in an increase in arterial pressure.[2,3] Bickerton and Buckley demonstrated in the early 1960s that Ang II, in addition to acting on peripheral cardiovascular structures, could also elicit a centrally mediated pressor response in the dog.[22] A common approach used to investigate the cardiovascular role of the central Ang

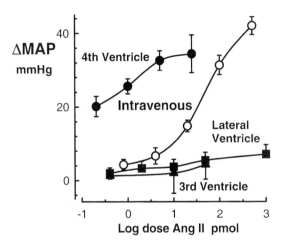

**FIGURE 1.** Average dose-response relationships from conscious rabbits given Ang II into the 4th ventricle (*filled circles, n = 7*), lateral ventricle (*filled squares, n = 9*), 3rd ventricle (*filled triangles, n = 5*), and intravenously (*open circles, n = 8*). *Vertical bars* are means ± SE and indicate between-animal variance. (Data from Head & Williams, with permission.[28])

system has been to administer Ang peptides into the cerebral ventricles. Early studies by Severs and colleagues showed a pressor response from perfusion of the lateral ventricle of anesthetized cats with Ang II.[23] Preventing the perfusate from leaving the third ventricle blocked the response, suggesting a site of action below the midbrain. Hoffman and Phillips examined the effects intraventricular administration of Ang II to conscious rats and found marked pressor and dipsogenic responses via the lateral ventricle as well as the anterior and posterior third ventricle.[24] In this species, however, the site of action involved the anterior ventral third ventricle (AV3V), which correlates well with the location of the receptors and is relatively close to the injection site.[25] Indeed, the administration of Ang II has often been used to test the patency of the ventricular cannula because the rat begins to drink shortly after the Ang administration.

Unlike the forebrain, the role of an Ang system in the brainstem has received relatively little attention until recently. Early studies showed that injecting Ang II into the fourth ventricle (4V) of rats produced no change in blood pressure, suggesting this region was not a major site of action for Ang,[24] despite high concentrations of Ang receptors in hindbrain areas such as the NTS and area postrema.[17] By contrast, we found that conscious rabbits are most sensitive to Ang II given into the 4V.[26,27] Bolus injections of Ang II produced dose-dependent increases in blood pressure with doses about 400 times lower than would be expected to increase blood pressure given intravenously (FIG. 1). The onset of the response was relatively quick within 1 min, and the response generally lasts only 5 min, depending on the dose.[28] Surprisingly, lateral ventricle or third ventricle injections of Ang II to conscious rabbits had little effect on blood pressure with doses as large as 1000 pmol (FIG. 1).[28] The rabbit also does not respond to chronic infusions of Ang into the lateral ventricle[29] nor do acute injections of Ang produce dipsogenic responses[30] as they do in the rat.

The receptors are $AT_1$ because the pressor response to Ang II administered into the 4V of conscious rabbits was completely blocked by low doses of the nonpeptide-selective antagonist losartan, but not affected by the $AT_2$ antagonist PD123319.[31] Vasoconstriction occurs in both the mesenteric and renal vascular beds but was accompanied by dilatation of the hindlimb vascular bed and a fall in heart rate, which opposed the vasoconstriction and reduced the observed pressor response.[28] However, the hindlimb dilatation changes to hindlimb vasoconstriction in sinoaortically denervated rabbits suggesting that it is predominantly due to a baroreflex response to the rise in blood pressure. Surprisingly, chronic baroreceptor denervation increased the sensitivity to Ang II administration into the 4V by approximately 1000-fold, suggesting that the Ang receptors that have been stimulated by 4V administration may become important when baroreflex mechanisms are suppressed such as in hypertension and heart failure.[26] The phenomenon that sinoaortic denervation profoundly increased the sensitivity to central Ang II has been observed in both rats with lateral ventricle administration and in rabbits with 4V injections.[27,32] In both species it involves an increase in the sensitivity of the hindlimb presympathetic vasomotor pathways to Ang. Thus, it is likely that the mechanism of the change in the muscle bed response to central Ang II from dilatation to constriction that we observed after sinoaortic denervation (SAD) is associated with this change in sensitivity to Ang II produced by baroreceptor denervation.

## EFFECTS OF INTRAVENTRICULAR ANGIOTENSIN ON SYMPATHETIC NERVE ACTIVITY

The importance of the sympathetic nervous system in mediating central cardiovascular effects of Ang has been recognized since the mid-1960s in all species studied, although relatively few studies have measured nerve activity directly.[3,23,27,33,34] Tobey and colleagues observed a marked increase in splanchnic nerve activity but no effect on renal sympathetic nerve activity (RSNA) following intraventricular administration of Ang II using anesthetized, sinoaortic denervated, vagotomized cats, suggesting there may be differential effects on sympathetic activity depending on the vascular bed.[35] A number of studies suggest that in the rat there is an important contribution to the pressor response by release of vasopressin.[36–39] However, direct recordings of RSNA do show a significant increase in RSNA concomitant with the pressor response following Ang II injected into the third ventricle.[40] In contrast to the rat, the pressor response observed with 4V Ang II given to conscious rabbits is predominantly due to sympathetic vasoconstriction because it is blocked by intravenous prazosin.[27] Using the same preparation, Dorward and Rudd observed that 4V administration of Ang II produced a transient increase in RSNA, but as blood pressure increased the RSNA was inhibited and returned to a level slightly above control, suggesting that the renal sympathoexcitatory effect of Ang II was under marked baroreceptor feedback inhibition.

While much has been written about the effect of circulating Ang on cardiac and sympathetic baroreflexes,[41] very few studies have examined the effect of intraventricular Ang on baroreflexes. In conscious rabbits Dorward and Rudd found that 4V Ang II produced a marked increase in RSNA excitation when the baroreceptors were unloaded with decreasing blood pressure.[42] Thus, the upper plateau of the MAP-

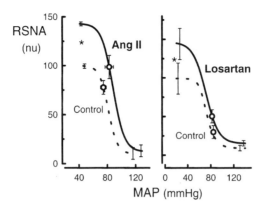

**FIGURE 2. Left panel:** Average mean arterial pressure (MAP, mm Hg)—renal sympathetic activity (RSNA-normalized units) baroreflex curves from six urethane anesthetized rabbits before (control, *dashed lines*) and during infusion of Ang II into the fourth ventricle (*solid line*). **Right panel:** Average MAP (mmHg)-RSNA (normalized units) curves from eight conscious rabbits before (control, *dashed lines*) and after 10 μg losartan into the fourth ventricle (losartan, *solid line*). *Circles* on curves represent resting values. *Error bars* indicate average SEM. (Adapted with permission from Saigusa & Head[43] and Bendle, Malpas & Head.[31])

RSNA curve was doubled, and the curve shifted to the right because of the increase in blood pressure. We observed a similar pattern of the effect of 4V Ang II on the RSNA baroreflex in urethane-anesthetized rabbits (FIG. 2), although the magnitude of the increase in the RSNA in response to the baroreceptor unloading was less.[43]

## CARDIOVASCULAR EFFECT OF BLOCKING ENDOGENOUS ANGIOTENSIN

There has been a great deal of interest in the cardiovascular role of the endogenous Ang system within the brain. Studies to block the endogenous brainstem Ang II have mainly used Ang peptide antagonists, which are based on the peptide sequence for Ang II, nonpeptide antagonists such as losartan, or inhibitors of the synthetic enzymes such as converting enzyme inhibitors. Dorward and Rudd examined the renal sympathetic and heart rate baroreceptor reflex effects of the antagonist Sar[1]Ile[8]Ang II administered into the 4V of rabbits. The antagonist had no effect on renal sympathetic reflexes while an Ang-converting enzyme inhibitor, enalaprilat, slightly enhanced maximal baroreflex sympathetic responses.[42] Possibly the Ang receptors that were activated by 4V administration were not being activated by endogenous Ang II in a conscious rabbit or the antagonists used were not effective. We therefore examined the actions of losartan on baroreceptor reflexes in conscious rabbits chronically implanted with a renal nerve–recording electrode for the measurement of RSNA (FIG. 2). The effect of Ang II on the RSNA baroreflex curve closely resembled the effect of chemoreceptor stimulation with hypoxia,[44,45] suggesting that endogenous Ang may be activated during chemoreceptor stimulation. Thus, baroreflex curves were also examined during hypoxia. The $AT_1$-receptor antagonist losartan increased resting RSNA during normoxia (FIG. 2) and also during the hypoxia regime.[31] In addition, the upper plateau of the RSNA-MAP was elevated by both Ang II and losartan during normoxia, but only Ang II shifted the curve to the right (FIG. 2). The elevation of the upper plateau was particularly marked when the hypocapnia that results from hyperventilation was prevented by the animal breathing 3% $CO_2$.[31] These results were surprising given that the receptor antagonist produced qualitatively similar effects to Ang itself and suggest that losartan is blocking a tonically active sympathoinhibitory action of endogenous Ang (FIG. 2, compare left and right panels). By contrast, the effects of trigeminal stimulation were not affected by losartan, suggesting that Ang normally modulates specific inputs to the presympathetic neurons, possibly by a presynaptic action. The action of losartan was most likely a specific effect because we observed similar changes with the angiotensin-converting enzyme inhibitor, enalapril.[46] Although at this stage we do not know the site of action of the sympathoinhibitory Ang pathways, possibilities include the CVLM and the NTS (see below).

## CHRONIC EFFECT OF ACTIVATION AND INHIBITION OF HINDBRAIN ANG RECEPTORS ON CARDIAC BAROREFLEXES

Studies concerning the cardiovascular role of central Ang II have predominantly involved *acute* administration of agonists and antagonists. However, perhaps even more important for the cardiovascular system is the impact of chronic activation or inhibition of central Ang II receptors. It has been known since the early 1980s that central infusion of Ang produces hypertension, and central inhibition of the renin-Ang system attenuates hypertension.[47,48] Despite many such subsequent studies, relatively few have examined cardiovascular reflex mechanisms. Chronic but not acute administration of $AT_1$-receptor antagonist EXP 3174 has been shown to normalize cardiac baroreflex function in SHR.[49] However, this does not only apply to hypertension; rabbits with pacing-induced heart failure have a central Ang II-mediated inhibition of cardiac baroreflex function mechanism involving the area postrema that can be restored by $AT_1$-receptor blockade.[50] Thus, the participation of central Ang II in inhibiting cardiac baroreflexes does not appear to occur in the normal animal but requires a long-term perturbation of the cardiovascular system such as hypertension or heart failure. Acute intraventricular administration of Ang II does not influence cardiac baroreflex mechanisms in either rats[49] or rabbits.[31,42,46,51]

We recently examined the effect of chronic activation or inhibition of central Ang II receptors on cardiac baroreflex function in conscious normotensive rabbits. Animals received a 4V infusion by osmotic minipump of either Ang II, losartan, or Ringer's solution for two weeks. Assessment of the HR baroreflex was performed by a single slow ramp rise and fall in blood pressure by intravenous infusion of phenylephrine and by caval balloon inflation, respectively. Ang II (100 ng/h) decreased cardiac baroreflex gain by –20% after one week and –37% after two weeks, while losartan (30 µg/h) increased baroreflex gain by +24% and +58% at these times (FIG. 3).[52] The intriguing feature of this study was that the effect of Ang II and losartan took the full two weeks to develop. Within a week of stopping the infusions, car-

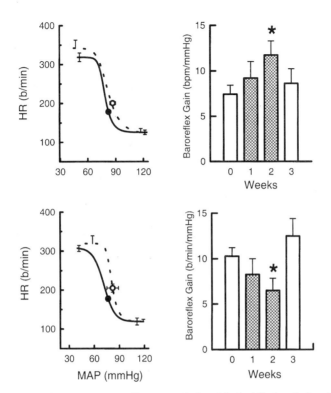

**FIGURE 3. Left:** Cardiac baroreflex curves before (*dashed line*) and after (*black line*) a two-week period of fourth ventricle infusion of angiotensin II (*upper panel*, 100 ng/h) or losartan (*lower panel, 30 μg/h*). *Circles* on curves are basal values. *Error bars* are average SEM. **Right:** Gain of the cardiac baroreflex before (week 0, *open bar*), during (week 1 and 2, *cross-hatched bars*), and after (week 3, *right open bar*) a two-week 4V infusion angiotensin II (*upper panel*, 100 ng/h) or losartan (*lower panel*, 30 μg/h). Control values are the average of the two control experiments (week 0). *$p < 0.05$ for comparison between control and treatment. (Adapted with permission from Gaudet, Godwin & Head.[52])

diac baroreflex gain had returned to control (FIG. 3). Ringer's solution or lower doses of Ang II or losartan did not modify the cardiac baroreflex function. Blood pressure and heart rate were not altered by any treatment nor was their variability affected as assessed by power spectral analysis.[52] These data indicate a novel long-term modulation of cardiac baroreflexes by endogenous Ang II, which is independent of the level of blood pressure. The reason for such a long time course is not clear because activation of neuronal $AT_1$ receptors by Ang II occurs relatively rapidly, due to a reduction in $K^+$ current via protein kinase C, raised intracellular $Ca^{2+}$, and stimulation of $Ca^{2+}$ current.[53] Possibly there is long-term regulation of the receptor or altered expression of $AT_1$ receptors. Another possibility may involve alteration to the levels of biosynthetic/degradative enzymes that in turn influence the levels and release of other peptides. Such is the case with converting enzyme inhibitors that prevent the formation of Ang II from Ang I, but also result in an increase in bradykinin levels. With prolonged infusions, it is possible that Ang II and losartan may access baroreflex integration sites in the NTS where they are known from studies in anesthetized rats to inhibit and facilitate the baroreflex gain, respectively.[54] In support of this is the observation that the effect of Ang II and losartan given chronically 4V altered the curvature parameter of the baroreflex without affecting the range parameter, which is precisely the manner in which these two agents influence the baroreflex when injected directly into the NTS.[41]

## MEDULLARY SITES OF ACTION OF ANGIOTENSIN

Intraventricular administration has been a useful tool particularly in conscious animals to help unravel the role of the Ang peptides within the CNS, but it is limited by agents given in this way, influencing large brain regions rather than specific nuclei. In order to determine the distribution of neurons within the medulla activated by infusion of Ang II into the 4V of conscious rabbits, we used the expression of Fos, the protein product of the immediate early gene c-fos, as a marker of neuronal activation in baroreceptor-intact and barodenervated animals.[55] Ang II induced a marked increase in the number of Fos-positive neurons in the NTS and in the rostral, intermediate, and caudal parts of the ventrolateral medulla with 30–75% of cells

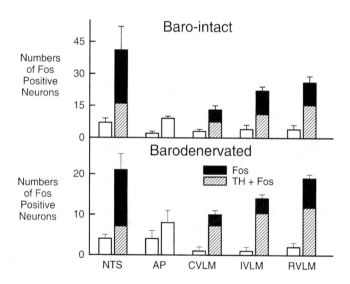

**FIGURE 4.** Number of Fos-positive neurons per section in different brain regions after fourth ventricle administration of 4–8 pmol/min Angiotensin II (*filled bars*) or Ringer's solution (*open bars*) in conscious baroreceptor intact (*upper panel*) or conscious sinoaortically denervated (*lower panel*) rabbits. The number of Fos-positive cells that contain tyrosine hydroxylase is shown by the *shaded bars*. NTS, nucleus of the solitary tract; AP, area postrema; CVLM, caudal ventrolateral medulla; IVLM, intermediate ventrolateral medulla; RVLM, rostral ventrolateral medulla. (Data adapted from Hirooka *et al.*[55])

double-labeled for Fos and tyrosine hydroxylase immunoreactivity[55] (FIG. 4). We found that the distribution of Fos-positive neurons closely correlated with the location of Ang II receptor binding sites as previously determined in the rabbit.[6]

## ANGIOTENSIN ACTIONS WITHIN THE ROSTRAL VENTROLATERAL MEDULLA

Microinjection techniques into the brain parenchyma have been widely used to limit drug action to small brain regions, but have been confined in most cases to anesthetized preparations. One of the most important regions in the medulla where Ang peptides are likely to have an action is the RVLM.[56,57] The RVLM is a major source of bulbospinal sympathetic drive to the preganglionic neurons in the spinal cord[58] and contains high Ang II receptor binding in the rabbit[6] and other species including the cat and dog.[59] The existence of ANG II immunoreactive fibers in the ventrolateral medulla[60] and extended neural processes of the RVLM neurons close to the ventral surface[61] suggests that Ang II may have a ready access to the RVLM neurons both from neural pathways and from cerebrospinal fluid. Allen and co-workers demonstrated that direct microinjection of Ang II into the subretrofacial pressor region in the RVLM of the cat resulted in a pressor response.[62] In the same year, Andreatta and colleagues suggested that the RVLM may contain a renin-Ang system because Ang I applied to the ventral surface of the brainstem of the cat produced an increase in blood pressure after conversion to Ang II.[63] They also provided the first evidence of tonically active Ang II in the RVLM of the anesthetized cat by showing that with the same topical application approach $Sar^1Ile^8Ang$ II decreased blood pressure. Sasaki and Dampney found that the sites that produced the greatest increase in blood pressure in the RVLM were also those containing the highest concentration of Ang receptors[64,65] and provided the first evidence of tonically active Ang II in the RVLM of the anesthetized baroreceptor-denervated rabbit by showing that injection of $Sar^1Thr^8Ang$ II decreased blood pressure and RSNA. We initially mapped various dorsal and ventral sites with microinjections of 1 pmol of Ang II and found that marked pressor responses were observed only when administered into a discrete region of the RVLM corresponding to the subretrofacial nucleus (FIG. 5). These findings were consistent with the findings of Sasaki and Dampney.[64,65] We found that injections as close as 1 mm from this region gave very much smaller pressor responses, suggesting that the Ang II-sensitive site is relatively small. Dose-response curves to Ang II in this region indicate that very low doses were required, with the half-maximal dose approximately 9 fmol. This was approximately 1000-fold less than that required by the 4V route.[66]

We also observed that local microinfusion of Ang II into the RVLM produced facilitation of the renal sympathetic baroreflex (FIG. 6, upper left), which was very similar to that produced by 4V administration (FIG. 2, left).[43] We found that glutamate infusions into the same region of the RVLM have similar effects to Ang, increasing blood pressure, resting RSNA, and the upper sympathetic baroreflex plateau without affecting the lower plateau (FIG. 6, upper right).[43] The similarity of its actions to those of glutamate suggest that it may directly excite sympathetic vasomotor cells in this region. Indeed, electrophysiological studies have shown that Ang appears to directly excite bulbospinal C1 neurons[67,68] by activating postsynaptic

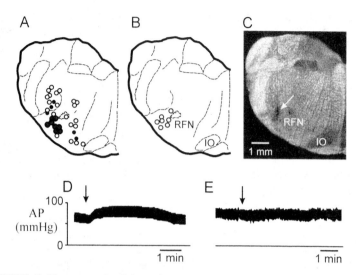

**FIGURE 5. Upper panels:** Schematic representation of coronal view of the rabbit medulla with *circles* showing distribution of injection sites in the RVLM at the level of the rostral tip of the inferior olive in anesthetized (**A**) and conscious (**B**) rabbits. *Open circles* indicate no change in arterial pressure (−5 to +5 mmHg), *small filled circles* represent pressor responses +6 to +15 mmHg, and *large filled circles* indicate pressor responses greater than 16 mmHg. (**C**) Photomicrograph of a coronal section of the brain stem at the same level showing a typical injection site in the RVLM (from a conscious rabbit experiment) and the tissue damage near the injection site. IO, inferior olive; RFN, retrofacial nucleus. *White arrow* shows the site of microinjection. **Bottom panels:** original recordings of arterial pressure (AP) responses to microinjections of Ang II into the RVLM from individual anesthetized (**D**) and conscious (**E**) rabbits. *Arrows* mark injection of 1 pmol (**D**) and 20 pmol (**E**) of Angiotensin II.

$AT_1$-receptors, resulting in a depolarization involving the closing of $K^+$ channels.[69] Administration of 10 pmol of the antagonist Sar[1]Ile[8]Ang II bilaterally into the sub-retrofacial region of anesthetized rabbits blocked the pressor response to locally applied Ang II and reduced the pressor responses to 4V Ang II by two-thirds.[66] This is perhaps the strongest evidence to suggest that the RVLM is the major site of action for Ang II given into the cerebrospinal fluid surrounding the brainstem, but the remaining response suggests that other sites make a small contribution.

While other studies have observed pressor responses to local application of Ang II to this region in cats, they have used higher doses than did our study.[62,63] Sasaki and Dampney have shown that Ang II and Ang III are equipotent when injected into the RVLM of the rabbit.[65] Ang 1–7 is some 50 times less potent, suggesting that in this species it is unlikely to be the active form. While the presence of $AT_1$-receptors is not so obvious in the ventrolateral medulla of the rat, a number of studies have shown pressor responses to microinjections of Ang II.[70,71] However, Santos and colleagues have shown evidence that Ang 1–7 is perhaps more important in the rat RVLM, possibly acting at a distinct receptor.[72–75]

Much interest exists as to whether there is a contribution to maintaining sympathetic tone by Ang II endogenously released in the RVLM. However, we did not ob-

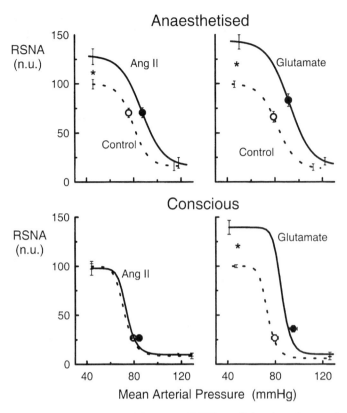

**FIGURE 6.** Average mean arterial pressure (MAP, mmHg) and renal sympathetic activity (RSNA-normalized units) curves before (control, *dashed lines*) and during infusion of Ang II (**left panels,** *solid line*) or glutamate (**right panels,** *solid line*) into the rostral ventrolateral medulla (RVLM) (*left, solid line*) from six urethane-anesthetized rabbits (**upper panels**) or in seven conscious rabbits (**lower panels**). *Circles* on each curve represent resting values. *Error bars* are average SEM calculated from analysis of variance indicating variation within animals. $*p < 0.05$. (Adapted with permission from Mayorov & Head.[51])

serve any change in blood pressure or nerve activity by giving an effective dose of Sar[1]Ile[8]Ang II. This contrasts the findings of other groups that found a marked reduction in blood pressure with this agent or with Sar[1]Thr[8]Ang II.[64,76–78] A recent study suggests, however, that this effect is not related to the blockade of Ang II receptors.[79] Presumably, this was an effect observed only at much higher doses used in these studies (100–1000 pmol) because we observed no effect on basal blood pressure using 10 pmol, but still had a complete blockade of the pressor response when Ang II was administered into the RVLM. Since we did not observe any attenuation of the glutamate response, the blockage by Sar[1]Ile[8]Ang II was likely to be specific.

Until recently, the ability to microinject into the RVLM was essentially confined to acute, anesthetized preparations because this area is close to the flexion point of the cervical spinal cord and is subject to movement in the conscious animal. The role of Ang peptides in the ventrolateral medulla and the role of the RVLM itself may be very much influenced by the anesthetized animal preparations. Indeed, a high degree of surgical stress is typically associated with microinjecting into the RVLM in the acute anesthetized preparation, and hormonal systems such as the renin-angiotensin system have been reported to become activated during anesthesia and surgery.[80] Because of the quiet nature of rabbits, we have found them a suitable animal for microinjection into the RVLM while they were conscious and sitting in a standard rabbit box otherwise unrestrained. We therefore developed a new cannula system which permitted us to make repeated bilateral microinjections into the RVLM of conscious rabbits.[81] We used this new technique to examine the role of Ang II in the RVLM while measuring RSNA at rest and during baroreflex responses. Bilateral microinjection of Ang II (10 and 20 pmol) into the RVLM did not change blood pressure or RSNA (FIG. 5). Histological analysis revealed that the injection sites were exactly in the same region as those that produced pressor responses in the anesthetized rabbits and also that the cannula system produced minimal damage (FIG. 5). We did observe that a higher dose of 30 pmol of Ang II gradually increased blood pressure by 8 mmHg, without affecting RSNA. The time course of the increase in blood pressure was slow, starting to increase within 0.5–1 min and reaching a peak within 4 min of completion of the injection. Bilateral microinfusion of Ang II (4 pmol/min for 20 min) did not affect resting blood pressure or RSNA.[51] During the infusion of Ang II, baroreflexes were examined but no effects were observed (FIG. 6, lower left).[51] At the same site glutamate produced an increase in blood pressure and increases in sympathetic activity and augmentation of the sympathetic baroreflex in a similar fashion to what was seen in the anesthetized animal (FIG. 6, compare upper right with lower right). By contrast, infusion of the same dose of Ang II into the 4V cerebrospinal fluid increased arterial blood pressure and RSNA by 22 and 34%, respectively, suggesting that sites other than the RVLM may be mediating these responses. We also determined the effects of blocking Ang receptors, with a specific antagonist. Pretreatment with Sar[1]Ile[8]Ang II into the RVLM did not change renal sympathetic baroreflex parameters. The lack of effect inhibiting Ang II receptors in the RVLM is consistent with our previous findings in anesthetized animals, but the lack of effect of Ang II itself is somewhat surprising.

One possibility is that the action of Ang II may depend very much on the state of excitatory inputs to the region, which is similar to the view expressed by Fontes and colleagues in the rat.[75] Fontes and colleagues had also developed a method for administration of agents into the RVLM, but in conscious rats.[74] They showed that Ang II and Ang 1–7 caused an increase in blood pressure while the peptide antagonist Sar[1]Ile[8]Ang II produced a small decrease in it. They observed an increase in blood pressure with two different AT$_1$-receptor antagonists;[74,75] this may be related to our observations that losartan produced an increase in sympathetic activity when given 4V to conscious rabbits.[31] One possibility is that the relatively large volume of 200 nl enabled the drug to block the sympathoinhibitory action of Ang in the CVLM. The other possibility is that the effect of Ang II depends on the synaptic inputs to the premotor cells. Electrophysiological studies have shown that Ang II increases input resistance of the vasomotor cell body which should have the effect of potentiating both excitatory and inhibitory synaptic inputs.[69] In support of this concept, Fontes and colleagues who showed that the AT$_1$-receptor antagonist CV-11974 produced an in-

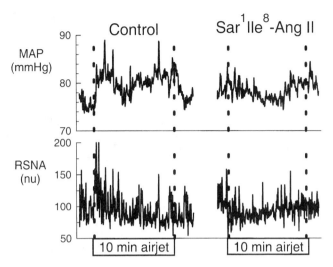

**FIGURE 7.** Average recordings of arterial blood pressure (mmHg, **upper panel**) and renal sympathetic nerve activity (RSNA, normalized units, **lower panel**) before (*left of dashed line*) and during (*between dashed lines*) 10 min airjet stress in four conscious rabbits prior to (control) and after treatment of the rostral ventrolateral medulla (RVLM) with the Ang II antagonist Sar[1]Ile[8]Ang II. Note that blockade of angiotensin II receptors in the RVLM blocked the pressor and RSNA response to airjet stress.

crease in blood pressure in normotensive rats (blocking a predominant depressor role of Ang peptides) also found that this drug produced a depressor response in the hypertensive transgenic rat harboring the mouse Ren-2 gene (blocking a predominant pressor response).[75] They suggested that the role of Ang peptides depends on the endogenous activity of the Ang system. In support of this we have recently found that blockade of Ang II receptors in the RVLM attenuated the renal sympathoexcitatory responses to airjet stress (FIG. 7).

## ANGIOTENSIN ACTIONS WITHIN THE CAUDAL VENTROLATERAL MEDULLA

Activation of the CVLM causes sympathoinhibition that is mediated by a short ascending inhibitory projection from the CVLM to the RVLM.[82] Electrophysiological studies show tonically active neurons in the CVLM inhibit the firing of sympathoexcitatory barosensitive neurons in the RVLM of the rabbit.[83] While the CVLM of the rabbit contains Ang II receptors,[6] relatively few studies have investigated the role of Ang receptors in this region. Microinjection of Ang II in the region of the A1 noradrenergic cells within the CVLM of the rabbit results in a depressor response.[84] The most extensive study was performed by Saigusa and colleagues who found that Ang II infusion in the CVLM of anesthetized rabbits decreased sympathetic activity and inhibited renal sympathetic baroreflexes while blockade of

CVLM Ang receptors increased the sympathetic baroreflex but did not alter blood pressure or RSNA.[85]

## ANGIOTENSIN ACTIONS WITHIN THE NUCLEUS TRACTUS SOLITARII

Within the medulla, the NTS has been the most extensively studied with respect to a likely site of action of Ang peptides. The NTS is the nucleus containing the primary termination of baroreceptor and chemoreceptor afferents[86] but, more importantly, in most species including human, cat, rabbit, and rat, the NTS contains the highest concentration of Ang receptors within the medulla.[6,60,87,88] Thus, it is not surprising that this nucleus has been suggested as a main region for Ang influencing baroreceptor afferent information[41,54] as well as the integration of chemoreceptor afferents.[54] In anesthetized rats, microinjection of Ang into the NTS produces pressor responses in nmol doses[70,89] and depressor responses at pmol doses,[70,90] and attenuates the baroreceptor reflex[91,92] through $AT_1$-receptors.[93] Our own studies in anesthetized rabbits are consistent with these findings since we observed mainly depressor responses to 1 pmol Ang II injected into the dorsomedial region.[66] This decrease may involve an increase in GABA release[94] and possibly the release of NO.[54] Conversely, blockade of the Ang II receptors increases blood pressure[70,95] or has no effect,[96] but appears to consistently increase the gain of the baroreflex.[96–98]

## CONCLUSION

In recent years we have made good progress in the understanding of the importance of Ang peptides and receptors within the brainstem to cardiovascular regulation. There is growing recognition from a variety of different studies that the effects of activating Ang II receptors in the RVLM, CVLM, and NTS appear to be very much dependent on the state of the animal and the activity of specific afferent information. This aspect may be a critically important mechanism for the adaptive ability of the CNS to respond with appropriate autonomic response patterns depending on the situation. The development of the microinjecting system for conscious animals opens the door to more fully investigate the neurotransmitter mechanisms within the RVLM without the constraints of anesthesia and will permit an investigation into the role of Ang peptides in mediating the circulatory responses to emotional and behavioral stimuli. For the most part, in conscious normal animals, there is relatively little indication of the sympathoexcitatory influence at the level of the RVLM, as shown by the observations that blockade of $AT_1$-receptors does not change blood pressure by very much and in some cases increases blood pressure. The latter finding indicates that in conscious animals the sympathoinhibitory influence of Ang is more evident than in the anesthetized preparation. This sympathoinhibition appears to be mainly mediated by an interaction with baroreceptor inhibitory and also chemoreceptor excitatory inputs into the vasomotor neurons because the sympathoinhibitory actions of Ang II are of greatest influence during hypoxia and hypotension. The specific ability to modulate synaptic inputs may be very much related to the linking of the $AT_1$ receptor to a $K^+$ channel. Studies in rats and rabbits suggest that the excitatory action of Ang II is normally under profound baroreceptor inhibition because the sensitivity to Ang is markedly increased in barodenervated animals and the sympathoexcitatory effect of Ang is most evident when baroreceptor input is reduced. Interestingly, baroreflexes themselves can be modulated by Ang peptides over several weeks of drug administration. The precise mechanism of this long-term action remains to be elucidated. Much evidence now shows that in situations where there is increased excitatory and decreased inhibitory inputs to the RVLM brainstem such as barodenervation, acute stress, hypertension, or heart failure, the importance of the sympathoexcitatory Ang system within the brainstem clearly becomes very evident.

## ACKNOWLEDGMENTS

These studies were supported by an Institute grant from the National Health and Medical Research Council of Australia. The authors wish to acknowledge the contribution of collaborators Jean-Luc Elghozi, Naomi Williams, Takeshi Saigusa, Robert Bendle, Elisabeth Lambert, Yoshitaka Hirooka, and Roger Dampney to the work described in this review.

## REFERENCES

1. GANONG, W.F. 1984. The brain renin-angiotensin system. Annu. Rev. Physiol. **46:** 17–31.
2. PHILLIPS, M.I. 1987. Functions of angiotensin in the central nervous system. Annu. Rev. Physiol. **49:** 413–435.
3. SEVERS, W.B. & A.E. DANIELS-SEVERS. 1973. Effects of angiotensin on the central nervous system. Pharmacol. Rev. **25:** 415–449.
4. MANN, J.F., P.W. SCHILLER, E.L. SCHIFFRIN, et al. 1981. Brain receptor binding and central actions of angiotensin analogs in rats. Am. J. Physiol. **241:** R124–R129.
5. MENDELSOHN, F.A.O., R. GUIRION, J.M. SAAVEDRA, et al. 1984. Autoradiographic localisation of angiotensin II receptors in rat brain. Proc. Natl. Acad. Sci. USA **81:** 1575–1579.
6. MENDELSOHN, F.A.O., A.M. ALLEN, J. CLEVERS, et al. 1988. Localisation of angiotensin II receptor binding in the rabbit brain *in vitro* autoradiography. J. Comp. Neurol. **270:** 372–384.
7. SIRETT, N.E., S.N. THORNTON & J.I. HUBBARD. 1979. Angiotensin binding and pressor activity in the rat ventricular system and midbrain. Brain Res. **166:** 139–148.
8. LANDAS, S., M.I. PHILLIPS, J.F. STAMLER & M.K. RAIZADA. 1980. Visualization of specific angiotensin II binding sites in the brain by fluorescent microscopy. Science **210:** 791–793.
9. WILLIAMS, J.L., K.L. BARNES, K.B. BROSNIHAN & C.M. FERRARIO. 1992. Area postrema—a unique regulator of cardiovascular function. News Physiol. Sci. **7:** 30–34.
10. HARDING, J.W., M.J. SULLIVAN, J.M. HANESWORTH, et al. 1988. Inability of [125I]Sar1, Ile8-angiotensin II to move between the blood and cerebrospinal fluid compartments. J. Neurochem. **50:** 554–557.
11. SCHELLING, P., J.S. HUTCHINSON, U. GANTEN, et al. 1976. Impermeability of the blood-cerebrospinal fluid barrier for angiotensin II in rats. Clin. Sci. Mol. Med. Suppl. **3:** 399s–402s.
12. UNGER, T., E. BADOER, D. GANTEN, et al. 1988. Brain angiotensin: pathways and pharmacology. Circulation **77:** I 40–I 54.
13. CHIU, A.T., W.F. HERBLIN, D.E. MCCALL, et al. 1989. Identification of angiotensin II receptor subtypes. Biochem. Biophys. Res. Commun. **165:** 196–203.
14. DUDLEY, D.T., R.L. PANEK, T.C. MAJOR, et al. 1990. Subclasses of angiotensin II binding sites and their functional significance. Mol. Pharmacol. **38:** 370–377.

15. IWAI, N. & T. INAGAMI. 1992. Identification of two subtypes in the rat type I angiotensin II receptor. FEBS Lett. **298:** 257–260.
16. ALDRED, G.P., S.Y. CHAI, K. SONG, et al. 1993. Distribution of angiotensin II receptor subtypes in the rabbit brain. Regul. Pept. **44:** 119–130.
17. SONG, K.F., A.M. ALLEN, G. PAXINOS & F.A.O. MENDELSOHN. 1991. Angiotensin-II receptor subtypes in rat brain. Clin. Exp. Pharmacol. Physiol. **18:** 93–96.
18. HEAD, G.A. 1994. Cardiac baroreflexes and hypertension. Clin. Exp. Pharmacol. Physiol. **21:** 791–802.
19. HEAD, G.A. 1995. Baroreflexes and cardiovascular regulation in hypertension. J. Cardiovasc. Pharmacol. **26** (Suppl. 2): S7–S16.
20. HEAD, G.A. & S.C. MALPAS. 1997. Baroreflex mechanisms in hypertension. Fundam. Clin. Pharmacol. **11** (Suppl. 1): 65s–69s.
21. FLORAS, J.S., M.O. HASSAN, J.V. JONES, et al. 1988. Consequences of impaired arterial baroreflexes in essential hypertension: effects on pressor responses, plasma noradrenaline and blood pressure variability. J. Hypertens. **6:** 525–535.
22. BICKERTON, R.K. & J.P. BUCKLEY. 1961. Evidence for a central mechanism in angiotensin induced hypertension. Proc. Soc. Exp. Biol. Med. **106:** 834–836.
23. SEVERS, W.B., A.E. DANIELS, H.H. SMOOKLER, et al. 1966. Interrelationship between angiotensin II and the sympathetic nervous system. J. Pharmacol. Exp. Ther. **153:** 530–537.
24. HOFFMAN, W.E. & M.I. PHILLIPS. 1976. Regional study of cerebral ventricle sensitive sites to angiotensin II. Brain Res. **110:** 313–330.
25. HOFFMAN, W.E. & M.I. PHILLIPS. 1976. The effect of subfornical organ lesions and ventricular blockade on drinking induced by angiotensin II. Brain Res. **108:** 59–73.
26. HEAD, G.A., J.-L. ELGHOZI & P.I. KORNER. 1988. Baroreflex modulation of central angiotensin II pressor responses in conscious rabbits. J. Hypertens. **6**(Suppl. 6): S505–S507.
27. ELGHOZI, J.-L. & G.A. HEAD. 1990. Spinal noradrenergic pathways and the pressor responses to central angiotensin II. Am. J. Physiol. **258:** H240–H246.
28. HEAD, G.A. & N.S. WILLIAMS. 1992. Hemodynamic effects of central angiotensin I, II and III in conscious rabbits. Am. J. Physiol. **263:** R845–R851.
29. WRIGHT, J.W., M.J. SULLIVAN, E.P. PETERSEN & J.W. HARDING. 1985. Brain angiotensin II and III binding and dipsogenicity in the rabbit. Brain Res. **358:** 376–379.
30. TARJAN, E., D.A. DENTON, M.I. MCBURNIE & R.S. WEISINGER. 1988. Water and sodium intake of wild and New Zealand rabbits following angiotensin. Peptides **9:** 677–679.
31. BENDLE, R.D., S.C. MALPAS & G.A. HEAD. 1997. Role of endogenous angiotensin II on sympathetic reflexes in conscious rabbits. Am. J. Physiol. **272:** R1816–R1825.
32. BARRON, K.W., A.J. TRAPANI, F.J. GORDON & M.J. BRODY. 1989. Baroreceptor denervation profoundly enhances cardiovascular responses to central angiotensin II. Am. J. Physiol. **257:** H314–H323.
33. SEVERS, W.B., J. SUMMY-LONG, J.S. TAYLOR & J.D. CONNOR. 1970. A central effect of angiotensin: release of pituitary pressor material. J. Pharmacol. Exp. Ther. **174:** 27–34.
34. KEIM, K.L. & E.B. SIGG. 1971. Activation of central sympathetic neurons by angiotensin II. Life Sci. **10:** 565–574.
35. TOBEY, J.C., H.K. FRY, C.S. MIZEJEWSKI, et al. 1983. Differential sympathetic responses initiated by angiotensin and sodium chloride. Am. J. Physiol. **245:** R60–R68.
36. KEIL, L.C., J. SUMMY-LONG & W.B. SEVERS. 1975. Release of vasopressin by angiotensin II. Endocrinology **96:** 1063–1065.
37. FISHER, L.A. & M.R. BROWN. 1984. Corticotropin-releasing factor and angiotensin II: comparison of CNS actions to influence neuroendocrine and cardiovascular function. Brain Res. **296:** 41–47.
38. BRUNER, C.A. & G.D. FINK. 1986. Neurohumoral contributions to chronic angiotensin-induced hypertension. Am. J. Physiol. **250:** H52–H61.
39. HAACK, D. & J. MOHRING. 1978. Vasopressin-mediated blood pressure response to intraventricular injection of angiotensin II in the rat. Pflugers Arch. **373:** 167–173.
40. STEELE, M.K., D.G. GARDNER, P.L. XIE & H.D. SCHULTZ. 1991. Interactions between ANP and ANG II in regulating blood pressure and sympathetic outflow. Am. J. Physiol. **260:** R1145–R1151.

41. AVERILL, D.B. & D.I. DIZ. 2000. Angiotensin peptides and baroreflex control of sympathetic outflow: pathways and mechanisms of the medulla oblongata. Brain Res. Bull. **51:** 119–128.

42. DORWARD, P.K. & C.D. RUDD. 1991. Influence of the brain renin-angiotensin system on renal sympathetic and cardiac baroreflexes in conscious rabbits. Am. J. Physiol. **260:** H770–H778.

43. SAIGUSA, T. & G.A. HEAD. 1993. Renal sympathetic baroreflex effects of angiotensin II infusions into the rostral ventrolateral medulla of the rabbit. Clin. Exp. Pharmacol. Physiol. **20:** 351–354.

44. IRIKI, M., P. DORWARD & P.I. KORNER. 1977. Baroreflex "resetting" by arterial hypoxia in the renal and cardiac sympathetic nerves of the rabbit. Pflugers Arch. **370:** 1–7.

45. IRIKI, M. & E. KOZAWA. 1983. Renal sympathetic baroreflex during normoxia and during hypoxia in conscious and in anesthetized rabbits. Pflugers Arch. **398:** 23–26.

46. GAUDET, E., S.J. GODWIN & G.A. HEAD. 1998. Role of central catecholaminergic pathways in the actions of endogenous ANG II on sympathetic reflexes. Am. J. Physiol. **44:** R1174–R1184.

47. OKUNO, T., S. NAGAHAMA, M.D. LINDHEIMER & S. OPARIL. 1983. Attenuation of the development of spontaneous hypertension in rats by chronic central administration of captopril. Hypertension **5:** 653–662.

48. FINK, G.D. & C.A. BRUNER. 1985. Hypertension during chronic peripheral and central infusion of angiotensin III. Am. J. Physiol. **249:** E201–E208.

49. BARTHOLOMEUSZ, B. & R.E. WIDDOP. 1995. Effect of acute and chronic treatment with the angiotensin II subtype 1 receptor antagonist EXP 3174 on baroreflex function in conscious spontaneously hypertensive rats. J. Hypertens. **13:** 219–225.

50. LIU, J.L., H. MURAKAMI, M. SANDERFORD, et al. 1999. ANG II and baroreflex function in rabbits with CHF and lesions of the area postrema. Am. J. Physiol. Heart Circ. Phy. **46:** H342–H350.

51. MAYOROV, D.N. & G.A. HEAD. 2001. Influence of rostral ventrolateral medulla on renal sympathetic baroreflex in conscious rabbits. Am. J. Physiol. **280:** R577–R587.

52. GAUDET, E., S.J. GODWIN & G.A. HEAD. 2000. Effects of central infusion of angiotensin II and losartan on baroreflex control of heart rate in rabbits. Am. J. Physiol. **278:** H558–H566.

53. SUMNERS, C., M.K. RAIZADA, J. KANG, D. LU & P. POSNER. 1994. Receptor-mediated effects of angiotensin II on neurons. Front. Neuroendocrinol. **15:** 203–230.

54. PATON, J.F. & S. KASPAROV. 2000. Sensory channel specific modulation in the nucleus of the solitary tract. J. Auton. Nerv. Syst. **80:** 117–129.

55. HIROOKA, Y., G.A. HEAD, P.D. POTTS, et al. 1996. Medullary neurons activated by angiotensin II in the conscious rabbit. Hypertension **27:** 287–296.

56. TAGAWA, T., M.A. FONTES, P.D. POTTS, et al. 2000. The physiological role of AT1 receptors in the ventrolateral medulla. Braz. J. Med. Biol. Res. **33:** 643–652.

57. HEAD, G.A. 1996. Role of AT1 receptors in the central control of sympathetic vasomotor function. Clin. Exp. Pharmacol. Physiol. **23:** S93–S98.

58. DAMPNEY, R. 1994. The subretrofacial vasomotor nucleus: anatomical, chemical and pharmacological properties and role in cardiovascular regulation. Prog. Neurobiol. **42:** 197–227.

59. SPETH, R.C., J.K. WAMSLEY, D.R. GEHLERT, et al. 1985. Angiotensin II receptor localization in the canine CNS. Brain Res. **326:** 137–143.

60. LIND, R.W., L.W. SWANSON & D. GANTEN. 1985. Organization of angiotensin II immunoreactive cells and fibers in the rat central nervous system. Neuroendocrinology **40:** 2–24.

61. BENARROCH, E.E., A.R. GRANATA, D.A. RUGGIERO, et al. 1986. Neurons of C1 area mediate cardiovascular responses initiated from ventral medullary surface. Am. J. Physiol. **250:** R932–R945.

62. ALLEN, A.M., R.A.L. DAMPNEY & F.A.O. MENDELSOHN. 1988. Angiotensin receptor binding and pressor effects in cat subretrofacial nucleus. Am. J. Physiol. **255:** H1011–H1017.

63. ANDREATTA, S.H., D.B. AVERILL, R.A. SANTOS & C.M. FERRARIO. 1988. The ventrolateral medulla. A new site of action of the renin-angiotensin system. Hypertension **11:** I163–I166.

64. SASAKI, S. & R.A.L. DAMPNEY. 1990. Tonic cardiovascular effects of angiotensin II in the ventrolateral medulla. Hypertension **15:** 274–283.
65. SASAKI, S., Y.W. LI & R.A.L. DAMPNEY. 1993. Comparison of the pressor effects of angiotensin-II and angiotensin-III in the rostral ventrolateral medulla. Brain Res. **600:** 335–338.
66. HEAD, G.A., N.S. WILLIAMS & S.J. GODWIN. 1990. Evidence for central renin angiotensin system controlling sympathetic tone in the rabbit. Proc. Aust. Physiol. Pharmacol. Soc. **21:** 41P.
67. LI, Y.W. & P.G. GUYENET. 1995. Neuronal excitation by angiotensin II in the rostral ventrolateral medulla of the rat *in vitro*. Am. J. Physiol. **37:** R272–R277.
68. CHAN, R.K.W., Y.S. CHAN & T.M. WONG. 1991. Responses of cardiovascular neurons in the rostral ventrolateral medulla of the normotensive wistar kyoto and spontaneously hypertensive rats to iontophoretic application of angiotensin-II. Brain Res. **556:** 145–150.
69. LI, Y.W. & P.G. GUYENET. 1996. Angiotensin II decreases a resting $K^+$ conductance in rat bulbospinal neurons of the C1 area. Circ. Res. **78:** 274–282.
70. MOSQUEDA-GARCIA, R., C.J. TSENG, M. APPALSAMY & D. ROBERTSON. 1990. Cardiovascular effects of microinjection of angiotensin-II in the brainstem of renal hypertensive rats. J. Pharmacol. Exp. Ther. **255:** 374–381.
71. MURATANI, H., D.B. AVERILL & C.M. FERRARIO. 1991. Effect of angiotensin-II in ventrolateral medulla of spontaneously hypertensive rats. Am. J. Physiol. **260:** R977–R984.
72. SILVA, L.C.S., M.A.P. FONTES, M.J. CAMPAGNOLESANTOS, *et al.* 1993. Cardiovascular effects produced by micro-injection of angiotensin-(1–7) on vasopressor and vasodepressor sites of the ventrolateral medulla. Brain Res. **613:** 321–325.
73. FONTES, M.A.P., L.C.S. SILVA, M.J. CAMPAGNOLESANTOS, *et al.* 1994. Evidence that angiotensin-(1–7) plays a role in the central control of blood pressure at the ventrolateral medulla acting through specific receptors. Brain Res. **665:** 175–180.
74. FONTES, M.A.P., M.C.M. PINGE, V. NAVES, *et al.* 1997. Cardiovascular effects produced by microinjection of angiotensins and angiotensin antagonists into the ventrolateral medulla of freely moving rats. Brain Res. **750:** 305–310.
75. FONTES, M.A.P., O. BALTATU, S.M. CALIGIORNE, *et al.* 2000. Angiotensin peptides acting at rostral ventrolateral medulla contribute to hypertension of TGR(MREN2)27 rats. Physiol. Genomics **2:** 137–142.
76. TAGAWA, T., J. HORIUCHI, P. POTTS & R.A.L. DAMPNEY. 1999. Sympathoinhibition after angiotensin receptor blockade in the rostral ventrolateral medulla is independent of glutamate and gamma-aminobutyric acid receptors. J. Autonom. Nerv. Syst. **77:** 21–30.
77. ITO, S. & A.F. SVED. 1996. Blockade of angiotensin receptors in rat rostral ventrolateral medulla removes excitatory vasomotor tone. Am. J. Physiol. **270:** R1317–R1323.
78. HIROOKA, Y., P.D. POTTS & R.A.L. DAMPNEY. 1997. Role of angiotensin II receptor subtypes in mediating the sympathoexcitatory effects of exogenous and endogenous angiotensin peptides in the rostral ventrolateral medulla of the rabbit. Brain Res. **772:** 107–114.
79. POTTS, P.D., A.M. ALLEN, J. HORIUCHI & R.A. DAMPNEY. 2000. Does angiotensin II have a significant tonic action on cardiovascular neuron in the rostral and caudal VLM. Am. J. Physiol. **279:** R1392–R1402.
80. CHERNOW, B., H.R. ALEXANDER, R.C. SMALLRIDGE, *et al.* 1987. Hormonal responses to graded surgical stress. Arch. Intern. Med. **147:** 1273–1278.
81. MAYOROV, D.M., S.L. BURKE & G.A. HEAD. 2001. Relative importance of rostral ventrolateral medulla in sympathoinhibitory action of rilmenidine in conscious and anesthetized rabbits. J. Cardiovasc. Pharmacol. **37:** 252–261.
82. CHALMERS, J. & P. PILOWSKY. 1991. Brainstem and bulbospinal neurotransmitter systems in the control of blood pressure. J. Hypertens. **9:** 675–694.
83. LI, Y.W., Z.J. GIEROBA, R.M. MCALLEN & W.W. BLESSING. 1991. Neurons in rabbit caudal ventrolateral medulla inhibit bulbospinal barosensitive neurons in rostral medulla. Am. J. Physiol. **261:** R44–R51.

84. ALLEN, A.M., F.A.O. MENDELSOHN, Z.J. GIEROBA & W.W. BLESSING. 1990. Vasopressin release following microinjection of angiotensin-II into the caudal ventrolateral medulla-oblongata in the anaesthetized rabbit. J. Neuroendocrinol. **2:** 867–873.
85. SAIGUSA, T., M. IRIKI & J. ARITA. 1996. Brain angiotensin II tonically modulates sympathetic baroreflex in rabbit ventrolateral medulla. Am. J. Physiol. **271:** H1015–H1021.
86. BERGER, A.J. 1979. Distribution of carotid sinus nerve afferent fibers to solitary tract nuclei of the cat using transganglionic transport of horseradish peroxidase. Neurosci. Lett. **14:** 153–158.
87. SONG, K., A.M. ALLEN, G. PAXINOS & F.A. MENDELSOHN. 1992. Mapping of angiotensin II receptor subtype heterogeneity in rat brain. J. Comp. Neurol. **316:** 467–484.
88. ALLEN, A.M., S.Y. CHAI, J. CLEVERS, et al. 1988. Localization and characterisation of angiotensin II receptor binding and angiotensin converting enzyme in the human medulla oblongata. J. Comp. Neurol. **269:** 249–264.
89. CASTO, R. & M.I. PHILLIPS. 1984. Cardiovascular actions of microinjections of angiotensin II in the brain stem of rats. Am. J. Physiol. **246:** R811–R816.
90. DIZ, D.I., K.L. BARNES & C.M. FERRARIO. 1984. Hypotensive actions of microinjections of angiotensin II into the dorsal motor nucleus of the vagus. J. Hypertens. **2:** 53–56.
91. CASTO, R. & M.I. PHILLIPS. 1986. Angiotensin II attenuates baroreflexes at nucleus tractus solitarius of rats. Am. J. Physiol. **250:** R193–R198.
92. PATON, J.F.R. & S. KASPAROV. 1999. Differential effects of angiotensin II on cardiorespiratory reflexes mediated by nucleus tractus solitarii: a microinjection study in the rat. J. Physiol. (Lond.) **521:** 213–225.
93. LUOH, H.F. & S.H. CHAN. 1998. Participation of AT1 and AT2 receptor subtypes in the tonic inhibitory modulation of baroreceptor reflex response by endogenous angiotensins at the nucleus tractus solitarii in the rat. Brain Res. **782:** 73–82.
94. KASPAROV, S. & J.F.R. PATON. 1999. Differential effects of angiotensin II in the nucleus tractus solitarii of the rat plausible neuronal mechanisms. J. Physiol. (Lond.) **521:** 227–238.
95. RETTIG, R., D.P. HEALY & M.P. PRINTZ. 1986. Cardiovascular effects of microinjections of angiotensin II into the nucleus tractus solitarii. Brain Res. **364:** 233–240.
96. CAMPAGNOLE-SANTOS, M.J., D.I. DIZ & C.M. FERRARIO. 1988. Baroreceptor reflex modulation by angiotensin II at the nucleus tractus solitarii. Hypertension **11:** I167–I171.
97. MATSUMURA, K., D.B. AVERILL & C.M. FERRARIO. 1998. Angiotensin II acts at AT1 receptors in the nucleus of the solitary tract to attenuate the baroreceptor reflex. Am. J. Physiol. **275:** R1611–R1619.
98. KASPAROV, S., J.W. BUTCHER & J.F.R. PATON. 1998. Angiotensin II receptors within the nucleus of the solitary tract mediate the developmental attenuation of the baroreceptor vagal reflex in pre-weaned rats. J. Auton. Nerv. Syst. **74:** 160–168.

# The Interaction of Angiotensin II and Osmolality in the Generation of Sympathetic Tone during Changes in Dietary Salt Intake

## An Hypothesis

VIRGINIA L. BROOKS, KARIE E. SCROGIN, AND DONOGH F. McKEOGH

*Departments of Physiology and Pharmacology, Oregon Health Sciences University, Portland, Oregon 97034, USA*

ABSTRACT: At rest, sympathetic nerves exhibit tonic activity which contributes to arterial pressure maintenance. Significant evidence suggests that the absolute level of sympathetic tone is altered in a number of physiologic and pathophysiologic states. However, the mechanisms by which such changes in sympathetic tone occur are incompletely understood. The purpose of this review is to present evidence that humoral factors are essential in these changes and to detail specifically an hypothesis for the mechanisms that underlie the changes in sympathetic tone that are produced during increases or decreases in dietary salt intake. It is proposed that the net effect of changes in dietary salt on sympathetic activity is determined by the balance between simultaneous and parallel sympathoinhibitory and sympathoexcitatory humoral mechanisms. A key element of the sympathoinhibitory mechanism is the chronic sympathoexcitatory effects of angiotensin II (ANG II). When salt intake increases, ANG II levels fall, and the sympathoexcitatory actions of ANG II are lost. Simultaneously, a sympathoexcitatory pathway is triggered, possibly via increases in osmolality which activate osmoreceptors or sodium receptors. In normal individuals, the sympathoinhibitory effects of increased salt predominate, sympathetic activity decreases, and arterial pressure remains normal despite salt and water retention. However, in subjects with salt-sensitive hypertension, it appears that the sympathoexcitatory effects of salt predominate, possibly due to an inability to adequately suppress the levels or actions of ANG II. The net result, therefore, is an inappropriate increase in sympathetic activity during increased dietary salt which may contribute to the hypertensive process.

KEYWORDS: Angiotensin II; Baroreceptor reflex; Salt-sensitive hypertension; Sodium chloride; Sympathetic nervous system

Sympathetic nerves exhibit tonic activity which is driven by spinally projecting neurons in the rostral ventrolateral medulla (RVLM) and which is required for the maintenance of peripheral resistance and thus arterial pressure (for reviews, see Refs. 1–

Address for correspondence: Virginia L. Brooks, Ph.D., Department of Physiology and Pharmacology, L-334, Oregon Health Sciences University, Portland, Oregon 97034. Voice: 503-494-5843; fax: 503-494-4352.

brooksv@ohsu.edu

3). The importance of such tone in pressure maintenance is indicated by the large depressor responses elicited by either acute inhibition of excitatory RVLM bulbospinal projections to preganglionic sympathetic neurons or by autonomic ganglionic blockade.[1–3] However, whether or how the absolute level of basal tone can be appropriately and chronically altered in order to contribute to the regulation of the long-term arterial pressure level is disputed. The purpose of this review is to present evidence that the tonic level of sympathetic activity can be altered homeostatically and that these changes may be mediated via the influence of humoral factors on the brain.

## SYMPATHETIC ACTIVITY CAN BE CHRONICALLY CHANGED

It has been proposed that maintenance of adequate blood flow to the tissues is ensured, in part, by day-to-day regulation of the so-called "effective arterial blood volume," which is that fraction of the extracellular fluid volume in the arteries that effectively perfuses the tissues.[4,5] The existence of an effective arterial blood volume which is homeostatically regulated independently of the total blood volume is suggested largely by physiological and pathophysiological states in which the effective blood volume varies independently of the total extracellular fluid volume. For example, in heart failure and in pregnancy, despite markedly increased total extracellular fluid volume, arterial blood volume or blood pressure can be decreased. It is hypothesized that the size of the effective arterial blood volume is sensed indirectly via changes in arterial pressure which trigger changes in the activity of baroreceptors in the arterial tree. When changes in arterial pressure are sensed, effector mechanisms are then evoked which act to bring arterial pressure and effective blood volume back towards normal.

The sympathetic nervous system is one effector mechanism that has been hypothesized to be important in the chronic maintenance of effective arterial blood volume or pressure via its actions on the kidney and also via regulation of total peripheral resistance.[4] However, if the contention that the sympathetic nervous system contributes to long-term arterial pressure regulation is correct, then it must be established that appropriate and sustained compensatory changes in sympathetic activity are produced in response to deviations in body fluid balance. For example, it would be predicted that states associated with chronic decreases in effective arterial blood volume or blood pressure should cause sympathetic activity to be chronically increased.

Whether or not sustained changes in effective arterial blood volume do elicit sustained changes in sympathetic activity has been frequently investigated. However, a major challenge to this area of research is that day-to-day changes in sympathetic activity cannot be accurately quantified.[6,7] Instead, indirect indices must be measured. Some of these include indices of neuronal activity such as the bursting frequency of superficial nerves in humans, plasma catecholamine levels and norepinephrine spillover, as well as the mRNA or protein levels of tyrosine hydroxylase or of the norepinephrine transporter, two proteins critical in the function of sympathetic nerves. Alternatively, some studies have quantified the net effects of sympathetic activation by measuring changes in total peripheral or regional resistances or the depressor response to ganglionic blockade. Finally, more recent studies have evaluated the activity of RVLM vasoactive neurons to assess sympathetic tone.

While no one study has unequivocally proven that sustained changes in sympathetic activity can be produced, the assessment and summation of an extensive literature utilizing these indirect indices reveals that sympathetic activity is increased in states associated with decreases in effective arterial blood volume or pressure, such as congestive heart failure, sodium or water depletion, or pregnancy.[4–8] Conversely, evidence suggests that increases in sodium intake are normally associated with decreases in sympathetic activity.[6] In addition to these homeostatic changes, sympathetic activity also appears to be chronically increased in some forms of human hypertension and some models of experimental hypertension.[6,9] Interestingly, recent microinjection studies probing activity of the RVLM report that nonspecific blockade of excitatory amino acid receptors with kynurenic acid has no effect in normal animals, but decreases arterial pressure in rats with Goldblatt hypertension[10] or in spontaneously hypertensive rats (SHRs).[11] Thus, these data support the conclusion that the tonic excitatory input to RVLM is increased in hypertensive models. Parallel results indicate that, in turn, output from RVLM to sympathetic preganglionic neurons is also elevated.[12] Collectively, therefore, a large body of evidence suggests that the tonic level of sympathetic outflow can be changed, at least in part via a change in the output of RVLM bulbospinal neurons. However, the mechanisms for these changes have not been delineated.

## MECHANISM FOR SUSTAINED CHANGES IN SYMPATHETIC ACTIVITY

### *The Baroreceptor Reflex?*

With the exception of the hypertensive models, it is important to to again emphasize that the sustained changes in sympathetic activity just described are teleologically appropriate; that is, effective arterial blood volume or arterial pressure are generally inversely related to the chronic level of sympathetic outflow, as is observed with the reflex changes in response to acute alterations in arterial pressure or volume. Therefore, it is tempting to suggest that these changes are mediated by the arterial baroreceptor reflex.[4,5] Nevertheless, there are two lines of evidence that argue against an exclusive or even necessary role for the arterial baroreceptors as mechano- or pressure sensors involved in mediating changes in basal sympathetic tone.[6,13] First, arterial baroreceptors rapidly reset or adapt to sustained changes in pressure[14–16]; that is, baroreceptor firing rates return towards their original level despite a continued change in pressure. Resetting begins within seconds to minutes, and is nearly complete within a few days. Second, the tonic level of sympathetic activity appears to be normal in arterial baroreceptor–denervated animals.[17] While removal of the tonic inhibitory input from arterial baroreceptor afferents initially produces profound sympathoexcitation, measurements of indirect indices of sympathetic outflow suggest that the level of activity eventually returns to normal. Furthermore, arterial or cardiac deafferentation does not prevent the increase in sympathetic activity produced by heart failure, as assessed by changes in plasma norepinephrine levels or the depressor response to ganglionic blockade.[18,19] These results suggest that not only can the normal basal level of sympathetic activity be set by a mechanism other than baroreceptor input, but also that changes in sympathetic activity can occur independently of this input. Therefore, given that baroreceptors rapidly adapt and thus cannot provide a sustained absolute signal that reflects the degree of arterial filling, and also that the tonic activity of sympathetic nerves can be chronically changed independently of baroreceptor input, it seems that the arterial baroreceptors alone cannot mediate long-term changes in sympathetic activity.

### Humoral Factors?

Since current evidence suggests that the arterial baroreceptor reflex does not mediate chronic changes in sympathetic outflow, then the signal must be relayed either by other neuronal afferents or by circulating factors. An accumulation of data indicates that humoral factors, which either chronically stimulate or inhibit sympathetic activity, may be important. In recent years, several hormones have been shown to be capable of sustained, non-adaptable modulation of sympathetic outflow. Experiments to test this concept have utilized primarily three approaches. First, chronic infusion of humoral agents, such as leptin,[20] or chronic inhibition of humoral production, such as sustained nitric oxide synthase blockade,[21] produce increases in indices of sympathetic activity. Secondly, genetically altered rodents that either are transgenic for or lack genes for specific proteins, such as ANF,[22] exhibit changes in the tonic level of sympathetic outflow. Finally, acute i.v. blockade of chronically elevated endogenous hormonal levels produces acute decreases or increases in sympathetic activity, suggesting that the hormones chronically support or suppress sympathetic activity. While these experimental approaches do not specifically delineate the mode of action of the hormones, either circulating in plasma in the classical sense or acting in brain as neurotransmitters or neuromodulators, nevertheless, they do support a role for these messenger substances in long-term control of sympathetic activity.

Using these approaches, abundant evidence has been gathered to indicate that angiotensin II (ANG II) is chronically sympathoexcitatory. First, while there is controversy as to whether the absolute level of sympathetic activity is increased when ANG II is chronically infused, because arterial pressure is increased in these studies, sympathetic activity relative to arterial pressure is clearly increased.[6,23] This shift to a higher pressure in the reflex relationship between arterial pressure and heart rate or sympathetic activity with chronic infusion of ANG II is not due to pressure-dependent baroreflex resetting. Instead, the relative increase is caused by a more direct effect of ANG II, since the increase rapidly reverses upon termination of ANG II infusion, even if the hypertension is maintained by infusion of another vasoconstrictor.[24] Similarly, heart rate increases are maintained, even when ANG II-induced hypertension is reversed by concurrent infusion of a vasodilator.[25] Second, acute blockade of the renin-angiotensin system in several physiological or pathophysiological states with decreased effective arterial blood volume and elevated endogenous ANG II levels (such as salt or water deprivation, pregnancy, and congestive heart failure) results in decreases in sympathetic activity and heart rate if arterial blood pressure is not allowed to fall.[6] Collectively, these data support the hypothesis that ANG II is capable of sustained sympathoexcitation.

ANG II not only supports the tonic level of sympathetic activity, but also appears to influence the magnitude of baroreflex-induced changes in sympathetic activity around this baseline. For example, in salt-deprived animals, acute ANG II blockade

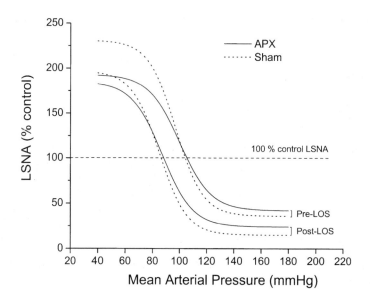

**FIGURE 1.** Effect of i.v. losartan administration on baroreflex control of lumbar sympathetic nerve activity (LSNA) in sodium-deprived rats with lesions of the area postrema (APX; *solid line*) or sham lesions (Sham; *dotted line*). Shown are curves before losartan (Pre-LOS) and after losartan (Post-LOS). Data are replotted from Xu *et al.*[27]

decreases sympathetic activity over the entire baroreflex range of arterial pressure levels[26–28] (Fig. 1). As a result, reflex curves are shifted to a lower pressure level, as if ANG II were setting the baseline tone around which the baroreflex operates. In addition, endogenous ANG II has been shown to contribute to the decreased reflex gain observed in animals with chronic heart failure[29–32] or with hypertension.[33,34]

The question of where ANG II acts to influence the tonic and reflex regulation of heart rate and sympathetic activity has received some attention. Because the peptide cannot cross the blood–brain barrier, it is feasible that circulating ANG II acts via circumventricular organs (CVO), many of which contain ANG II binding sites. Lesions of the area postrema, a CVO in the medullary region, have been reported to block the action of ANG II type 1 (AT1) antagonists to enhance baroreflex gain in SHRs[35] and in rabbits with pacing-induced heart failure.[31] Thus, circulating ANG II may act at this site to decrease reflex gain, possibly via connections with nucleus tractus solitarius. On the other hand, the area postrema may not be not required for the action of ANG II to reset the baroreflex, since area postrema lesions fail to prevent the ability of AT1 blockade to shift reflex curves to a lower pressure level in conscious salt-deprived rats[27] (Fig. 1) or anesthetized SHRs.[35] Thus, the site of action of circulating ANG II to increase sympathetic activity relative to pressure is unknown. However, the subfornical organ is a likely candidate, given its high sensitivity to ANG II and the anatomical circuitry that exists between the SFO and sympathetic preganglionic neurons.[36,37] On the other hand, the AT1 antagonist losartan can cross the blood–brain barrier (BBB)[38,39] and many studies which demonstrated decreased sympathetic activity after ANG II receptor blockade used losartan. Thus, it is also possible that AT1 antagonists are lowering sympathetic activity partially via an action in brain regions with an intact barrier. Indeed, in salt-deprived rats, the sympathoinhibitory effect of losartan takes several minutes to be maximized,[26,27] consistent with the idea that the antagonist acts both by blocking receptors behind the BBB as well as readily accessible receptors in CVOs. In support of this hypothesis, DiBona *et al.*[40] recently reported that acute AT1 blockade of RVLM produces greater decreases in RSNA and blood pressure in sodium-deprived rats compared to rats on a normal or high salt diet. Thus, ANG II may contribute to long-term control of sympathetic outflow via both CVOs and sites behind the BBB. The reader is referred to other chapters in this volume for a more complete discussion of the actions of ANG II or ANG II-like peptides in brain on tonic and reflex regulation of sympathetic outflow.

In summary, it appears that humoral factors can influence the absolute level of sympathetic tone and that, in the case of ANG II, they can participate in a reflex which evokes appropriate changes in the tonic level of sympathetic outflow during chronic changes in body fluid balance. More specifically, evidence suggests that decreases in effective arterial blood volume are associated with increased ANG II, which chronically supports sympathetic outflow. The remainder of this review will focus on the specific alterations that occur during changes in salt intake in normal animals, and how salt-sensitive hypertension is produced when these normal responses are disrupted.

## CHANGES IN SYMPATHETIC OUTFLOW DURING CHANGES IN SALT INTAKE: AN HYPOTHESIS

Our working hypothesis for how dietary salt influences the sympathetic nervous system is summarized in FIGURE 2. According to this hypothesis, when salt intake is increased, sympathetic activity is inhibited through one set of mechanisms (*left*), and simultaneously stimulated through different parallel mechanisms (*right*). The corollary hypothesis is that a decrease in salt intake would have the opposite effects on the two parallel mechanisms. Thus, the net effect of dietary salt on the tonic level of sympathetic outflow is determined by the balance between stimulatory and inhibitory signals.

## EFFECTS OF INCREASED SALT INTAKE ON THE SYMPATHETIC NERVOUS SYSTEM

### *Sympathoinhibitory Mechanisms*

The sympathoinhibitory mechanism includes the chronic sympathoexcitatory action of ANG II. As described in the previous section and as summarized in numerous reviews,[13,23,32,41] there is now abundant evidence that this peptide hormone can produce sustained activation of the sympathetic nervous system. However, when salt intake increases, the positive salt balance is sensed not by arterial baroreceptors, but

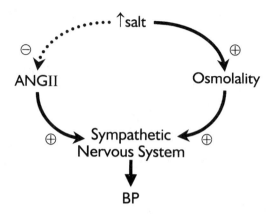

**FIGURE 2.** Hypothesis for how increases in dietary salt influence the tonic level of sympathetic outflow. See text for details of the hypothesis.

instead in part by the kidney, presumably via the renal baroreceptor and macula densa, which triggers the decreases in renin and ANG II that signals the brain to lower the tonic level sympathetic outflow. Conversely, when salt intake decreases, increased ANG II levels promote sympathoexcitation. In support of this inhibitory mechanism is evidence that angiotensin blockade lowers sympathetic activity relative to arterial blood pressure in low-salt animals; this sympathoinhibitory action of angiotensin blockade is markedly reduced in animals on a normal salt diet and is absent in high-salt animals.[26–28,42] Collectively, therefore, the literature indicates that increased salt intake, by virtue of its ability to inhibit Ang II production, tends to chronically reduce sympathetic activity.

### Sympathoexcitatory Mechanisms

While the inverse relationship between salt intake and plasma ANG II levels causes increased dietary salt to inhibit sympathetic activity via one mechanism, indirect evidence suggests that sympathetic tone is simultaneously stimulated in normal animals via a parallel series of mechanisms. For example, in one set of studies, increased dietary salt was found to increase excitability of RVLM, the sympathetic tone generator. In the original report by Pawloski-Dahm and Gordon,[43] the pressor response to RVLM glutamate microinjection was increased in normal rats drinking 0.9% sodium chloride compared to rats drinking tap water. The augmented pressor response was mediated by sympathetic activation, since it was prevented by ganglionic blockade. Moreover, the enhanced pressor responses could not be explained by increased vascular reactivity, since phenylephrine injection and spinal cord stimulation produced the same increase in pressure in saline- and water-drinking rats. In follow-up studies, Ito et al.[44] reported that the enhanced pressor responses to RVLM glutamate microinjection were also observed in rats consuming 8% salt in the food. The increased responsivity was not restricted to glutamate, since enhanced responses to other excitatory substances, carbachol and DOPA, were also observed.

While increased dietary salt evokes mechanisms that may tend to activate the sympathetic nervous system, it also appears that decreased dietary salt has effects that tend to inhibit sympathetic activity. In the report of Ito *et al.*[44] the pressor responses of rats on a low salt diet to RVLM injection of glutamate were reduced. Another hint that some aspect of decreased salt intake is inhibitory is that in sodium-deficient rats after ANG II blockade and normalization of arterial pressure, lumbar and renal sympathetic activity are markedly suppressed relative to baseline.[42] A similar suppression is observed for other variables regulated by the baroreflex, such as heart rate, and plasma ACTH and vasopressin levels.[42,45,46] Because basal and reflex increases in heart rate, vasopressin, and ACTH are similar before ANG II blockade,[42,45,46] it appears that some aspect of a low salt diet suppresses these variables, and high ANG II levels return them back to control. Thus, during a low salt intake, the tonic level of activity of sympathetic activity, heart rate, vasopressin and ACTH may be determined by the balance between an inhibitory effect of the low salt diet and the excitatory effect of ANG II.

The mechanism by which increased dietary salt activates sympathoexcitatory mechanisms (or decreased salt intake is sympathoinhibitory) is unknown; however, one hypothesis (FIG. 2) is that salt-induced changes in body fluid osmolality or in extracellular fluid sodium chloride concentrations activate pathways which tend to excite the nervous system during increased salt intake and suppress it during low salt intake. There are data that make this an attractive hypothesis: osmoreceptors have been established as one of the major sensors of the status of body fluid balance and are exquisitely sensitive to small changes in osmolality. In addition, osmoreceptors have been shown to be nonadaptive. Verbalis and colleagues[47,48] demonstrated that the setpoint of the relationship between plasma osmolality and plasma vasopressin secretion is not significantly altered in rats made chronically hyponatremic.

Critical to the hypothesis that osmolality chronically and directly influences sympathetic activity is the demonstration that there is a direct relationship between salt intake and plasma osmolality or sodium/chloride concentrations. Such a relationship has been observed in dog studies in which increased salt intake has been produced by i.v. infusion[49–51]; however, most reports utilizing rats suggest that changes in salt intake do not significantly affect plasma sodium concentration (e.g. Refs. 52–54). Nevertheless, a potential concern with these studies is that longitudinal measurements within rats have not been performed; the effects of salt intake on plasma sodium concentration have been deduced from between-group comparisons. Therefore, we recently studied the changes in plasma sodium and chloride concentrations within rats during the transition from a low to a high salt diet. A particular emphasis was placed on changes in plasma sodium and chloride concentrations during the dark phase of the day-night cycle, when the rats are actively eating and drinking.[55] Our results document a significant 1–4% increase in plasma sodium chloride levels, with largest difference occurring at night. Similar results have been observed in several longitudinal human studies .[56, 57]

Therefore, there is evidence that increased dietary salt intake does increase plasma sodium and chloride concentration, but the increases are small. A critical question then becomes whether such small increases in plasma sodium or osmolality can produce sustained sympathoexcitation. We have recently investigated this question in rats made hyperosmotic by water deprivation.[58] We found that when osmolality was normalized with i.v. infusion of 5% dextrose in water, lumbar sympathetic nerve activity (LSNA) and arterial pressure decreased. These data suggest that the increased osmolality produced by water deprivation supports the tonic level of sympathetic activity. Moreover, the sensitivity of LSNA to changes in osmolality is high; decreases in osmolality of only 1% were sufficient to decrease LSNA by 5–10%. Nevertheless, further experiments are required to determine whether a similar sympathoexcitatory effect of increased osmolality exists in animals on a high salt diet.

## SIMULTANEOUS INHIBITORY AND EXCITATORY EFFECTS OF INCREASED DIETARY SALT: WHAT IS THE BOTTOM LINE?

If increases in dietary salt can both excite and inhibit the nervous system system via different parallel pathways, then what is the net effect of changes in salt intake on sympathetic activity? The answer to this question must rely on the indirect measures of the tonic level of sympathetic outflow. Nevertheless, what evidence is available indicates that changes do occur, and that the net effect of salt on sympathetic outflow is different in normotensive versus salt-sensitive hypertensive animals.

### Normal Animals

Increases in salt intake produce net salt retention, an expansion of extracellular fluid volume and an increase in cardiac output.[6] Arterial pressure does not increase, however, because of a simultaneous decrease in total peripheral resistance. Measurement of indirect indices of sympathetic outflow suggest that the systemic vasodilation may be due in part to decreases in sympathetic activity. For example, numerous studies generally indicate an inverse relationship between salt intake and plasma norepinephrine concentration or norepinephrine spillover (for reviews, see Refs 6 and 8). In addition, we have found that increased dietary salt decreases the mRNA and protein levels of tyrosine hydroxylase in several sympathetic ganglia[59] (FIG. 3). Because sustained increases in the firing of postganglionic neurons is associated with increases in tyrosine hydroxylase mRNA and protein levels,[60–62] these data also indirectly suggest that sympathetic activity decreases in normal animals consuming a high salt diet. Thus, the net effect of salt in normal animals appears to be sympathoinhibition, which contributes to arterial pressure maintenance in the face of extracellular fluid expansion. As indicated above, it is likely that decreases in ANG II mediate at least part of the decreases in sympathetic activity produced.

### Salt-Sensitive Hypertension

In a subset of humans with essential hypertension and in a number of experimental models of hypertension, increased dietary salt increases arterial pressure (TABLE 1). Interestingly, in these models, there is also evidence that the hypertensive effect of salt is mediated by increased sympathetic activity or a failure to decrease sympathetic activity when salt intake is increased. The mechanism for the net sympathoexcitation has not been definitively established. However, if it assumed that the tonic level of sympathetic outflow is determined by the balance between distinct, parallel sympathoexcitatory and sympathoinhibitory mechanisms, then an explana-

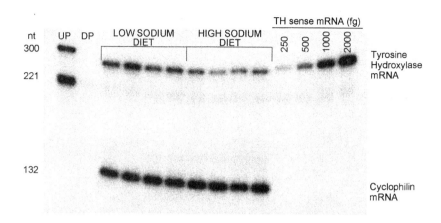

**FIGURE 3.** Representative ribonuclease protection assay autoradiogram showing that adrenal tyrosine hydroxylase (TH) mRNA levels are higher in four rats on a low-sodium (<0.1%) diet compared to four rats on a high-sodium (8%) diet. *Lanes*: UP, incubated undigested probes; DP, ribonuclease digested probes; experimental samples (8 lanes); standard curve with increasing amounts of TH sense mRNA shown on *right*. Bands are for TH and cyclophilin, the housekeeping gene used to control for differences in total RNA loading. See Brooks *et al.*[66] for details of assay method and quantification.

**TABLE 1. Salt-sensitive hypertension with elevated sympathetic activity**

| |
| --- |
| *SHR* (Oparil *et al.*, 1988[67]; Ono *et al.*, 1997[68]) |
| *Dahl rats* (Mark, 1991 [69]) |
| *DOC-salt rats* (Takeda and Bunag, 1980[70]; Fink *et al.*, 1987 [71]; Gavras and Gavras, 1989[72]) |
| *ANG II-induced hypertension* (Bruner & Fink, 1986[73]; Luft *et al.*, 1989[74]; Cox & Bishop, 1991[75]; Blaine *et al.*, 1998[23]) |
| *Human essential hypertension* (Fujita *et al.*, 1980[76]; Campese *et al.*, 1982[77]; Dichtchekenian *et al.*, 1989[78]) |
| *mRen-2 transgenic rats* (Li *et al.*, 1998[79]) |
| *ANP knockout mice* (Melo *et al.*, 1999[22]) |

tion for salt-sensitive hypertension logically follows. In these individuals, the sympathoexcitatory effects of salt may predominate, due either to an enhancement of the sympathoexcitatory effects of dietary salt or to an attenuation of the sympathoinhibitory mechanisms.

In many cases the problem appears to be a failure of the sympathoinhibitory mechanism due to insufficient suppression of the levels or actions of ANG II. Indirect evidence to support this possibility is that in each of the hypertensive models delineated in TABLE 1, the renin-angiotensin system is malfunctional (see Ref. 13

and the references in TABLE 1). A more direct test of this possibility, however, would be to determine whether increased dietary salt increases arterial blood pressure and sympathetic activity in animals in which ANG II levels were not allowed to fall. Krieger and Cowley investigated the hemodynamic basis of salt-sensitive hypertension produced in dogs in which ANG II was clamped at normal levels.[51,63] They found that increased salt increased cardiac output as in control animals, but the normal decrease in peripheral resistance did not occur. Instead, total peripheral resistance and arterial pressure increased. A key question is why net vasodilation is transformed into net vasoconstriction in animals with clamped ANG II levels. The answer is not known, but studies in rats suggest that the normal decrease in sympathetic activity does not occur when salt intake is increased in animals with clamped or elevated plasma ANG II levels.[64,65]

## CONCLUSIONS

Evidence is presented to support the hypothesis that appropriate, long-term changes in the tonic level of sympathetic outflow occur in response to deviations in body fluid balance and that they are mediated by changes in circulating factors rather than the arterial baroreflex. During increases in dietary sodium chloride intake, for example, it is proposed that basal sympathetic tone is determined by the balance between parallel humoral sympathoexcitatory and sympathoinhibitory mechanisms. The sympathoinhibitory mechanism includes decreases in the sympathoexcitatory peptide, ANG II. Simultaneously, a sympathoexcitatory pathway may be triggered, possibly via increases in osmolality and/or other unidentified mechanisms. In normotensive animals, the sympathoinhibitory effects of salt predominate, sympathetic activity decreases, and arterial pressure remains normal despite salt and water retention. On the other hand, in subjects with salt-sensitive hypertension, it appears that the sympathoexcitatory actions of salt dominate, possibly due to an attenuation of the decreases in the levels or actions of ANG II.

## ACKNOWLEDGMENTS

We are grateful for the technical assistance of Eugene Grygielko and Kathy Clow and for suggestions made by Alan Sved during preparation of the manuscript. This work was supported in part by grants from the NIH (HL35872 to V.L.B.) and from the American Heart Association, National (K.E.S.) and Northwest Affiliate (D.F.M.).

## REFERENCES

1. DAMPNEY, R.A.L. 1994. Functional organization of central pathways regulating the cardiovascular system. Physiol. Rev. **74:** 323–364.
2. GUYENET, P.G. 1990. Role of the ventral medulla oblongata in blood pressure regulation. *In* Central Regulation of Autonomic Functions. A.D. Loewy & K.M. Spyer, Eds.: 145–167. Oxford University Press. New York.

3. KUMADA, M., N. TERUI & T. KUWAKI. 1990. Arterial baroreceptor reflex: its central and peripheral neural mechanisms. Prog. Neurobiol. **35:** 331–361.
4. SCHRIER, R.W. 1990. Body fluid volume regulation in health and disease: a unifying hypothesis. Ann. Intern. Med. **113:** 155–159.
5. ROSE, B.D. 1994. Regulation of the effective circulating volume. *In* Clinical Physiology of Acid-Base and Electrolyte Disorders, 4th ed. B.D. Rose, Ed. :235–260. McGraw-Hill. New York.
6. BROOKS, V.L. & J.W. OSBORN. 1995. Hormonal-sympathetic interactions in long-term regulation of arterial pressure: an hypothesis. Am. J. Physiol. **268:** R1343–R1358.
7. ESLER, M., G. JENNINGS, G. LAMBERT, *et al.* 1990. Overflow of cathecholamine neurotransmitters to the circulation: source, fate and functions. Physiol. Rev. **70:** 963–985.
8. VOLLMER, R.R. 1984. Effects of dietary sodium on sympathetic nervous system control of cardiovascular function. J. Auton. Pharmacol. **4:** 133–144.
9. GOLDSTEIN, D.S. 1983. Plasma catecholamines and essential hypertension: an analytical review. Hypertension **5:** 86–99.
10. BERGAMASCHI, C., R.R. CAMPOS, N. SCHOR & O.U. LOPES. 1995. Role of the rostral ventrolateral medulla in maintenance of blood pressure in rats with Goldblatt hypertension. Hypertension **26:** 1117–1120.
11. ITO, S., K. KOMATSU, K. TSUKAMOTO & A.F. SVED. 2000. Excitatory amino acids in the rostral ventrolateral medulla support blood pressure in spontaneously hypertensive rats. Hypertension **35:** 413–417.
12. MURATANI, H., C.M. FERRARIO & D.B. AVERILL. 1993. Ventrolateral medulla in spontaneously hypertensive rats: Role of angiotensin II. Am. J. Physiol. (Reg. Integ. Comp. Physiol.) **264:** R388–R395.
13. BROOKS, V.L. 1997. Interactions between angiotensin II and the sympathetic nervous system in the long-term control of arterial pressure. Clin. Exp. Pharmacol. Physiol. **24:** 83–90.
14. ANDRESEN, M.C. & M. YANG. 1989. Arterial baroreceptor resetting: contributions of chronic and acute processes. Clin. Exp. Pharmacol. Physiol. **15:** 19–30.
15. KORNER, P.I. 1989. Baroreceptor resetting and other determinants of baroreflex properties in hypertension. Clin. Exp. Pharmacol. Physiol. **15:** 45–64.
16. KRIEGER, E.M. 1989. Arterial baroreceptor resetting in hypertension. Clin. Exp. Pharmacol. Physiol. **15:** 3–17.
17. SVED, A.F., A.M. SCHREIHOFER & C.K. KOST, JR. 1997. Blood pressure regulation in baroreceptor-denervated rats. Clin. Exp. Pharmacol. Physiol. **24:** 77–82.
18. LEVETT, J.M., C.C. MARINELLI, D.D. LUND, *et al.* 1994. Effects of β-blockade on neurohumoral responses and neurochemical markers in pacing-induced heart failure. Am. J. Physiol. (Heart Circ. Physiol.) **266:** H468–H475.
19. BRANDLE, M., K.P. PATEL, W. WANG & I.H. ZUCKER. 1996. Hemodynamic and norepinephrine responses to pacing-induced heart failure in conscious sinoaortic-denervated dogs. J. Appl. Physiol. **81:** 1855–1862.
20. HALL, J.E., M.W. BRANDS, D.A. HILDEBRANDT, *et al.* 2000. Role of sympathetic nervous system and neuropeptides in obesity hypertension. Braz. J. Med. Biol. Res. **33:** 605–618.
21. SANDER, M., P.G. HANSEN & R.G. VICTOR. 1995. Sympathetically mediated hypertension caused by chronic inhibition of nitric oxide. Hypertension **26:** 691–695.
22. MELO, L.G., A.T. VERESS, C.K. CHONG, *et al.* 1999. Salt-sensitive hypertension in ANP knockout mice is prevented by AT1 receptor antagonist losartan. Am. J. Physiol. **277:** R624–R630.
23. BLAINE, E.H., J.T.CUNNINGHAM, E.M. HASSER, *et al.* 1998. Angiotensin hypertension. Clin .Exp. Pharmacol. Physiol. **25:** S16–S20.
24. BROOKS, V.L. 1995. Chronic infusion of angiotensin II resets baroreflex control of heart rate by an arterial pressure-independent mechanism. Hypertension **26:** 420–424.
25. BROOKS, V.L., K.R. ELL & R.M. WRIGHT. 1993. Pressure-independent baroreflex resetting produced by chronic infusion of angiotensin II in rabbits. Am. J. Physiol. **265:** H1275–H1282.
26. XU, L. & V.L. BROOKS. 1997. Sodium intake, angiotensin II receptor blockade and baroreflex function in conscious rats. Hypertension **29:** 450–457.

27. XU, L., J.P. COLLISTER, J.W. OSBORN & V.L. BROOKS. 1998. Endogenous angiotensin II supports lumbar sympathetic activity in conscious, sodium deprived rats: role of area postrema. Am. J. Physiol. **275:** R46–R55.
28. DIBONA, G.F., S.Y. JONES & L.L. SAWIN. 1996. Effect of endogenous angiotensin II on renal nerve activity and its arterial baroreflex regulation. Am. J. Physiol. **271:** R361–R367.
29. DIBONA, G.F., S.Y. JONES & V.L. BROOKS. 1995. ANG II receptor blockade and arterial baroreflex regulation of renal nerve activity in cardiac failure. Am. J. Physiol. **269:** R1189–R1196.
30. MURAKAMI, H., J.-L. LIU & I.H. ZUCKER. 1997. Angiotensin II enhances baroreflex control of sympathetic outflow in heart failure. Hypertension **29:** 564–569.
31. LIU, J.-L., H. MURAKAMI, M. SANDERFORD, et al. 1999. ANG II and baroreflex function in rabbits with CHF and lesions of the area postrema. Am. J. Physiol. **277:** H342–H350.
32. GOLDSMITH, S.R. 1999. Angiotensin II and sympathoactivation in heart failure. J. Cardiac Failure **5:** 139–145.
33. KUMAGAI, H., D.B. AVERILL, M.C. KHOSLA & C.M. FERRARIO. 1993. Role of nitric oxide and angiotensin II in the regulation of sympathetic nerve activity in spontaneously hypertensive rats. Hypertension **21:** 476–484.
34. AVERILL, D.B. & D.I. DIZ. 2000. Angiotensin peptides and baroreflex control of sympathetic outflow: pathways and mechanisms of the medulla oblongata. Brain Res. Bull. **51:** 119–128.
35. MATSUMURA, K., D.B. AVERILL & C.M. FERRARIO. 1999. Role of AT1 receptors in area postrema on baroreceptor reflex in spontaneously hypertensive rats. Brain Res. **850:** 166–172
36. FERGUSON, A.V. & J.S. BAINS. 1997. Actions of angiotensin in the subfornical organ and area postrema: implications for long term control of autonomic output. Clin. Exp. Pharmacol. Physiol. **24:** 96–101.
37. FERGUSON, A.V. & D.L.S. WASHBURN. 1998. Angiotensin II: a peptidergic neurotransmitter in central autonomic pathways. Progr. Neurobiol. **54:** 169–192.
38. LI, Z., J.S. BAINS & A.V. FERGUSON. 1993. Functional evidence that the angiotensin antagonist losartan crosses the blood-brain barrier in the rat. Brain Res. Bull. **30:** 33–39.
39. ZHUO, J., K. SONG, A. ABDELRAHMAN & F.A.O. MENDELSOHN. 1994. Blockade by intravenous losartan of AT1 angiotensin II receptors in rat brain, kidney and adrenals demonstrated by in vitro autoradiography. Clin. Exp. Pharmacol. Physiol. **21:** 557–567
40. DIBONA, G.F. & S.Y. JONES. 2000. Dietary sodium intake influences responses to injection of angiotensin antagonists into RVLM. FASEB J. **14:**A624 [abstract].
41. DIBONA, G.F. 1999. Central sympathoexcitatory actions of angiotensin II: role of type 1 angiotensin II receptors. J. Am. Soc. Nephrol.**10:** S90–S94.
42. XU, L. & V.L. BROOKS. 1996. ANG II chronically supports renal and lumbar sympathetic nerve activity in sodium deprived, conscious rats. Am. J. Physiol. **271:** H2591–H2598.
43. PAWLOSKI-DAHM, C.M. & F.J. GORDON. 1993. Increased dietary salt sensitizes vasomotor neurons of the rostral ventrolateral medulla. Hypertension **22:** 929–933.
44. ITO, S., F.G. GORDON & A.F. SVED. 1999. Dietary salt intake alters cardiovascular responses evoked from the rostral ventrolateral medulla. Am. J. Physiol. **276:** R1600–R1607.
45. BROOKS, V.L. & I.A. REID. 1986. Interaction between angiotensin II and the baroreceptor reflex in the control of adrenocorticotropic hormone secretion and heart rate in conscious dogs. Circ. Res. **58:** 816–828.
46. BROOKS, V.L., L.C. KEIL & I.A. REID. 1986. Role of the renin-angiotensin system in the control of vasopressin secretion in conscious dogs. Circ. Res. **58:** 829–838.
47. VERBALIS, J.G., E.F. BALDWIN & A.G. ROBINSON. 1986. Osmotic regulation of plasma vasopressin and oxytocin after sustained hyponatremia. Am. J. Physiol. **250:** R444–R451.
48. VERBALIS, J.G. & J. DOHANICS. 1991. Vasopressin and oxytocin secretion in chronically hyposmolar rats. Am. J. Physiol. **261:** R1028–R1038.

49. HALL, J.E., A.C. GUYTON, M.J. SMITH & T.G. COLEMAN. 1980. Blood pressure and renal function during chronic changes in sodium intake: role of angiotensin. Am. J. Physiol. **239:** F271–F280.
50. KRIEGER, J.E. & A.W. COWLEY, JR. 1990. Prevention of salt angiotensin II hypertension by servo control of body water. Am. J. Physiol. **258:** H994–H1003.
51. KRIEGER, J.E., J.-F. LIARD & A.W. COWLEY, JR. 1990. Hemodynamics, fluid volume, and hormonal responses to chronic high-salt intake in dogs. Am. J. Physiol. **259:** H1629–H1636.
52. HUANG, B.S. & F.H.H. LEENEN. 1992. Dietary Na, age, and baroreflex control of heart rate and renal sympathetic nerve activity in rats. Am. J. Physiol. **262:** H1441–H1448.
53. TARJAN, E., A. SPAT, T. BALLA & A. SZEKELY. 1980. Role of the renin-angiotensin system in the adaptation of aldosterone biosynthesis to sodium restriction in the rat. Acta Endocrinologica **94:** 381–388.
54. WHITESCARVER, S.A., B.J. HOLTZCLAW, J.H. DOWNS, *et al.* 1986. Effect of dietary chloride on salt-sensitive and renin-dependent hypertension. Hypertension **8:** 56–61.
55. GRYGIELKO, E.T., B. FOOTE & V.L. BROOKS. 1999. Increased salt intake elevates plasma sodium and chloride concentrations at night. FASEB J. **13:** A772 [abstract].
56. KAWANO, Y., K. YOSHIDA, M. KAWAMURA, *et al.* 1992. Sodium and noradrenaline in cerebrospinal fluid and blood in salt-sensitive and non-salt-sensitive essential hypertension. Clin. Exp. Pharmacol. Physiol. **19:** 235–241.
57. ROOS, J.C., H.A. KOOMANS, E.J. DORHOUT MEES & I.M.K. DELAWI. 1985. Renal sodium handling in normal humans subjected to low, normal, and extremely high sodium supplies. Am. J. Physiol. (Renal Fluid Electrolyte Physiol.) **249:** F941–F947.
58. SCROGIN, K.E., E.T. GRYGIELKO & V.L. BROOKS. 1999. Osmolality: a physiological long-term regulator of lumbar sympathetic nerve activity and arterial pressure. Am. J. Physiol. **1276:** R1579–R1586.
59. SILLIMAN, T.L., L. XU, J.A. RESKO & V.L. BROOKS. 1995. Sodium deprivation increases tyrosine hydroxylase mRNA in rat adrenals and celiac ganglia. Soc. Neurosci. Abstr. **21:** 1406.
60. BIGUET, N.F., A.R. RITTENHOUSE, J. MALLET & R.E. ZIGMOND. 1989. Preganglionic nerve stimulation increases mRNA levels for tyrosine hydroxylase in the rat superior cervical ganglion. Neurosci.Lett. **104:** 189–194.
61. SCHALLING, M., P.E. STIEG, C. LINDQUIST, *et al.* 1989. Rapid increase in enzyme and peptide mRNA in sympathetic ganglia after electrical stimulation in humans. Proc. Natl. Acad. Sci.USA **86:** 4302–4305.
62. STACHOWIAK, M.K., R. SEBBANE, E.M. STRICKER *et al.* 1985. Effect of chronic cold exposure on tyrosine hydroxylase mRNA in rat adrenal gland. Brain Res. **359:** 356–359.
63. KRIEGER, J.E., R.J. ROMAN & A.W. COWLEY, JR 1989. Hemodynamics and blood volume in angiotensin II salt-dependent hypertension in dogs. Am. J. Physiol. **257:** H1402–H1412.
64. SATO, Y., E. OGATA & T. FUJITA. 1991. Role of chloride in angiotensin II-induced salt-sensitive hypertension. Hypertension **18:** 622–629.
65. KATAHIRA, K., H. MIKAMI, T. OGIHARA, *et al.* 1989. Synergism of intraventricular NaCl infusion and subpressor angiotensins in rats. Am. J. Physiol. **256:** H1–H8.
66. BROOKS, V.L., T.A. HUHTALA, T.L. SILLIMAN & W.C. ENGELAND. 1997. Water deprivation and rat adrenals mRNAs for tyrosine hydroxylase and the norepinephrine transporter. Am. J. Physiol. **272:** R1897–R1903.
67. OPARIL, S., Y.-F. CHEN, Q.C. MENG, *et al.* 1988. The neural basis of salt sensitivity in the rat: altered hypothalamic function. Am. J. Med. Sci. **295:** 360–369.
68. ONO, A., T. KUWAKI, M. KUMADA& T. FUJITA. 1997. Differential central modulation of the baroreflex by salt loading in normotensive and spontaneously hypertensive rats. Hypertension **29:** 808–814.
69. MARK, A.L. 1991. Sympathetic neural contribution to salt-induced hypertension in Dahl rats. *Hypertension* **17:** I86–I90.
70. TAKEDA, K. & R.D. BUNAG. 1980. Augmented sympathetic nerve activity and pressor responsiveness in DOCA hypertensive rats. Hypertension **2:** 97–101.
71. FINK, G.D., C.M. PAWLOSKI, M.L. BLAIR& M.L. MANGIAPANE. The area postrema in deoxycorticosteone-salt hypertension in rats. Hypertension **9:** III206 III209.

72. Gavras, H. & I. Gavras. 1989. Salt-induced hypertension: the interactive role of vasopressin and of the sympathetic nervous system. J. Hypertension 7: 601–606.
73. Bruner, C.A. & G.D. Fink. 1986. Neurohumoral contributions to chronic angiotensin-induced hypertension. Am. J. Physiol. 250: H52–H61.
74. Luft, F.C., C.S. Wilcox, T. Unger, et al. 1989. Angiotensin-induced hypertension in the rat. Sympathetic nerve activity and prostaglandins. Hypertension 14: 396–403.
75. Cox, B.F. & V.S. Bishop. 1991. Neural and humoral mechanisms of angiotensin-dependent hypertension. Am. J. Physiol. 261: H1284–H1291.
76. Fujita, T., W.L. Henry, F.C. Bartter, et al. 1980. Factors influencing blood pressure in salt-sensitive patients with hypertension. Am. J. Med. 69: 334–344.
77. Campese, V.M., M.S. Romoff, D. Levitan, et al. 1982. Abnormal relationship between sodium intake and sympathetic nervous system activity in salt-sensitive patients with essential hypertension. Kidney Int. 21: 371–378.
78. Dichtchekenian, V., D.M.C. Sequeira, A. Andriollo, et al. 1989. Salt sensitivity in human essential hypertension: effect of renin-angiotensin and sympathetic nervous system blockade. Clin. Exp. Theory Pract. A11: 379–387.
79. Li, P., M. Morris, C.M. Ferrario, et al. 1998. Cardiovascular, endocrine, and body fluid-electrolyte responses to salt loading in REN-2 transgenic rats. Am. J. Physiol. 275: H1130–H1137.

# Peripheral and Central Interactions between the Renin-Angiotensin System and the Renal Sympathetic Nerves in Control of Renal Function

GERALD F. DiBONA

*Departments of Internal Medicine and Physiology, University of Iowa College of Medicine, and the Veterans Administration Medical Center, Iowa City, Iowa 52242, USA*

ABSTRACT: Increases in renal sympathetic nerve activity (RSNA) regulate the functions of the nephron, the vasculature, and the renin-containing juxtaglomerular granular cells. As increased activity of the renin-angiotensin system can also influence nephron and vascular function, it is important to understand the interactions between RSNA and the renin-angiotensin system in the control of renal function. These interactions can be intrarenal, that is, the direct (via specific innervation) and indirect (via angiotensin II) contributions of increased RSNA to the regulation of renal function. The effects of increased RSNA on renal function are attenuated when the activity of the renin-angiotensin system is suppressed or antagonized with angiotensin-converting enzyme inhibitors or angiotensin II–type $AT_1$ receptor antagonists. The effects of intrarenal administration of angiotensin II are attenuated following renal denervation. These interactions can also be extrarenal, that is, in the central nervous system, wherein RSNA and its arterial baroreflex control are modulated by changes in activity of the renin-angiotensin system. In addition to the circumventricular organs, the permeable blood–brain barrier of which permits interactions with circulating angiotensin II, there are interactions at sites behind the blood–brain barrier that depend on the influence of local angiotensin II. The responses to central administration of angiotensin II type $AT_1$ receptor antagonists, into the ventricular system or microinjected into the rostral ventrolateral medulla, are modulated by changes in activity of the renin-angiotensin system produced by physiological changes in dietary sodium intake. Similar modulation is observed in pathophysiological models wherein activity of both the renin-angiotensin and sympathetic nervous systems is increased (e.g., congestive heart failure). Thus, both renal and extrarenal sites of interaction between the renin-angiotensin system and RSNA are involved in influencing the neural control of renal function.

KEYWORDS: Renin-angiotensin system; Renal sympathetic nerves; Renal function; Angiotensin II

Address for correspondence: Gerald F. DiBona, M.D., Department of Internal Medicine, University of Iowa College of Medicine, 200 Hawkins Drive, Iowa City, Iowa 52242. Voice: 319-339-7195; fax: 319-339-7023.

gerald dibona@uiowa.edu

The renal sympathetic nerves innervate the tubules, the vessels and the juxtaglomer-ular granular cells of the kidney.[1,2] In this way, changes in renal sympathetic nerve activity (RSNA) directly influence the functions of these innervated renal effector units. Increases in RSNA decrease urinary sodium and water excretion by increasing renal tubular water and sodium reabsorption throughout the nephron, decrease renal blood flow and glomerular filtration rate by constricting the renal vasculature, and increase activity of the renin-angiotensin system (angiotensin II, ANG II) via stim-ulating renin release from juxtaglomerular granular cells. ANG II, via direct actions on ANG II $AT_1$ receptors located on tubular and vascular segments, can also increase renal tubular sodium and chloride and water reabsorption and constrict the renal vas-culature.[3] Thus, it is important to understand the interactions between the renal sym-pathetic nerves and the renin-angiotensin system in the control of renal function. These interactions can be intrarenal, that is, the direct (via specific innervation) and indirect (via angiotensin II) contributions of increased renal sympathetic nerve ac-tivity to the regulation of renal function. These interactions can also be extrarenal, that is, in the central nervous system, where RSNA and its arterial baroreflex control are modulated by changes in activity of the renin-angiotensin system.

## INTRARENAL INTERACTIONS

An important starting point was the observation that intrarenal generation of ANG II facilitated renal venous outflow of norepinephrine during renal sympathetic nerve stimulation, an effect which was blocked by an ANG II receptor antagonist.[4] This suggested a presynaptic action of ANG II on renal sympathetic nerve terminals to enhance norepinephrine release.

Subsequently, administration of the angiotensin-converting enzyme inhibitor (ACEI), captopril, or an ANG II receptor antagonist attenuated the antinatriuretic re-sponse to either low-frequency electrical or reflex renal sympathetic nerve stimula-tion in anesthetized rats consuming a normal dietary sodium intake.[5,6] When renin-angiotensin system activity was stimulated by low dietary sodium intake, captopril completely eliminated the antinatriuretic response.[7] When renin-angiotensin system activity was suppressed by high dietary sodium intake, the antinatriuretic responses were absent but could be restored to (but not greater than) normal by ANG II given in nonpressor doses which did not affect baseline renal hemodynamic and excretory function. These results suggested that a certain degree of renin-angiotensin system activity was necessary to optimize release of norepinephrine from renal sympathetic nerve terminals (presynaptic action). Another possible sequence was that renin was released following stimulation of $\beta_1$ adrenoceptors on renin-containing juxtaglom-erular granular cells by the norepinephrine released from renal sympathetic nerve terminals; the subsequently formed ANG II could have either a presynaptic action or a postsynaptic action on ANG II receptors located on tubules.

This was clarified by determining the effects of ANG II on rat proximal tubular chloride and water reabsorption before and after renal denervation.[8] Following renal denervation, the effect of ANG II to increase proximal tubular chloride and water reabsorption was decreased by approximately 75%. This suggests that only a very small portion of ANG II's effect, approximately 25%, can be ascribed to a direct action on ANG II receptors located on proximal tubules and the majority of the effect is dependent on intact renal innervation. This indicates that an important action of ANG II in the kidney is to facilitate the release of norepinephrine from renal sympathetic nerve terminals via a presynaptic site of action. Further studies showed that the ANG II's presynaptic effect was tonic in that, in kidneys with intact innervation, the ANG II $AT_1$ receptor antagonist, losartan, decreased proximal tubular chloride and water reabsorption.[9] The $\alpha_1$ adrenoceptor antagonist, prazosin, decreased proximal tubular chloride and water reabsorption to a similar extent as losartan, and the effects of losartan and prazosin were additive.

These presynaptic effects of ANG II are also found in the renal vasculature.[10,11] Losartan dose-dependently decreased the renal vasoconstrictor response to renal sympathetic nerve stimulation, but not to injection of norepinephrine.

These observations suggest that ANG II has an important presynaptic action on renal sympathetic nerve terminals on both renal tubular epithelial cells and vessels to facilitate the release of norepinephrine. This ANG II facilitation of norepinephrine release is manifest as a greater effect on renal tubular sodium reabsorption, urinary sodium excretion, and blood flow when ANG II is present in normal (but not increased) amounts and a lesser effect when ANG II is decreased or absent.

A physiological role for this facilitatory effect of ANG II on renal neuroeffector junctions has been more difficult to observe in conscious animals. Urinary sodium excretion was similar in the denervated and contralateral innervated kidney of conscious dogs subjected to modest dietary sodium restriction during control, ACEI, and ACEI plus ANG II infusion periods.[12] Although no interaction was seen between RSNA (i.e., the innervated kidney) and ANG II, the similar urinary sodium excretion from innervated and denervated kidneys during the control period may suggest that basal RSNA was not increased by the degree of sodium restriction used to levels comparable to those seen during low-frequency renal sympathetic nerve stimulation, where such an interaction has been observed. Similarly, when nonhypotensive hemorrhage was used to produce reflex increases in RSNA in conscious dogs, the associated antinatriuretic response was unaffected by renal arterial administration of either an ACEI (captopril) or losartan.[13] As renal denervation blocked the antinatriuretic response to this maneuver, it may be taken that RSNA is increased in this setting. While increases in RSNA that produce antinatriuresis will also increase renin secretion rate, it appears that, in conscious conditions, this increase is not sufficient to markedly influence the magnitude of the antinatriuretic response.

Studies in this context involving reflex activation of RSNA in human subjects have not been explored. However, it is known that the antinatriuretic response to norepinephrine infusion is attenuated by treatment with an ACEI (enalapril).[14] This suggests that the norepinephrine infusion, which slightly increased arterial pressure and decreased renal blood flow, was stimulating renin release and the derived ANG II was contributing to the antinatriuretic response. As the increase in arterial pressure would have reflexly decreased RSNA, the ANG II, rather than acting presynaptically to facilitate norepinephrine release from renal sympathetic nerve terminals, was more likely having an effect on tubular renal ANG II receptors to increase renal tubular sodium reabsorption.

## CENTRAL ACTIONS

There is substantial evidence that ANG II, in addition to its peripheral actions, contributes to the regulation of arterial pressure and intravascular volume via actions on several brain sites.[15,16] The distribution of type 1 ($AT_1$) and type 2 ($AT_2$) ANG II receptors in the brain of several species, including man, has been examined using both non-peptide $AT_1$ and $AT_2$ receptor antagonists in autoradiographic binding studies and *in situ* hybridization histochemistry for expression of $AT_1$ and $AT_2$ receptor mRNA.[17–21] ANG II receptor binding sites are found within discrete areas of the forebrain and the brainstem, which are importantly involved in regulation of RSNA. This can occur via direct projections to sympathetic preganglionic neurons in the intermediolateral column (IML) of the spinal cord or by participation in major reflexes that modulate RSNA (e.g. arising from peripheral arterial and cardiac baroreceptors, chemoreceptors, and somatic receptors).

A hormonal-sympathetic reflex model for the long-term control of arterial pressure has been proposed.[22–24] A critical element of the model is that chronic increases in ANG II produce sustained increases in peripheral sympathetic nerve activity. Acute increases in circulating ANG II concentration affect sympathetic nervous system activity via actions on the brain, sympathetic ganglia, and sympathetic nerve endings.[25] However, how chronic increases in ANG II influence peripheral sympathetic nerve activity is unclear. Two general pathways may be considered: one that deals with the effects of circulating ANG II on the central nervous system and a second that deals with the central nervous system effects of ANG II originating within the central nervous system.

### *Circulating ANG II Increases Peripheral (Renal) Sympathetic Nerve Activity*

As to the site of action of circulating ANG II within the central nervous system, there are a limited number of specialized central nervous system areas wherein the normal blood–brain barrier is lacking, thus enabling ready access to circulating ANG II. These are called circumventricular organs (CVO) and consist (*inter alia*) of subfornical organ (SFO), organum vasculosum of the lamina terminalis (OVLT), median eminence (ME), and area postrema (AP).[17–20] Of these, substantial evidence supports the importance of the SFO and AP as major sites of action of circulating ANG II in the central nervous system.[26,27] Both sites contain ANG II immunoreactive nerve terminals and predominant $AT_1$ receptor mRNA and $AT_1$ receptor binding sites.[17–21] Projections from the SFO to the paraventricular nucleus (PVN) and from there to both the medulla and the IML provide the connectivity for modulation of peripheral SNA by the SFO.[27]

The AP is an important site at which circulating ANG II modulates peripheral sympathetic nerve activity.[26] Ablation of the AP prevents hypertension due to chronic intravenous administration of ANG II, a hypertensive model known to be caused by increased neurogenic pressor activity. The beneficial effects of intravenous $AT_1$ receptor antagonist on the impaired arterial baroreflex control of both heart rate and RSNA in rabbits with pacing-induced heart failure were abolished by lesions of the AP.[28] The major established efferent connections of the AP are the NTS and the lateral parabrachial nucleus (PBN), both of which provide substantial input to sympathetic preganglionic neurons in the IML of the spinal cord. Lesions of the lateral

PBN also impair chronic ANG II–induced hypertension.[29] Losartan injected into RVLM attenuated the increases in MAP, HR, and RSNA produced by injection of bicuculline into the PVN,[30] suggesting that the excitatory input into the RVLM arising from PVN is mediated by ANG II $AT_1$ receptors. It has been reported that electrical activation of the AP both excites[31] and inhibits[32] neurons in the RVLM which provide input to sympathetic preganglionic neurons in the IML of the spinal cord, and anatomic studies support the existence of such connections. Thus, circulating ANG II activation of AP may increase peripheral sympathetic nerve activity via an excitatory direct connection from AP to RVLM.

The blood–brain barrier would prevent access of circulating ANG II to the RVLM.[33] However, there is indirect evidence that circulating ANG II can activate RVLM neurons. Using an *in vivo* microdialysis technique, an intravenous ANG II infusion (subpressor) was shown to increase the release of glutamate, the excitatory amino acid neurotransmitter, from the RVLM.[34] More importantly, intravenous administration of an angiotensin-converting enzyme inhibitor decreased basal arterial pressure as well as the basal rate of glutamate release. Prevention of the reduction in arterial pressure with intravenous administration of ANG II also prevented the decrease in glutamate release.[35]

In summary, there is strong evidence to indicate that circulating ANG II can increase peripheral sympathetic nerve activity and that this can be influenced by physiological alterations in the level of activity of the endogenous renin-angiotensin system (i.e, alterations in dietary sodium intake). A major central nervous system site of action whereby circulating ANG II increases peripheral SNA is the AP; an additional site is the SFO. These effects are mediated by $AT_1$ receptors. There is preliminary evidence that circulating ANG II and the level of activity of the endogenous renin-angiotensin system can influence the activity of neurons in RVLM. These central nervous system sites have efferent pathways which result in activation of sympathetic preganglionic neurons in the IML of the spinal cord.

## ANG II of Central Nervous System Origin Increases Peripheral (Renal) Sympathetic Nerve Activity

It has been considered that ANG II fulfills the criteria to be considered a peptidergic neurotransmitter within the central nervous system.[18] Here, ANG II of central nervous system origin would act on brain sites involved in the regulation of peripheral sympathetic nerve activity. These brain sites, not being CVOs, would not be affected by circulating ANG II.[33] However, the concentration of ANG II at the synapse is not known and microinjections may deliver pharmacological or subthreshold concentrations, thus failing to mimic the *in vivo* situation. However, such studies do identify functional ANG II receptors, characterize their postsynaptic effects and, with the use of pharmacological antagonists, classify the ANG II receptor type.

Two mechanisms of action whereby ANG II of central nervous system origin acting on brain sites may increase peripheral sympathetic nerve activity have received attention. One postulates an inhibition of arterial baroreflex regulation of peripheral sympathetic nerve activity wherein neuronal ANG II originating from the paraventricular nucleus (PVN) and released in the nucleus tractus solitarius (NTS) inhibits neurotransmitter release at the first synapse in the arterial baroreflex pathway via presynaptic $AT_1$ receptors. In the NTS, ANG II injection decreases,[36] whereas the nonselective peptide ANG II receptor antagonist [Sar$^1$, Thr$^8$]ANG II increases,[37] arterial baroreflex gain.

A second mechanism of action postulates that ANG II originating from neurons in the PVN and released in the NTS, RVLM, or IML leads to activation of sympathetic preganglionic neurons. The RVLM plays a central role in the autonomic neural control of the circulation, including arterial baroreflex regulation of peripheral sympathetic nerve activity.[38–40] The RVLM contains ANG II immunoreactive nerve terminals, predominant AT$_1$ receptor mRNA and AT$_1$ receptor binding sites which, however, are less in rat compared to rabbit or man.[20,21] Microinjection of ANG II into the RVLM increases arterial pressure[41] and/or peripheral sympathetic nerve activity[42] and facilitates arterial baroreflex modulation of RSNA[43]; these effects of exogenous ANG II are blocked by AT$_1$ but not by AT$_2$ receptor blockers.[40]

Experimental strategies used to differentiate these two general pathways relates to the administration of agonists and antagonists of the renin-angiotensin system. Initial studies utilized intravenous ANG II infusions and a variety of methods, each with unique advantages and disadvantages, to measure peripheral sympathetic nerve activity, that is, ganglionic blockade, plasma norepinephrine concentrations, or turnover and recordings of peripheral SNA in both conscious and anesthetized animals.[23] The results were variable, with increases, decreases, and no change having been reported. A confounding factor was the change in arterial pressure induced by the intravenous ANG II infusion, which, via pressure-dependent resetting of the arterial baroreflex regulation of peripheral sympathetic nerve activity, could complicate the analysis of the results. When arterial baroreflex regulation of heart rate and plasma norepinephrine concentration were compared during similar increases in arterial pressure produced by intravenous ANG II or phenylephrine infusion, it was evident that there was an additional pressure-independent effect of ANG II to increase heart rate and plasma norepinephrine concentration at any level of arterial pressure.[44,45]

These studies with exogenous ANG II produce limited insight into the effects of endogenous ANG II on peripheral sympathetic nerve activity. Through the use of physiological interventions such as alterations in dietary sodium content[46–48] to manipulate endogenous ANG II or animal models characterized by increased endogenous ANG II such as normal birth,[49,50] congestive heart failure,[51–58] and hypertension[59,60] together with agents that interrupt the renin-angiotensin system (angiotensin-converting enzyme inhibitor, ANG II AT$_1$ receptor antagonist), important information on the effects of endogenous ANG II on peripheral sympathetic nerve activity has emerged.

A general finding is that when alterations in arterial pressure are prevented either by intracerebroventricular (icv) administration of the agent or restoration of arterial pressure with infusion of appropriate vasoactive substances, agents that interrupt the renin-angiotensin system decrease the basal level of peripheral sympathetic nerve activity and shift the arterial baroreflex regulation of peripheral sympathetic nerve activity to a lower level of arterial pressure. This is exemplified in the results from icv administration of losartan, a non-peptide selective ANG II AT$_1$ receptor antagonist, to rats consuming low, normal or high dietary sodium.[46,53] Plasma renin activity (PRA) in low-sodium-diet rats was increased, while it was decreased in high-sodium-diet rats relative to normal-sodium-diet rats. While icv losartan did not affect basal levels of mean arterial pressure in the three dietary groups, it decreased basal RSNA in the low and normal, but not the high dietary sodium groups. The arterial baroreflex relationship between RSNA and mean arterial pressure is shifted leftward to a lower level of mean arterial pressure (arterial pressure at midpoint of curve) following icv losartan administration in the low and normal, but not the high dietary sodium groups. Similar results and conclusions were obtained using intravenous administration of losartan with restoration of arterial pressure by intravenous methoxamine infusion.[46] Thus, the effect is a lower level of RSNA for a given level of mean arterial pressure. These results indicate that the level of endogenous ANG II tonically supports the level of RSNA and resets the arterial baroreflex regulation of RSNA to a higher level of arterial pressure. The effect is proportional to the degree of activation of the renin-angiotensin system, being greatest during low-sodiumdiet (high PRA), least during high-sodium diet (low PRA), and tonic during normal-sodium diet (normal PRA).

While the strategy of icv administration obviates the problems related to changes in arterial pressure produced by iv administration, it does not completely localize the source and brain site of action of the ANG II. With icv losartan administration, it is still possible that the losartan could be diffusing via the ventricular system to those brain sites to which circulating ANG II has ready access by virtue of absence of normal blood–brain barrier function. A more direct approach in this regard is the selective and specific microinjection of losartan into candidate brain sites that are situated behind a normal blood–brain barrier.

Since circulating ANG II does not have direct access to the RVLM, endogenous ANG II excitation is likely derived from either angiotensinergic neural inputs (*vide supra*) or from paracrine secretion of angiotensin peptides within the brain stem. More significant, therefore, are the findings that microinjection of ANG II receptor blockers into the RVLM produce decreases in arterial pressure and/or peripheral sympathetic nerve activity. Such observations suggest that endogenous ANG II causes tonic excitation of RVLM neurons with increased peripheral sympathetic nerve activity. Many of these studies employed nonselective (peptide) ANG II receptor blockers, which have partial agonist properties, and did not include measurements of peripheral sympathetic nerve activity. In the anesthetized rat, microinjection of high doses of losartan, a selective non-peptide $AT_1$ receptor blocker, into the RVLM increased resting arterial pressure and splanchnic sympathetic nerve activity (effects ascribed to the potassium salt) and blocked the pressor and sympathoexcitatory responses to microinjection of ANG II into the RVLM.[61] These results raised the possibility that tonic excitation of RVLM neurons is mediated by $AT_1$ receptors, likely being stimulated by endogenous ANG II. In the anesthetized rabbit with basal RSNA elevated by the stress of surgery and anesthesia, neither resting arterial pressure nor RSNA were affected by losartan or PD123319, a selective non-peptide $AT_2$ receptor blocker, but were significantly decreased by the peptidic non-selective ANG II receptor blocker, [Sar[1], Thr[8]]ANG II.[62] Losartan but not PD123319 blocked the pressor and sympathoexcitatory responses to microinjection of ANG II and ANG III. These results suggest that the tonic sympathoexcitation produced by endogenous angiotensin peptides in the rabbit RVLM are mediated by receptors other than $AT_1$ or $AT_2$ receptors, possibly being stimulated by endogenous angiotensin peptides other than ANG II or ANG III. Evidence in support of ANG (1-7) as an endogenous angiotensin peptide in RVLM derives from studies in conscious[63] and anesthetized[64] rats showing that RVLM microinjection of A-779 (D-Ala7-angiotensin [1-7]), a selective blocker of ANG (1-7) receptors, decreased resting arterial pressure (no measurements of peripheral sympathetic nerve activity). These responses to A-779 are similar to those observed with RVLM microinjection of [Sar$^1$, Thr$^8$]ANG II.[65-67] There was no effect (anesthetized) or a pressor effect (conscious) with $AT_1$ or $AT_2$ receptor blockers. Thus, studies in both rabbits and rats suggest a role for ANG(1-7).

However, in anesthetized rabbits and rats, the depressor and sympathoinhibitory responses after bilateral microinjections of either [Sar$^1$, Thr$^8$]ANG II or [Sar$^1$, Ile$^8$]ANG II were unchanged after prior selective blockade of $AT_1$ or ANG (1-7) receptors.[68] These results suggest that the depressor and sympathoinhibitory responses to nonselective peptidic ANG II receptor antagonists are operating via mechanisms that are independent of $AT_1$ or ANG (1-7) receptors.

Physiological alterations in endogenous angiotensin II activity (as produced by changes in dietary sodium intake) have a distinct modulatory effect on the responses to microinjection of ANG II $AT_1$ receptor antagonists (losartan, candesartan) into the RVLM.[69] Losartan and candesartan decreased heart rate, mean arterial pressure, and RSNA dose-dependently; the responses were significantly greater in low than in high-sodium-diet rats. A-779 did not affect mean arterial pressure, heart rate, or RSNA in either low- or high-sodium-diet rats. In low-sodium-diet rats, the lowest dose of candesartan decreased the basal level of RSNA (but not mean arterial pressure) and reset arterial baroreflex control of RSNA to a lower level of arterial pressure. Rats with congestive heart failure are characterized by increases in both renin-angiotensin system activity and RSNA as well as by defective arterial baroreflex regulation of RSNA (i.e., lower gain). In CHF rats, the lowest dose of candesartan decreased the basal level of RSNA (but not mean arterial pressure) and improved the arterial baroreflex gain of RSNA toward normal.

These results support the view that angiotensin peptides of brain origin may have a local paracrine or autocrine action on sites that regulate RSNA and its arterial baroreflex control. That this action is influenced by alterations in dietary sodium intake, long known to modulate activity of the circulating renin-angiotensin system, suggests a potentially important compensatory adaptation in the overall neural regulation of renal function.

## ACKNOWLEDGMENTS

This work was supported by National Institutes of Health Grants DK 15843, DK 52617, and HL 55006, and by the Department of Veterans Affairs.

## REFERENCES

1. DiBona, G.F. & U.C. Kopp. 1997. Neural control of renal function. Physiol. Rev. **77:** 75–197.
2. DiBona, G.F. & U.C. Kopp. 2000. Neural control of renal function. *In* The Kidney: Physiology and Pathophysiology. D.W. Seldin & G. Giebisch, Eds.: 981–1006. Lippincott Williams & Wilkins. New York.

3. HALL, J.E. & M.W. BRANDS. 2000. The renin-angiotensin-aldosterone systems: renal mechanisms and circulatory homeostasis. *In* The Kidney: Physiology and Pathophysiology. D.W. Seldin & G. Giebisch, Eds.: 1009–1046. Lippincott Williams & Wilkins. New York.

4. BÖKE, T. & K.U. MALIK. 1983. Enhancement by locally generated angiotensin II of release of the adrenergic transmitter in the isolated rat kidney. J. Pharmacol. Exp. Ther. **226:** 900–907.

5. HANDA, R.K. & E.J. JOHNS. 1985. Interaction of the renin-angiotensin system and the renal nerves in the regulation of rat kidney function. J. Physiol. **369:** 311–321.

6. HANDA, R.K. & E.J. JOHNS. 1987. The role of angiotensin II in the renal responses to somatic nerve stimulation in the rat. J. Physiol. **393:** 425–436.

7. JOHNS, E.J. 1987. The role of angiotensin II in the antidiuresis and antinatriuresis induced by stimulation of the sympathetic nerves to the rat kidney. J. Auton. Pharmacol. **7:**205–214.

8. LIU, F.-Y. & M.G. COGAN. 1988. Angiotensin II stimulation of hydrogen secretion in the rat early proximal tubule. J. Clin. Invest. **82:** 601–607.

9. WONG, K.R., C.A. BERRY & M.G. COGAN. 1996. Alpha$_1$ adrenergic control of chloride transport in the rat S1 convoluted tubule. Am. J. Physiol. **270:** 1049–1056.

10. WONG, P.C., S.D. HART & P.B.M.W.M. TIMMERMANS. 1991. Effect of angiotensin II antagonism on canine renal sympathetic nerve function. Hypertension **17:** 1127–1134.

11. WONG, P.C., R. BERNARD & P.B.M.W.M. TIMMERMANS. 1992. Effect of blocking angiotensin II receptor subtypes on rat sympathetic nerve function. Hypertension **19:** 663–667.

12. MIZELLE, L.L., J.E. HALL & L.L. WOODS. 1988. Interactions between angiotensin II and renal nerves during chronic sodium deprivation. Am. J. Physiol. **255:** F823–F827.

13. NELSON, L.D. & J.L. OSBORN. 1993. Neurogenic control of renal function in response to graded nonhypotensive hemorrhage in conscious dogs. Am. J. Physiol. **264:** R661–R667.

14. LANG, C.C., A.R. RAHMAN, D.J. BALFOUR & A.D. STRUTHERS. 1993. Enalapril blunts the antinatriuretic effect of circulating noradrenaline in man. J. Hypertens. **11:**565–571.

15. WRIGHT, J.W. & J.W. HARDING. 1997. Regulatory role of brain angiotensins in the control of physiological and behavioral processes. Brain Res. Rev. **17:** 227–262.

16. DiBONA, G.F. 1999. Central sympathoexcitatory actions of angiotensin II: role of type 1 angiotensin II receptors. J. Am. Soc. Nephrol. **10:** S90–S94.

17. LENKEI, Z., M. PALKOVITS, P. CORVOL & C. LLORENS–CORTÈS. 1997. Expression of angiotensin type-1 (AT1) and type-2 (AT2) receptor mRNAs in the adult rat brain: a functional neuroanatomical review. Frontiers Neuroendocrinol. **18:** 383–439.

18. FERGUSON, A.V. & D.L.S. WASHBURN. 1998. Angiotensin II: a peptidergic neurotransmitter in central autonomic pathways. Prog. Neurobiol. **54:** 169–192.

19. WRIGHT, J.W. & J.W. HARDING. 1997. Important roles for angiotensin III and IV in the brain renin-angiotensin system. Brain Res. Rev. **25:** 96–124.

20. SONG, K., A.M. ALLEN, G. PAXINOS & F.A.O. MENDELSOHN. 1992. Mapping of angiotensin II receptor heterogeneity in rat brain. J. Comp. Neurol. **316:** 467–484.

21. MACGREGOR, D.P., C. MURONE, K. SONG, A.M. ALLEN, G. PAXINOS & F.A.O. MENDELSOHN. 1995. Angiotensin II receptor subtypes in the human central nervous system. Brain Res. **675:** 231–240.

22. BROOKS, V.L. & J.W. OSBORN. 1995. Hormonal-sympathetic interactions in long-term regulation of arterial pressure: an hypothesis. Am. J. Physiol. **268:** R1343–R1358.

23. BROOKS, V.L. 1997. Interactions between angiotensin II and the sympathetic nervous system in the long-term control of arterial pressure. Clin. Exp. Pharmacol. Physiol. **24:** 83–90.

24. OSBORN, J.W. 1997. Hormones as long-term error signals for the sympathetic nervous system: importance of a new perspective. Clin. Exp. Pharmacol. Physiol. **24:** 109–115.

25. REID, I.A. 1992. Interactions between ANG II, sympathetic nervous system and baroreceptor reflexes in regulation of blood pressure. Am. J. Physiol. **262:** E763–E778.

26. FINK, G.F. 1997. Long-term sympathoexcitatory effect of angiotensin II: a mechanism of spontaneous and renovascular hypertension. Clin. Exp. Pharmacol. Physiol. **24:** 91–95.
27. FERGUSON, A.V. & J.S. BAINS. 1997. Actions of angiotensin in the subfornical organ and area postrema: implications for long term control of autonomic output. Clin. Exp. Pharmacol. Physiol. **24:** 96–101.
28. LIU, J.-L., H. MURAKAMI, M. SANDERFORD, V.S. BISHOP & I.H. ZUCKER. 1999. ANG II and baroreflex function in rabbits with CHF and lesions of the area postrema. Am. J. Physiol. **277:**H342–H350.
29. FINK, G.D., C.M. PAWLOSKI, L. OHMAN & J.R. HAYWOOD. 1991. Lateral parabrachial nucleus and angiotensin II induced hypertension. Hypertension **17:** 1177–1184.
30. TAGAWA, T. & R.A.L. DAMPNEY. 1999. $AT_1$ receptors mediate excitatory inputs to rostral ventrolateral medulla pressor neurons from hypothalamus. Hypertension **34:** 1301–1307.
31. WILSON, C.G. & A.C. BONHAM. 1994. Area postrema excites and inhibits sympathetic related neurons in rostral ventrolateral medulla in rabbit. Am. J. Physiol. **266:** H1075–H1086.
32. SUN, M.-K. & K.M. SPYER. 1990. GABA-mediated inhibition of medullary vasomotor neurones by area postrema stimulation in rats. J. Physiol. **436:** 669–684..
33. VAN HOUTON, M., E.L. SCHIFFRIN, J.F.E. MANN, B.I. POSNER AND R. BOUCHER. 1980. Radioautographic localization of specific binding sites for blood born angiotensin II in rat brain. Brain Res. **86:** 480–485.
34. MORIGUCHI, A., H. MIKAMI, A. OTSUKA, K. KATAHIRA, K. KOHARA & T. OGIHARA. 1995. Amino acids in the medulla oblongata contribute to baroreflex modulation by angiotensin II. Brain Res. Bull. **36:** 85–89.
35. KATAHIRA, K., H. MIKAMI, A. OTSUKA, A. MORIGUCHI, K. KOHARA, K. HIGASHIMORI, N. OKUDA, M. NAGANO, R. MORISHITA & T. OGIHARA. 1994. Differential control of vascular tone and heart rate by different amino acid neurotransmitters in the rostral ventrolateral medulla of the rat. Clin. Exp. Pharmacol. Physiol. **21:** 545–556.
36. CASTO, R. & M.I. PHILLIPS. 1986. Angiotensin II attenuates baroreflexes at nucleus tractus solitarius of rats. Am. J. Physiol. **250:** R193–R198.
37. CAMPAGNOLE-SANTOS, M.J., D.I. DIZ & C.M. FERRARIO. 1988. Baroreceptor reflex modulation by angiotensin II at the nucleus tractus solitarii. Hypertension **11**(Suppl I): I167–I171.
38. DAMPNEY, R.A.L. 1994. Functional organization of central pathways regulating the cardiovascular system. Physiol. Rev. **74:** 323–364.
39. DAMPNEY, R.A.L. 1994. The subretrofacial vasomotor nucleus: anatomical, chemical and pharmacological properties and role in cardiovascular regulation. Prog. Neurobiol. **42:**197–227.
40. DAMPNEY, R.A.L., Y. HIROOKA, P.D. POTTS & G.A. HEAD. 1996. Functions of angiotensin peptides in the rostral ventrolateral medulla. Clin. Exp. Pharmacol. Physiol. **23** (Suppl 23): S105–S111.
41. ALLEN, A.M., R.A.L. DAMPNEY & F.A.O. MENDELSOHN. 1988. Angiotensin receptor binding and pressor effects in cat subretrofacial nucleus. Am. J. Physiol. **255:** H1011–H1017.
42. SASAKI, S. & R.A.L. DAMPNEY. 1990. Tonic cardiovascular effects of angiotensin II in the ventrolateral medulla. Hypertension **15:** 274–283.
43. SAIGUSA, T. M. IRIKI & J. ARITA. 1996. Brain angiotensin II tonically modulates sympathetic baroreflex in rabbit ventrolateral medulla. Am. J. Physiol. **271:** H1015–H1021.
44. BROOKS, V.L. K.R. ELL & R.M. WRIGHT. 1993. Pressure-independent baroreflex resetting produced by chronic infusion of angiotensin II in rabbits. Am. J. Physiol. **265:** H1275–H1282.
45. BROOKS, V.L. 1995. Chronic infusion of angiotensin II resets baroreflex control of heart rate by an arterial pressure-independent mechanism. Hypertension **26:** 420–424.
46. DIBONA, G.F., S.Y. JONES & L.L. SAWIN. 1996. Effect of endogenous angiotensin II on renal nerve activity and its arterial baroreflex regulation. Am. J. Physiol. **271:** R361–R367.

47. Xu, L. & V.L. Brooks. 1996. ANG II chronically supports renal and lumbar sympathetic nerve activity and heart rate in sodium-deprived conscious rats. Am. J. Physiol. **271:** H2591–H2598.
48. Xu, L. & V.L. Brooks. 1997. Sodium intake, angiotensin II blockade and baroreflex function in conscious rats. Hypertension **29:** 450–457.
49. Segar, J.L., J.E. Masursky & J.E. Robillard. 1994. Changes in ovine renal sympathetic nerve activity and baroreflex function at birth. Am. J. Physiol. **267:** H1824–H1832.
50. Segar, J.L., D.C. Merrill & J.E. Robillard. 1994. Role of endogenous ANG II on resetting arterial baroreflex during development. Am. J. Physiol. **266:** H52–H59.
51. DiBona, G.F., S.Y. Jones & V.L. Brooks. 1995. ANG II receptor blockade and arterial baroreflex regulation of renal nerve activity in heart failure. Am. J. Physiol. **269:** R1189–R1196.
52. DiBona, G.F., S.Y. Jones & L.L. Sawin. 1998. Effect of endogenous angiotensin II on renal nerve activity and its cardiac baroreflex regulation. J. Am. Soc. Nephrol. **9:** 1983–1989,1998.
53. DiBona, G.F., S.Y. Jones & L.L. Sawin. 1998. Angiotensin receptor antagonist improves cardiac reflex control of renal sodium handling in heart failure. Am. J. Physiol. **274:** H636–H641.
54. Murakami, H., L. Liu & I.H. Zucker. 1997. Angiotensin II blockade enhances baroreflex control of sympathetic outflow in heart failure. Hypertension **29:** 564–569.
55. Ma, R., I.H. Zucker & W. Wang. 1997. Central gain of the cardiac sympathetic afferent reflex in dogs with heart failure. Am. J. Physiol. **273:** H2664–H2771.
56. Dibner-Dunlap, M., M.L. Smith, T. Kinugawa & M.D. Thames. 1996. Enalaprilat augments arterial and cardiopulmonary baroreflex control of sympathetic nerve activity in patients with heart failure. J. Am. Coll. Cardiol. **27:** 358–364.
57. Grassi, G., B.M. Caetano, G. Seravalle, A. Lanfranchi, M. Pozzi, A. Morganti, S. Carugo S & G. Mancia. 1997. Effects of chronic ACE inhibition on sympathetic nerve traffic and baroreflex control of circulation in heart failure. Circulation **96:** 1173–1179.
58. Heesch, C.M., M.E. Crandall & J.A. Turbek. 1996. Converting enzyme inhibitors cause pressure-independent resetting of baroreflex control of sympathetic outflow. Am. J. Physiol. **270:** R728–R737.
59. Takishita, S., H. Muratani, S. Sesoko, H. Teruya, M. Tozawa, K. Fukiyama & Y. Inada. 1994. Short-term effects of angiotensin II blockade on renal blood flow and sympathetic nerve activity in awake rats. Hypertension **24:** 445–450.
60. Averill, D.B., T. Tsuchihashi, M.C. Khosla & C.M. Ferrario. 1994. Losartan, nonpeptide angiotensin II-type 1 (AT1) receptor antagonist, attenuates pressor and sympathoexcitatory responses evoked by angiotensin II and L-glutamate in rostral ventrolateral medulla. Brain Res. **665:** 245–252.
61. Hirooka, Y., P.D. Potts & R.A.L. Dampney. 1997. Role of angiotensin II receptor subtypes in mediating the sympathoexcitatory effects of exogenous and endogenous angiotensin peptides in the rostral ventrolateral medulla. Brain Res. **772:** 107–114.
62. Fontes, M.A.P, L.C.S. Silva, M.J. Campagnole-Santos, M.C. Khosla, P.G. Guertzenstein, R.A.S. Santos. 1994. Evidence that angiotensin plays a role in the central control of blood pressure at the ventrolateral medulla acting through specific receptors. Brain Res. **665:** 175–180.
63. Fontes, M.A., M.C. Pinge, V. Naves, M.J. Campagnole-Santos, O.U. Lopes, M.C. Khosla & R.A.S. Santos. 1997. Cardiovascular effects produced by microinjection of angiotensins and angiotensin antagonists into the ventrolateral medulla of freely moving rats. Brain Res. **750:** 305–310.
64. Sasaki, S. & R.A.L. Dampney. 1990. Tonic cardiovascular effects of angiotensin II in the ventrolateral medulla. Hypertension **15:** 274–283.
65. Hirooka, Y. & R.A.L. Dampney. 1995. Endogenous angiotensin within the rostral ventrolateral medulla facilitates the somatosympathetic reflex. J. Hypertens. **13:** 747–754.
66. Saigusa, T., M. Iriki & J. Arita. 1996. Brain angiotensin II tonically modulates sympathetic baroreflex in rabbit ventrolateral medulla. Am. J. Physiol. **271:** H1015–H1021.

67. POTTS, P.D., A.M. ALLEN, J. HORIUCHI & R.A.L. DAMPNEY. 2000. Does angiotensin II have a significant tonic action on cardiovascular neurons in the rostral and caudal RVLM. Am. J. Physiol. **279:** R1392–R1402.
68. DIBONA, G.F. & S.Y. JONES. 2001. Sodium intake influences hemodynamic and neural responses to angiotensin receptor blockade in rostral ventrolateral medulla. Hypertension **37:** 1114–1123.

# Renal Arterial Pressure Variability

## A Role in Blood Pressure Control?

B. NAFZ AND P. B. PERSSON

*Johannes-Müller-Institut für Physiologie, Humboldt Universität (Charité),*
*10117 Berlin, Germany*

ABSTRACT: It is becoming generally appreciated that blood pressure (BP) fluctuations can have major pathophysiological importance in hypertensives.
Nonetheless, little is known regarding the influence of short-term changes in
BP on kidney function, a crucial control element for long-term BP regulation.
This overview summarizes first efforts to unravel the importance of BP dynamics on renal function. It seems that the kidney is not only an important control
element in the BP regulation network; the renal vascular bed may also be very
susceptible to BP oscillations, which can occur, for example, from baroreflex
malfunction.

KEYWORDS: Arterial blood pressure; Hypertension; Nitric oxide; Renal blood
flow; Renin; Blood pressure oscillations

## GENERAL IMPORTANCE OF BLOOD PRESSURE VARIATIONS

To maintain adequate blood flow to the organs, blood pressure (BP) and vascular
resistance are controlled by a complex regulatory network, which establishes a
crucial element for normal function of the cardiovascular system.[1] The known interactions between the many, still not fully understood, components of this system
apparently improve overall cardiovascular performance. Most of these control elements respond to very specific stimuli within a relatively narrow input range. For
instance, renal excretory function and the renin-angiotensin system depend on perfusion pressure as a control input. It seems, therefore, likely that excessive variations
in BP may perturb their regulation and thus compromise cardiovascular performance
under these conditions. Hence, it is not surprising that the organism is equipped with
potent BP-buffering mechanisms, such as the arterial baroreceptor reflex, which
maintain BP fluctuations within tight boundaries. The afferent branch of this reflex
consists of stretch receptors located in the carotid sinus region and the aortic arch,
while the effector side of the reflex is mediated by the sympathetic and parasympathetic nervous system.[2] Consequently, this reflex can serve to buffer BP fluctuations
that are detected by the carotid sinus and aortic arch region, whereas remote changes
in BP or blood flow, for example, within the vascular tree of the kidney, remain
largely unaffected. Such local changes in hemodynamics are known to induce the

Address for correspondence: P. B. Persson, Johannes-Müller-Institut für Physiologie, Humboldt Universität (Charité), Tucholskystrasse 2, D-10117 Berlin, Germany. Voice: +49-30-450-
528162; fax: +49-30-450-528972.

pontus.persson@charite.de

release of vasoactive substances from the endothelium. One of them, nitric oxide (NO), has been suggested to act as a local buffer for BP fluctuations because fixing NO levels in conscious rats significantly enhances BP variability between 0.2 and 0.6 Hz.[3] Furthermore, genetically induced impairment of the endothelial NO system elevates BP and also enhances short-term BP oscillations in mice.[4]

There have been a vast number of studies in recent years focusing on the description of BP oscillations in order to quantify various aspects of cardiovascular control. Among these applications, the possibility of using spectral analysis of BP as a tool for quantifying baroreflex sensitivity or sympathetic and vagal tone has attracted the most attention.[5] In spite of the widespread investigations on the origin of BP variability, astonishingly little is known about the importance of BP waves for cardiovascular control. Remarkably, it has been recognized early that changes in the dynamic properties of BP commonly coincide with hypertension. This may be explained by the fact that several BP buffers play also an important role in the regulation of mean BP. For instance, surgical or pharmacological interruption of the baroreceptor reflex enhances short-term BP oscillations and can also elevate 24-h BP in conscious animals.[1] It is well accepted that the average level of arterial BP establishes a major determinant of future cardiovascular complications in hypertension.[6] To a large degree, high BP seems to be responsible for cardiovascular disease, which is the principal cause of death in industrialized nations.[7] Interestingly, recent investigations show that the dynamic properties of BP are of significance for the development of hypertension-related end-organ damage in patients.[6,8] In fact, changes in the dynamic properties of BP, which usually coincide with hypertension, seem to establish an independent risk factor for cardiovascular complications. In light of these results, it seems of great importance to clarify to which extent BP variability modulates mechanisms, for example, renal sodium and water handling, which can play a crucial role in the development of hypertension.

## BLOOD PRESSURE VARIABILITY TO THE KIDNEY

In particular, renal function may depend critically on oscillating perfusion pressure. The kidney is protected from slow variations in BP by at least two mechanisms guaranteeing blood flow and filtration rate autoregulation: the myogenic response of vascular smooth muscles and the tubuloglomerular feedback mechanism. A conventional autoregulation diagram plots blood flow versus perfusion pressure. In a certain range, renal blood flow reveals little or no pressure-dependency.

It must be kept in mind, however, that this classical plot of the blood flow autoregulation is derived from experiments that employed stepwise reductions in renal perfusion pressure. Thus, this description is only valid for very slow changes in BP. Due to time constants of the underlying mechanisms, the time course of an initial stimulus can gain major influence on the response of the system to that stimulus. It seems therefore plausible that the influence of faster BP fluctuations on RBF cannot be correctly described by the classical model of renal autoregulation. To clarify the characteristics of regulating systems at different stimulating frequencies, a spectral analysis in the frequency domain has been shown to be a very helpful tool.[9,10] This approach can be of particular benefit for autoregulation studies of renal blood flow since, as mentioned above, the kidney has two potent autoregulatory mechanisms. As these two autoregulatory instruments operate in different frequency ranges, it is possible to discern the individual autoregulatory potencies[10,11] and, thus, to quantify the individual effects of both autoregulatory mechanisms. Most importantly, the transfer function provides information as to which oscillations can override both mechanisms of autoregulation. A transfer function between renal arterial pressure and renal blood flow indicates to which extent and at what frequencies changes in pressure will alter blood flow to the kidney. Accordingly, the transfer function characterizes renal autoregulation in the frequency domain.[10–15] The gain is calculated by dividing the cross-spectral estimates by the corresponding autospectral values. The entire transfer function is then obtained by plotting each gain over the respective frequency. There are two frequency domains within which autoregulation takes place: a fast mechanism at 0.1–0.2 Hz, recognized by the decrease of the gain below this frequency, and a slower one around 0.03 Hz, characterized by a peak of high gain.[9] The faster mechanism probably corresponds to the myogenic response, whereas the slower one reflects the tubuloglomerular feedback. The latter conclusion has been substantiated by observations of similar fluctuations of tubular flow and chloride concentration.[16] Furthermore, the oscillations are abolished by ureter ligation[17] or furosemide.[18,19] Below 0.01 Hz, a plateau of low gain is attained. This level reflects the autoregulatory efficiency. Thus, the two control elements of the kidney act as high-pass filters; that is, oscillations that occur above a certain frequency cannot be buffered. Consequently, these rapid blood pressure oscillations will lead to similar changes in renal blood flow, which can have important consequences for maintaining medullary osmolarity and renal NO synthesis. The latter two are assumed to be closely intertwined with long-term BP control: First, renal medullary osmolarity is important in relation to pressure diuresis. According to the renal/body-fluid–pressure-control concept, fluid and electrolyte excretion is crucial for long-term BP regulation (see Refs. 1 and 20 for review). In line with this hypothesis, several investigators reported that an impaired capability of the kidney to form adequate amounts of urine induces hypertension.[21] The renal medulla has a very high osmotic pressure, which is crucial for the fluid and electrolyte reabsorption that contributes to the formation of a concentrated urine. Increased medullary blood flow may wash out the osmotic gradient within the renal medulla and thereby blunt the ability of the kidney to form a concentrated urine.[22] Therefore, if BP oscillations induce changes in renal medullary hemodynamics, then longer-term BP may be affected via a change in renal fluid and sodium excretion.

A second pathway for connecting renal function to systemic BP may also be affected by variations of BP and kidney blood flow: the renal NO system. NO formation has been seen as a crucial element in mediating pressure natriuresis,[23] particularly since the acute relationship between renal BP and sodium excretion is blunted by NO inhibition.[24] The renal medulla is enriched in immunoreactive NO synthase (NOS) protein and NOS enzymatic activity when compared with the renal cortex.[25] Particularly high NOS activity is present in the inner medullary collecting ducts, while less NOS activity is located in glomeruli and vasa recta. The latter sites, though, should be of more importance for pressure natriuresis. It is remarkable that changes in BP causing enhanced sodium excretion lead to likewise changes in renal medullary NO activity.[26] The importance of the renal medullary NO system for BP control is underscored by experiments employing selective renal medullary NOS inhibition. This maneuver diminishes sodium and water excretion and leads to hypertension.[27] It seems likely that spontaneous BP oscillations, which are not effectively buffered by RBF autoregulation, augment intrarenal shear stress. This would take place at the level of the vascular wall. Shear stress, in turn, is known to enhance the liberation of NO along the renal vascular tree *in vitro*. Thus, again, one may expect a profound impact of BP oscillations on medullary blood flow, on renal excretory function, and on longer-term BP regulation.[25,28]

Finally, the renin-angiotensin system interactions with BP are well known and are probably of great importance in long-term BP control.[29] BP regulation by renin takes place via the direct vasoconstrictor effects of angiotensin II and via the influence on renal fluid and sodium handling. A previous study employing BP oscillations to the kidney shed light on the importance of renal blood flow versus renal perfusion pressure for the release of renin.[30] Renal perfusion pressure and renal blood flow were dissociated by impinging BP oscillations within the resonance frequency of renal autoregulation. In consequence, maximum blood flow occurred at minimal BP. It was found that BP is the dominant factor for renin release, with blood flow playing only a minor role. Taking this study into account, it may seem as if BP oscillations to the kidney may have an important effect on renin release, although oscillations in blood flow have no effect. This could be underscored by the particular relationship between BP and renin release. The renin stimulus response curve describing this relationship is not linear, but is characterized by a threshold pressure below which renin release markedly increases. Above this threshold, only a meager effect of BP on renin release is found. BP oscillations slightly below the threshold pressure for renin release should thus lead to greater renin release: The drops in BP markedly enhance renin release, whereas the BP increments do not attenuate renin release to the same extent.

## EFFECT OF ENHANCING BP OSCILLATIONS TO THE KIDNEY

The following experiments were carried out to clarify whether enhanced BP variability may affect renal functions. The working hypothesis was that normally occurring BP oscillations cannot be completely buffered by the mechanisms of kidney blood flow autoregulation. Thus, the resulting blood flow variability may modify certain functions of this organ.

As shown in FIGURE 1, BP oscillations (BPO) of 0.1 Hz elicit concurrent changes in renal cortical and medullary blood flow. Thus, the premise that BP oscillations at this frequency can override renal blood flow autoregulation is warranted. This experiment was performed in the rat using the laser-Doppler technique; therefore, local renal blood flow could only be estimated by the laser-Doppler flux signal (for details of the measurement, see Ref. 31).

The upcoming protocols were done in adult, chronically instrumented, pure-bred beagles,[32] which could move freely and undisturbed in their kennels during the experiments. Data recording, control of renal BP, continuous urine sampling, and blood sampling were done via a swivel system from an adjacent room. Catheters were advanced via the femoral arteries into the abdominal aorta, where they were placed distally and proximally to both renal arteries, respectively. An inflatable cuff

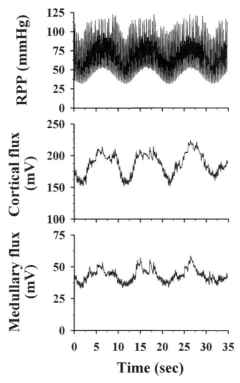

**FIGURE 1.** Induced BPO with a frequency of 0.1 Hz override the renal blood flow autoregulation and reach the renal medulla. RPP: renal perfusion pressure.

was positioned around the aorta, above the origin of the renal arteries and between the tips of the catheters. Finally, a bladder catheter was implanted to allow continuous urine collection. The cuff and the distal catheter were connected to an electropneumatic pressure control system that was able to reduce and to oscillate renal BP around a preset level with high precision.

Three protocols were done. The first was a 24-h time control. In a second protocol, acute Goldblatt hypertension was induced by reduction of mean renal BP to 85 mmHg. The last protocol was designed to determine the influence of BP variations on the onset of Goldblatt hypertension. To this end, renal BP was oscillated sinusoidally over 24 h with a frequency of 0.1 Hz (amplitude $\pm$ 10 mmHg) around the same mean pressure as in the second protocol, that is, 85 mmHg.

The 24-h mean value of BP was $110 \pm 3$ mmHg during control. The static reduction of renal arterial BP to 85 mmHg increased systemic BP by almost 60 mmHg at the end of the 24-h recording period (FIG. 2, $p < 0.01$). This BP increase was markedly attenuated by superimposing 0.1-Hz oscillations. In this protocol, BP increased by only half as much as seen during static BP reduction (FIG. 2, $p < 0.01$).

The static BP reduction decreased urine flow to roughly half of the control values ($p < 0.01$). Superimposing 0.1-Hz BP oscillations restored urine flow to near control

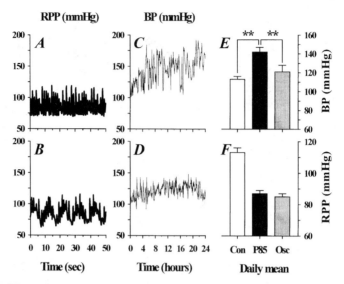

**FIGURE 2.** Original recordings of RPP (A: P85; B: Osc) and systemic BP (C: P85; D: Osc). P85 elevated mean systemic BP to about 150 mmHg (E, black bar vs. white bar). This hypertensive effect was attenuated (E, gray bar) when mean RPP oscillated around the same value of ≈85 mmHg (F). $**p < 0.01$

values. Changes in sodium and potassium excretion behaved similarly. Static renal BP reduction diminished sodium excretion to 20% of control ($p < 0.01$). When renal BP was oscillated at this reduced pressure, sodium excretion became twice as high as during static reduction of renal BP; however, control levels were not reached.

As shown in a recent publication,[32] these data obtained in renovascular hypertensive dogs demonstrate a pronounced antihypertensive effect of BP oscillations to the kidney. This may rely on changes in intrarenal microcirculation. BP oscillations induce changes in local blood flow, which presumably modulate physical forces along the nephron. Moreover, it is plausible that these BP oscillations interfere with the local release of many vasoactive substances (e.g., prostaglandins and kinins), thereby changing local hemodynamics and kidney function.

Interestingly, 0.1-Hz oscillations in muscle sympathetic nerve activity and RR interval have been reported to be markedly attenuated during heart failure and blunted during severe heart failure in humans.[33] Provided that the patterns of muscle sympathetic nerve activity and RR interval are mirrored by corresponding BP oscillations, one may speculate that BP oscillations facilitate excretion of fluid and electrolytes, thereby improving the prognosis of these patients.

The induced renal BP oscillations augment shear stress at the vascular wall. Endothelial shear stress stimulates NO release from arteries, thereby inducing vasodilatation and changes in intrarenal hemodynamics. Urinary $NO_3$ excretion was used as a marker for NO production. Unfortunately, the direct assessment of renal NO is still not possible in freely moving animals. Thus, we aimed at obtaining greatest accuracy by performing all experiments during the post-reabsorptive state when in-

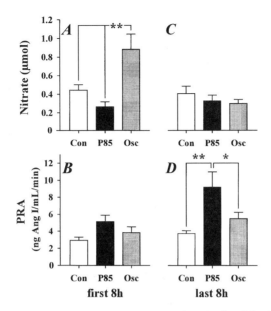

**FIGURE 3.** Osc doubled renal $NO_3$ excretion during the first 8 h of the experiments **(A)**, while the influence on acute changes of PRA was less pronounced **(B)**. In face of the 24-h reduction of RPP, $NO_3$ excretion returned to normal **(C)**, whereas Osc induced a significant reduction in PRA versus P85 **(D)**. $*p < 0.05$, $**p < 0.01$; C and D: mean values of last 8 h of the experiments.

fluences of food composition on urinary $NO_3$ are least. Furthermore, a very specific mass spectrometric analysis, instead of the Griess-Ilosvay reaction, was used. This avoids possible interference with most physiological $NO_x$ compounds. A stimulation in NO liberation was detectable only during the first 8 h of the experiments (FIG. 3). Thus, the prolonged antihypertensive effect of BP waves cannot be explained by a direct effect of the enhanced NO release.

Plasma renin activity in the oscillation protocol was about 30% less than that seen with static pressure reduction. This may indicate an important role of the renin system in the observed antihypertensive effect. In light of the aforementioned stimulus-response curve of pressure-dependent renin release, the finding of an attenuated renin release in this protocol is surprising: a pronounced influence of renal BP on renin release has been detected only below 90 mmHg.[34] Thus, the minima of the BP oscillations lead to pressure-dependent stimulation in renin release, whereas maxima in renal BP cannot reduce renin release to the same extent. Therefore, if one assumes that possible hysteresis effects can be neglected, one would expect higher PRA during Osc than during P85. Evidently, the BP waves exerted a major influence on renin release in the freely moving dog. This suggests that the sustained antihypertensive effect of Osc on renovascular hypertension may at least in part be mediated by lowered PRA. In contrast to the prolonged effect on PRA, the stimulation of NO generation seems to be important only during the first 8 h of our experiments.

## CONCLUSIONS

By chronically oscillating renal BP around a reduced mean pressure, it was found that these BP waves enhance daily sodium and fluid excretion and attenuate the BP elevation during the onset of renal hypertension. Variations in BP at the frequency chosen for this study are largely unaffected by renal autoregulation and thus lead to concomitant changes in renal blood flow. Since renal medullary blood flow plays a key role in controlling BP and water-electrolyte balance, it is not surprising that these oscillations in perfusion pressure evoke profound effects on renal excretory function. The BP waves also blunted pressure-dependent renin release, which may have contributed significantly to the antihypertensive effect.

## ACKNOWLEDGMENTS

These studies were supported by the German Research Foundation.

## REFERENCES

1. PERSSON, P.B. 1996. Modulation of cardiovascular control mechanisms and their interaction. Physiol. Rev. **76:** 193–244.
2. KIRCHHEIM, H.R. 1976. Systemic arterial baroreceptor reflexes. Physiol. Rev. **56:** 100–176.
3. NAFZ, B., C.D. WAGNER & P.B. PERSSON. 1997. Endogenous nitric oxide buffers blood pressure variability between 0.2 Hz and 0.6 Hz in the conscious rat. Am. J. Physiol. **272:** H632–H637.
4. STAUSS, H.M., A. GÖDECKE, R. MROWKA et al. 1999. Enhanced blood pressure variability in eNOS knockout mice. Hypertension **33:** 1359–1363.
5. PERSSON, P.B. 1997. Spectrum analysis of cardiovascular time series. Am. J. Physiol. **273:** R1201–R1210.
6. SYTKOWSKI, P.A., R.B. D'AGOSTINO, A.J. BELANGER & W.B. KANNEL. 1996. Secular trends in long-term sustained hypertension, long-term treatment, and cardiovascular mortality: the Framingham Heart Study 1950 to 1990. Circulation **93:** 697–703.
7. WHELTON, P.K. 1994. Epidemiology of hypertension. Lancet **344:** 101–106.
8. MANCIA, G., A. FRATTOLA, G. PARATI et al. 1994. Blood pressure variability and organ damage. J. Cardiovasc. Pharmacol. **24**(suppl. A): S6–S11.
9. HOLSTEIN-RATHLOU, N.H. & D.J. MARSH. 1994. Renal blood flow regulation and arterial pressure fluctuations: a case study in nonlinear dynamics. Physiol. Rev. **74:** 637–681.
10. WITTMANN, U., B. NAFZ, H. EHMKE et al. 1995. Frequency domain of renal autoregulation in the conscious dog. Am. J. Physiol. **269:** F317–F322.
11. HOLSTEIN-RATHLOU, N.H., A.J. WAGNER & D.J. MARSH. 1991. Tubuloglomerular feedback dynamics and renal blood flow autoregulation in rats. Am. J. Physiol. **260:** F53–F68.
12. BASAR, E. & C. WEISS. 1968. Analyse des Frequenganges druckinduzierter Änderungen des Stromwiderstandes isolierter Rattennieren. Pflüg. Arch. **304:** 121–135.
13. SAKAI, T., E. HALLMAN & D.J. MARSH. 1986. Frequency domain analysis of renal autoregulation in the rat. Am. J. Physiol. **250:** F364–F373.
14. CHEN, Y.M. & N.H. HOLSTEIN-RATHLOU. 1993. Differences in dynamic autoregulation of renal blood flow between SHR and WKY rats. Am. J. Physiol. **264:** F166–F174.
15. CHON, K.H., Y.M. CHEN, N.H. HOLSTEIN-RATHLOU et al. 1993. On the efficacy of linear system analysis of renal autoregulation in rats. IEEE Trans. Biomed. Eng. **40:** 8–20.
16. HOLSTEIN-RATHLOU, N.H. & D.J. MARSH. 1989. Oscillations of tubular pressure, flow, and distal chloride concentration in rats. Am. J. Physiol. **256:** F1007–F1014.

17. DANIELS, F., W. ARENDSHORST & R. ROBERDS. 1990. Tubuloglomerular feedback and autoregulation in spontaneously hypertensive rats. Am. J. Physiol. **258:** F1479–F1489.
18. AJIKOBI, D.O., P. NOVAK, F.C. SALEVSKY & W.A. CUPPLES. 1996. Pharmacological modulation of spontaneous renal blood flow dynamics. Can. J. Physiol. Pharmacol. **74:** 964–972.
19. JUST, A., U. WITTMANN, H. EHMKE & H.R. KIRCHHEIM. 1998. Autoregulation of renal blood flow in the conscious dog and the contribution of the tubuloglomerular feedback. J. Physiol. (Lond.) **506:** 275–290.
20. COWLEY, A.W., JR. 1992. Long-term control of arterial blood pressure. Physiol. Rev. **72:** 231–300.
21. GUYTON, A.C. 1991. Blood pressure control—special role of the kidney and body fluids. Science **252:** 1813–1816.
22. COWLEY, A.W. 1997. Role of the renal medulla in volume and arterial pressure regulation. Am. J. Physiol. **273:** R1–R15.
23. GRANGER, J.P. & B.T. ALEXANDER. 2000. Abnormal pressure-natriuresis in hypertension: role of nitric oxide. Acta Physiol. Scand. **168**(1): 161–168.
24. FORTEPIANI, L.A., E. RODRIGO, M.C. ORITZ et al. 1999. Pressure natriuresis in nitric oxide–deficient hypertensive rats: effect of antihypertensive treatments. J. Am. Soc. Nephrol. **10:** 21–27.
25. WU, F., F. PARK, A.W. COWLEY, JR. & D.L. MATTSON. 1999. Quantification of nitric oxide synthase activity in microdissected segments of the rat kidney. Am. J. Physiol. **276:** F874–F881.
26. MAJID, D.S., K.E. SAID & S.A. OMORO. 1999. Responses to acute changes in arterial pressure on renal medullary nitric oxide activity in dogs. Hypertension **34:** 832–836.
27. MATTSON, D.L., S. LU, K. NAKANISHI et al. 1994. Effect of chronic medullary nitric oxide inhibition on blood pressure. Am. J. Physiol. **266:** H1918–H1926.
28. MATTSON, D.L. & F. WU. 2000. Control of arterial blood pressure and renal sodium excretion by nitric oxide synthase in the renal medulla. Acta Physiol. Scand. **168:** 149–154.
29. EHMKE, H., P.B. PERSSON & H.R. KIRCHHEIM. 1987. A physiological role for pressure-dependent renin release in long-term blood pressure control. Pflüg. Arch. **410:** 450–456.
30. NAFZ, B., H. BERTHOLD, H. EHMKE et al. 1997. Flow versus pressure in the control of renin release in conscious dogs. Am. J. Physiol. **273:** F200–F205.
31. NAFZ, B., K. BERGER, C. RÖSSLER & P.B. PERSSON. 1998. Kinins modulate the sodium-dependent autoregulation of renal medullary blood flow. Cardiovasc. Res. **40:** 573–579.
32. NAFZ, B., E. SEELIGER, H.W. REINHARDT & P.B. PERSSON. 2000. Antihypertensive effect of 0.1 Hz blood pressure oscillations to the kidney. Circulation **101:** 553–557.
33. VAN DE BORNE, P., N. MONTANO, M. PAGANI et al. 1997. Absence of low-frequency variability of sympathetic nerve activity in severe heart failure. Circulation **95:** 1449–1454.
34. FINKE, R., R. GROSS, E. HACKENTHAL et al. 1983. Threshold pressure for the pressure-dependent renin release in the autoregulating kidney of conscious dogs. Pflüg. Arch. **399:** 102–110.

# Rhythmicities in Sympathetic Discharge: A Signal of Cardiorespiratory Integration in Developing Animals

BRUCE W. HUNDLEY,[a] ANTHONY L. SICA,[b] AND PHYLLIS M. GOOTMAN[a]

[a]Department of Physiology and Pharmacology, State University of New York, Downstate Medical Center, Brooklyn, New York 11203, USA

[b]Department of Medicine, Division of Pulmonary Medicine, Long Island Jewish Medical Center of Albert Einstein College of Medicine, New Hyde Park, New York 11040, USA

ABSTRACT: We have been pursuing various avenues of investigation to elucidate the postnatal maturation of neural regulation of cardiovascular and respiratory integration. In this paper we present our results from a systematic analysis of age-related modulations of sympathetic (SYMP) activity with respect to experimental alterations in baroreceptor afferent inputs. The three age groups of piglets were chosen based on different responses to a complex stimulus, i.e., the Valsalva maneuver. Postnatal maturation of SYMP activity was examined by spectral analysis of SYMP discharge using cross-power, full and partial coherence. Three general oscillations were observed in spontaneous SYMP discharges in the 0–30 Hz range. We divided that range into five frequency bands (0–2, 2–6, 6–12, 12–20, 20–30 Hz), which included periodicities in phase with both central respiratory activity and the cardiac cycle. Spectral analyses of SYMP activity after either baroreceptor activation (phenylephrine) or deactivation (nitroprusside) revealed that respiratory modulation was age-related across all frequencies while baroreceptor modulation was usually age-related within three of the five frequency bands. These results lead to questions concerning the possible role of the autonomic nervous system and/or central interactions between the respiratory and SYMP rhythm generators in the etiology of sudden infant death syndrome (SIDS).

KEYWORDS: Piglet; Neonate; Power spectra; Coherence; Sympathetic; Valsalva maneuver; Baroreceptor sensitivity; Partialization

## INTRODUCTION

Although cardiovascular reflex responses tend to be similar across species in the adult, the rates of maturation of cardiovascular responses can differ markedly among species.[1,2] We have chosen to study the subprimate model, *Sus scrofa,* because of similarities to human development.[3] We had found in adult mammals, in addition to the cardiac and respiratory modulation of sympathetic (SYMP) discharge reported

Address for correspondence: Dr. Phyllis M. Gootman, Dept. of Physiology and Pharmacology, Box 31, SUNY–Downstate Medical Center, 450 Clarkson Avenue, Brooklyn, NY 11203. Voice: 718-270-1232; fax: 718-270-3103.

gootman@hscbklyn.edu

early in the twentieth century,[4] a 10-Hz rhythm[5,6] and, occasionally, a higher frequency approximately 30 Hz in cervical sympathetic nerve activity.[7,8] A question raised regarding the level or degree of autonomic regulation in the neonate led us to conduct similar studies in neonatal swine.[9–12] Spontaneous SYMP periodicities have been observed in these studies: 2–30 Hz oscillations in phase with the central respiratory cycle and oscillations in phase with the cardiac cycle.[10–14] This report presents our more recent results concerning age-related alterations of the spontaneous frequencies found in SYMP activity in neonates occurring in response to baroreceptor manipulation. The results from these studies should extend our knowledge of the possible role of the autonomic nervous system in the etiology of sudden infant death syndrome (SIDS).[15]

Evaluation of the age-related changes in cardiovascular regulation was obtained previously with the fictive Valsalva maneuver.[10] We reported[10] that SYMP activity did not change in the two-week-old piglet, while blood pressure continued to fall and no heart rate responses were observed. At 4 weeks, SYMP activity increased initially and the blood pressure fall was arrested; heart rate increased. It was at 7 weeks that the full adult Valsalva response was obtained. While phrenic (PHR) nerve activity remained quiescent throughout the Valsalva maneuver, both SYMP nerves showed high-frequency activity. Quantitation of the Valsalva responses at different ages in a series of animals is shown in FIGURE 1. Prior to 10 days of postnatal life, neither the tachycardia or Valsalva ratio[16] changed from one. From 10 days to 20 days of postnatal life, piglets showed a falling tachycardia ratio; however, the Valsalva ratio remained at one. The Valsalva ratio began to change after 21 days of postnatal life. Using the criteria for cardiovascular change found with the tachycardia and Valsalva ratios and the changes in SYMP activity between the three ages, piglets could now be classified into three postnatal age groups for the present study.

## METHODS

Piglets ($n = 18$) were anesthetized with Saffan (18 mg/kg, i.v.), tracheotomized, and ventilated on 100% $O_2$, as detailed extensively in our earlier studies.[9–14] Nerves (cervical sympathetic [CS], splanchnic [SPL], and phrenic [PHR]) were exposed, desheathed, cut, immersed in paraffin oil, and the central crushed end placed on bipolar platinum electrodes to measure monophasic activity. Intratracheal pressure (ITP), aortic pressure (AoP), and electrocardiogram (ECG) were also measured simultaneously, and all signals were stored on FM tapes for offline analysis.

Prior to these studies, piglets were classified into age groups (FIG. 1) according to their Valsalva and tachycardia ratios. Valsalva and tachycardia ratios were calculated[10,16] from fictive Valsalva maneuvers[10] and were graphed, and a polynomial equation was found to fit the age-related changes observed. The tachycardia ratio is derived by dividing the pre-Valsalva maneuver cardiac rate by the cardiac rate during the Valsalva maneuver. The Valsalva ratio is derived by dividing the cardiac rate during the Valsalva maneuver by the cardiac rate immediately following the Valsalva maneuver (bradycardia at Stage 4). Animals less than 10 days of age exhibited no change in either Valsalva or tachycardia ratios (Group I). Animals 11–20 days of age exhibited changes in the tachycardia ratio, but had no bradycardia at Stage 4 of

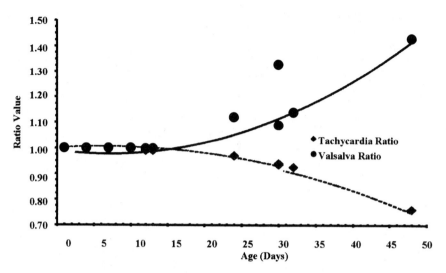

**FIGURE 1.** Valsalva and tachycardia ratios were calculated[10,16] from fictive Valsalva maneuvers,[10] were graphed, and a polynomial equation found to fit the age-related changes observed. The tachycardia ratio was derived by dividing the pre-Valsalva maneuver cardiac rate by the cardiac rate during the Valsalva maneuver. The Valsalva ratio was derived by dividing the cardiac rate during the Valsalva maneuver by the cardiac rate immediately following the Valsalva maneuver (bradycardia at Stage 4).

the Valsalva maneuver (Group II). Animals >21 days of age (Group III) began to develop bradycardias in Stage 4 of the Valsalva maneuver.

After surgery, anesthesia was reduced to 4–6 mg/kg i.v. for one hour before baseline measurements were recorded. After baseline measurements were recorded, the following protocols were performed: (1) Phenylephrine (PE, 20 µg/kg i.v.) was given as a bolus. Parameters were recorded for five minutes prior to the infusion (baseline control) to five minutes after the elevated AoP returned to baseline levels. (2) Nitroprusside (NP, 30 µg/kg i.v.) was given as a bolus. Parameters were recorded for five minutes prior to the infusion (baseline control) to five minutes after the lowered AoP returned to baseline levels.

Offline analyses consisted of filtering the nerve activities from 3–40 Hz (Kronhite filters) and digitizing all measured parameters on a computer (RC electronics A/D board, 128 samples per second). Event markers were placed either randomly (50 random event triggers), or at the peak of systole (200 event triggers), or at the onset and offset of PHR nerve discharge, inspiration (I) and expiration (E), respectively, (normally 30 event triggers for each phase). All signals were first averaged from each event marker. The means and trends were subtracted, the signals were smoothed by a Hamming window function, and autopower spectral densities were computed from each event trigger. Power spectral density is the power spectrum normalized to power per second by dividing the power spectrum by the sample time. Secondary analysis included computation of cross-spectral densities and coherence. Tertiary analysis consisted of mathematical removal of AoP from the cross-power density and coherence functions (delineation of baroreceptor activity).

### Random Triggered Spectra

Baseline power spectral densities were obtained using data synchronized to randomly placed triggers. Such spectra represent activity not triggered by either cardiac or respiratory events, but are obtained as a standard when results are unknown. This is a standard engineering practice when amplification is unknown and an evaluation of the amplifier gain (baroreceptor sensitivity) is wanted because a random sample of sufficient sample time will include all the known frequencies being measured. The total area under the random triggered spectrum was therefore set to 100% random mean value (% RMV). Since there were at least 50 random spectra averaged under baseline conditions, the resulting spectrum is the mean individual random triggered spectrum (hence random mean spectrum), and the total power under this spectrum is set as the standard (100% RMV). All other power spectra were normalized to this random triggered mean spectrum for evaluation of the activity change in association with the cardiac or respiratory cycle, and baroreceptor activation or deactivation. The spectra were then separated into the three age groups (1–10 days, Group I; 11–20 days, Group II; and >21 days, Group III) for statistical analysis.

Cross power and coherence spectra were calculated from CS and SPL activities.[17] Cross-power spectrum represents oscillations that are common to both CS and SPL activities. Cross-power spectral density is the cross power divided by the sample time. Cross power essentially is the product of two or more autopower spectra and the cosine of the phase angle between the autopower spectra. Cross-spectral density is a filter in that only the common components of two or more autopower spectra will show peaks. Coherence spectrum estimates the probability that two signals are derived from the same source.

Partialization procedures were carried out on CS and SPL cross power and coherence calculations.[17] Partialization is the mathematical removal of a component present in individual nerve spectra; in this case, baroreceptor-related inputs. This removal of baroreceptor-related inputs would leave only respiratory and brainstem oscillators as contributors to the cross power. Surgical denervation of the carotid sinus and vagus nerves was used to verify the mathematical subtraction.

Nonparametric statistical tests were used. The Kruskal-Wallis test (a nonparametric ANOVA) was performed between each age group in each protocol to determine the age-related significance of the measured parameters. Paired Wilcoxon rank tests were performed between protocol and baseline spectra to test for significant changes between control and protocols.

Baroreceptor sensitivity (gain) was calculated by dividing the change in baroreceptor-related SYMP power by the associated change in mean aortic pressure (AoP). Units therefore are given as % RMV/mmHg AoP. The level for statistical significance was established at $p < 0.05$ for all comparisons.

## RESULTS

### Respiratory Modulation of Baroreceptor-related SYMP Activity

Power spectra, relative to a random mean power spectra, were categorized according to age and event trigger. FIGURE 2 presents typical SYMP spectra. CS activ-

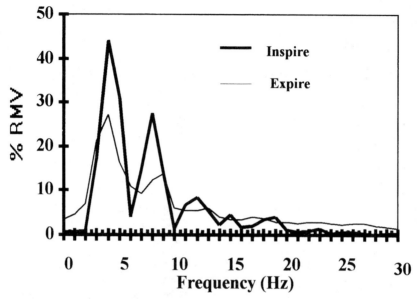

**FIGURE 2.** Power spectral densities of CS activity during inspiration (Inspire) and expiration (Expire). Power is expressed as % of random mean spectra value (% RMV). (Adapted from Gootman *et al.*[10] with permission.)

ity was at control baseline levels for two events, I and E. CS power spectra showed clearly demarcated peaks at specific frequencies. These frequency bands have been identified as related to the central respiratory cycle, the cardiac cycle, and the "brainstem" 10 Hz SYMP generator. The area under each frequency band was calculated and then compared. In general, CS and SPL power was significantly greater during I than E for every protocol (Wilcoxon paired rank test).[10]

In FIGURE 3, secondary (cross power and coherence of CS and SPL nerve activities, top) and tertiary (cross power and coherence partialized with respect to AoP to show overall respiratory modulation, middle) analyses, and the difference spectra (cross power minus partialized cross power, or coherence minus partialized coherence, bottom), revealed age-related significance within several frequency ranges (Kruskal-Wallis test). Statistically significant age-related differences were present in the 2–6 Hz range of both total cross power (top left) and baroreceptor-related cross power (bottom left). Overall coherence showed a trend toward age-related significance ($p < 0.1$) in the 6–12 Hz band (10 Hz oscillator band). Partialized coherence (primarily respiratory-related, middle right) showed distinct age-related significance in three bands: the 2–6 Hz band, the 6–12 Hz band, and the 12–20 Hz band: Group II (11- to 20-day-old) piglets consistently demonstrated the highest respiratory-related coherence, while Group III piglets (> 21 days of age) showed the least coherence. These results, especially with respect to the two-week-old group, support our earlier studies of activation of neurons in the nucleus tractus solitarius (NTS) at this age.[18]

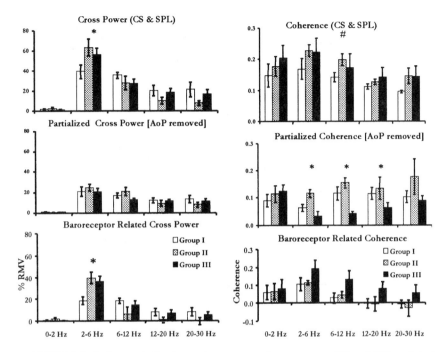

**FIGURE 3. Left top:** AoP-triggered average total cross power (CS and SPL activity) per frequency band in the three age groups. **Left middle:** Average cross power totals (CS and SPL activity) following partialization (removal of baroreceptor inputs by mathematical denervation, thus leaving respiratory-related cross power). **Left bottom:** AoP-triggered average baroreceptor-related cross power totals (CS and SPL activity) per frequency band. **Right top:** Average coherence value (CS and SPL activity) per frequency band for the three age groups. **Right middle:** Average coherence value (CS and SPL activity) per frequency band after partialization (respiratory-related coherence). **Right bottom:** Average baroreceptor-related coherence value (CS and SPL activity) per frequency band. *, Age-related significance ($p < 0.05$, Kruskal-Wallis test); #, age-related trend toward significance ($p < 0.1$, Kruskal Wallis test).

## Baroreceptor Reflexes

With the use of phenylephrine (PE) to elevate AoP, or nitroprusside (NP) to lower AoP, the baroreceptors could be activated or deactivated. Respiratory-related partialized cross power revealed age-related significance ($p < 0.05$) in three frequency ranges: the 2–6 Hz range, the 12–20 Hz range, and the 20–30 Hz range. In all but the 20–30 Hz range, Group II piglets continued to exhibit the greatest power. The change in cross power (difference of PE minus the control spectra, FIG. 4) showed age-related significant changes in SYMP cross power in three major frequency bands: the 0–2 Hz, 2–6 Hz, and 12–20 Hz ranges. Within the respiratory-related partialized cross power difference (middle of FIG. 4), age-related significance was identified in the three aforementioned frequency ranges. All SYMP power changed significantly from control (Wilcoxon paired rank test).

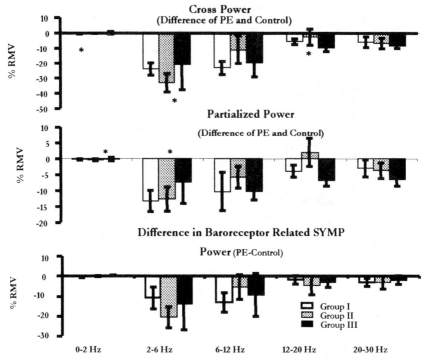

**FIGURE 4. Top:** Difference of AoP-triggered cross-power totals (CS and SPL activity) per frequency band. (Difference is subtraction of AoP-triggered control totals [CS and SPL activity] from PE protocol values). **Middle:** Difference of AoP-triggered partialized cross-power totals (CS and SPL activity) per frequency band. **Bottom:** Difference of AoP-triggered average baroreceptor-related cross-power totals (CS and SPL activity) per frequency band. See FIGURE 3 for further explanations.

With the elevation of AoP, coherence (left graphs of FIG. 5) showed significant age-related differences in most frequency bands. Age-related coherence was greatest in Group III piglets for all frequency bands. Respiratory-related partialized coherence showed age-related significance in three frequency bands: the 0–2 Hz band, the 2–6 Hz band, and the 12–20 Hz band. Group II respiratory-related SYMP activity had the greatest coherence in frequencies <12 Hz. Group I (1–10-day-old) piglets had the highest respiratory-related coherence for frequencies >12 Hz. Group II piglets showed increases in respiratory-related coherence differences (middle right of FIG. 5), while Group III piglets showed decreases. Examination of the respiratory-related SYMP cross power to AoP elevation suggested that Group II was the most resistant to hypertensive apnea[1,14] that also frequently occurred. In baroreceptor-related coherence, age-related significance was found in three frequency bands: the 2–6 Hz band, the 6–12 Hz band, and the 12–20 Hz band. In all frequency bands of baroreceptor-related coherence, Group III piglets had the greatest coherence, thus showing that Group III piglets exhibit the tightest coupling of SYMP activity to

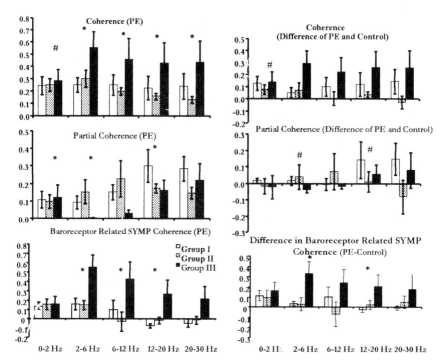

**FIGURE 5. Left top:** AoP-triggered average coherence totals (CS and SPL activity) per frequency band for the three age groups after elevation of AoP by pharmacological means (PE, 20 μg/kg i.v. bolus). **Left middle:** AoP-triggered partialized average coherence totals (CS and SPL activity) per frequency band. **Left bottom:** AoP-triggered average baroreceptor-related coherence totals (CS and SPL activity) per frequency band. **Right top:** Difference of AoP-triggered coherence totals (CS and SPL activity) per frequency band. (Difference is subtraction of AoP-triggered control totals [CS and SPL activity] from PE protocol values). **Right middle:** Difference of AoP-triggered partialized coherence totals (respiratory-related CS and SPL activity) per frequency band. **Right bottom:** Difference of AoP-triggered average baroreceptor-related coherence totals (CS and SPL activity) per frequency band. See FIGURE 3 for further explanations.

baroreceptor activity. To further exemplify this point, the differences in coherence between PE and control (right bottom of FIG. 5) showed a significant age-related increase in baroreceptor-related coherence for the 2–6 Hz and 12–20 Hz frequency bands. These results suggest that central respiratory modulation may fluctuate in importance while baroreceptor inputs increase with age.

The average total baroreceptor-related cross power for each age group is shown in FIGURE 6. Within each age group, average total baroreceptor-related cross power was significantly different with respect to either increases in AoP (PE) or decreases in AoP (NP) [FIG. 6, top]. The bottom graph of FIGURE 6 reveals that the influence of baroreceptor inputs was significantly greater during I than E for each age group, regardless of experimental manipulation.

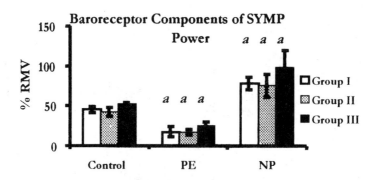

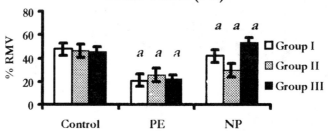

**FIGURE 6.** Average baroreceptor-related cross-power totals for all age groups during Control, PE, and NP protocols. Spectras triggered from peak of systole (*top*) and (*bottom*) as difference between I totals and E totals. *a*, Denotes significant change in power from control ($p < 0.05$, Wilcoxon paired rank test).

While cross power significantly declined with an elevation in AoP (Wilcoxon paired rank test), the decline uncovered the strong respiratory influence on SYMP activity in the Group II piglets and the strong baroreceptor influence on SYMP activity in the Group III piglets.

The following two figures (FIGS. 7 and 8) present the changes in baroreceptor sensitivity (gain) depending upon AoP level and phase within the central respiratory cycle. Mean AoP is given on the *Y*-axis and baroreceptor-related SYMP power is given on the *X*-axis. The steeper the slope, the less sensitive the baroreflex. FIGURE 7 shows the baroreceptor sensitivity of SYMP activity triggered from the peak of systole. With an elevation in AoP (left), Group III animals were the most sensitive to changes in mean AoP, while Group II piglets were the least sensitive. With a depression in mean AoP (FIG. 7, right), Group II piglets were the most sensitive to changes in mean AoP, while animals 1–10 days old were the least sensitive. FIGURE 8 shows the baroreceptor sensitivity of SYMP activity triggered during inspiration. The baroreflex was the most sensitive in Group III animals (>21 days of age). For increased mean AoP, Group I piglets (<10 days old) were the least sensitive to AoP changes. For decreased mean AoP, Group II piglets (11–20 days old) were the least

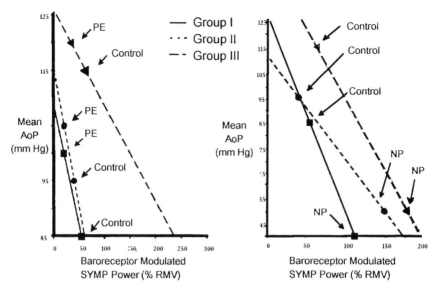

**FIGURE 7.** Baroreceptor sensitivity of the SYMP system calculated from baroreceptor-related cross-power spectra (CS and SPL activity) triggered from peak systole. Slope of lines (sensitivity) were derived by dividing change of SYMP power by change in mean AoP. **Left:** Difference from PE and control. **Right:** Difference from NP and control. NOTE: The steeper the slope, the less sensitive the baroreceptor sensitivity.

sensitive to AoP changes. The baroreflex in Group III piglets (triggered from expiration, not shown) was the most sensitive during elevation in mean AoP. The baroreflex in Group III piglets were least sensitive during a decline in mean AoP.

Respiratory phase had a great influence on the sensitivity of the baroreflex. With little cross power developed during E (generally 20–25% of that during I), a large change in AoP must occur before a significant change in baroreceptor-related SYMP cross power will occur. During I, when SYMP activity is greatest, age factors become relevant, that is, the older the animal, the more sensitive the piglet is to changes in mean AoP.

## DISCUSSION

We examined baroreceptor modulation of SYMP outflows from two levels of the spinal cord to determine whether such modulation differed with development. Spectral analyses of preganglionic SYMP activity in response to alterations in baroreceptor afferent inputs permitted examination of sensitivity changes as a function of age uncomplicated by maturational changes at the effector, for example, neuromuscular cleft, transmitter release, and neuroeffector coupling. Our results revealed that baroreceptor sensitivity, as measured by change in mean AoP versus change in SYMP power, varied both as a function of postnatal age and phase of the central respiratory cycle. Two major factors revealed by our analyses were (1) the lack of a

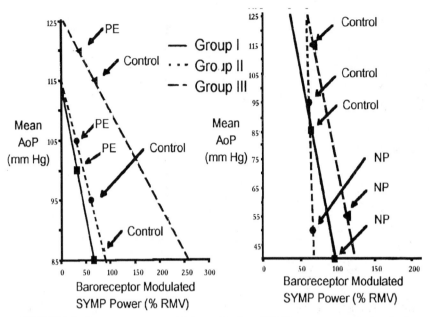

**FIGURE 8.** Baroreceptor sensitivity of the SYMP system calculated from baroreceptor-related cross-power spectra (CS and SPL activity) triggered from I. The slope of the lines (sensitivity) was derived from the changes in SYMP power and changes in mean AoP. **Left:** Difference from PE and control. **Right:** Difference from NP and control.

monotonic relationship of SYMP activity with postnatal age, that is, the circa 2-week-olds (Group II) tended to show responses either smaller than the youngest group or larger than the oldest, and (2) the importance of location within the central respiratory cycle. Nevertheless, the effects of baroreceptor inputs were greatest in the most mature animals.

Since we also wanted to document the commonality between SYMP outflows from different spinal levels, analytic techniques of cross power and coherence were essential for our examination of postnatal changes in SYMP activity. Both cross-power spectral density and coherence analyses were used to define the commonality of two signals. If two signals have similar peaks at a given frequency in their autospectra, then an equivalent peak in the cross power would be prominent at that given frequency. Coherence is a probability function that determines if two signals at a given frequency are derived from the same or similar source(s), that is, it reveals the degree of linear dependence between two signals. Partialized cross power and partialized coherence were particularly useful for removal of a signal noninvasively, for example, AoP (baroreceptor-related components), from two SYMP preganglionic nerves. Such removal (mathematically or surgically) unmasked signals that were minimized by the influence of a dominant input; in this case, baroreceptor afferent inputs. Subtracting the partialized spectra from the full spectra derived baroreceptor-related spectra.

Total cross power showed that a significant increase in amplitude at the cardiac frequency (2–6 Hz) occurred in the circa 2-week-old group (FIG. 4, top left). Furthermore, the baroreceptor-related cross power was not totally modulated by respiratory phase in this age group (FIG. 5, bottom left). In the oldest piglets, baroreceptor-related cross power showed a small decrease from that of the circa 2-week-old group; in addition, the baroreceptor-related cross power showed respiratory phase modulation.[10] On the other hand, there was no difference in baroreceptor-related coherence with respect to respiratory phase (FIG. 5, bottom right).

While there were no respiratory-related cross power differences in AoP-triggered spectra, a trend toward greater power in the circa 2-week-old group between the respiratory phases (FIGS. 4 and 5, left, middle) was observed. On the other hand, respiratory-related coherence (I- and E-triggered) was significantly age-related (FIG. 4, right, middle). A disproportionate increase in respiratory-related coherence occurred in the circa 2-week-old group, suggesting SYMP rhythm-generating networks were strongly influenced by central respiratory inputs at this age. The oldest group had the greatest baroreceptor-related cross power and coherence (FIG. 8), suggesting that SYMP activity becomes entrained to baroreceptor inputs later during postnatal development than central respiratory inputs. These results, especially with respect to the 2-week-old group, support our earlier studies of activation of neurons in NTS at this age.[18]

When AoP was pharmacologically increased (PE, FIG. 6), respiratory modulation of SYMP activity was shown to be significantly age-related (FIG. 6, left middle). Again the circa 2-week-old group had the greatest respiratory-related cross power. Furthermore, with comparisons of differences in cross power between PE and control (Fig. 6, right, top and middle) several frequency bands showed significant age-related cross power differences for both overall power and respiratory-related cross power. When AoP was pharmacologically decreased (FIG. 8, NP), respiratory-related SYMP activity was again greatest in the circa 2-week-old piglets, while the greatest baroreceptor modulation was again seen in the oldest group. Examination of the respiratory-related SYMP cross power to AoP elevation (FIG. 6, middle) suggested that the circa 2-week-old group was the most resistant to hypertensive apnea[1,14] that also frequently occurred.

Age-related significance of coherence for all frequency bands occurred with AoP elevation (FIG. 7, left top). Respiratory-related SYMP coherence (FIG. 7, left middle) was significantly age-related within several frequency bands, the greatest coherence occurring in the circa 2-week-old group at frequencies up to, and including, the circa 10 Hz band. At higher frequencies, the 1-week-old group had the greatest coherence while the older groups were more chaotic. The baroreceptor-related SYMP coherence (FIG. 7, left bottom) continued to be both significantly age-related and greatest in the oldest group. Examination of the frequency bands (FIG. 7, right bottom) showed significant increases in the oldest group's baroreceptor-related coherence; no change occurred in the younger groups. These results suggest that central respiratory modulation may fluctuate in importance while baroreceptor inputs increase with age.

The results presented support the view that these age groups in piglets are the significant ages for investigation of postnatal maturation of SYMP development. We have examined the effector responses, for example, regional blood flows, to alterations in AoP as well as to hypoxia, and our results frequently showed that the circa 2-week-old group did not fit into a monotonic pattern of postnatal maturation.[1,3] The question, therefore, that needed to be answered was, Is this age difference also observed when looking, not at the effector responses, but rather at the outflow of the regulatory system, that is, SYMP preganglionic activity?

Examination of the baroreceptor gain (mean AoP vs. baroreceptor-related SYMP cross power) revealed complexities with respect to age, sensitivity, and location within the respiratory cycle (FIGS. 7 and 8). In summary, the oldest group of piglets was the most sensitive to alterations in AoP, especially during I. For falls in AoP, elicited by NP, sensitivity was greatest in the circa 2-week-olds during E. Thus, baroreceptor gain was effected not just by age, but also by time of measurement with respect to the respiratory phases. This may explain the controversy as to whether baroreceptor sensitivity (gain) increases or decreases with maturation. Because the I-phase shortens with age, more baroreceptor measurements would tend to occur during E (a time of decreased overall power) in the older animals, resulting in the possibly erroneous result of an age-related decrease in gain.[19] Thus, respiratory modulation of SYMP activity should be considered when examining either directional or age-related changes in baroreceptor function.

Baroreceptor manipulation resulted in little change in coherence between SYMP outflows from different spinal levels. Since changes in AoP are common in the neonate, an infant who has an immature response (for age) due to an imbalance in autonomic outflow—for example, to the heart, or within the brainstem integrating system—may be susceptible to a catastrophic outcome.[15,20,21] It has been documented that many SIDS victims are found dead after being laid down to sleep. Arousals from sleep elevate blood pressure,[22–24] thus putting a susceptible infant at risk.

We have postulated that failure in SYMP and/or parasympathetic outflow, for example, loss of coherence between SYMP outflows to the vasculature and the heart, could lead to sudden death. Our results to date with experimental imbalance of autonomic innervation of the heart have shown decreased heart rate variability with denervation of one or more cardiac autonomic nerves.[25] In addition, electrocardiographic pauses seem to occur spontaneously following chronic denervation of the right vagus[26] or either of the major cardiac SYMP nerves.[27] Baroreceptor stimulation (pharmacologically induced with PE) elicited ventricular bigemini in autonomically imbalanced hearts.[28–30] These results, combined with the present results, suggest that failure of normal postnatal autonomic nervous system development might be important in the etiology of SIDS.

## ACKNOWLEDGMENTS

This work was supported by USPHS grants from NIH: HL-20864 and HD-28931. The authors acknowledge the invaluable assistance of Nancy M. Buckley, M.D., in the preparation of this manuscript.

Most of the material in this paper was included in a thesis submitted by B.W.H. in partial fulfillment of the requirements for the Ph.D. degree at State University of New York, Downstate Medical Center, Brooklyn, New York.

# REFERENCES

1. GOOTMAN, P.M. 1991. Developmental aspects of reflex control of the circulation. *In* Reflex Control of the Circulation. J.P. Gilmore and I.H. Zucker, Eds.: 965–1027. CRC Press. Boca Raton, FL.
2. SICA, A.L., B.W. HUNDLEY, D.A. RUGGIERO & P.M. GOOTMAN. 2000. The sympathetic nervous system of the developing mammal. *In* Respiratory-Circulatory Interactions in Health and Disease. S.M.S. Scharf, S.M. Pinsky and M.P. Magder, Eds.: 145–182. Marcel Dekker. New York.
3. GOOTMAN, P.M. 1986. Development of central autonomic regulation of cardiovascular function. *In* Developmental Neurobiology of the Autonomic Nervous System. P.M. Gootman, Ed.: 279–325. Humana Press. Clifton, NJ.
4. ADRIAN, E.D., D.W. BRONK & G. PHILLIPS. 1932. Discharges in mammalian sympathetic nerves. J. Physiol. **74:** 115–133.
5. COHEN, M.I. & P.M. GOOTMAN. 1969. Spontaneous and evoked oscillations in respiratory and sympathetic discharge. Brain Res. **16:** 265–268.
6. COHEN, M.I. & P.M. GOOTMAN. 1970. Periodicities in efferent discharge of splanchnic nerve of the cat. Am. J. Physiol. **218:** 1092–1101.
7. GOOTMAN, P.M. & M.I. COHEN. 1971. Evoked potentials produced by electrical stimulation of medullary vasomotor regions. Exp. Brain Res. **13:** 1–14.
8. GOOTMAN, P.M. & M.I. COHEN. 1973. Periodic modulation (cardiac and respiratory) of spontaneous and evoked sympathetic discharge. Acta Physiol. Pol. **24:** 99–109
9. GOOTMAN, P.M., H.L. COHEN, S.M. DiRUSSO, *et al.* 1984. Characteristics of spontaneous efferent splanchnic discharge in neonatal swine. *In* Catecholamines: Part A: Basic and Peripheral Mechanisms. E. Usdin, A. Dahlstrom, J. Engel and A. Carlsson, Eds.: 369–374. Alan R. Liss. New York.
10. GOOTMAN, P.M., M.R. GANDHI, A.M. STEELE, *et al.* 1991. Respiratory modulation of sympathetic activity in neonatal swine. Am. J. Physiol. **261:** R1147–R1154.
11. GOOTMAN, P.M., B.W. HUNDLEY & A.L. SICA. 1996. The presence of coherence in sympathetic and phrenic activities in a developing mammal. Acta Neurobiol. Exp. **56:** 137–145.
12. GOOTMAN, P.M., A.L., SICA, A.M. STEELE, *et al.* 1991. Interrelationships between the respiratory and sympathetic rhythm generating systems in neonates as revealed by alterations in afferent inputs. *In* Cardiorespiratory and Motor Coordination. H.-P. Koepchen and T. Huopaniemi, Eds.: 26–32. Springer-Verlag. Berlin, Germany.
13. GOOTMAN, P.M., B.W. HUNDLEY, A.L. SICA & N. GOOTMAN.1995. Coherence of efferent sympathetic activity and phrenic discharge in a neonatal animal: relation to SIDS. *In* Sudden Infant Death Syndrome. New Trends in the Nineties. T.O. Rognum, Ed.: 235–241. Scandinavian University Press. Stockholm.
14. GOOTMAN, P.M., A.L. SICA, A.M. STEELE, *et al.* 1988. Spontaneous efferent preganglionic sympathetic (SYMP) activity in neonatal swine. *In* Progress in Catecholamine Research, Part A: Basic Aspects and Peripheral Mechanisms. A. Dahlstrom, R.H. Belmaker and M. Sandler, Eds.: 449–453. Alan R. Liss. New York.
15. GOOTMAN, P.M., N. GOOTMAN & A.L. SICA. 1996. A neuro-cardiac theory for sudden infant death syndrome: role of the autonomic nervous system. J. SIDS & Infant Mortality **1:** 169–182.
16. LEVIN, A.B. 1966. A simple test of cardiac function based upon the heart rate changes induced by the Valsalva maneuver. Am. J. Cardiol. **18:** 90–99.
17. JENKINS, G.M. & D.G. WATTS. 1998. Spectral Analysis and Its Applications. Holden-Day. Oakland, CA.
18. SICA, A.L., P.M. GOOTMAN & D.A. RUGGIERO. 1999. $CO_2$-induced expression of *c-fos* in the nucleus of the solitary tract and the area postrema of developing swine. Brain Res. **837:** 106–116.
19. SEGAR, J.L. 1997. Ontogeny of the arterial and cardiopulmonary baroreflex during fetal and postnatal life. Am. J. Physiol. **273:** R457–R471.
20. HARPER, R.M. & R. BANDLER. 1998. Finding the failure mechanism in sudden infant death syndrome. Nature Med. **4:** 157–158.

21. MENY, R.G., J.G. CARROLL, M.T. CARBONE & D.H. KELLY. 1994. Cardiorespiratory recordings from infants dying suddenly and unexpectedly at home. Pediatrics **93:** 44–49.
22. HORNER, R.L. 1956. Autonomic consequences of arousal from sleep-mechanisms and implications. Sleep **19:** S193–S195.
23. HORNER, R.L. D. BROOKS, L.F. KOZAR, *et al.* 1995. Immediate effects of arousal from sleep on cardiac autonomic outflow in the absence of breathing in dogs. J. Appl. Physiol. **79:** 151–162.
24. CHONG, A., N. MURPHY & T. MATTHEWS. 2000. Effect of prone sleeping on circulatory control in infants. Arch. Dis. Child. **82:** 253–256.
25. LIPSITZ, L.A, S.M. PINCUS, R.J. MORIN, *et al.* 1997. Preliminary evidence for the evolution in complexity of heart rate dynamics during autonomic maturation in neonatal swine. J. Auton. Nerv. Syst. **65:** 1–9.
26. KHAN, M.S., N. ZHAO, A.L. SICA, *et al.* 2001. Changes in R-R and Q-T interval following cardiac vagotomy in neonatal swine. Exp. Biol. Med. **226:** 32–36.
27. ZHAO, N., M. KHAN, S. INGENITO, *et al.* 2001. Electrocardiographic changes during postnatal development in conscious swine with cardiac autonomic imbalance. Auton. Neurosci. **88:** 167–174.
28. ZHAO, N., M.S. KHAN, S. INGENITO, *et al.* 1998. Effects of chronic right or left stellectomy on electrocardiographic responses to baroreceptor stimulation in developing swine [abstract]. Pediatr. Res. **43:** 28A.
29. ZHAO, N., A.L. SICA, M.S. KHAN, *et al.* 1998. Baroreceptor stimulation in chronic, cardiac sympathetic-denervated developing swine [abstract]. Neurosci. Abstr. **24:** 623.
30. KHAN, M.S., N. ZHAO, S. INGENITO, *et al.* 1999. Chronic cardiac vagotomy or stellectomy on ECG responses to baroreceptor stimulation in neonatal swine [abstract]. FASEB J. **13:** A453.

# The Regulation of Sympathetic Outflow in Heart Failure

## The Roles of Angiotensin II, Nitric Oxide, and Exercise Training

IRVING H. ZUCKER, WEI WANG, RAINER U. PLIQUETT, JUN-LI LIU, AND KAUSHIK P. PATEL

*Department of Physiology and Biophysics, University of Nebraska Medical Center, Omaha, Nebraska 68198-4575, USA*

ABSTRACT: Sympatho-excitation is a hallmark of the chronic heart failure (CHF) state. It has long been assumed that this sympatho-excitation is mediated by a reduction in sensory input from cardiopulmonary and arterial baroreceptors. However, recent data suggest that these reflexes may only be important in the initiation of the sympatho-excitatory state and may not be necessary for the sustained increase in sympathetic nerve activity (SNA) in CHF. Two humoral factors that can influence SNA are nitric oxide (NO) and angiotensin II (AngII). Animals with CHF exhibit a downregulation in central gene expression for the neuronal isoform of nitric oxide synthase (nNOS). In addition, blockade of AngII receptors in combination with NO donation reduces SNA in animals with CHF, while NO donation alone has no effect on SNA. Chronic exercise training (EX) reduces both plasma AngII and SNA in rabbits with CHF while improving baroreflex function. Blockade of $AT_1$ receptors enhances baroreflex function in non-EX CHF rabbits, but has little effect in EX CHF rabbits. These data suggest that the sympatho-excitatory state that is typical of CHF is, in part, due to changes in AngII and NO. Depressed baroreflex function and the elevated SNA can be improved by EX in animals with CHF.

KEYWORDS: Sympatho-excitation; Chronic heart failure; Sympathetic nerve activity; Angiotensin II; Nitric oxide; Exercise training

## INTRODUCTION

Clinical studies have clearly shown an activation of the sympathetic nervous system in the chronic heart failure (CHF) state. The degree of sympatho-excitation is prognostic for survival in the CHF state.[1,2] The regulation of sympathetic outflow in the setting of CHF is a complex issue that has been of interest to both clinicians and basic scientists for some time. It has become increasingly apparent that the concept of a reduction in the sensitivity of sympatho-inhibitory reflexes does not completely explain the chronic elevation in sympathetic outflow in this disease state.[3,4] It has

Address for correspondence: Irving H. Zucker, Ph.D., Department of Physiology and Biophysics, University of Nebraska Medical Center, 984575 Nebraska Medical Center, Omaha, NE 68198-4575. Voice: 402-559-7161; fax: 402-559-4438.

izucker@unmc.edu

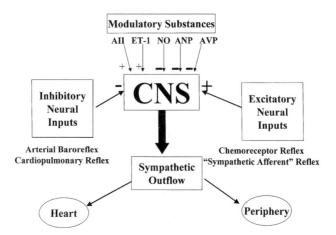

**FIGURE 1.** A schematic overview of the neurohumoral regulation of sympathetic outflow. Important inhibitory and excitatory cardiovascular reflexes regulate sympathetic outflow to the heart and peripheral circulation on a moment-to-moment basis. However, a variety of humoral factors can modulate sympathetic outflow and "fine-tune" the system. Many of these humoral agents are abnormal-regulated in the heart failure state.

long been known that even chronic sino-aortic denervation does not increase sympathetic outflow or arterial pressure.[5] Investigators have therefore searched for alternative explanations to account for the sympatho-excitation in CHF.

A schematic of the possible control mechanisms that may be important in CHF is depicted in FIGURE 1. In addition to the classical negative feedback of arterial and cardiopulmonary baroreflexes, there are both positive-feedback, sympatho-excitatory reflexes and humoral regulatory mechanisms that modulate sympathetic outflow centrally. The most likely candidates for this modulation are angiotensin II (AngII) and endothelin-1 (ET-1), both of which are sympatho-excitatory, and vasopressin, atrial natriuretic peptide, and nitric oxide (NO), which are sympatho-inhibitory.

This laboratory has concentrated on several aspects of sympathetic regulation in the CHF state. In this review, we summarize the role of NO, AngII, and ET-1 in the sympatho-excitation of CHF. In addition, we describe an important role for exercise training (EX) in the modulation of these control systems in experimental CHF.

## THE ROLE FOR ANGIOTENSIN II

AngII modulates sympathetic function at several loci. These include classical neurotransmitter function in several areas of the central nervous system, enhancement of ganglionic transmission, facilitation of norepinephrine release presynaptically, and modulation of the postjunctional effects of norepinephrine.[6] In recent studies from this and other laboratories, it has been shown that blockade of the AngII type-1 receptors ($AT_1$) reduces sympathetic tone and enhances arterial baroreflex function.[7,8] In rabbits with pacing-induced CHF, administration of losartan intra-

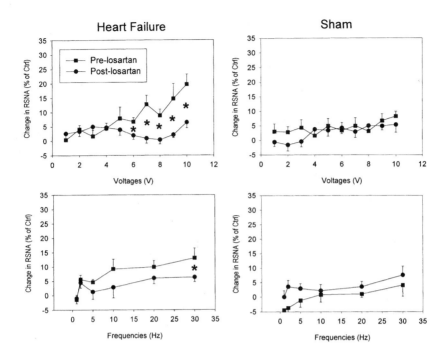

**FIGURE 2.** Responses of RSNA to cardiac "sympathetic afferent" stimulation before and after intracerebroventricular injection of losartan (0.125 mg/kg) in heart failure **(left)** and sham dogs **(right)**. *$p < 0.05$ compared to pre-losartan. (Reproduced from Ma *et al.*,[9] with permission.)

venously normalized arterial baroreflex control of both heart rate and renal sympathetic nerve activity (RSNA)[7]. In similar studies by DiBona *et al.*,[8] it was shown that central administration of losartan reduced RSNA and improved baroreflex function in rats with chronic myocardial infarction–induced CHF.

In recent experiments carried out in dogs with pacing-induced CHF, Ma *et al.*[9] showed that both central and peripheral administration of losartan normalized the enhanced cardiac "sympathetic afferent" reflex (FIG. 2). The fact that AngII may be causal in the sympatho-excitatory process in CHF is supported by clinical studies using angiotensin-converting enzyme (ACE) inhibitors that have shown a decrease in plasma norepinephrine[10] and improvement in arterial baroreflex function in the CHF state.[11,12] Furthermore, administration of enalapril to animals with CHF increased myocardial $\beta$-adrenoreceptor density,[13] suggesting a lower interstitial norepinephrine concentration. In the latter studies, it is not possible to dissociate clinical improvement in the CHF state from direct effects of AngII reduction. However, in recent studies from this laboratory, we showed that exercise training (EX) of rabbits with CHF resulted in a decrease in plasma AngII and resting RSNA in spite of little improvement in several parameters of cardiac function.[14] In addition, Wang and Ma have recently reported a significant increase in the cerebrospinal fluid concentration of AngII in dogs with pacing-induced heart failure.[15]

It seems clear from the above discussion and from a wealth of clinical and animal data that blockade of AngII generation or $AT_1$ receptors plays a role in the effective management of patients with CHF and that modulation of sympathetic tone may be one of the mechanisms involved in clinical improvement.[16–18]

## THE ROLE OF ENDOTHELIN-1

Endothelin-1 (ET-1) is a 21-amino-acid peptide originally isolated from endothelial cells,[19] but now known to be elaborated by many tissues and to be involved in the pathophysiology of a variety of disease states.[20] While this peptide possesses extremely potent vasoconstrictor effects, it also has been shown to exert growth and neural effects.[21] ET-1 has been shown to be elevated both in patients with CHF and in animal models of CHF.[22–25] Only recently has ET-1 been implicated as a sympatho-excitatory substance.[26] In spontaneously hypertensive, stroke-prone rats, Nakamura et al.[27] demonstrated that central administration of the $ET_A$ receptor antagonist BQ-123 reduced RSNA. In a recent study by Moe et al.,[28] carried out in dogs with pacing-induced CHF, an apparent sympatho-inhibitory effect was observed after $ET_A$ blockade. In a recent study from this laboratory, we observed similar effects following chronic administration of the $ET_A$ receptor antagonist PD156707.[29] As can be seen in FIGURE 3, plasma norepinephrine increased to extremely high levels in placebo-treated dogs with CHF. However, in dogs given PD156707, plasma norepinephrine increased during the first week of pacing and then leveled off so that the difference between this group and the placebo group reached significance after 1 week of treatment. This sympatho-inhibitory effect occurred despite little improvement in myocardial function. It was not clear from this study if the sympatho-inhibition in response to $ET_A$ receptor blockade may have been due to activation of $ET_B$ receptors by the elevated ET-1 levels seen in the $ET_A$ receptor–blocked dogs. Since $ET_B$ receptor activation can increase NO synthesis,[30,31] it is possible that the effect of $ET_A$ blockade is mediated by the sympatho-inhibitory effects of NO (discussed below). However, a proposed beneficial action arising from $ET_B$ receptor stimulation would be of minor significance since the nonspecific receptor antagonist L-754142 also induced a reduction in RSNA.[32] On the other hand, several studies have shown significant improvement in myocardial function in experimental and human CHF.[33–35] Therefore, it is still not completely clear if the decrease in sympathetic outflow is mediated by a direct effect of endothelin blockade on central mechanisms or due to improvement in the CHF state.[20]

## THE ROLE OF NITRIC OXIDE

Since the discovery of NO gas as the endothelial-dependent relaxing factor,[36] this substance has been shown to participate in diverse biological actions that may be important in the regulation of many organ systems. NO has been implicated as a neuromodulatory substance that has effects on a variety of central pathways including the regulation of sympathetic tone.[37] The role played by central NO in the modulation of sympathetic outflow has just begun to be investigated. In recent studies from our laboratories, it has been shown that the neuronal isoform of nitric oxide synthase

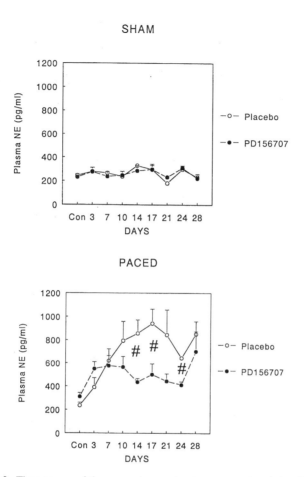

**FIGURE 3.** Time course of the mean changes in plasma norepinephrine (NE) level in (**left**) sham-operated, nonpaced dogs and (**right**) paced dogs given either placebo or PD156707. A significantly greater increase in plasma NE level was observed in the paced dogs given placebo versus PD156707. *Significant from the control period. #Significant from placebo. (Reproduced from McConnell *et al.*,[29] with permission.)

(nNOS) is substantially reduced in animals with experimental CHF.[38,39] Since NO is sympatho-inhibitory in the hypothalamus and medulla,[40–42] a decrease in the synthesis of NO may lead to chronic increases in sympathetic outflow in the CHF state. In an attempt to determine if blockade of the NO system increases RSNA, we administered L-nitro-arginine methyl ester (L-NAME) to conscious, chronically instrumented normal rabbits.[43] We were surprised that this substance did not result in an increase in resting RSNA, despite the fact that we normalized the increase in arterial pressure with a concomitant infusion of hydralazine. Several other studies had reported increases in sympathetic outflow when NO synthesis was blocked either systemically or centrally.[44–46] However, a human study reported by Hansen and coworkers[47] showed that short-term administration of L-nitro-monomcthyl arginine

# 436 ANNALS NEW YORK ACADEMY OF SCIENCES

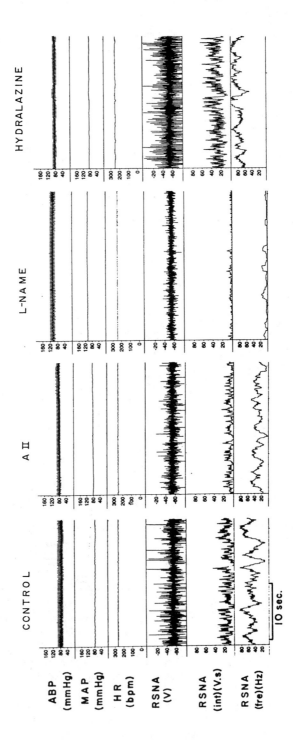

**FIGURE 4.** An original recording from one rabbit in the control state, during the infusion of angiotensin II (AII), after the infusion of AII plus L-NAME, and during hydralazine infusion. All increased MAP and decreased RSNA. Addition of L-NAME caused a further increase in MAP and almost complete abolition of RSNA. When MAP was returned to control by hydralazine, RSNA increased to a level markedly higher than control. ABP, pulsatile arterial pressure; int, integrated; fre, frequency. (Reproduced from McConnell *et al.*,[43] with permission.)

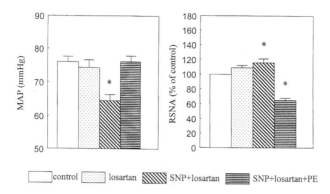

**FIGURE 5.** Mean data of arterial pressure and RSNA from CHF rabbits given SNP and losartan followed by normalization of arterial pressure with PE. *Significantly different from control. (Reproduced from Liu and Zucker,[50] with permission.)

did not increase muscle sympathetic nerve activity (MSNA). In fact, MSNA decreased as arterial pressure rose. This suggested that the change in MSNA followed a baroreflex pattern. A subsequent study by this group has shown that more prolonged administration of an NOS inhibitor does, indeed, result in sympatho-excitation,[48] indirectly establishing the concept of NO as a sympatho-inhibitory substance in humans.

While administration of L-NAME to conscious rabbits resulted in a decrease in RSNA as arterial pressure rose[43] (i.e., a baroreflex function), we found that, if we infused a low dose of AngII prior to administration of L-NAME, RSNA was increased significantly above baseline levels when arterial pressure was normalized (FIG. 4). This suggests that NO and AngII interact in such a way as to be mutually inhibitory[49] with regard to sympathetic outflow: That is, AngII acts as a sympatho-excitatory substance that potentiates the effects of NO blockade in normal animals. If this is true, we would expect AngII blockade combined with replacement of a source of NO in animals with CHF to result in a sympatho-inhibition. Therefore, in a subsequent study,[50] we infused sodium nitroprusside (SNP) into conscious rabbits with CHF in the presence and absence of AngII receptor blockade with losartan. As shown in FIGURE 5, the combination of AngII receptor blockade and infusion of low-dose SNP resulted in a significant suppression in RSNA in rabbits with CHF when arterial pressure was normalized. This did not occur in normal rabbits. These data strongly suggest that the reduction in NO synthesis in animals with CHF amplifies the sympatho-excitatory effects of AngII. These data are consistent with the observation described above of an increase in central AngII in the CHF state, thus favoring a higher sympathetic tone.

## THE ROLE OF EXERCISE TRAINING

The cardiovascular and neural adjustments to chronic EX represent a complex integrative and adaptive response. Patients with CHF have limited exercise capacity,

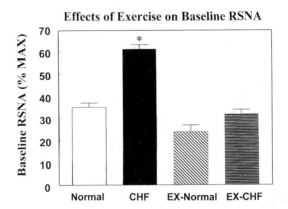

**FIGURE 6.** Baseline RSNA expressed as a percent of maximum nerve activity in each group of rabbits. Animals with CHF had significantly higher RSNA compared with normal (EX Normal) rabbits or EX CHF rabbits; $*p < 0.01$. (Reproduced from Liu et al.,[14] with permission.)

which is, in part, due to a reduced cardiac output, but may also be due to peripheral vasoconstriction and muscle wasting induced by alterations in the neurohumoral environment in this disease state.[51] It has been shown that long-term regular EX of patients with CHF increases the quality of life as well as survival.[52,53] EX also has been shown to upregulate eNOS and endothelial-dependent responses in the coronary circulation of dogs with CHF.[54–56] Finally, EX lowers arterial pressure in hypertensives[57–59] most likely through an NO-dependent mechanism. It therefore seemed reasonable to investigate the role of EX on RSNA and baroreflex function in the CHF state.

Rabbits with pacing-induced CHF underwent treadmill EX for a period of approximately 1 month while they developed CHF.[14] Four groups of animals were examined: a normal group that was not EX, a normal group that was EX trained, a CHF non-EX group, and a CHF EX group. Resting RSNA was evaluated in the conscious state following 3–4 weeks of EX in each group. As can be seen in FIGURE 6, resting RSNA was significantly higher in the CHF non-EX group. EX in the CHF group reduced RSNA to levels not different from the normal group. EX of normal rabbits had little effect on RSNA. In addition, FIGURE 7 shows that arterial baroreflex control of both heart rate and RSNA was significantly enhanced in EX CHF animals. The mechanism for the EX effect on RSNA is not precisely known. However, this study also found a decrease in circulating AngII in EX rabbits with CHF. If this is reflected in the central nervous system, it is conceivable that a decrease in AngII would reduce RSNA.

On the other hand, modulation of the NO system in the peripheral circulation and in the central nervous system during EX may also contribute to the sympatho-inhibition in CHF animals. In a recent study, we reported that EX in rabbits with CHF prevented the downregulation of NADPH diaphorase–positive neurons in the PVN.[60] Because it has been shown that NO has its inhibitory effect on RSNA via the release of the inhibitory neurotransmitter GABA,[41] it is conceivable that one mech-

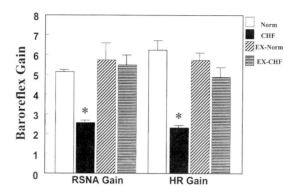

**FIGURE 7.** The mean data taken from the baroreflex curves for the regulation of heart rate and RSNA in EX and non-EX normal and CHF rabbits. (Data taken from Liu *et al.*[14])

anism by which EX reduces sympathetic outflow is via an NO-dependent GABA-ergic pathway in synergy with a reduction in AngII.

## SUMMARY

In this review, we have tried to promote the idea that the regulation of sympathetic outflow in the CHF state is regulated by neurohumoral mechanisms in addition to a decrease in the sensitivity of the traditional negative-feedback reflexes (the arterial baroreflex and cardiopulmonary reflexes of vagal origin). It is becoming increasingly clear that substances that are elevated in the CHF state also participate in the chronic sympatho-excitation.

AngII and ET-1 are sympatho-excitatory substances that have been shown to be elevated in both animals and humans with CHF. Because these two potent vaso-constrictor agents also have autonomic effects, they should be considered a primary target for CHF therapy. Indeed, ACE inhibitors and $AT_1$ receptor antagonists have been widely used in the medical management of patients with CHF. ET-1 antagonists are currently undergoing clinical trials and will most likely be added to the armamentarium of drugs used in the treatment of CHF.

Data are now being accrued that point to reduced NO as a maladaptive mechanism in the CHF state. Certainly, the use of NO donors and gene therapy for the enhancement of the expression of nNOS and eNOS may be beneficial in CHF. In the central nervous system, these enzymes may be important regulators of sympathetic outflow in combination with changes in central AngII and perhaps ET-1.

Exercise training is rapidly becoming an important therapeutic tool for the rehabilitation of CHF patients. An overview of the interaction between the AngII and NO systems in the central nervous system and the role of EX on sympathetic outflow is schematized in FIGURE 8. The mechanisms by which EX improves survival and enhances quality of life in CHF are not completely understood. Animal experiments have shed light on these mechanisms. EX reduces RSNA and improves arterial baroreflex function in animals with CHF. At the same time, it reduces AngII

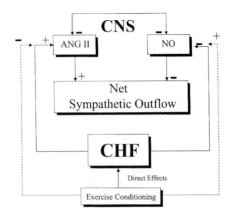

**FIGURE 8.** A summary of the roles played by AngII and NO in the control of sympathetic outflow in the CHF state. AngII and NO are mutually inhibitory within the CNS. Activation of the renin-AngII system in the brain or periphery may lead to an increase in net sympathetic outflow, while upregulation of the NO system may lead to sympatho-inhibition. While exercise conditioning may have direct beneficial effects on the heart and peripheral circulation, it may also upregulate the production of central NO by reducing AngII levels and preventing the downregulation of nNOS in the CHF state.

levels and increases the production of both eNOS in endothelial cells and nNOS in the central nervous system. Therefore, modulation of NO synthesis and the interaction of NO with AngII in the central nervous system may be an important mechanism for the regulation of sympathetic nerve activity in CHF.

## ACKNOWLEDGMENTS

We acknowledge the expert technical assistance of Johnnie F. Hackley and Pamela Curry in many of the studies described in this review. Many of the studies described herein were supported by grants from the National Institutes of Health (Nos. R37 HL-38690 and PO1 HL-62222) and a grant from the Shrike-Hlavac Trust.

## REFERENCES

1. COHN, J.N., T.B. LEVINE, M.T. OLIVARI *et al.* 1984. Plasma norepinephrine as a guide to prognosis in patients with chronic congestive heart failure. N. Engl. J. Med. **311:** 819–823.
2. FERGUSON, D.W., W.J. BERG & J.S. SANDERS. 1990. Clinical and hemodynamic correlates of sympathetic nerve activity in normal humans and patients with heart failure: evidence from direct microneurographic recordings. J. Am. Coll. Cardiol. **16:** 1125–1134.
3. BRÄNDLE, M., K. PATEL, W. WANG & I.H. ZUCKER. 1996. Hemodynamic and norepinephrine responses to pacing-induced heart failure in conscious sino-aortic denervated dogs. J. Appl. Physiol. **81:** 1855–1862.
4. LEVETT, J.M., C.C. MARINELLI, D.D. LUND *et al.* 1994. Effects of β-blockade on neurohumoral responses and neurochemical markers in pacing-induced heart failure. Am. J. Physiol. Heart Circ. Physiol. **266:** H468–H475.

5. COWLEY, A.W., JR., J.F. LIARD & A.C. GUYTON. 1973. Role of the baroreceptor reflex in daily control of arterial blood pressure and other variables in dogs. Circ. Res. **32:** 564–576.
6. REID, I.A. 1992. Interactions between ANG II, sympathetic nervous system, and baroreceptor reflexes in regulation of blood pressure. Am. J. Physiol. Endocrinol. Metab. **262:** E763–E778.
7. LIU, J-L., H. MURAKAMI, M. SANDERFORD *et al.* 1999. Ang II and baroreflex function in rabbits with CHF and lesions of the area postrema. Am. J. Physiol. Heart Circ. Physiol. **277:** H342–H350.
8. DIBONA, G.F., S.Y. JONES & V.L. BROOKS. 1995. ANG II receptor blockade and arterial baroreflex regulation of renal nerve activity in cardiac failure. Am. J. Physiol. Regul. Integr. Comp. Physiol. **269:** R1189–R1196.
9. MA, R., H.D. SCHULTZ & W. WANG. 1997. Central gain of the cardiac sympathetic afferent reflex in dogs with heart failure. Am. J. Physiol. Heart Circ. Physiol. **273:** H2664–H2671.
10. TURINI, G.A., H.R. BRUNNER, M. GRIBIC *et al.* 1979. Improvement of chronic congestive heart-failure by oral captopril. Lancet **1:** 1213–1215.
11. DIBNER-DUNLAP, M.E., M.L. SMITH, T. KINUGAWA & M.D. THAMES. 1996. Enalaprilat augments arterial and cardiopulmonary baroreflex control of sympathetic nerve activity in patients with heart failure. J. Am. Coll. Cardiol. **27:** 358–364.
12. EGAN, B.M., M.J. FLEISSNER, K. STEPNIAKOWSKI *et al.* 1993. Improved baroreflex sensitivity in elderly hypertensives on lisinopril is not explained by blood pressure reduction alone. J. Hypertens. **11:** 1113–1120.
13. FORSTER, C., G.O. NAIK & G. LAROSA. 1994. Myocardial beta-adrenoceptors in pacing-induced heart failure: regulation by enalapril? Can. J. Physiol. Pharmacol. **72:** 667–672.
14. LIU, J-L., S. IRVINE, I.A. REID *et al.* 2000. Chronic exercise reduces sympathetic nerve activity in rabbits with pacing-induced heart failure: a role for angiotensin II. Circulation **102:** 1854–1862.
15. WANG, W. & R. MA. 2000. Cardiac sympathetic afferent reflexes in heart failure. Heart Failure Rev. **5:** 57–71.
16. FRANCIS, G.S. 1989. The relationship of the sympathetic nervous system and the renin angiotensin system in congestive heart failure. Am. Heart J. **118:** 642–648.
17. HAMROFF, G., S.D. KATZ, D. MANCINI *et al.* 1999. Addition of angiotensin II receptor blockade to maximal angiotensin-converting enzyme inhibition improves exercise capacity in patients with severe congestive heart failure. Circulation **99:** 990–992.
18. HOLTZ, J. 1993. Pathophysiology of heart failure and the renin-angiotensin-system. Basic Res. Cardiol. **88**(Suppl. 1): 183–201.
19. YANAGISAWA, M., H. KURIHARA, S. KIMURA *et al.* 1988. A novel potent vasoconstrictor peptide produced by vascular endothelial cells. Nature **332:** 411–415.
20. LÜSCHER, T.F. & M. BARTON. 2000. Endothelins and endothelin receptor antagonists: therapeutic considerations for a novel class of cardiovascular drugs. Circulation **102:** 2434–2440.
21. MASAKI, T. 1993. Endothelins: homeostatic and compensatory actions in the circulatory and endocrine systems. Endocr. Rev. **14:** 256–268.
22. CLAVELL, A., A. STINGO, K. MARGULIES *et al.* 1993. Physiological significance of endothelin: its role in congestive heart failure. Circulation **87**(Suppl. 5): V45–V50.
23. KOBAYASHI, T., T. MIYAUCHI, S. SAKAI *et al.* 1999. Expression of endothelin-1 ET-A and ET-B receptors, and ECE and distribution of endothelin-1 in failing rat heart. Am. J. Physiol. Heart Circ. Physiol. **276:** H1197–H1206.
24. LOVE, M.P. & J.J.V. MCMURRAY. 1996. Endothelin in congestive heart failure. Basic Res. Cardiol. **91**(Suppl. 1): 21–29.
25. TOMODA, H. 1993. Plasma endothelin-1 in acute myocardial infarction with heart failure. Am. Heart J. **125:** 667–672.
26. DAMON, D.H. 1998. Postganglionic sympathetic neurons express endothelin. Am. J. Physiol. Regul. Integr. Comp. Physiol. **274:** R873–R878.
27. NAKAMURA, K., S. SASAKI, J. MORIGUCHI *et al.* 1999. Central effects of endothelin and its antagonists on sympathetic and cardiovascular regulation in SHR-SP. J. Cardiovasc. Pharmacol. **33:** 876 882.

28. MOE, G.W., A. ALBERNAZ, G.O. NAIK et al. 1998. Beneficial effects of long-term selective endothelin type A receptor blockade in canine experimental heart failure. Cardiovasc. Res. **39:** 571–579.
29. McCONNELL, P.I., C.E. OLSON, K.P. PATEL et al. 2000. Chronic endothelin blockade in dogs with pacing-induced heart failure: possible modulation of sympathoexcitation. J. Cardiac Failure **6:** 56–65.
30. HIRATA, Y., T. EMORI, S. EGUCHI et al. 1993. Endothelin receptor subtype B mediates synthesis of nitric oxide by cultured bovine endothelial cells. J. Clin. Invest. **91:** 1367–1373.
31. PERNOW, J. & A. MODIN. 1993. Endothelial regulation of coronary vascular tone in vitro: contribution of endothelin receptor subtypes and nitric oxide. Eur. J. Pharmacol. **243:** 281–286.
32. ZUCKER, I.H., J-L. LIU, K.G. CORNISH & Y-T. SHEN. 1999. Chronic endothelin-1 blockade reduces sympathetic nerve activity in rabbits with heart failure [abstract]. Neuroscience **25:** 1953.
33. ONISHI, K., M. OHNO, W.C. LITTLE & C.P. CHENG. 1999. Endogenous endothelin-1 depresses left ventricular systolic and diastolic performance in congestive heart failure. J. Pharmacol. Exp. Ther. **288:** 1214–1222.
34. SPINALE, F.G., D. WALKER, R. MUKHERJEE et al. 1999. Concomitant endothelin receptor subtype-A blockade during the progression of pacing-induced congestive heart failure in rabbits: beneficial effects on left ventricular and myocyte function. Circulation **95:** 1918–1929.
35. SÜTSCH, G., O. BERTEL & W. KIOWSKI. 1997. Acute and short-term effects of the nonpeptide endothelin-1 receptor antagonist bosentan in humans. Cardiovasc. Drugs Ther. **10:** 717–725.
36. PALMER, R.M., A.G. FERRIGE & S. MONCADA. 1987. Nitric oxide release accounts for the biological activity of endothelium-derived relaxing factor. Nature **327:** 524–526.
37. GARTHWAITE, J. & C.L. BOULTON. 1995. Nitric oxide signaling in the central nervous system. Annu. Rev. Physiol. **57:** 683–706.
38. PATEL, K.P., K. ZHANG, I.H. ZUCKER & T.L. KRUKOFF. 1996. Decreased gene expression of neuronal nitric oxide synthase in hypothalamus and brainstem of rats in heart failure. Brain Res. **734:** 109–115.
39. ZHANG, K., I.H. ZUCKER & K.P. PATEL. 1998. Altered number of diaphorase (NOS) positive neurons in the hypothalamus of rats with heart failure. Brain Res. **786:** 219–225.
40. MA, S., F.M. ABBOUD & R.B. FELDER. 1995. Effects of L-arginine-derived nitric oxide synthesis on neuronal activity in nucleus tractus solitarius. Am. J. Physiol. Regul. Integr. Comp. Physiol. **268:** R487–R491.
41. ZHANG, K. & K.P. PATEL. 1998. Effect of nitric oxide within the paraventricular nucleus on renal sympathetic nerve discharge: role of GABA. Am. J. Physiol. Regul. Integr. Comp. Physiol. **275:** R728–R734.
42. ZHANG, K., W.G. MAYHAN & K.P. PATEL. 1997. Nitric oxide within the paraventricular nucleus mediates changes in renal sympathetic nerve activity. Am. J. Physiol. Regul. Integr. Comp. Physiol. **273:** R864–R872.
43. LIU, J-L., H. MURAKAMI & I.H. ZUCKER. 1998. Angiotensin II–nitric oxide interaction on sympathetic outflow in conscious rabbits. Circ. Res. **82:** 496–502.
44. SAKUMA, I., H. TOGASHI, M. YOSHIOKA et al. 1992. $N^G$-Methyl-L-arginine, an inhibitor of L-arginine-derived nitric oxide synthesis, stimulates renal sympathetic nerve activity in vivo: a role for nitric oxide in the central regulation of sympathetic tone. Circ. Res. **70:** 607–611.
45. TODA, N., Y. KITAMURA & T. OKAMURA. 1993. Neural mechanism of hypertension by nitric oxide synthase inhibitor in dogs. Hypertension **21:** 3–8.
46. TOGASHI, H., I. SAKUMA, M. YOSHIOKA et al. 1992. A central nervous system action of nitric oxide in blood pressure regulation. J. Pharmacol. Exp. Ther. **262:** 343–347.
47. HANSEN, J., T.N. JACOBSEN & R.G. VICTOR. 1994. Is nitric oxide involved in the tonic inhibition of central sympathetic outflow in humans? Hypertension **24:** 439–444.
48. SANDER, M., P.G. HANSEN & R.G. VICTOR. 1995. Sympathetically mediated hypertension caused by chronic inhibition of nitric oxide. Hypertension **26:** 691–695.

49. KIRCHHEIM, H.R., A. JUST & H. EHMKE. 1998. Physiology and pathophysiology of baroreceptor function and neuro-hormonal abnormalities in heart failure. Basic Res. Cardiol. **93**(Suppl. 1): 1–2.
50. LIU, J-L. & I.H. ZUCKER. 1999. Regulation of sympathetic nerve activity in heart failure—a role for nitric oxide and angiotensin II. Circ. Res. **84**: 417–423.
51. HAMBRECHT, R., S. GIELEN, A. LINKE *et al.* 2000. Effects of exercise training on left ventricular function and peripheral resistance in patients with chronic heart failure. JAMA **283**: 3095–3101.
52. BELARDINELLI, R., D. GEORGIOU, G. CIANCI & A. PURCARO. 1999. Randomized, controlled trial of long-term moderate exercise training in chronic heart failure—effects on functional capacity, quality of life, and clinical outcome. Circulation **99**: 1173–1182.
53. COATS, A.J. 1999. Exercise training for heart failure—coming of age. Circulation **99**: 1138–1140.
54. WANG, J., M.S. WOLIN & T.H. HINTZE. 1993. Chronic exercise enhances endothelium-mediated dilation of epicardial coronary artery in conscious dogs. Circ. Res. **73**: 829–838.
55. WANG, J., G.H. YI, M. KNECHT *et al.* 1997. Physical training alters the pathogenesis of pacing-induced heart failure through endothelium-mediated mechanisms in awake dogs. Circulation **96**: 2683–2692.
56. ZHAO, G., X.P. ZHANG, X.B. XU *et al.* 1997. Short-term exercise training enhances reflex cholinergic nitric oxide–dependent coronary vasodilation in conscious dogs. Circ. Res. **80**: 868–876.
57. ARVOLA, P., X.M. WU, M. KÄHÖNEN *et al.* 1999. Exercise enhances vasorelaxation in experimental obesity associated hypertension. Cardiovasc. Res. **43**: 992–1002.
58. HAGBERG, J.M., J.J. PARK & M.D. BROWN. 2000. The role of exercise training in the treatment of hypertension: an update. Sports Med. **30**: 193–206.
59. SOMERS, V.K., J. CONWAY, J. JOHNSTON & P. SLEIGHT. 1991. Effects of endurance training on baroreflex sensitivity and blood pressure in borderline hypertension. Lancet **337**: 1363–1368.
60. ZUCKER, I.H., K.P. PATEL & J-L. LIU. 2000. Exercise training normalizes central nitric oxide synthase activity in rabbits with chronic heart failure: relation to sympathetic tone [abstract]. FASEB J. **102**: 236.

# Neurohumoral Regulation in Ischemia-Induced Heart Failure

## Role of the Forebrain

ROBERT B. FELDER, JOSEPH FRANCIS, ROBERT M. WEISS, ZHI-HUA ZHANG, SHUN-GUANG WEI, AND ALAN KIM JOHNSON

*Research Service, Department of Veterans Affairs Medical Center, and Departments of Internal Medicine and Psychology, University of Iowa, Iowa City, Iowa 52242, USA*

ABSTRACT: Congestive heart failure (CHF) is characterized by neurohumoral excitation. Increased sympathetic drive and activation of the renin-angiotensin-aldosterone system (RAAS), with vasoconstriction and volume retention, are hallmarks of the CHF syndrome. Treatment strategies have targeted the peripheral influences of these two systems, but have not addressed the central mechanisms that drive them. We monitored the development of CHF following coronary ligation in adult Sprague-Dawley rats. Left ventricular dysfunction characteristic of CHF was confirmed by echocardiography, and the CHF syndrome was validated by measurements of circulating hormones, sodium appetite, thirst, renal sodium and water retention, and renal sympathetic nerve activity (RSNA). In CHF rats, neuronal activity in the hypothalamic paraventricular nucleus (PVN), which mediates downstream effects of forebrain circumventricular organs, was increased and was inhibited by blocking components of the RAAS at the forebrain level. Forebrain (AV3V) lesions and intracarotid (forebrain directed) injections of agents (captopril, losartan, spironolactone) that block RAAS substantially attenuated the behavioral and physiological manifestations of CHF. Intravenous losartan and captopril, in doses that lower arterial pressure, increased RSNA. These findings demonstrate an important role for RAAS-activated forebrain mechanisms in CHF and suggest that the central neural mechanisms driving sympathetic nerve activity and volume retention may persist and promote the progression of CHF despite treatments directed toward the peripheral influences of RAAS.

KEYWORDS: Rat; Angiotensin; Aldosterone; Paraventricular nucleus; Anteroventral third ventricle; Baroreflex; Sympathetic nerve activity

Congestive heart failure (CHF) is the common outcome of a variety of cardiovascular diseases, including myocardial infarction, that ultimately result in left ventricular dysfunction with dilation of the left ventricle and a requirement for increased left ventricular filling to sustain adequate cardiac output. The humoral and autonomic

Address for correspondence: Robert B. Felder, M.D., Professor, Division of Cardiovascular Diseases, Department of Internal Medicine, University of Iowa College of Medicine, Iowa City, IA 52242. Voice: 319-356-3642; fax: 319-353-6343.
robert-felder@uiowa.edu

mechanisms called into play to sustain cardiac output under these conditions are the same ones that are activated by hypovolemia; the renin-angiotensin-aldosterone system (RAAS) and the sympathetic nervous system work in tandem to restore intravascular volume and arterial pressure and to divert blood flow to critical organs. In clinical scenarios like hemorrhage, in which the stimulus activating these physiological defenses is transient, the RAAS and the sympathetic nervous system adequately support the circulation through an acute challenge and are finally inactivated by negative feedback mechanisms. A necessary condition for recovery of homeostasis is normal function of end-organs responding to these compensatory neurohumoral mechanisms. In CHF, the impaired cardiac function that triggers these mechanisms persists, preventing restoration of normal cardiovascular function. Thus, mechanisms favoring volume retention and vasoconstriction continue, and what began as an adaptive physiological response to an acute stressor evolves into a major detrimental influence on long-term prognosis.

The most successful recent innovations in the medical treatment of CHF have targeted the peripheral manifestations of augmented neurohumoral drive.[1] Despite the obligatory involvement of the central nervous system in many of the physiological (e.g., sympathetic drive, vasopressin release) and behavioral (e.g., thirst, sodium appetite) aspects of CHF, only a few studies have focused on the importance of central neural mechanisms to the heart failure syndrome. We have begun to address this issue using the rat model of ischemia-induced CHF, which simulates the most common cause of heart failure in Western societies.

In initial studies,[2] we systematically examined the neurohumoral characteristics of ischemia-induced CHF. Adult male Sprague-Dawley rats were instrumented with chronic jugular venous cannulas and maintained in metabolic cages for 6 weeks. At the end of the first week, after baseline measurements had been obtained, coronary ligation (CL) or sham CL was performed to induce CHF. The severity of left ventricular dysfunction, the substrate for CHF, was assessed by echocardiography performed under light anesthesia at 2–3 weeks following CL. Compared with their sham-operated littermates (SHAM), rats with CL (CHF) had pathognomonic signs of CHF, including reduced left ventricular (LV) ejection fractions, increased LV end-diastolic volumes, and strikingly increased LV volume/mass indices. At the conclusion of the 6-week protocol, the CHF rats also had higher LV end-diastolic pressures than the SHAM rats. Postmortem exam revealed increased heart/body weight and lung/body weight ratios in the CHF rats.

The humoral markers increased in the CHF rats, consistent with a state of generalized neurohomoral excitation. Plasma renin activity (PRA), presumably driven by underperfusion of the kidneys and by increased sympathetic activity, increased early and peaked 2 weeks after CL. Arginine vasopressin (AVP, also known as antidiuretic hormone), released from forebrain in response to activation of the RAAS and also to reductions in baroreceptor input,[3] increased within the first week, but peaked 3 weeks after CL. Atrial natriuretic factor (ANF), released from the heart in proportion to the severity of LV dilatation, had already reached a steady-state level within 1 week after CL.

Considered in a functional context, PRA is the rate-limiting step in the formation of angiotensin II (ANG II), which elicits peripheral vasoconstriction and sodium and water retention, but also activates the forebrain to stimulate thirst, sodium appetite,

AVP release, and sympathetic drive.[4–6] AVP is another potent vasoconstrictor, in addition to its effects on the kidney to retain free water. ANF counters the effects of ANG II both centrally and peripherally, but appears to be a weaker system that can be overcome by the effects of an overactive RAAS.[7]

Measures of volume regulation in these same animals, presumably reflecting the outcome of interactions among these humoral modulators, were generally more stable. Coincident with the early rise in PRA, CHF rats demonstrated increased ingestion of 1.8% NaCl solution (available as an alternate fluid choice), decreased urine output, and decreased urinary sodium excretion within the first week after CL. Intake of 1.8% NaCl remained high and urine volume remained low for the remainder of the 6-week study protocol. Urinary sodium excretion returned toward normal in the second week and then tended to decrease again gradually over the remainder of the 6-week protocol. The overall effect was an accumulation of extracellular fluid volume in the CHF rats, manifested by increased lung/body weight ratio and the presence of pleural effusions and ascites.

Recordings of renal sympathetic nerve activity (RSNA) were made in these same rats in the conscious state after completion of the metabolic cage protocol (about 6 weeks after CL or sham CL). RSNA was higher in the CHF rats whether analyzed as rectified and integrated nerve activity or as burst frequency within the integrated tracing. Waveform analysis of the average integrated RSNA signal on a beat-by-beat basis revealed substantially higher RSNA in the CHF rats. The conscious CHF rats had slightly lower arterial pressures and slightly higher heart rates than the sham-operated controls, measured in the conscious state. Baroreflex testing, using intravenous nitroprusside and phenylephrine to lower and raise arterial pressure, respectively, revealed blunted baroreflex regulation of heart rate and RSNA in the CHF compared with the SHAM rats, as others have shown.[8–10]

From these initial experiments, in which sequential measurements of neuroactive circulating peptides, indices of volume regulation, and sympathetic nerve activity were obtained from the same animals over a 6-week interval following induction of CHF, we concluded that ischemia-induced CHF in the rat mimicked many of the features of human heart failure and that the early stages in the development of CHF in this model were characterized by marked adaptive fluctuations in the circulating neurohumoral milieu. These comprehensive initial studies, clearly demonstrating activation of central neural mechanisms driving thirst, sodium appetite, AVP release, and RSNA, provided the basis for our further studies of the role of central neural mechanisms in CHF.

In considering regions of the central nervous system that might contribute to the development of CHF, the forebrain seems a likely candidate. Extrapolating from previous work in normal rats, it is known that blood-borne ANG II can act upon AT1 receptors in circumventricular organs in the forebrain, which lack a blood-brain barrier, to increase thirst, sodium appetite, the release of arginine vasopressin (AVP), and sympathetic drive.[4–6] Notably, these are among the key physiological processes that are deranged in CHF, as demonstrated in our rat model. In a seminal study that called attention to the potential importance of forebrain mechanisms in CHF, Patel and colleagues[11] demonstrated that rats with ischemia-induced CHF had increased metabolic activity in the paraventricular nucleus of the hypothalamus (PVN), a major downstream relay site for forebrain circumventricular organs activated by the

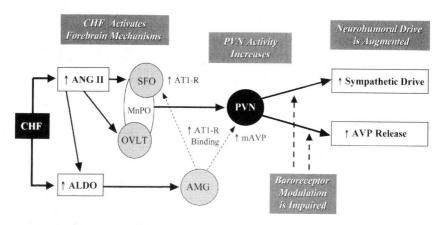

**FIGURE 1.** Proposed role of the forebrain in heart failure. In the normal rat circulating angiotensin II (ANG II) exerts central effects via AT1 receptors (AT1-R) in forebrain circumventricular organs lacking a blood-brain barrier. Activation of neurons in the subfornical organ (SFO) and the organum vasculosum of the lamina terminalis (OVLT) by circulating ANG II increases thirst, sodium appetite, and sympathetic nerve activity. The paraventricular nucleus of hypothalamus (PVN) is an important projection site mediating the downstream effects of SFO and OVLT on sympathetic nerve activity and vasopressin release. Circulating aldosterone (ALDO) activates neurons in the medial amygdala that influence sodium appetite and volume regulation. ALDO also increases the binding of ANG II to AT1 receptors in SFO and PVN, and increases message for AVP in magnocellular neurons. In the CHF rat we propose that these forebrain mechanisms are enhanced by high circulating levels of ANG II and ALDO, and possibly by enhanced brain RAAS activity, to promote neurohumoral excitation and volume retention. These influences may be amplified by blunting of baroreflex mechanisms that normally restrain sympathetic drive and AVP release.

RAAS.[5] In direct recordings from PVN neurons,[12] we have demonstrated for the first time that the spike activity of a random sampling of PVN neurons is higher in CHF rats than in SHAM or normal rats.

A working hypothesis concerning the involvement of the CNS in heart failure, based upon the known influences of RAAS on the forebrain in normal animals and the increased activity of PVN neurons in CHF, is illustrated in FIGURE 1. The high circulating levels of ANG II in CHF, acting upon AT1 receptors in the subfornical organ (SFO) and the organum vasculosum of the lamina terminalis (OVLT), induce thirst and sodium appetite and excite downstream PVN neurons that increase sympathetic drive and the production and release of AVP. Aldosterone (ALDO), also present in high serum concentrations in CHF,[13,14] acts on mineralocorticoid receptors (MR) in amygdala (AMG) to promote sodium appetite,[15,16] increases the binding of ANG II to AT1 receptors in the SFO and PVN,[17] and increases message for the production of AVP in PVN.[18] Since AT1 receptors in the brain increase in response to higher circulating levels of ANG II,[19] and ALDO increases the binding of ANG II to AT1 receptors,[17] the anticipated effect is an RAAS-mediated, dramatic increase in the influence of this region of the brain in CHF.

We have conducted several tests of the hypothesis that the forebrain contributes substantially to the pathophysiology of CHF. These initial studies have addressed in a preliminary manner the involvement of forebrain mechanisms in CHF and provide a basis for more definitive future studies.

In the *first* test of the hypothesis, we examined the effects of manipulating key central elements of the RAAS on the state of neuronal excitation in the PVN of CHF rats.[12] We delivered either the selective AT1 receptor antagonist losartan (100–200 µg/kg) or the angiotensin-converting enzyme inhibitor captopril (50 µg/kg) to the forebrain, using intracarotid injections ipsilateral to sites of PVN neuronal recording. Intracarotid (ICA) injections in the rat selectively target the ipsilateral forebrain[20] and have the distinct advantage of activating forebrain mechanisms by the normal blood-borne route. Interestingly, we found that losartan, which competitively blocks the AT1 receptors mediating the central effects of ANG II, and captopril, which blocks conversion of angiotensin I to ANG II by angiotensin-converting enzyme (ACE), both significantly reduced the activity of PVN neurons in CHF rats. The losartan data are compatible with the hypothesis that blood-borne ANG II activates AT1 receptors in forebrain circumventricular organs to drive PVN neurons. The captopril data argue strongly for an alternative hypothesis: if the activity of central is ACE increased in CHF, the intrinsic brain RAAS may produce the increased ANG II that activates AT1 receptors to enhance PVN neuronal activity. Of course, both mechanisms may be operative. It is notable that reductions in PVN neuronal activity by losartan and captopril were also observed in the SHAM rats, suggesting that the RAAS normally exerts a tonic facilitatory influence on the excitability of PVN neurons. Thus, this influence is not unique to the CHF syndrome, but it may be exaggerated in that setting.

In the *second* test of our hypothesis we examined the effects of eliminating forebrain influences on the development of CHF.[21] To accomplish this, we took advantage of the known effect of lesions in the anteroventral third ventricular (AV3V) region to block forebrain-mediated responses to blood-borne ANG II.[4] Rats that had fully recovered from the AV3V lesion (or a sham procedure) performed 4 weeks earlier were kept in metabolic cages for 2 weeks before and 2 weeks after CL or sham CL. CHF was again confirmed by echocardiographic criteria. The sham-lesioned CHF rats had altered sodium and water intake and excretion as described before in the initial studies characterizing the CHF model. In the AV3V-lesioned CHF rats, in contrast, sodium intake decreased rather than increasing after CL, urine sodium excretion was normal, and urine volume actually increased. In other words, the compensatory mechanisms expected in the early stages of CHF were absent or even reversed. In the sham CL group, these variables were not affected by the presence of an AV3V lesion. In a separate group of animals not kept in metabolic cages, the effects of the AV3V lesion on sympathetic drive were studied.[22] The AV3V lesion reduced RSNA in both CHF and sham CL groups.

A notable finding of this study was that the AV3V-lesioned CHF rats had a dramatic reduction in survival after week 2. In contrast, the AV3V-lesioned rats that underwent sham CL survived well beyond 2 weeks. The requirement of the failing LV for high filling pressures to sustain an adequate cardiac output may help explain this dramatic difference in survival: the AV3V-lesioned CL rats lack the central volume regulatory mechanisms needed to meet this requirement. Of course, the AV3V lesion may interrupt other critical forebrain pathways related to stress (e.g., ACTH release), but the seemingly normal survival pattern of the AV3V-lesioned animals undergoing the same surgery without CL argues against that interpretation.

The AV3V lesioning studies findings suggest two conclusions: (1) the forebrain is an essential component in the early adjustments of fluid regulation and sympathetic drive in CHF, and (2) forebrain mechanisms, whether related to regulation of fluid volume or sympathetic drive or other critical adaptive processes, are essential to survival in CHF. It may be that the same mechanisms that are viewed as maladaptive and worthy of therapeutic intervention in established CHF are necessary initial adaptations to myocardial injury and hemodynamic insufficiency.

The *third* test of our hypothesis was a more subtle intervention in the workings of the forebrain, selectively inhibiting the influence of one component of the RAAS. ALDO released from the zona glomerulosa of the adrenal gland by circulating ANG II is present in high levels in CHF.[13,14] ALDO has multiple peripheral effects, an important one being the facilitation of sodium retention by the kidney. As mentioned earlier, ALDO also has central nervous system effects that complement these peripheral effects, acting on MR in medial amygdala to increase sodium appetite, increasing the binding of ANG II to AT1 receptors in SFO and PVN, and increasing the message for AVP production in PVN. These influences may facilitate the effectiveness of blood-borne ANG II[23] and perhaps of ANG II produced in SFO and other forebrain sites that have all the elements of brain RAAS. In addition, ICV ALDO elicits a sympathetically mediated pressor response,[24] suggesting that central MR might directly influence the level of sympathetic discharge in CHF.

Attention was called to the important role of ALDO in CHF by the recently published Randomized Aldactone Evaluation Study (RALES),[25] which found that addition of the MR antagonist spironolactone (SL) to the regimens of CHF patients on otherwise stable medical treatment substantially reduced morbidity and mortality. The RALES study was terminated early because of those findings, but the mechanism for the favorable influence of SL was not elucidated.

We examined the possibility that at least some of the beneficial effects of SL might be attributed to its influences on central MR regulating fluid balance and/or sympathetic drive.[26] Rats were implanted with Alzet® minipumps that delivered SL (100 ng/h) either centrally (ICV) or peripherally (IP) for 1 month following CL or sham CL. CHF in the CL rats was confirmed by echocardiographic criteria. Volume regulation in CHF rats treated either ICV or IP with the ethanol vehicle was the same as that in the untreated CHF rats in our initial studies characterizing the CHF model. During the first week of ICV SL treatment CHF rats had decreased intake of 1.8% saline and normalized urine volume and urine sodium excretion; these beneficial effects were maintained throughout the 4-week treatment protocol. The sham-operated animals also had an initial reduction in salt intake that was not sustained. After 2 weeks of treatment, the CHF rats treated with IP SL demonstrated similar improvement in the measured parameters of fluid balance. This unexpected finding suggests that even low doses of peripherally administered SL may eventually saturate central MR. In CHF rats treated with SL by either route, examined at the end of the 4-week treatment protocol, RSNA was reduced and baroreflex sensitivity was improved (but not normalized). Since central MR effects on renal function have been shown previously to be dependent upon intact renal nerves,[27] it seems likely that the seemingly remote beneficial effects of central MR blockade on renal sodium and water handling observed in this study were related to these reductions in renal nerve activity—in effect, a central "diuretic" effect.

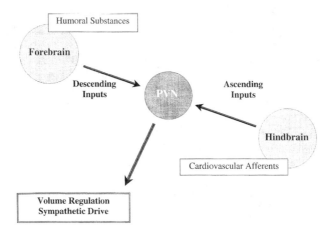

**FIGURE 2.** The paraventricular nucleus of hypothalamus (PVN) may play a pivotal role in CHF. PVN neuronal activity is increased in the rat model of CHF. PVN activity may be affected by descending excitatory influences from forebrain circumventricular organs activated by circulating peptides such as angiotensin II, or by ascending excitatory influences from brain stem regions activated by cardiovascular afferent information.

The data from the SL studies indicate that central neural interventions specifically targeting the central receptors (MR) for one component of the RAAS can effect important changes in volume regulation and sympathetic drive in CHF. The beneficial effect of MR blockade on the prognosis of CHF patients treated with SL may well be related to its central nervous system effects.

Taken together, the results of the studies summarized here indicate that neural activity in the forebrain is accentuated in CHF and that forebrain mechanisms are linked to the development or maintenance of CHF. However, they do not provide definitive insights into the stimulus activating the forebrain in CHF. The PVN, which by its location and its connectivity[5,28–30] seems likely to play a pivotal role, is a target of ascending projections from the hindbrain and of descending projections from the forebrain regions activated by RAAS, emphasized in this paper (FIG. 2). Baroreceptor inputs, which have their first synapse in the hindbrain and which when activated inhibit both sympathetic drive and AVP release,[3] clearly influence the activity of PVN neurons.[6] The well-recognized blunting of these inhibitory inputs in CHF[9,10] may well contribute to the augmented PVN neuronal activity. Recent evidence suggests that sympathoexcitatory inputs ascending from chemoreceptors[31,32] and cardiac sympathetic afferents[33,34] may also contribute. All of these peripheral afferent inputs affect regions of the hindbrain that project to PVN and may affect its function in CHF. Whether the activation of this region of the hypothalamus is dependent primarily upon renin-angiotensin-aldosterone mechanisms acting through forebrain or upon ascending excitatory (or blunted inhibitory) inputs from hindbrain— or more likely a combination of the two—remains to be determined. It is interesting in this regard that the hexokinase study in CHF rats by Patel et al.[11] did not show augmented metabolism in the SFO, a principal target of blood-borne ANG II .

Finally, although forebrain effects of ANG II on fluid balance are well established, the potential significance of the forebrain effects of ANG II on sympathetic drive in CHF may be debated. In anesthetized normal rats with baroreceptors intact, stimulation of the forebrain with ICV ANG II produces only a modest increase in arterial pressure,[35] probably mediated in part by AVP release. We found that activation of the forebrain RAAS with ICA ANG I in intact rats elicits a pressor response, but a *decrease* in RSNA,[36] and ICA captopril or losartan decreases arterial pressure and *increases* RSNA. Only after sectioning the carotid sinus and aortic depressor nerves was it possible to demonstrate the anticipated directionally similar changes in RSNA and arterial pressure. In CHF, in which the baroreflexes are blunted, the combination of diminished baroreceptor inhibition and increased PVN neuronal activity may favor a more prominent role of the forebrain in driving sympathetic nerve activity. Importantly, however, we have observed that sufficient baroreflex response remains to augment the already exaggerated RSNA in response to peripherally administered AT1 receptor blockade.[37] This observation may have clinical significance, since systemically administered ACE inhibitors and AT1 receptor blockers may have the adverse initial effect of increasing sympathetic drive.

In summary, this work provides evidence that forebrain mechanisms are prominently involved in the pathophysiology of heart failure. Our work and that of others[8,38–40] suggests that selectively manipulating the central nervous system targets of the RAAS can have a substantial beneficial influence on the peripheral manifestations of CHF. Moreover, peripheral pharmacological manipulations of the RAAS may have unexpected effects to promote fluid retention and sympathetic drive. Thus, developing strategies to more specifically target central neural mechanisms is an important goal of future heart failure research.

## ACKNOWLEDGMENTS

The authors wish to thank Kathy Zimmerman, RDMS/RDCS, for her diligent and expert assistance in the performance of the echocardiograms, and Terry Beltz for his excellent technical support in the AV3V lesioning studies. Support for this project was provided by a VA Merit Review (to R. B. Felder), AHA Grant-in-Aid 96-010430 (to R. M. Weiss), and Cardiovascular Interdisciplinary Research Fellowship NIH Grant HL 07121 (to J. Francis).

## REFERENCES

1. FRANCIS, G.S. 1998. Neurohumoral activation and progression of heart failure: hypothetical and clinical considerations. J. Cardiovasc. Pharmacol. **32:** S16–S21.
2. FRANCIS, J. *et al.* 2000. Neurohumoral consequences of congestive heart failure (CHF) in rats (Abstr.). Soc. Neurosci. Abstr. **26:** 823.
3. THAMES, M.D. & P.G. SCHMID. 1981. Interaction between carotid and cardiopulmonary baroreflexes in control of plasma ADH. Am. J. Physiol. **241:** H431–H434.
4. BRODY, M.J. & A.K. JOHNSON. 1980. Role of the anteroventral third ventricle region in fluid and electrolyte balance, arterial pressure regulation, and hypertension. *In* Frontiers in Neuroendocrinology, pp. 249–292. Raven Press. New York.
5. MCKINLEY, M.J., G.L. PENNINGTON & B.J. OLDFIELD. 1996. Anteroventral wall of the third ventricle and dorsal lamina terminalis: headquarters for control of body fluid homeostasis? Clin. Exp. Pharmacol. Physiol. **23:** 271–281.

6. JOHNSON, A.K. & R.L. THUNHORST. 1997. The neuroendocrinology of thirst and salt appetite: visceral sensory signals and mechanisms of central integration. Front. Neuroendocrinol. **18:** 292–353.
7. VILLARREAL, D. & R.H. FREEMAN. 1991. ANF and the renin-angiotensin system in the regulation of sodium balance: longitudinal studies in experimental heart failure. J. Lab. Clin. Med. **118:** 515–522.
8. DIBONA, G.F., S.Y. JONES & V.L. BROOKS. 1995. ANG II receptor blockade and arterial baroreflex regulation of renal nerve activity in cardiac failure. Am. J. Physiol. **269:** R1189–R1196.
9. THAMES, M.D. *et al.* 1993. Abnormalities of baroreflex control in heart failure. J. Am. Coll. Cardiol. **22:** 56A–60A.
10. ZUCKER, I.H. & W. WANG. 1991. Reflex control of renal sympathetic nervous activity in heart failure. Herz **16:** 82–91.
11. PATEL, K.P., P.L. ZHANG & T.L. KRUKOFF. 1993. Alterations in brain hexokinase activity associated with heart failure in rats. Am. J. Physiol. **265:** R923–R928.
12. ZHANG, Z.H. *et al.* 2000. The brain renin angiotensin system contributes to hyperexcitability of hypothalamic paraventricular nucleus neurons in congestive heart failure (Abstr.). Circulation **102:** 349.
13. ZANNAD, F. 1995. Aldosterone and heart failure. Eur. Heart J. **16:** 98–102.
14. PITT, B. 1995. "Escape" of aldosterone production in patients with left ventricular dysfunction treated with an angiotensin converting enzyme inhibitor: implications for therapy. Cardiovasc. Drugs Ther **9:** 145–149.
15. DE NICOLA, A.F., C. GRILLO & S. GONZALEZ. 1992. Physiological, biochemical, and molecular mechanisms of salt appetite control by mineralocorticoid action in brain. Braz. J. Med. Biol. Res. **25:** 1153–1162.
16. JOHNSON, A.K. *et al.* 1999. The extended amygdala and salt appetite. Ann. N.Y. Acad. Sci. **877:** 258–280.
17. DE NICOLA, A.F. *et al.* 1993. Effects of deoxycorticosterone acetate (DOCA) and aldosterone on Sar1–angiotensin II binding and angiotensin-converting enzyme binding sites in brain. Cell. Mol. Neurobiol. **13:** 529–539.
18. GRILLO, C.A. *et al.* 1998. Increased expression of magnocellular vasopressin mRNA in rats with deoxycorticosterone-acetate induced salt appetite. Neuroendocrinology **68:** 105–115.
19. WILSON, K.M., C. SUMNERS & M.J. FREGLY. 1988. Effects of increased circulating angiotensin II (AII) on fluid exchange and binding of AII in the brain. Brain Res. Bull. **20:** 493–501.
20. HAYWOOD, J.R. *et al.* 1980. The area postrema plays no role in the pressor action of angiotensin in the rat. Am. J. Physiol. **239:** H108–H113.
21. FRANCES, J. *et al.* 2000. Effects of anterior third ventricle lesioning on heart failure (Abstr.). Physiologist **43:** 286.
22. WEI, S. *et al.* 2001. Anterior third ventricle (AV3V) lesioning attenuates sympathetic drive and improves baroreflex responses in heart failure (Abstr.). FASEB J. **15:** A469.
23. WILSON, K.M. *et al.* 1986. Mineralocorticoids modulate central angiotensin II receptors in rats. Brain Res. **382:** 87–96.
24. GOMEZ-SANCHEZ, E.P. 1997. Central hypertensive effects of aldosterone. Front. Neuroendocrinol. **18:** 440–462.
25. PITT, B. *et al.* 1999. The effect of spironolactone on morbidity and mortality in patients with severe heart failure: Randomized Aldactone Evaluation Study Investigators. N. Engl. J. Med. **341:** 709–717.
26. FRANCIS, J. *et al.* 2000. Influences of central mineralocorticoid receptors on congestive heart failure (Abstr.). Circulation **102:** II-105.
27. RAHMOUNI, K. *et al.* 1999. Brain mineralocorticoid receptor control of blood pressure and kidney function in normotensive rats. Hypertension **33:** 1201–1206.
28. SWANSON, L.W. & H.G. KUYPERS. 1980. The paraventricular nucleus of the hypothalamus: cytoarchitectonic subdivisions and organization of projections to the pituitary, dorsal vagal complex, and spinal cord as demonstrated by retrograde fluorescence double-labeling methods. J. Comp. Neurol. **194:** 555–570.

29. McKellar, S. & A.D. Loewy. 1981. Organization of some brain stem afferents to the paraventricular nucleus of the hypothalamus in the rat. Brain Res. **217:** 351–357.
30. Porter, J.P. & M.J. Brody. 1985. Neural projections from paraventricular nucleus that subserve vasomotor functions. Am. J. Physiol. **248:** R271–R281.
31. Sun, S.Y. *et al.* 1999. Enhanced peripheral chemoreflex function in conscious rabbits with pacing-induced heart failure. J. Appl. Physiol. **86:** 1264–1272.
32. Sun, S.Y. *et al.* 1999. Enhanced activity of carotid body chemoreceptors in rabbits with heart failure: role of nitric oxide. J. Appl. Physiol. **86:** 1273–1282.
33. Ma, R., I.H. Zucker & W. Wang. 1997. Central gain of the cardiac sympathetic afferent reflex in dogs with heart failure. Am. J. Physiol. **273:** H2664–H2671.
34. Ma, R., I.H. Zucker & W. Wang. 1999. Reduced NO enhances the central gain of cardiac sympathetic afferent reflex in dogs with heart failure. Am. J. Physiol. **276:** H19–H26.
35. Barron, K.W. *et al.* 1989. Baroreceptor denervation profoundly enhances cardiovascular responses to central angiotensin II. Am. J. Physiol. **257:** H314–H323.
36. Wei, S.G. *et al.* 2000. Forebrain angiotensin converting enzyme activity influences renal sympathetic discharge in anesthetized rat (Abstr.). Soc. Neurosci. Abstr. **26:** 1950.
37. Wei, S. *et al.* 2000. AT1 receptor blockade with losartan in heart failure: central vs. peripheral influences on sympathetic drive (Abstr.). Psysiologist **43:** 286.
38. Sato, T. *et al.* 1998. The brain is a possible target for an angiotensin-converting enzyme inhibitor in the treatment of chronic heart failure. J. Cardiac Failure **4:** 139–144.
39. Zhang, W., B.S. Huang & F.H. Leenen. 1999. Brain renin-angiotensin system and sympathetic hyperactivity in rats after myocardial infarction. Am. J. Physiol. **276:** H1608–H1615.
40. Liu, J.L. & I.H. Zucker. 1999. Regulation of sympathetic nerve activity in heart failure: a role for nitric oxide and angiotensin II. Circ. Res. **84:** 417–423.

# Regulation of Sympathetic Nervous System Function after Cardiovascular Deconditioning

EILEEN M. HASSER[a] AND JULIA A. MOFFITT[b]

[a]Dalton Cardiovascular Research Center and Department of Veterinary Biomedical Sciences, University of Missouri, Columbia, Missouri 65211, USA

[b]The Cardiovascular Center and Department of Psychology, University of Iowa, Iowa City, Iowa 52242, USA

ABSTRACT: Humans subjected to prolonged periods of bed rest or microgravity undergo deconditioning of the cardiovascular system, characterized by resting tachycardia, reduced exercise capability, and a predisposition for orthostatic intolerance. These changes in cardiovascular function are likely due to a combination of factors, including changes in control of body fluid balance or cardiac alterations resulting in inadequate maintenance of stroke volume, altered arterial or venous vascular function, reduced activation of cardiovascular hormones, and diminished autonomic reflex function. There is evidence indicating a role for each of these mechanisms. Diminished reflex activation of the sympathetic nervous system and subsequent vasoconstriction appear to play an important role. Studies utilizing the hindlimb-unloaded (HU) rat, an animal model of deconditioning, evaluated the potential role of altered arterial baroreflex control of the sympathetic nervous system. These studies indicate that HU results in blunted baroreflex-mediated activation of both renal and lumbar sympathetic nerve activity in response to a hypotensive stimulus. HU rats are less able to maintain arterial pressure during hemorrhage, suggesting that diminished ability to increase sympathetic activity has functional consequences for the animal. Reflex control of vasopressin secretion appears to be enhanced following HU. Blunted baroreflex-mediated sympathoexcitation appears to involve altered central nervous system function. Baroreceptor afferent activity in response to changes in arterial pressure is unaltered in HU rats. However, increases in efferent sympathetic nerve activity for a given decrease in afferent input are blunted after HU. This altered central nervous system processing of baroreceptor inputs appears to involve an effect at the rostral ventrolateral medulla (RVLM). Specifically, it appears that tonic $GABA_A$-mediated inhibition of the RVLM is enhanced after HU. Augmented inhibition apparently arises from sources other than the caudal ventrolateral medulla. If similar alterations in control of the sympathetic nervous system occur in humans in response to cardiovascular deconditioning, it is likely that they play an important role in the observed tendency for orthostatic intolerance. Combined with potential changes in vascular function, cardiac function, and hypovolemia, the predisposition for orthostatic intolerance following cardiovascular deconditioning would be markedly enhanced by blunted ability to reflexly activate the sympathetic nervous system.

KEYWORDS: Hindlimb unloading; Baroreflex; Ventrolateral medulla; GABA; Microgravity; Bed rest; Vasopressin; Fos

Address for correspondence: Eileen M. Hasser, Ph.D., Dalton Cardiovascular Research Center, University of Missouri, Columbia, MO 65211.Voice: 573-882-6125.
HasserE@missouri.edu

## INTRODUCTION

Humans exposed to prolonged bed rest or microgravity experience a number of adverse consequences, including muscle atrophy and weakness, bone demineralization, and cardiovascular dysfunction. Upon initial exposure to bed rest or microgravity there is a shift of body fluids centrally. This central shift of fluids results in diuresis and natriuresis, and a reduction in plasma volume and blood volume.[1–5] Upon return to an upright posture or to a normal gravitational environment, humans exhibit signs of cardiovascular deconditioning, including resting tachycardia, reduced exercise capacity, and a tendency for orthostatic intolerance.[4–8] Cardiovascular deconditioning prolongs recovery time following bed rest and poses potential dangers to astronauts, who may have to react quickly and forcefully upon return to a 1-$g$ environment.

Hindlimb unloading (HU) in rodents is an animal model used to simulate exposure to bed rest or microgravity in humans. Responses to HU include an initial central shift in fluids, diuresis, natriuresis, and reduced plasma volume and blood volume.[5,9] Importantly, upon removal from hindlimb unloading, rats exhibit typical signs of deconditioning: resting tachycardia, reduced exercise capability, and effects consistent with orthostatic intolerance.[10–12]

Reduced orthostatic tolerance is a hallmark of cardiovascular deconditioning. Orthostatic stress produces a decrease in cardiac output that is normally compensated by reflex increases in heart rate and total peripheral resistance in order to maintain adequate cerebral perfusion. There are a number of potential mechanisms that could account for orthostatic intolerance after bed rest or microgravity. These include hypovolemia, cardiac changes resulting in inadequate maintenance of stroke volume, vascular dysfunction, and diminished autonomic reflex function. There is evidence indicating a role for each of these mechanisms in orthostatic intolerance after cardiovascular deconditioning.[13–17] In this review, we will focus on altered reflex control of neuroendocrine function.

## ARTERIAL BAROREFLEX FUNCTION AND DECONDITIONING

Adequate compensation for an orthostatic challenge requires appropriate baroreflex responses.[18,19] These responses include reflexly mediated inhibition of the parasympathetic nervous system, increases in sympathetic nervous system activity, activation of the renin angiotensin system, and increased release of vasopressin. Thus, during orthostatic stress arterial pressure is maintained because decreases in stroke volume and cardiac output are balanced by reflex increases in heart rate and total peripheral resistance.[19] Although vagally mediated changes in heart rate provide rapid adjustments, sympathetically mediated increases in vascular resistance appear to be the most important compensation for orthostatic stress.[19,20] Thus, it is possible that decreased arterial baroreflex function—in particular, baroreflex control of the sympathetic nervous system—could contribute to the predisposition for orthostatic intolerance observed following cardiovascular deconditioning.

Studies evaluating baroreflex control of heart rate in humans following cardiovascular deconditioning have produced variable results. Much of this work suggests that carotid baroreflex control of heart rate is blunted after head-down bed rest or microgravity.[7,21–26] However, Crandall *et al.*[27] reported that although the carotid barore-ceptor reflex is diminished, the aortic baroreceptor reflex is enhanced. This results in no change in overall baroreflex control of heart rate. In addition, most of the stud-ies in humans have used protocols that evaluated primarily parasympathetic nervous system effects on heart rate,[7,21,23,25,26] and thus provide relatively little information concerning control of the sympathetic nervous system.

Several studies evaluating orthostatic tolerance suggest that baroreflex control of sympathetic outflow is attenuated following deconditioning. Buckey and colleagues[6] showed that astronauts who were unable to complete a stand test after flight had decreases in cardiac output and stroke volume similar to those who com-pleted the test. However, the nonfinishers were not able to further increase total pe-ripheral resistance. It is logical to hypothesize that this reduced capacity for vasoconstriction may be due to diminished activation of the sympathetic nervous system. Support for this concept is provided by the fact that norepinephrine release is less in astronauts who were subject to presyncope.[28] Similarly, Shoemaker and colleagues[29] reported that following deconditioning due to head-down bed rest, sympathetic nerve discharge in response to head up-tilt is attenuated. Taken together, these studies suggest that overall baroreflex control of heart rate is unaltered by car-diovascular deconditioning, but that reflex control of the sympathetic nervous sys-tem may be attenuated.

Studies using the hindlimb unloaded rat model of cardiovascular deconditioning have also produced variable results. While baroreflex control of heart rate may be attenuated after 24 h of HU,[30] alterations in the cardiac component of baroreflex function appear to be normalized after 9–14 days.[31,32] However, data from these studies do not indicate whether baroreflex control of sympathetic nerve activity to the vasculature is altered following HU.

## BAROREFLEX FUNCTION FOLLOWING HINDLIMB UNLOADING

As discussed above, sympathetically mediated increases in peripheral vascular resistance are of primary importance in compensating for orthostatic stress.[19,20] In addition, orthostatic-intolerant astronauts demonstrate diminished increases in pe-ripheral resistance[6] and norepinephrine.[28] Therefore, we hypothesized that cardio-vascular deconditioning results in impaired arterial baroreflex control of sympathetic nervous system activity. In addition, previous studies indicate that blood flow redistribution during exercise is altered following HU in rats.[12,33] The inade-quate redistribution of blood flow during exercise following HU appears to be asso-ciated with exaggerated increases in sympathetic outflow in working muscle and attenuated increases in sympathetic nervous system activity in inactive tissue beds.[34] These findings led us to further hypothesize that deconditioning due to HU results in a differential effect on baroreflex control of sympathetic activity to the viscera versus skeletal muscle. To test this hypothesis, we evaluated the effect of HU on ar-terial baroreflex-mediated changes in heart rate and on renal or lumbar sympathetic nerve activity (RSNA or LSNA) in conscious rats.[35] Rats were subjected to HU for 14 days by elevating the hindlimbs using a modification of a procedure previously described.[36] Control rats received a partial HU apparatus and were maintained on normal cage activity. On the 13th day of the protocol, rats were instrumented with

**TABLE 1. Resting hemodynamic parameters, body weights, and muscle weights**

| | | MAP (mmHg) | HR (bpm) | Body Weight (g) D1 | Body Weight (g) D14 | Soleus Wt. (mg) | Soleus/BW (×10³) |
|---|---|---|---|---|---|---|---|
| | $n$ | | | | | | |
| Control | 16 | $104 \pm 2$ | $354 \pm 7$ | $371 \pm 16$ | $383 \pm 12$ | $160 \pm 0.01$ | $0.42 \pm .001$ |
| HU | 16 | $109 \pm 3$ | $398 \pm 11^a$ | $405 \pm 16$ | $373 \pm 13^b$ | $91 \pm 0.01^a$ | $0.24 \pm .001^a$ |

NOTE: Values are mean $\pm$ SE. $^a p < 0.01$ from control; $^b p < 0.01$ from D1. Body weight was measured pre-hindlimb unloading on day 1 (D1), and post-hindlimb unloading on day 14 (D14); all other variables were measured on D14. HU, hindlimb unloaded; MAP, mean arterial pressure; HR, heart rate; BW, body weight. (Data reprinted with permission from Moffitt et al.[35])

catheters for recording arterial pressure and for drug injection, and with electrodes for recording RSNA or LSNA. Animals were returned to HU or to cage activity as soon as they had recovered adequately from anesthesia. After a 24-h recovery period, animals were removed from HU or from their cage and placed in a cage lined with the animal's own bedding. We studied rats in the horizontal position in order to simulate resumption of upright posture after a period of bed rest or return to a 1-$g$ environment after spaceflight. Baroreflex function was evaluated in conscious rats by increasing or decreasing arterial pressure over 2–3 minutes using increasing rates of infusion of the $\alpha_1$ agonist phenylephrine and the vasodilator nitroprusside, respectively. Reflex changes in heart rate and LSNA or RSNA in response to changes in pressure were fit to a sigmoid logistic function.[37]

Baseline hemodynamic parameters, muscle weight, and body weight before and after experimental procedures in control and HU rats are shown in TABLE 1. Resting mean arterial pressure was unaltered by HU, whereas resting heart rate was significantly elevated. Soleus muscle weight was significantly reduced. Resting tachycardia and soleus muscle atrophy confirm the efficacy of the HU procedure.[36]

Effects of HU on baroreflex control of RSNA, evaluated as a percentage of baseline, and gain of the reflex are shown in FIGURE 1. Sympathoinhibition in response to increases in arterial pressure was unaltered by 14 days of HU. In contrast, reflex activation of RSNA during decreases in arterial pressure was significantly attenuated. Maximum %RSNA during a hypotensive stimulus was significantly diminished in HU rats ($204 \pm 11.9\%$ baseline) as compared to control ($342 \pm 30.6\%$ baseline). In addition, ANOVA revealed that RSNA was reduced compared to control rats over a pressure range of 40–95 mmHg. Maximum gain of baroreflex control of RSNA was reduced in HU rats, and gain was diminished over a range of pressures of 80–110 mmHg. Thus, the ability to increase sympathetic nervous system activity to the kidneys was significantly attenuated by cardiovascular deconditioning. Importantly, this blunted reflex sympathoexcitation was evident at arterial pressures near the basal pressure.

Effects of HU on baroreflex control of LSNA were similar to those observed with RSNA (data not shown). While inhibition of LSNA during increases in arterial pressure was unaltered following HU, reflex activation of LSNA was markedly attenuated. This attenuated ability to reflexly increase LSNA is reflected in a decreased maximum LSNA during hypotension and reduced LSNA over a pressure range of 40–90 mmHg. Maximum gain and gain over a pressure range of 65–110 mmHg also

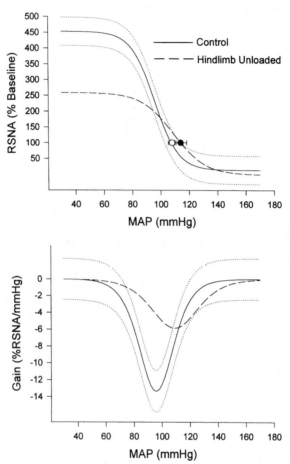

**FIGURE 1. (Top)** Mean baroreflex curves describing reflex control of renal sympathetic nerve activity (RSNA) expressed as a percentage of baseline activity. Hindlimb-unloaded rats ($n = 8$) exhibited a significant attenuation in the ability to increase RSNA in response to a decrease in MAP compared to control rats ($n = 8$). *Symbols* indicate percent baseline RSNA and resting MAP for control (*open circle*) and HU (*solid circle*) animals. **(Bottom)** Mean curves illustrating the instantaneous gain of baroreflex control of LSNA for HU ($n = 8$) and control ($n = 8$) rats. *Dotted lines* represent mean values for control animals $\pm 1$ LSD ($\alpha = 0.05$). Any points outside the dotted lines should be considered significantly different from control animal values. (Data reprinted with permission from Moffitt *et al.*[35])

were reduced. In contrast to effects of HU on baroreflex control of sympathetic nerve activity, reflex control of heart rate was unaltered. Thus, it appears that baroreflex regulation of sympathetic activity to the kidneys and to skeletal muscle is attenuated in a similar fashion by cardiovascular deconditioning due to HU, while reflex control of heart rate is unaffected.

Reduced arterial baroreflex activation of sympathetic outflow to the vasculature, if it occurs in humans, would likely have significant consequences related to control of the cardiovascular system following deconditioning. The ability to increase peripheral vascular resistance is important in compensation for orthostatic stress, and attenuated sympathoexcitation would limit vasoconstriction. Thus, diminished baroreflex function is likely to contribute to orthostatic intolerance after bed rest or spaceflight.

In conscious animals, the response to hemorrhage mimics the effects of orthostatic stress. In the initial stages of blood loss, arterial pressure is well maintained. Pressure maintenance is due to baroreflex-mediated increases in sympathetic nervous system activity, heart rate, and peripheral vascular resistance.[38] At some critical point in blood loss, pressure rapidly declines in association with sympathoinhibition and global vasodilation. We conducted preliminary experiments to test the hypothesis that the ability to compensate for acute hemorrhage is blunted in HU rats.[39] Rats were subjected to HU or maintained on normal cage activity as described above. They were then chronically instrumented for recording arterial pressure, heart rate, and LSNA. Experiments were conducted in conscious rats in the horizontal position. Control rats exhibited the typical biphasic response to hemorrhage. In HU rats, the initial reflex sympathoexcitation during blood loss was blunted. In addition, arterial pressure began to decline earlier in hemorrhage, and the blood loss required to decrease mean arterial pressure to 40 mmHg was significantly reduced. Thus, blunted reflex sympathoexcitation in HU rats is associated with reduced ability to compensate for acute blood loss. These data provide further support for the concept that altered baroreflex function may contribute to orthostatic intolerance following cardiovascular deconditioning.

In addition to sympathetic activation, the reflex response to hypotensive stimuli includes increased release of the vasoconstrictor hormone vasopressin.[40] Additional preliminary studies[41] evaluated reflex release of vasopressin in HU rats. Control and HU rats were chronically instrumented for recording arterial pressure and heart rate in the conscious state. They were then subjected to administration of 15 or 25 mg/kg diazoxide i.v. to produce dose-dependent decreases in arterial pressure, or to saline vehicle. After 90 minutes, animals were anesthetized and decapitated, and trunk blood was collected for measurement of plasma vasopressin concentration. Baseline vasopressin levels appear to be elevated following HU. The depressor response to diazoxide was similar in both groups. However, reflex increases in vasopressin appeared to be greater in HU rats. These data are consistent with studies in astronauts (J.M. Fritsch-Yelle, unpublished data), in which astronauts who became presyncopal exhibited greater vasopressin release. Thus, it appears that although cardiovascular deconditioning is associated with blunted reflex sympathoexcitation in response to hypotension,[35] reflex increases in plasma vasopressin may be enhanced. The role of enhanced vasopressin secretion in the response to orthostatic stress following cardiovascular deconditioning is unclear. In addition, the mechanisms responsible for differential effects of deconditioning on reflex control of the sympathetic nervous system and of vasopressin release are not clear.

## SITE OF ALTERED BAROREFLEX FUNCTION

Mechanisms responsible for orthostatic intolerance following cardiovascular deconditioning may be related in part to attenuated baroreflex function. Studies in both humans and animals report changes in baroreflex function following cardiovascular deconditioning.[22,24,30,42] In addition, previous data indicate a significant attenuation in the ability of HU rats to increase lumbar and renal sympathetic nervous system activity in response to hypotensive stimuli.[35] The mechanisms responsible for baroreflex dysfunction following cardiovascular deconditioning could involve several factors. Changes at a number of different points within the baroreflex arc could lead to an attenuated ability to regulate efferent vasomotor function in response to changes in arterial pressure. Specifically with regard to HU, changes in baroreflex regulation of sympathetic nervous system activity may be due to impairments in baroreceptor function (altering afferent input) or possibly a change within the central nervous system processing of baroreceptor afferent information. By using a simple design whereby changes in baroreceptor afferent input are related to sympathetic efferent output during changes in arterial pressure, the central nervous system processing component of the arterial baroreflex arc can be isolated. Conclusions can then be drawn with regard to which component(s) is altered and is thus responsible for the impairment in baroreflex control of sympathetic nervous system activity following HU. Studies using this design were employed to investigate these potential mechanisms following cardiovascular deconditioning. Animals were randomly assigned to

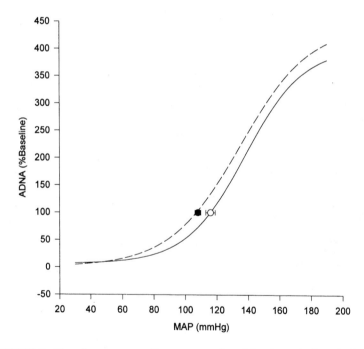

**FIGURE 2.** Mean baroreceptor afferent curves describing control of aortic depressor nerve activity (ADNA) expressed as a percentage of baseline activity. *Symbols* indicate percent baseline ADNA and resting MAP for control (*open circle*) and HU (*solid circle*) animals. HU ($n = 9$) and control groups ($n = 7$) exhibited a similar ADNA response to increases and decreases in MAP. (Data reprinted with permission from Moffitt *et al.*[43])

HU or normal cage environment. Following 14 days of the HU or control intervention animals were anesthetized with inactin. Aortic baroreceptor nerve discharge (ADNA, baroreceptor afferent activity) and renal sympathetic nervous system activity (RSNA) were recorded simultaneously in response to increases and decreases in arterial pressure elicited through infusion of phenylephrine and sodium nitroprusside, respectively.

Similar to previous results, maximum baroreflex-elicited increases in RSNA were attenuated following HU in anesthetized rats (C: $144 \pm 4.9$ vs. HU: $122 \pm 3.8\%$ baseline). However, there were no differences in the sigmoid relationship between ADNA and MAP between control animals and HU animals (FIG. 2). These data suggest that overall baroreceptor function is normal after HU. Mean arterial pressure at threshold ($P_{th}$; C: $66 \pm 4.1$ vs. HU: $64 \pm 2.4$ mmHg) and maximum ($P_{max}$; C: $172 \pm 2.4$ vs. $174 \pm 2.4$ mmHg) ADNA were not different, further indicating that cardiovascular deconditioning does not effect the afferent component of the arterial baroreflex. Upon relating the sigmoid relationships describing baroreceptor afferent input to efferent sympathetic nerve output, a linear relationship between these factors results. The slope of this linear response is indicative of the capacity of the central nervous system to integrate baroreceptor afferent signals and coordinate an appropriate efferent vasomotor response. Upon raising pressure with infusion of phenylephrine, the slope of the central nervous system response was not significantly different between control and HU rats (FIG. 3, right panel). However, when MAP was lowered, the slope of the central nervous system integrative response was significantly lower in HU compared to control animals (FIG. 3, left panel; C: $-0.40 \pm 0.04$ vs. HU: $-0.18 \pm 0.04$). Thus, for any given decrease in ADNA during a hypotensive stimulus, the increase in RSNA was less. Taken together, results from this study suggest that there is no change in the afferent limb of the arterial baroreflex. However, central nervous system integration of the afferent response is attenuated, resulting in a reduced ability to increase RSNA in response to hypotension following HU. These results point

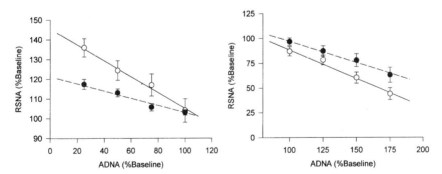

**FIGURE 3.** Central integration of baroreceptor afferent activity was analyzed by comparing mean linear regression lines fit to data expressing the percent change in RSNA to the percent change in ADNA in response to decreases (**left panel**) and increases (**right panel**) in arterial pressure in HU (*closed symbols, dashed lines*) and control (*open symbols, solid lines*) groups. Central integration of baroreceptor afferent activity was significantly attenuated during hypotension in HU rats. (Data reprinted with permission from Moffitt *et al.*[43])

to the potential mechanism responsible for baroreflex dysfunction following cardio-vascular deconditioning being located within the central nervous system.

## POTENTIAL CENTRAL NERVOUS SYSTEM ALTERATIONS

The above data indicate that arterial baroreflex activation of the sympathetic ner-vous system is blunted following cardiovascular deconditioning.[35] This appears to be due to altered central nervous system processing of baroreceptor afferent input rather than an alteration in the baroreceptors themselves.[43] Changes in central ner-vous system processing of the baroreflex could involve many different regions of the brain. However, likely sites of altered function are those specifically involved in the baroreflex arc. Baroreflex control of sympathetic nervous system activity appears to involve at least three synapses. Arterial baroreceptor afferents terminate in the nu-cleus tractus solitarius (NTS).[44] From the NTS, there is an excitatory synapse in the caudal ventrolateral medulla (CVLM). The CVLM then sends an inhibitory, GABAergic projection to the rostral ventrolateral medulla (RVLM), which is the pri-mary controller of baroreflex-mediated changes in sympathetic nervous system ac-tivity.[45] To assess potential central nervous system sites of altered baroreflex function, we used immunocytochemistry for Fos,[46] the protein product of the early response gene, c-fos. Fos is involved in initiating genomic effects related to synaptic activation[47] and has been used extensively to examine regions of the central nervous system involved in cardiovascular regulation. Control and HU rats were chronically instrumented with catheters for recording arterial pressure and heart rate and for drug injection, as described above. Conscious animals were given saline vehicle or an intravenous injection of hydralazine (10 mg/kg) to produce a sustained hypoten-sive response. After 90 min, rats were deeply anesthetized with pentobarbital and killed, and their brains were prepared for evaluation of Fos immunoreactivity. The depressor response to hydralazine was similar in control and HU rats. Fos immu-noreactivity in the RVLM is shown in FIGURE 4. In response to saline infusion, the number of Fos-positive nuclei was small and was similar in both groups of animals (FIG. 4A and 4B). In response to hypotension, the number of Fos-positive nuclei in the RVLM was increased in both groups. However, the increase in Fos immunoreac-tivity was markedly less in HU rats as compared to control animals (FIG. 4C and 4D; C:18.3 ± 3.7 vs. HU: 7.7 ± 1.8). These data are consistent with activation of RVLM sympathoexcitatory neurons in both groups of animals. However, they suggest that excitation of RVLM sympathetic neurons during hypotension may be reduced in HU rats. Thus, it appears that at least a portion of blunted baroreflex control of the sym-pathetic nervous system may involve altered function at the level of the RVLM.

The RVLM is a primary site involved in maintaining basal sympathetic tone and in mediating reflex changes in sympathetic nervous system activity.[48] Bilateral inhi-bition of this region produces profound sympathoinhibition and hypotension, while stimulation of the RVLM results in increases in sympathetic nervous system activity and arterial pressure.[49–51] Sympathoexcitatory neurons in the RVLM are tonically active and receive both excitatory and inhibitory inputs.[52] The primary tonic inhibi-tion of RVLM neurons is mediated by the neurotransmitter γ-amino butyric acid (GABA) acting at $GABA_A$ receptors.[53] A large proportion of this GABAergic inhi-bition originates in neurons in the CVLM, although sources other than the CVLM

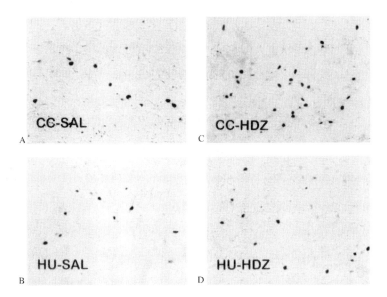

**FIGURE 4.** Relative levels of c-fos activiation in the RVLM in HU and control rats at baseline in response to saline injection (SAL) and in response to hypotension elicited through hydralazine administration (HDZ). Data indicate an increase in the number of c-fos–positive nuclei from baseline to hypotension in control rats and an attenuation in the number of c-fos–positive nuclei in HU rats during hypotension.

provide additional GABAergic inputs.[53,54] Important excitatory inputs appear to be mediated by an angiotensin-like transmitter and glutamate.[55,56]

Following cardiovascular deconditioning due to HU in rats, Fos immunocytochemistry (FIG. 4) suggests that activation of RVLM neurons in response to hypotensive stimuli is diminished. Reduced activation of RVLM neurons following HU could be due to a reduction in excitatory inputs to the RVLM, or enhanced inhibition of RVLM neurons. To examine these possibilities, we evaluated the effects of blockade of excitatory or inhibitory inputs at the level of the RVLM. Preliminary studies examined the arterial pressure and sympathetic nervous system response to blockade of an angiotensin-like transmitter using sarthran. Rats were subjected to either 14 days of HU or maintained on normal cage activity. They were anesthetized with inactin and instrumented with arterial and venous catheters and recording electrodes for RSNA. Rats were then placed in a stereotaxic apparatus and the brain stems exposed for microinjection into the ventrolateral medulla. Localization of the RVLM was verified by a pressor and sympathoexcitatory response to microinjection of glutamate (10 mM, 30 nL). As shown by others,[55] bilateral microinjection of sarthran (50 mM, 90 nL) produced a depressor response and sympathoinhibition. The response to sarthran was similar in control and HU rats. These preliminary data indicate that the reduced ability to activate the sympathetic nervous system due to cardiovascular deconditioning is not likely due to diminished angiotensin-like excitation at the level of the RVLM.

Further studies[57,58] evaluated the possibility that HU resulted in altered GABAergic mechanisms at the RVLM. We hypothesized that $GABA_A$ inhibition of RVLM
neurons is enhanced following HU. We further hypothesized that greater GABAergic input from the CVLM is responsible for increased $GABA_A$ receptor inhibition in
the RVLM. Control and 14-day HU rats were anesthetized with inactin and instrumented with arterial and venous catheters and recording electrodes for RSNA. Rats
were placed in a stereotaxic apparatus and the brain stems exposed for microinjection into the RVLM or CVLM. Localization of the RVLM and CVLM was verified
by a pressor and sympathoexcitatory response, and depressor response and sympathoinhibition, respectively, to microinjection of glutamate (10 mM, 30 nL). Overall tonic $GABA_A$ inhibition of the RVLM initially was evaluated by bilateral
microinjection of the $GABA_A$ receptor antagonist bicuculline (5 mM, 90 nL) into the
RVLM. Bilateral administration of bicuculline produced large increases in arterial
pressure and RSNA in both groups of animals. The pressor response and sympathoexcitation were greater in HU rats, suggesting enhanced $GABA_A$-mediated inhibition
of the RVLM after HU. To test whether this augmented $GABA_A$ inhibition is due to
inputs from the CVLM, neurons in the CVLM were inhibited by bilateral microinjection of kainic acid at a dose that produces depolarization blockade. Kainic acid
injection resulted in similar increases in arterial pressure and RSNA in both groups
of animals. Contrary to our hypothesis, these data suggest that inputs from the
CVLM to RVLM are unaltered following HU. At the peak of the excitatory response
to inhibition of the CVLM, bicuculline was microinjected bilaterally into the RVLM.
This was done to block any remaining $GABA_A$ inhibition of the RVLM after removal
of CVLM inputs. This subsequent injection of bicuculline produced a further increase in pressure and RSNA in both groups of animals. The pressor and sympathoexcitatory responses to bicuculline after CVLM inhibition were enhanced in HU rats.
Taken together, these data are consistent with the hypothesis that following cardiovascular deconditioning due to HU in rats there is augmented tonic $GABA_A$-mediat-
ed inhibition of sympathoexcitatory neurons in the RVLM. This enhanced $GABA_A$
inhibition appears to originate from sources other than the CVLM.

## SUMMARY

Cardiovascular deconditioning in humans subjected to prolonged bed rest or microgravity is characterized by resting tachycardia, reduced exercise capacity, and a
predisposition for orthostatic intolerance. There are a number of potential mechanisms that could contribute to orthostatic intolerance due to deconditioning, including hypovolemia, reduced cardiac function, and impaired vascular function. There is
evidence that each of these factors is involved. This paper has focused on the possible contribution of altered control of the autonomic nervous system. Studies examining baroreflex control of heart rate in both humans and animals have produced
variable results. However, reflex activation of the sympathetic nervous system to the
vasculature, producing vasoconstriction, appears to be a primary factor involved in
adequate compensation for orthostatic stress.
    Studies using the HU rat, an animal model for deconditioning, evaluated the po-
tential role of altered control of the sympathetic nervous system. These studies indicate that arterial baroreflex-mediated activation of sympathetic nervous system

activity both to the kidney and to skeletal muscle in response to a hypotensive stimulus is reduced in HU rats. This diminished ability to increase sympathetic activity appears to have functional consequences for the animal, because HU rats exhibit a decreased ability to maintain arterial pressure during hemorrhage. In contrast, reflex control of vasopressin secretion appears to be enhanced following HU. Blunted baroreflex-mediated activation of the sympathetic nervous system appears to involve altered central nervous system function. Baroreceptor afferent activity in response to changes in arterial pressure is unaltered in HU rats. However, increases in efferent sympathetic nerve activity for a given decrease in afferent input are blunted after HU, suggesting altered central nervous system processing of baroreceptor afferent input. This altered central nervous system processing of baroreceptor inputs appears to involve an effect at the RVLM. Specifically, it appears that tonic $GABA_A$-mediated inhibition of the RVLM is enhanced after HU. Augmented inhibition apparently arises from sources other than the CVLM.

If similar alterations in control of the sympathetic nervous system occur in humans in response to cardiovascular deconditioning, it is likely that they play an important role in the observed tendency for orthostatic intolerance. Compensation for orthostatic stress requires increases in total peripheral resistance. Blunted ability to reflexly increase sympathetic nervous system activity to the vasculature would reduce the capability for increasing peripheral resistance and thus diminish the overall ability to produce adequate compensation. Combined with potential changes in vascular function, cardiac function, and hypovolemia, the predisposition for orthostatic intolerance following cardiovascular deconditioning would be markedly enhanced.

## REFERENCES

1. CHOBANIAN, A.V., R.D. LILLE, A. TERCYAK & P. BLEVINS. 1974. The metabolic and hemodynamic effects of prolonged bed rest in normal subjects. Circulation **49:** 551–559.
2. CONVERTINO, V.A., J. HUNG, D. GOLDWATER & R.F. DEBUSK. 1982. Cardiovascular responses to exercise in middle-aged men after 10 days of bedrest. Circulation **65**(1): 134–140.
3. HUNG, J., D. GOLDWATER, V.A. CONVERTINO, et al. 1983. Mechanisms for decreased exercise capacity after bedrest in normal middle-aged men. Am. J. Cardiol. **51:** 344–348.
4. SALTIN, B., G. BLOMQVIST, J.H. MITCHELL, et al. 1968. Response to exercise after bed rest and after training. Circulation **38**(5) S-7: 7(1)–7(78).
5. TAYLOR, H.L., A. HENSCHEL, J. BROZEK & A. KEYS. 1949. Effects of bed rest on cardiovascular function and work performance. J. Appl. Physiol. **2**(5): 223–239.
6. BUCKEY, J.C., L.D. LANE, B.D. LEVINE, et al. 1996. Orthostatic intolerance after spaceflight. J. Appl. Physiol. **81:** 7–18.
7. FRITSCH-YELLE, J.M., J.B. CHARLES, M.M. JONES 1994. Spaceflight alters autonomic regulation of arterial pressure in humans. J. Appl. Physiol. **77**(4): 1776–1783.
8. LEVINE, B.D., L.D. LANE, D.E. WATENPAUGH, et al. 1996. Maximal exercise performance after adaptation to microgravity. J. Appl. Physiol. **81:** 686–694.
9. SHELLOCK, F.G., H.J.C. SWAN & S.A. RUBIN. 1985. Early central venous pressure changes in the rat during two different levels of head-down suspension. Aviat. Space. Environ. Med. **56:** 791–795.
10. MARTEL, E., P. CHAMPEROUX, P. LACOLLEY, et al. 1996. Central hypervolemia in the conscious rat: a model of cardiovascular deconditioning. J. Appl. Physiol. **80:** 1390–1396.

11. OVERTON, J.M., C.R. WOODMAN & C.M. Tipton. 1989. Effect of hindlimb suspension on $VO_2$ max and regional blood flow responses to exercise. J. Appl. Physiol. **66**(2): 653–659.
12. WOODMAN, C.R., L.A. SEBASTIAN & C.M. TIPTON. 1995. Influence of simulated microgravity on cardiac output and blood flow distribution during exercise. J. Appl. Physiol. **79**: 1762–1768.
13. CONVERTINO, V.A., D.F. DOERR, D.A. LUDWIG & J. VERNIKOS. 1994. Effect of simulated microgravity on cardiopulmonary baroreflex control of forearm vascular resistance. Am. J. Physiol. **266** (Regul. Integr. Comp. Physiol. **35**): R1962–R1969.
14. DELP, M.D., M. BROWN, M.H. LAUGHLIN & E.M. HASSER. 1995. Rat aortic vasoreactivity is altered by old age and hindlimb unloading. J. Appl. Physiol. **78**(6): 2079–2086.
15. GREENLEAF, J.E., J. VERNIKOS, C.E. WADE & P.R. BARNES. 1992. Effect of leg exercise training on vascular volumes during 30 days of 6 degrees head-down bed rest. J. Appl. Physiol. **72**: 1887–1894.
16. LEVINE, B.D., J.H. ZUCKERMANN & J.A. PAWELCZYK. 1997. Cardiac atrophy after bedrest deconditioning: a nonneural mechanism for orthostatic intolerance. Circulation **96**: 517–525.
17. SHOEMAKER, J.K., C.S. HOGEMAN, D.H. SILBER, et al. 1998. Head-down-tilt bed rest alters forearm vasodilator and vasoconstrictor responses. J. Appl. Physiol. **84**: 1756–1762.
18. BLOMQVIST, C.G. & H L. STONE. 1983. Cardiovascular adjustments to gravitational stress. *In* Handbook of Physiology. J.T. Shepherd & F.M. Abboud, Eds.: 1025 1057. American Physical Society. Bethesda, MD.
19. ROWELL, L.B. 1993. Human cardiovascular control: 36–254. Oxford University Press. New York.
20. TYDEN, G. 1977. Aspects of cardiovascular reflex control in man. Acta. Physiol. Scand. **S448**: 1–62.
21. CONVERTINO, V.A., D.F. DOERR, D.L. ECKBERG, et al. 1990. Head-down bed rest impairs vagal baroreflex responses and provokes orthostatic hypotension. J. Appl. Physiol. **68**(4): 1458–1464.
22. COOKE, W.H., J.E. AMES IV, A.A. CROSSMAN, et al. 2000. Nine months in space: effects on human autonomic cardiovascular regulation. J. Appl. Physiol. **89**: 1039–1045.
23. ECKBERG, D.L. & J.M. FRITSCH. 1991. Human autonomic responses to actual and simulated weightlessness. J. Clin. Pharmacol. **31**: 951–955.
24. ECKBERG, D.L. & J.M. FRITSCH. 1992. Influence of ten-day head-down bedrest on human carotid baroreceptor-cardiac reflex function. Acta. Physiol. Scand. **144**(S604): 69–76.
25. ENGELKE, K.A., D.F. DOERR & V. A. CONVERTINO. 1996. Application of acute maximal exercise to protect orthostatic tolerance after simulated microgravity. Am. J. Physiol. **271** (Regul. Integr. Comp. Physiol. **40**): R837–R847.
26. FRITSCH, J M., J.B. CHARLES, B.S. BENNETT, et al. 1992. Short-duration spaceflight impairs human carotid baroreceptor-cardiac reflex responses. J. Appl. Physiol. **73**(2): 664–671.
27. CRANDALL, C.G., K.A. ENGELKE, V.A. CONVERTINO & P.B. RAVEN. 1994. Aortic baroreflex control of heart rate after 15 days of simulated microgravity. J. Appl. Physiol. **77**(5): 2134–2139.
28. FRITSCH-YELLE, J.M., P.A. WHITSON, R.L. BONDAR & T. E. BROWN. 1996. Subnormal norepinephrine release relates to presyncope in astronauts after spaceflight. J. Appl. Physiol. **81**: 2134–2141.
29. SHOEMAKER, J.K., C.S. HOGEMAN & L. SINOWAY. 2000. Contributions of MSNA and stroke volume to orthostatic intolerance following bed rest. Am. J. Physiol. **277** (Regul. Integr. Comp. Physiol. **46**): R1084–R1090.
30. MARTEL, E., P. LACOLLEY, P. CHAMPEROUX, et al. 1994. Early disturbance of baroreflex control of heart rate after tail suspension in conscious rats. Am. J. Physiol. **267** (Heart Circ. Physiol. **36**): H2407–H2412.
31. BRIZZEE, B.L. & B.R. WALKER. 1990. Altered baroreflex function after tail suspension in the conscious rat. J. Appl. Physiol. **69**(6): 2091–2096.

32. FAGETTE, S., M. LO, C. GHARIB & G. GAUQUELIN. 1995. Cardiovascular variability and baroreceptor reflex sensitivity over a 14-day tail suspension in rats. J. Appl. Physiol. **78**(2): 717–724.
33. MCDONALD, K.S., M.D. DELP & R.H. FITTS. 1992. Fatigability and blood flow in the rat gastrocnemius-plantaris-soleus after hindlimb suspension. J. Appl. Physiol. **73**(3): 1135–1140.
34. WOODMAN, C.R., L.A. SEBASTIAN & C.M. TIPTON. 1994. Influence of simulated microgravity on regional sympathetic nervous system activity during heavy submaximal exercise. (Abstr.) FASEB J. **8**: A262.
35. MOFFITT, J.A., C.M. FOLEY, J.C. SCHADT, et al. 1998 Attenuated baroreflex control of sympathetic nerve activity after cardiovascular deconditioning in rats. Am. J. Physiol. **274** (Regul. Integr. Comp. Physiol. **43**): R1397–R1405.
36. JASPERS, S.R. & M.E. TISCHLER. 1984. Atrophy and growth failure of rat hindlimb muscles in tail-cast suspension. J. Appl. Physiol. **57**(5): 1472–1479.
37. KENT, B.B., J.W. DRANE, B. BLUMENSTEIN & J.W. MANNING. 1972. A mathematical model to assess changes in the baroreceptor reflex. Cardiology **57**: 295–310.
38. SCHADT, J.C. & J. LUDBROOK. 1991. Hemodynamic and neurohumoral responses to acute hypovolemia in conscious animals. Am. J. Physiol. (Heart Circ. Physiol.) **260**: H305–H318.
39. HASSER, E.M., J.A. MOFFITT, J.A. SMITH, et al. 1998. Response to hemorrhage in hindlimb unloaded rats. (Abstr.) FASEB J. **12**: A693.
40. SCHILTZ, J.C., G.E. HOFFMAN, E.M. STRICKER & A.F. SVED. 1997. Decreases in arterial pressure activate oxytocin neurons in conscious rats. Am. J. Physiol. Regul. Comp. Physiol. **273**: R1474–R1483.
41. HASSER, E.M., M.J. SULLIVAN & J.T. CUNNINGHAM. 2000. Reflex control of vasopressin release following hindlimb unloading. (Abstr.) Soc. Neurosci. In Press.
42. ZHANG, L.-F. 1994. Experimental studies on effects of simulated weightlessness on myocardial function and structure. J. Gravit. Pysiol. **1**: 133–136.
43. MOFFITT, J.A., J.C. SCHADT & E.M. HASSER. 1999. Central nervous system dysfunction following cardiovascular deconditioning. Am. J. Physiol. **277** (Heart Circ. Physiol. **6**): H2280–H2289.
44. SELLER, H. 1991. Central baroreceptor reflex pathways. In Baroreceptor Reflexes. P.B. Persson & H.R. Kirchheim, Eds.: 45–74. Springer-Verlag. Berlin.
45. DAMPNEY, R.A.L. 1994. Functional organization of central pathways regulating the cardiovascular system. Physiol. Rev. **74**: 323–364.
46. MOFFITT, J.A., E.M. HASSER, K.S. CURTIS, et al. 1998. Attenuated cFos expression in the rostral ventrolateral medulla (RVLM) of hindlimb unloaded rats after hydralazine treatment. (Abstr.) FASEB J. **12**: A63.
47. DRAGUNOW, M. & R. FAULL. 1989. The use of c-fos as a metabolic marker in neuronal pathway tracing. J. Neurosci. Methods **29**: 261–265.
48. DAMPNEY, R.A.L. 1994. The subretrofacial vasomotor nucleus: anatomical, chemical and pharmacological properties and role in cardiovascular regulation. Prog. Neurobiol. **42**: 197–227.
49. GUYENET, P.G. 1990. Role of the ventral medulla oblongata in blood pressure regulation. In Central Regulation of Autonomic Functions. A.D. Loewy & K.M. Spyer, Eds.: 145–167. Oxford University Press. New York.
50. MEDINA, A., N. BODICK, A.L. GOLDBERGER, et al. 1997. Effects of central muscarinic-1 receptor stimulation on blood pressure regulation. Hypertension **29**: 828–834.
51. ROSS, C.A., D.A. RUGGIERO, D.H. PARK, et al. 1984. Tonic vasomotor control by the rostral ventrolateral medulla: effect of electrical or chemical stimulation of the area containing c1 adrenaline neurons on arterial pressure, heart rate, and plasma catecholamines and vasopressin. J. Neurosci. **4**: 474–494.
52. MORRISON, S.F. & D.J. REIS. 1991. Responses of sympathetic preganglionic neurons to rostral ventrolateral medullary stimulation. Am. J. Physiol. **261** (Regul. Integr. Comp. Physiol. **30**): R1247–R1256.
53. LI, Y.-W., Z.J. GIEROBA, R.M. MCALLEN & W.W. BLESSING. 1991. Neurons in rabbit caudal ventrolateral medulla inhibit bulbospinal barosensitive neurons in rostral medulla. Am. J. Physiol. **261** (Regul. Integr. Comp. Physiol. **30**): R44–R51.

54. SMITH, J.K. & K.W. BARRON. 1990. GABAergic responses in ventrolateral medulla in spontaneously hypertensive rats. Am. J. Physiol. **258** (Regul. Integr. Comp. Physiol. **27**): R450–R456.
55. ITO, S. & A. F. SVED. 1996. Blockade of angiotensin receptors in rat rostral ventrolateral medulla removes excitatory vasomotor tone. Am. J. Physiol. **270** (Regul. Integr. Comp. Physiol. **39**): R1317–R1323.
56. ITO, S. & A.F. SVED. 1997. Tonic glutamate-mediated control of rostral ventrolateral medulla and sympathetic vasomotor tone. Am. J. Physiol. **273** (Regul. Integr. Comp. Physiol. **42**): R487–R494.
57. MOFFITT, J.A., C.M. HEESCH & E.M. HASSER. 1998. Increased GABAergic influence on rostral ventrolateral medulla neurons following hindlimb unloading. (Abstr.) SFN **24:** 372.
58. MOFFITT, J.A., C.M. HEESCH & E.M. HASSER. 1999. GABA$_A$ influences on the rostral ventrolateral medulla (RVLM) following hindlimb unloading. (Abstr.) FASEB J. **13:** A124.

# Dynamic Modulation of Baroreflex Sensitivity in Health and Disease

GIANFRANCO PARATI, MARCO DI RIENZO, AND GIUSEPPE MANCIA

*Istituto Scientifico Ospedale San Luca, Istituto Auxologico Italiano, 20149 Milano, Italy*

*LaRC, Centro di Bioingengeria, Fondazione Pro Juventute, Milano, Italy*

*Centro di Fisiologia Clinica e Ipertensione, Ospedale Maggiore, Milano, Italy*

*Clinica Medica, Università di Milano-Bicocca, Ospedale San Gerardo, Monza, Milano, Italy*

ABSTRACT: Assessment of arterial baroreflex function in humans through laboratory tests has provided a great deal of information of pathophysiological and clinical relevance. Indeed, the sensitivity of the baroreceptor–heart rate reflex quantified through these laboratory methods was shown to predict the risk of cardiovascular events and death from myocardial infarction, heart failure, and in diabetic patients. This traditional approach, however, does not provide information on daily life baroreflex cardiovascular control. Modern techniques, based on computer analysis of spontaneous blood pressure and heart rate fluctuations, are now available and allow baroreflex sensitivity to be assessed under real-life conditions with no need for external stimulation. In particular, these methods offer the possibility of investigating the dynamic modulation of baroreflex sensitivity occurring either on a minute-to-minute basis or over 24 hours.

KEYWORDS: Arterial baroreflex; Sequence technique; Spectral analysis; Blood pressure variability; Heart rate variability; Essential hypertension; Acute myocardial infarction

The arterial baroreflex is a mechanism of fundamental importance for cardiovascular homeostasis, and its impairment may play an adverse role in several diseases.[1–5] The clinical relevance of a baroreflex dysfunction, particularly alterations in arterial baroreflex control of heart rate, is supported by the evidence of an inverse relation between baroreflex sensitivity and the risk of mortality after myocardial infarction[3–9] and also by studies showing that interventions that improve baroreflex sensitivity (BRS), such as physical training[8,10] or β-adrenergic receptor blockade,[1,7,11] may also beneficially influence a patient's prognosis.[7,8]

The evidence for this has been obtained mostly through laboratory methods aimed at assessing arterial baroreflex function through the application of an external

Address for correspondence: Dr. Gianfranco Parati, Istituto Scientifico Ospedale San Luca, Istituto Auxologico Italiano, via Spagnoletto, 3 20149 Milano, Italy. Voice: +39-02-582161; fax +39-02-058216712.

gianfranco.parati@unimib.it

parati@auxologico.it

**TABLE 1. Laboratory methods for assessing baroreflex sensitivity in humans**[a]

| |
|---|
| Carotid sinus massage |
| Electrical stimulation of carotid sinus nerves |
| Anesthesia of carotid sinus nerves and vagi |
| Occlusion of common carotid artery |
| Valsalva maneuver |
| Head-up tilting |
| Lower body negative pressure application |
| Intravenous bolus injection of vasoactive agents with no (or little) direct effect on the heart |
| Intravenous stepwise infusion of vasoactive agents |
| Assessment of reflex changes in muscle sympathetic nerve activity induced by BP changes following vasoactive drug infusion |
| Neck chamber technique |

[a]From Parati et al.[23] Reproduced by permission.

stimulus to the subject under evaluation. These techniques, which provide a "spot" quantification of baroreflex sensitivity obtained under standardized conditions, include relatively nonspecific tests such as the Valsalva maneuver,[12] head-up tilting, lower body negative pressure application, and more specific methods such as the intravenous injection of vasoactive drugs with little or no direct effect on the heart, and a number of neck chamber devices. (TABLE 1). The intravenous (i.v.) bolus injection of a small dose of a pressor agent free from any major direct effect on the heart was one of the pioneering methods used to assess the sensitivity of baroreflex control of heart rate in humans. Smyth and coworkers used angiotensin II (later substituted with the more vasoselective agent phenylephrine) to increase systolic blood pressure and reflexively lengthen pulse interval. According to this popular method, the slope of the regression line fitting the systolic blood pressure and the reflex pulse interval changes (usually with a lag of one beat) is taken as a measure of BRS (expressed in ms/mmHg). The same approach was later employed to assess BRS when pulse interval was shortened following a reduction in systolic blood pressure induced by an i.v. bolus injection of a vasodilator agent such as nitroglycerine.[1,13,14] The disadvantages of this method are that only the reflex heart rate responses can be quantified, and the responses almost entirely depend on baroreflex modulation of parasympathetic control of the heart, since they are virtually abolished by atropine.[1] Its advantages include a greater methodological simplicity compared to head-up tilting and lower body negative pressure application and a higher specificity, as shown by the disappearance of the reflex heart rate responses following baroreceptor denervation in animals.[3,4,6,15,16] A later version of this technique is the "steady state" method proposed by Korner et al.,[17] which is based on a prolonged infusion of either a vasopressor (e.g., phenylephrine) or a vasodepressor (e.g., sodium nitroprusside) agent to induce stepwise and sustained increases or reductions in blood pressure, respectively, and plateau reflex changes in heart rate.

A common drawback of all drug injection-based methods is that the injected drugs may modify the tension of smooth muscle cells in the carotid and aortic walls, thereby altering baroreceptor activity not only through changes in blood pressure but also through unquantifiable mechanical distortion.[18] Another drawback is that all vasoactive drugs currently employed may stimulate other receptor populations (e.g., cardiopulmonary receptors); may act also in the central nervous system, thus altering autonomic control and baroreflex sensitivity; or may exert a direct stimulating effect on the sinus node.[19] The vasoactive drug infusion can also be used to assess reflex changes in muscle sympathetic nerve activity, thus allowing the sensitivity of the baroreflex control of efferent muscle sympathetic nerve activity to be quantified.[20] The neck chamber technique[1,21,22] consists of the use of a rigid chamber sealed around the subject's neck, in which the air pressure is increased or reduced in a graded fashion, resulting into graded and quantifiable reductions or increases in carotid transmural pressure. The key advantage of this method is that it allows not only heart rate but also blood pressure modulation by arterial baroreceptors to be specifically investigated. Its major disadvantage is that only carotid baroreceptor function is assessed, and the effect of carotid baroreceptor involvement is counteracted by the aortic baroreflex.[23] An additional disadvantage is that pressure changes produced within a neck chamber are not fully transmitted through the neck tissues to the carotid baroreceptors, the rate of transmission being about 80% for positive and only about 60% for negative pressure application.[22,24] Finally, correct use of a neck chamber device requires careful training of the subject under investigation, in order to prevent possible emotional reactions to the applied changes in pneumatic pressure around the neck, which might blunt the reflex changes in heart rate and blood pressure. Nevertheless, with this method important information on the sensitivity of baroreflex control of blood pressure and systemic vascular resistance, as well as on its resetting under conditions of normal and high blood pressure, has been obtained.[1,25,26] It has further allowed us to demonstrate that baroreflex alterations in

**TABLE 2. Advantages and limitations of laboratory methods for assessing baroreflex sensitivity in humans[a]**

**Advantages**

    Assessment of baroreflex function under standardized and controlled conditions

    Information of proved physiological and clinical value provided

**Limitations**

    Data collected in an artificial and at times stressful laboratory environment

    Only spot quantifications of baroreflex sensitivity obtained

    No information on daily life behavioral modulation of baroreflex sensitivity

    Most stimuli are not specific for the baroreflex

    Nonphysiological nature of laboratory stimuli (baroreflex function explored over a much wider range of stimulus intensities than that associated with spontaneous blood pressure fluctuations)

    A closed-loop mechanism such as the baroreflex assessed in a quasi-open-loop condition (i.e., by assuming the the SBP effects on RR interval are not simultaneously accompanied by effects of RR interval on SBP)

    Limited reproducibility of the responses to most laboratory methods

[a]From Parati *et al.*[23] Reproduced by permission.

disease may have different effects on the control of heart rate and vascular resistance.[1,2,26] More recently, computer-operated application of sinusoidal changes in
pneumatic pressure around the neck at variable frequencies has allowed us to develop a deeper insight into the role of the arterial baroreflex in the genesis of blood pressure fluctuations obtained.[27] The advantages and disadvantages of the above-
mentioned laboratory methods are summarized in TABLE 2.[28,29]

## MODERN TECHNIQUES FOR THE ANALYSIS OF SPONTANEOUS BAROREFLEX MODULATION OF HEART RATE

An important step forward in the investigation of the arterial baroreflex in humans has been achieved by the development of techniques that analyze the sensitivity of "spontaneous" baroreflex control of heart rate.[28,30] These techniques do not
require any external intervention with the subject under evaluation. Moreover, they
can be used not only to assess BRS in standardized laboratory conditions, but also
to investigate the dynamic features of baroreflex modulation of heart rate in daily
life.[28,30,31] These methods, which are listed in TABLE 3, are all based on the combined computer analysis of spontaneous blood pressure and heart rate fluctuations,
thereby allowing us to assess the baroreflex as it operates in response to blood pressure variations spontaneously occurring in daily life. This justifies the use of the
term "spontaneous baroreflex" function when referring to the data so obtained.[32]
From among the methods most commonly employed for spontaneous baroreflex
analysis, in this paper we focus on the "sequence technique," the spectral method
based on calculation of the "α coefficient," and the methods based on mathematical
modeling, through autoregressive and moving average techniques (ARMA) of the
mutual interactions between systolic blood pressure and RR interval that physiologically occur under closed-loop conditions.

### The Sequence Method

The "sequence" method is based on the computer identification in the time domain of spontaneously occurring sequences of four or more consecutive beats, characterized by either a progressive rise in systolic blood pressure and lengthening of
RR interval (+RR/+SBP sequences) or by a progressive decrease in systolic blood
pressure and shortening of RR interval (−RR/−SBP sequences; FIG. 1).[11,23,33–39]

**TABLE 3. Methods for assessing spontaneous baroreflex function[a]**

Sequence technique (sequences of beats where spontaneous SBP changes are coupled
with baroreflex-mediated RR interval changes)

RR interval–SBP cross correlation

Modulus of RR interval–SBP transfer function at 0.1 Hz

Squared ratio of RR interval/SBP spectral powers at 0.1 and 0.3 Hz ("α" coefficient)

Closed-loop RR interval–SBP transfer function (ARMA modeling)

Statistical dependence of RR interval on SBP fluctuations

[a]From Parati et al.[23] Reproduced by permission.

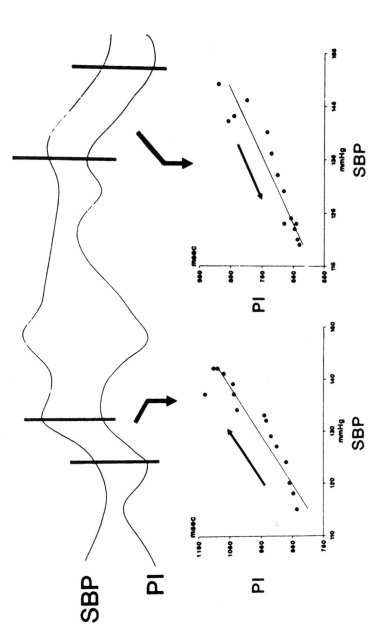

**FIGURE 1.** Scheme illustrating the method for spontaneous baroreflex analysis based on assessment of hypertension/bradycardia and hypotension/tachycardia sequences. In the **upper panel** a schematic drawing exemplifies changes in systolic blood pressure (SBP) and pulse interval (PI, the reciprocal of heart rate) as a function of time (on the horizontal axis). The corresponding regression lines between changes in SBP and changes in PI are also shown in the **lower panels**. (From Parati *et al.*[28] Reproduced by permission.)

The slope of the regression line between systolic blood pressure and RR interval values within any of these sequences is taken as an index of the sensitivity of the arterial baroreflex modulation of heart rate (BRS), as is done in the laboratory method based on i.v. injection of vasoactive drugs. The sequence technique has the advantage of allowing separate assessment of the reflex effects of daily life increases and of reductions in systolic blood pressure, and thus of the effects of spontaneously occurring baroreceptor stimulation and deactivation. The sequence method is based on relatively strict threshold criteria (only sequences of at least a four-beat duration are considered, and this is done only if consecutive SBP and RR interval changes are equal to or greater than a preselected threshold, usually 1 mmHg and 5 ms, respectively), and therefore the assessment of BRS is characterized by a remarkable specificity. The correlation coefficients between SBP and PI values within a sequence were invariably found to be higher than 0.85. The experimental demonstration that the RR interval changes observed in each sequence in response to the spontaneous changes in SBP are actually dependent on the baroreflex has been provided in cats by showing the almost complete disappearance of these sequences after sino-aortic denervation (SAD).[34] The specificity of spontaneous beat-by-beat interactions between systolic blood pressure and RR interval within a sequence in reflecting baroreflex influences rather than chance coupling was further supported by the data obtained via surrogate data analysis,[40] that is, by comparing a set of biological SBP and RR interval data with isospectral and isodistribution surrogate data sets. Finally, the sequence technique has been compared in individual subjects with laboratory methods based on i.v. injection of phenylephrine or nitroglycerine.[28,32,41] In most cases high correlation coefficients between the average estimates of BRS obtained through the two techniques were found. The absolute figures of BRS quantified by the two methods were not superimposable, however, presumably because the aspects of the baroreflex influences on the sinus node they address are somewhat different.[23,28,30,32,40] For example, as mentioned above, vasoactive drugs can induce changes in the mechanical properties of the arterial wall where baroreceptors are located, which may interfere with physiological baroreceptor stimulation (thereby resulting in a greater stimulus for reflex changes in heart rate at any given blood pressure alteration as compared with spontaneously occurring systolic blood pressure changes of the same magnitude).[41,42] It is also well known that BRS is different at the extremes compared to that around the linear portion of the stimulus–response curve encompassing the set point. Indeed, a theoretical advantage of the drug injection methods is the possibility of quantifying BRS in different portions of the stimulus–response curve; this advantage, however, is seldom exploited, because the current application of this technique is based on the computation of BRS over a wide range of blood pressure values, including those around the set point and those approaching baroreceptor saturation and threshold. Conversely, because the blood pressure changes characterizing a sequence are usually small, this method, in most instances, does not provide a "full-range" analysis of BRS.[23,32] Differences between the results obtained by these two methods for assessing the baroreflex should thus be expected, and their use should be regarded not as an alternative but as complementary approaches to evaluating baroreflex function. A much better agreement between these methods can be found when the reflex RR interval lengthening in response to SBP increases induced by phenylephrine and the reflex RR interval

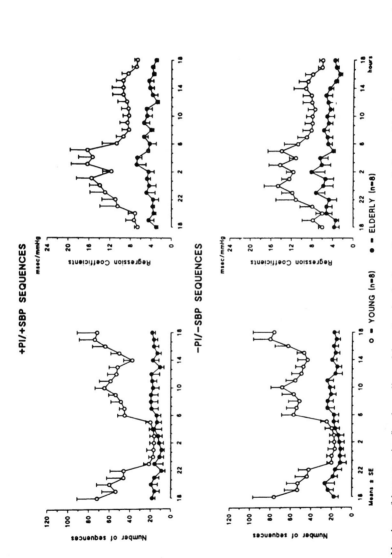

**FIGURE 2.** Number of hypertension/bradycardia and hypotension/tachycardia sequences (**left panels**) and sequence regression coefficients (**right panels**). Data are shown as average hourly values (±SE) for a group of young and a group of elderly individuals. (From Parati *et al.*[36] Reproduced by permission.)

shortening in response to SBP reductions induced by nitroglycerine are both considered, and the tangent to the sigmoidal baroreflex curve so obtained at a point corresponding to subject's resting blood pressure level is drawn. In such a case, the BRS values provided by the sequence slope and those provided by computing the slope of the tangent to the whole sigmoidal baroreflex curve obtained by the vasoactive drug bolus injection methods were almost identical.[32]

The results provided by the studies in which the sequence technique has been employed under daily life conditions have documented the high degree of variability that physiologically characterizes BRS under different behavioral conditions.[11,23,32–39] Variations in BRS are particularly pronounced when the sleep–wakefulness cycle is taken into account. The typical pattern of spontaneous baroreflex modulation of heart rate over 24 hours obtained in separate groups of young and elderly subjects is shown in FIGURE 2. Besides the occurrence of a minute-to-minute variability, BRS in young persons showed a clear-cut fluctuation between day and night, with the lowest values during the day and the highest values during the night. In elderly subjects, BRS was not only on average lower than in young persons over the whole 24-hour period, but it also displayed a loss of the physiological day–night difference. In part this may reflect a reduction in the degree of daytime physical activity with aging, but it may also be caused by a multifold impairment of baroreflex heart rate modulation in elderly subjects.[23,36]

### Recent Progress with the Sequence Technique

The sequence technique also allows us to quantify the number of times in daily life when the baroreflex is effective in overcoming nonbaroreflex influences acting on the sinus node (central neural influences, humoral factors, respiration, etc.). This is done by calculating the ratio between the number of +RR/+SBP or −RR/−SBP sequences and the total number of SBP ramp-like changes, in order to derive the so-called baroreflex effectiveness index (BEI). This index provides more specific information on baroreflex activation than the simple calculation of the number of sequences within any given recording period, as the latter may depend not only on the responsiveness of the baroreflex to spontaneous SBP fluctuations, but also on the degree of spontaneous SBP variability itself. In a preliminary application of this approach to 24 blood-pressure recordings, it was found that only a limited fraction of SBP ramp changes occurring over the 24 hours is coupled by baroreflex-mediated linear RR interval modulation, suggesting that the quantification of BEI adds important complementary information to BRS in the quantification of spontaneous baroreflex function.[43]

From a methodological point of view, it should be noticed that the sequence method requires beat-to-beat monitoring of SBP coupled with an ECG to obtain a precise assessment of RR interval–SBP relationships. If computer scanning of the BP signal is done at a sufficiently high sampling frequency and if the systolic peak of each BP waveform is reconstructed by interpolation, RR interval can be indirectly estimated from the blood pressure signal (by quantifying the interval between consecutive systolic peaks, i.e., the pulse interval) with a degree of accuracy that in most cases is comparable to that of RR interval detection from an ECG.[44,45] A further simplification of the technical requirements for application to humans of the sequence technique, as well as other modern techniques, is also possible because reliable

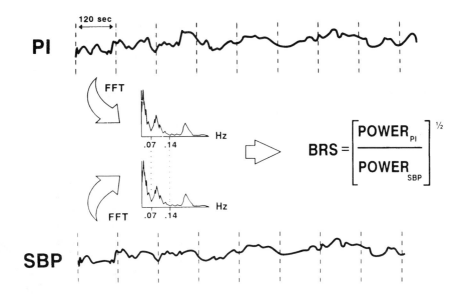

**FIGURE 3.** Schematic drawing illustrating how baroreflex sensitivity can be assessed in the frequency domain by calculation of the α coefficient. BRS: baroreflex sensitivity; SBP: systolic blood pressure; PI: pulse interval; FFT: fast Fourier transform. (From Parati *et al.*[23] Reproduced by permission.)

continuous SBP recordings, both at rest and under ambulatory conditions, can now be obtained from noninvasive devices.[46–49]

### The Spectral Technique (α Coefficient)

Previous observations[50,51] have led to the use of the spectral technique to assess spontaneous BRS on the basis of the subdivision of the recorded BP and RR interval signals into short segments, ranging from of 128 to 1024 beats. The quantification for each segment is accomplished by either the fast Fourier transform (FFT) or autoregressive modeling of the RR interval and SBP spectral powers in the frequency regions around 0.1 Hz (the so-called "low frequency" [LF]) and at the respiratory frequency (high frequency [HF], around 0.2 and 0.3 Hz). These regions have been selected because RR interval and SBP signals are linearly related, as is shown by their high coherence (>0.5). BRS is then calculated as the square root of the ratio between RR interval and SBP powers and is referred to as the "α coefficient," in the respective frequency regions (FIG. 3).[52,53] Similar to what has been done for the sequence method, the specificity of the spectral index of BRS has been assessed in conscious cats in which continuous blood pressure and heart rate recordings were obtained before and after sino-aortic denervation (SAD).[54,55] As expected, arterial baroreceptor denervation induced a reduction in overall RR interval variance that was particularly evident around 0.1 and 0.3 Hz. SBP spectral powers, conversely, changed differently in different frequency regions: SBP overall variance and the power of its very low frequency components increased, its power around 0.1 Hz markedly decreased, whereas the power around the respiratory frequency did not change. These modifications in SBP and RR interval powers were accompanied by a significant reduction of the α coefficient computed both for the 0.1 Hz (αLF) and the HF (αHF) regions. These observations thus validate the α coefficient as a measure of BRS in the frequency domain. Additional evidence supporting the assessment of BRS through calculation of the α coefficient has been obtained by demonstrating a relatively close correlation between α coefficient values and the estimates of BRS obtained by i.v. bolus injection of phenylephrine or nitroglycerine.[41,53]

Compared to the sequence technique, the interpretation of the α coefficient is more complex, however. First, when assessing the squared ratio of RR interval to SBP powers, the phase relationship between these variables is disregarded. Thus it cannot be taken for granted that the changes in RR interval associated with changes in SBP powers included in the calculation of the α coefficient are causally related. Second, the α coefficient is commonly computed by taking a high (>0.5) RR interval–SBP coherence value as a marker of RR–SBP coupling by the baroreflex. After SAD, however, the number of signal segments in which the HF coherence between RR interval and SBP powers was >0.5 remained high, although the magnitude of the RR spectral power was drastically reduced, as mentioned above. This indicates that in the HF band of the coupling between RR interval and SBP may also be due to non-baroreflex central or peripheral mechanisms.[55] This may lead to the provocative conclusion that high RR interval–SBP coherence may not necessarily guarantee a high specificity of the α coefficient in quantifying spontaneous BRS.

### Comparison of the Sequence and α Coefficient Methods

A common advantage of all the available methods for spontaneous baroreflex analysis is high reproducibility of the estimate of the average BRS that characterizes a given specific condition compared to traditional laboratory methods. At the same time, most of these methods provide detailed information on the physiological minute-to-minute variability of heart-rate baroreflex modulation. This advantage (see below) is particularly evident for the sequence technique, which allows the consideration of individual sequences of a few beats' duration, whereas for the calculation of the α coefficient a time window of at least 128 or 256 beats is required (see below). Besides this common advantage, the sequence and the spectral techniques are each characterized by a number of individual features.[23] The sequence approach makes use of spontaneous ramplike SBP transients, whereas the spectral approach focuses on SBP rhythmic oscillations. If we consider the frequency content of these patterns, it is evident that the αLF and αHF coefficients are estimates of the baroreflex response to SBP rhythmic modulations occurring at specific frequencies. This allows us to assess only the effects of vagal modulation when focusing on respiratory components (HF), or the effects of both sympathetic and parasympathetic modulation (with a predominance of the former in selected conditions) when focusing on the 0.1-Hz components.[56,57] On the other hand, the RR interval–SBP sequence technique focuses on BP and RR interval changes with a wider frequency content, and thus the

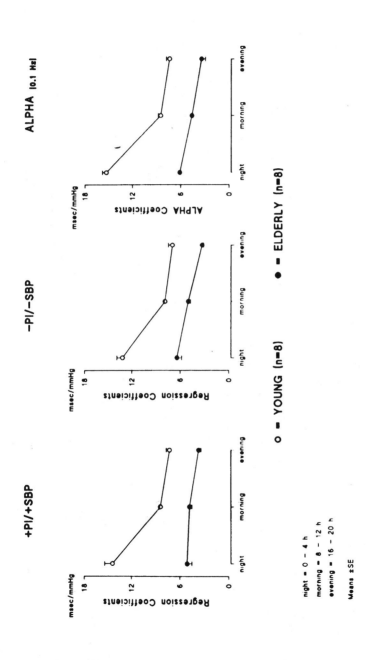

**FIGURE 4.** Time-domain and frequency-domain estimates of spontaneous baroreflex sensitivity. Data are shown as average values (±SE) of 4 hours selected in the morning, evening, and night for separate groups of 8 young and 8 elderly persons. **Left panel:** regression coefficients of hypertension/bradycardia sequences (+PI/+SBP); **middle panel:** regression coefficients of hypotension/tachycardia sequences (−PI/−SBP); **right panel:** α coefficients computed in the frequency region around 0.1 Hz. (From Parati *et al.*[36] Reproduced by permission.)

BRS estimation obtained by computing the sequence slope is a sort of "comprehensive" index of the baroreflex control of heart rate averaged over several frequencies.

Moreover, the RR interval–SBP sequences occur unevenly over time, because they are related to daily-life behavior. In spite of their irregular occurrence, however, the number of RR–SBP baroreflex sequences observed over each hour of a 24-h blood-pressure recording is high enough to obtain reliable hourly BRS estimates, and thus provides a detailed estimation of the day–night BRS profile.[35]

On the other hand, the occurrence of rhythmic SBP oscillations at the respiratory frequency and around 0.1 Hz is much more regular, so that the spectral approach provides an even estimation of BRS throughout the recording period, even when short recording periods are considered.[42] A final difference is that the sequence method, at variance from the spectral one, offers a separate assessment of the reflex RR interval changes induced by baroreceptor stimulation (+RR/+SBP sequences) and baroreceptor deactivation (−RR/−SBP sequences), which can be of interest in clinical conditions such as the obstructive sleep apnea syndrome.[37]

In spite of the methodological differences described, the quantification of the BRS parameters based on computation of $\alpha$ coefficient (which is estimated over time windows of at least a few minutes, see above) is surprisingly similar to that obtained by the sequence method when averaging the data from three to four sequences. This is the case when assessing the effects of sino-aortic denervation in animals, after which either time-domain and frequency-domain indices of baroreflex sensitivity are markedly reduced.[30,34,55] This is also the case when comparing average BRS data obtained by time-domain- and frequency-domain-based methods in subjects of different ages[36,38] and in diabetic patients with or without laboratory evidence of autonomic dysfunction,[58] either over the 24 hours or over shorter recordings in a clinical environment (FIG. 4).

### Autoregressive, Moving Average Modeling Techniques

The modern approaches to the spontaneous baroreflex analysis discussed here derive BRS estimates from the direct quantification of the effects of SBP changes on RR interval changes, under the assumption that the whole RR variability, or at least the fraction of RR interval variability that is linearly related to SBP variability, depends on baroreflex mechanisms. Moreover, these techniques do not include in the calculation the consequences of the physiological closed-loop nature of the interaction between SBP and RR interval changes. Thus, to better cope with this complex interaction, other methods have been proposed that evaluate the arterial baroreflex function through mathematical modeling of cardiovascular regulatory mechanisms. In this instance, biological signals are used to identify the parameters of a preselected mathematical model of the baroreflex that might account for the inherent complexity of the closed-loop BP–RR interval interactions, where not only changes in BP induce reflex changes in RR interval (*BP→RR feedback*), but also where, at the same time, changes in RR interval are responsible for changes in BP mediated through changes in cardiac output (*RR→BP feedforward*). The picture is even more complex if we consider that BP values at any given time point also depend on the BP values at previous times, this also being the case for HR values. Finally, BP and HR values are

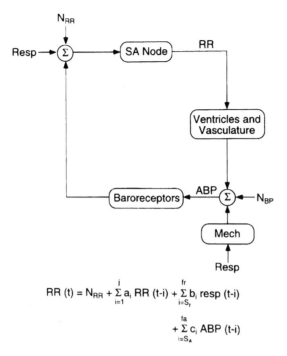

$$RR\,(t) = N_{RR} + \sum_{i=1}^{j} a_i\, RR\,(t\text{-}i) + \sum_{i=S_r}^{fr} b_i\, resp\,(t\text{-}i)$$

$$+ \sum_{i=S_A}^{fa} c_i\, ABP\,(t\text{-}i)$$

**FIGURE 5.** Schematic drawing illustrating the reciprocal interactions between blood pressure (BP) and heart rate (HR) fluctuations, including the reflex effects of BP on HR (baroreflex feedback) and the mechanical effects of HR on BP (mechanical feedforward). NBP and NHR refer to "noise" factors (i.e., factors independent of HR and BP) respectively acting on BP and HR. (From Parati *et al.*[28] Reproduced by permission.)

simultaneously affected by respiratory activity as well as by a number of other external or internal influences considered as "noise" factors, that is, factors not specifically accounted for in the model (FIG. 5).[23,59] Once a mathematical model has been analytically defined in order to take all the considered mechanisms into account, the gain of the transfer function between systolic blood pressure and heart rate (a quantification of baroreflex sensitivity), as well as the delay and the time constants that characterize baroreflex control of cardiovascular variables, can be derived by proper handling of the equations that describe the model. The accuracy of these estimates depends on how well the unavoidable simplifications inherent in the mathematical model fit the physiological complexity of cardiovascular control mechanisms.

An example of these models is represented by the method based on a closed-loop analysis that simultaneously considers the BP→RR interval feedback, the RR interval→BP feedforward, the effects of previous BP or RR interval values on their respective values actually measured at a given time point, and the concomitant effects of respiration on both BP and RR interval variability, by a trivariate *autoregressive moving average* (ARMA) approach applied to the analysis of continuous BP, RR interval, and respiratory activity recordings.[59,60]

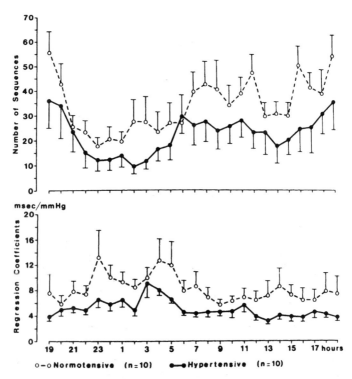

**FIGURE 6.** Hourly number of hypertension/bradycardia sequences (+PI/+SBP) **(upper panel)** and hourly values of the regression coefficients of these sequences **(lower panel)**. Data are shown as average values (±SE) for a group of 10 normotensive and a group of 10 hypertensive persons. (From Parati *et al.* [23] Reproduced here as modified by permission).

## SPONTANEOUS BAROREFLEX SENSITIVITY IN
## HEALTH AND DISEASE

Data obtained by either time and frequency domain methods for assessing spontaneous BRS have provided a large body of information on daily life baroreflex function in health and disease. They have offered detailed evidence on the fast and marked changes in BRS associated with changes in behavioral conditions as well as in particular situations such as under general anesthesia during surgery.[23,28] Analysis of 24-h ambulatory beat-to-beat blood pressure recordings by these techniques has also allowed the description of the day and night reduction in BRS in hypertensive or aged subjects compared to normotensive or young persons[35,36] (FIG. 6 and FIG. 2). These methods have been particularly helpful in demonstrating that aging is responsible not only for a reduction in average BRS values, but also for the loss of the physiological day–night modulation in the effectiveness of baroreflex heart rate modulation, an alteration that reaches its maximal severity in patients with primary autonomic failure.[61] Finally, the specificity and sensitivity of these techniques have

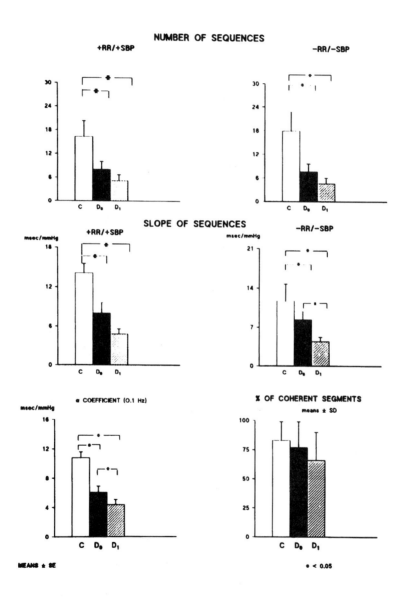

**FIGURE 7.** Time- and frequency-domain estimates of the baroreceptor–heart rate reflex in control subjects (C) ($n = 24$) and diabetic patients without (D0) ($n = 20$) or with (D1) ($n = 32$) autonomic dysfunction in classical laboratory tests. *$p < 0.05$. (From Frattola *et al.*[58] Reproduced by permission.)

provided data on the impairment of BRS associated with cigarette smoking (an impairment that escapes recognition when traditional laboratory methods are employed)[54] and on the changes in baroreflex function that characterize patients with obstructive sleep apnea syndrome.[37]

Assessment of spontaneous BRS has also been performed in diabetic patients with or without clinical evidence of autonomic dysfunction, as documented by the classical Ewing tests. The results have shown that both time and frequency domain methods can identify very early impairment of baroreflex control of heart rate at a time when traditional laboratory tests still yield normal results[58] (FIG. 7), emphasizing the superiority of these techniques over traditional laboratory procedures in the early detection of autonomic abnormalities, which may carry a higher risk of morbidity and mortality.[38,62]

## CONCLUSIONS

The data summarized in this brief review article have clearly shown that different methods for assessing BRS in humans may offer different and complementary perspectives on cardiovascular autonomic control. In fact, there is probably no gold standard among methods for assessing baroreflex sensitivity, either in the laboratory or in daily life, as each of them focuses on specific aspects of baroreflex cardiovascular modulation. It should be emphasized, however, that modern techniques for spontaneous baroreflex analysis have more recently provided us with a much deeper insight into the features of daily-life baroreflex control of heart rate,[23,31,35,51,53,59,63] adding to the information provided over the last 40 years by classical laboratory methods. In spite of their important advantages, techniques for spontaneous baroreflex sensitivity assessment also have some limitations. One of them is that, by focusing on arterial baroreflex control of heart rate, they cannot provide direct information on spontaneous baroreflex control of sympathetic activity, peripheral resistance, and blood pressure, unless complex mathematical models are developed.

Moreover, whether the richer amount of information provided by methods for the assessment of spontaneous baroreflex sensitivity might further improve the prognostic evaluation of patients with diseases characterized by an impairment of autonomic cardiovascular control needs to be tested in large-scale longitudinal studies.

## REFERENCES

1. MANCIA, G. & A.L. MARK. 1983. Arterial baroreflexes in humans. *In* J.T. Shepherd & F.M. Abboud, Eds.: 755–793. Handbook of Physiology, Section 2: The Cardiovascular System IV, Vol.3, part 2. American Physiologic Society. Bethesda, MD.
2. MANCIA, G., G. GRASSI & A.U. FERRARI. 1997. Reflex control of the circulation in experimental and human hypertension. *In* Handbbok of Hypertension, Vol. 17. Pathophysiology of Hypertension. A. Zanchetti & G. Mancia, Eds.: 568–601. Elsevier Science B.V. Amsterdam.
3. BRISTOW, J.D., A.J. HONOUR, G.W. PICKERING, *et al.* 1969. Diminished baroreflex sensitivity in high blood pressure. Circulation **39:** 48–54.
4. OSCULATI, G., G. GRASSI, C. GIANNATTASIO, *et al.* 1990. Early alterations of the baroreceptor control of heart rate in patients with acute myocardial infarction. Circulation **81:** 939–948.

5. ECKBERG, D., M. DRABINSKI & E. BRAUNWALD. 1971. Defective cardiac parasympathetic control in patients with heart disease. N. Engl. J. Med. **285:** 877–883.
6. SCHWARTZ, P.J., A. ZAZA, M. PALA, *et al.* 1988. Baroreflex sensitivity and its evolution during the first year after acute myocardial infarction. J. Am. Coll. Cardiol. **12:** 629–636.
7. LA ROVERE, M.T., T.J. BIGGER, F.I. MARCUS, *et al.* for the ATRAMI (Autonomic Tone and Reflexes After Myocardial Infarction) Investigators. 1998. Baroreflex sensitivity and heart rate variability in prediction of total cardiac mortality after myocardial infarction. Lancet **351:** 478–484.
8. HULL, S.S., E. VANOLI, P.B. ADAMSON, *et al.* 1994. Exercise training confers anticipatory protection from sudden death during acute myocardial ischemia. Circulation **89:** 548–552.
9. HOHNLOSER, S.H., T. KLINGENHEBEN, A. VAN DE LOO, *et al.* 1994. Reflex versus tonic vagal activity as a prognostic parameter in patients with sustained ventricular tachycardia and ventricular fibrillation. 1994. Circulation **89:** 1068–1073.
10. BILLMAN, G.E., P. J. SCHWARTZ & H.L. STONE. 1984. The effects of daily exercise on susceptibility to sudden cardiac death. Circulation **69:** 1182–1189.
11. PARATI, G., E. MUTTI, M. DI RIENZO, *et al.* 1994. Beta-adrenergic blocking treatment and 24-hour baroreflex sensitivity in essential hypertensive patients. Hypertension **23**(part 2): 992–996.
12. KORNER, P.I., A.M. TOMKIN & J.B. UTHER. 1976. Reflex and mechanical circulatory effects of graded Valsalva maneuvers in normal man. J. Appl. Physiol. **40:** 434–440.
13. SMYTH, H.S., P. SLEIGHT & G.W. PICKERING. 1969. Reflex regulation of arterial pressure during sleep in man: a quantitative method of assessing baroreflex sensitivity. Circ. Res. **24:** 109–121.
14. PICKERING, T.G., B. GRIBBIN & P. SLEIGHT. 1972. Comparison of the reflex heart rate responses to rising and falling arterial pressure in man. Cardiovasc. Res. **6:** 277–283.
15. LUDBROOK, J., I.B. FARIS, J. IANNOS & G. JAMIESON. 1980. Sine-wave evocation of the carotid baroreceptor reflex in conscious rabbits. *In* Arterial Baroreceptors and Hypertension. P. Sleight, Ed.: 39–44. Oxford University Press. Oxford, U.K.
16. GRIBBIN, B., T.G. PICKERING, P. SLEIGHT & R. PETO. 1971. Effect of age and high blood pressure on baroreflex sensitivity in man. Circ. Res. **29:** 424–431.
17. KORNER, P.I., M.J. WEST, J. SHAW & J.B. UTHER. 1974. "Steady-state" properties of the baroreceptor–heart rate reflex in essential hypertension in man. Clin. Exp. Pharmacol. Physiol. **1:** 65–76.
18. BERGEL, D.H., I.S. ANAND, D.E. BROOKS, *et al.* 1980. Carotid sinus nerve mechanics and baroreceptor function in the dog. *In* Arterial Baroreceptors and Hypertension. P. Sleight, Ed.: 1–5. Oxford University Press. Oxford, U.K.
19. MUSIALEK, P., M. LEI, H.F. BROWN, *et al.* 1997. Nitric oxide can increase heart rate by stimulating the hyperpolarization-activated inward current, I(f). Circ. Res. **81:** 60–68.
20. WALLYN, G.B. 1979. A quantitative study of muscle nerve sympathetic activity in resting normotensive and hypertensive subjects. Hypertension **1:** 67–77.
21. ECKBERG, D.L., M.S. CAVANAUGH, A.L. MARK & F.M. ABBOUD. 1975. A simplified neck suction device for activation of carotid baroreceptors. J. Lab. Clin. Med. **85:** 167–173.
22. LUDBROOK, J., G. MANCIA, A. FERRARI & A. ZANCHETTI. 1977. The variable neck-chamber method for studying the carotid baroreflex in man. Clin. Sci. Mol. Med. **53:** 165–171.
23. PARATI, G., M. DI RIENZO & G. MANCIA. 2000. How to measure baroreflex sensitivity: from the cardiovascular laboratory to daily life. J. Hypertens. **18:** 7–19.
24. PARATI, G. & G. MANCIA. 1992. The neck chamber technique. G. Ital. Cardiol. **22:** 511–516.
25. ECKBERG, D.L. 1979. Carotid baroreflex function in young men with borderline blood pressure elevation. Circulation **59:** 632–636.
26. MANCIA, G., J. LUDBROOK, A. FERRARI, *et al.* 1978. Baroreceptor reflexes in human hypertension. Circ. Res. **43:** 170–177.
27. BATH, E., L.E. LINDBLAD & B.G. WALLIN. 1981. Effects of dynamic and static neck suction on muscle nerve sympathetic activity, heart rate and blood pressure in man. J. Physiol. **311:** 551–564.

28. PARATI, G., S. OMBONI, A. FRATTOLA, et al. 1992. Dynamic evaluation of the barore-flex in ambulant subjects. In Blood Pressure and Heart Rate Variability. M. Di Rienzo, G. Mancia, G. Parati, et al., Eds.: 123–137. IOS Press. Amsterdam.

29. PARATI, G., G. POMIDOSSI, A.J. RAMIREZ, et al. 1985. Variability of the haemodynamic responses to laboratory tests employed in assessment of neural cardiovascular regulation in man. Clin. Sci. 69: 533–540.

30. PARATI, G., M. DI RIENZO, P. CASTIGLIONI, et al. 1995. Daily-life baroreflex modula-tion: new perspectives from computer analysis of blood pressure and heart rate vari-ability. In Computer Analysis of Cardiovascular Signals. M. Di Rienzo, G. Mancia, G. Parati, et al., Eds.: 209–218. IOS Press. Amsterdam.

31. PARATI, G., M. DI RIENZO & G. MANCIA. 1996. Neural cardiovascular regulation and 24-hour blood pressure and heart rate variability. In Time-Dependent Structure and Control of Arterial Blood Pressure. Ann. N.Y. Acad. Sci. 783: 47–63.

32. PARLOW, J., J.P. VIALE, G. ANNAT, et al. 1995. Spontaneous cardiac baroreflex in humans: comparison with drugs-induced responses. Hypertension 25: 1058–1068.

33. DI RIENZO, M., G. BERTINIERI, G. MANCIA & A. PEDOTTI. 1985. A new method for evaluating the baroreflex role by a joint pattern analysis of pulse interval and systolic blood pressure series. Med. Biol. Eng. Comput. 23(Suppl. I): 313–314.

34. BERTINIERI, G., M. DI RIENZO, A. CAVALLAZZI, et al. 1988. Evaluation of baroreceptors reflex by blood pressure monitoring in unanesthetized cats. Am. J. Physiol. 254: H377–H383.

35. PARATI, G., M. DI RIENZO, G. BERTINIERI, et al. 1988. Evaluation of the baroreceptor-heart rate reflex by 24-hour intra-arterial blood pressure monitoring in humans. Hypertension 12: 214–222.

36. PARATI, G., A. FRATTOLA, M. DI RIENZO, et al. 1995. Effects of aging on 24 hour dynamic baroreceptor control of heart rate in ambulant subjects. Am. J. Physiol. 268 (Heart Circ. Physiol. 37): H1606–H1612.

37. PARATI, G., M. DI RIENZO, M. BONSIGNORE, et al. 1997. Autonomic cardiac regulation in obstructive sleep apnea syndrome: evidence from spontaneous baroreflex analysis during sleep. J. Hypertens. 15: 1621–1626.

38. PARATI, G., M. DI RIENZO, P. CASTIGLIONI, et al. 1997. Spontaneous baroreflex sensi-tivity: from the cardiovascular laboratory to patient's bedside. In Frontiers of Blood Pressure and Heart Rate Analysis. M. Di Rienzo, G. Mancia, G. Parati, et al., Eds.: 219–240. IOS Press. Amsterdam.

39. IELLAMO, F., R.I. HUGHSON, F. CASTRUCCI, et al. 1994. Evaluation of spontaneous baroreflex modulation of sinus node during isometric exercise in healthy humans. Am. J. Physiol. 267(Heart Circ. Physiol. 36): H994–H1001.

40. BLEBER, A.B., Y. YAMAMOTO & R.L. HUGHSON. 1995. Methodology of spontaneous baroreflex relatioship assessed by surrogate date analysis. Am. J. Physiol. 268 (Heart Circ. Physiol. 37): H1682–H1687.

41. PITZALIS, M.V., F. MASTROPASQUA, A. PASSANTINO, et al. 1998. Comparison between noninvasive indices of baroreceptor sensitivity and the phenylephrine method in post-myocardial infarction patients. Circulation 97(14): 1362–1367.

42. DI RIENZO, M., G. PARATI, G. MANCIA, et al. 1997. Investigating baroreflex control of circulation using signal processing techniques. New approaches for evaluating the baroreflex function. IEEE Eng. Med. Biol. 10: 86–95.

43. DI RIENZO, M., G. PARATI, R. TORDI, et al. 1998. Developments in the analysis of spon-taneous baroreflex function. Proceedings of the Workshop on Computer Analysis of Blood Pressure and Heart Rate Variability. 20th Annual Conference of the IEEE Engineering in Medicine and Biology Society, Hong Kong. p. 5.

44. DI RIENZO, M., P. CASTIGLIONI, G. MANCIA, et al. 1989. Twenty-four-hour sequential spectral analysis of arterial blood pressure and pulse interval in free-moving sub-jects. IEEE Trans. 36: 1066–1075.

45. PARATI, G., P. CASTIGLIONI, M. DI RIENZO, et al. 1990. Sequential spectral analysis of 24-hour blood pressure and pulse interval in humans. Hypertension 16: 414–421.

46. PARATI, G., R. CASADEI, A. GROPPELLI, et al. 1989. Comparison of finger and intra-arterial blood pressure monitoring at rest and during laboratory testing. Hypertension 13: 647–655.

47. IMHOLZ, B.P.M., G. LANGEWOUTERS, G.A. VAN MONTFRANS, *et al.* 1993. Feasibility of ambulatory continuous 24-h finger arterial pressure recording. Hypertension **21:** 65–73.

48. OMBONI, S., G. PARATI, A. FRATTOLA, *et al.* 1993. Spectral and sequence analysis of finger blood pressure variability: comparison with analysis of intra-arterial recordings. Hypertension **22:** 22–26.

49. OMBONI, S., G. PARATI, P. CASTIGLIONI, *et al.* 1998. Estimation of blood pressure variability from 24-hour ambulatory finger blood pressure. Hypertension **32:** 52–58.

50. DE BOER, R.W., J.M. KAREMAKER & J. STRACKEE. 1987. Haemodynamic fluctuations and baroreflex sensitivity in humans: a beat-to-beat model. Am. J. Physiol. **253** (Heart Circ. Physiol. **22**): H680–H689.

51. ROBBE, H.W.J., L.J.M. MULDER, H. RUDDEL, *et al.* 1987. Assessment of baroreceptor reflex sensitivity by means of spectral analysis. Hypertension **10:** 538–543.

52. CERUTTI, S., G. BASELLI, S. CIVARDI, *et al.* 1987. Spectral analysis of heart rate and arterial blood pressure variability signals for physiological and clinical purposes. *In* Proceedings of Computers in Cardiology.: 435–438. IEEE Press. Los Alamitos, CA.

53. PAGANI, M., V. SOMERS, R. FURLAN, *et al.* 1988. Changes in autonomic regulation induced by physical training in mild hypertension. Hypertension **12:** 600–610.

54. DI RIENZO, M., P. CASTIGLIONI, G. PARATI, *et al.* 1996. Effects of sino-aortic denervation on spectral characteristics of blood pressure and pulse interval variability: a wide-band approach. Med. Biol. Eng. Comp. **34:** 133–141.

55. DI RIENZO, M., P. CASTIGLIONI, G. PARATI, *et al.* 1997. Critical appraisal of indices for the assessment of baroreflex sensitivity. Meth. Inform. Med. **36:** 246–249.

56. MALLIANI, A., M. PAGANI, F. LOMBARDI & S. CERUTTI. 1991. Cardiovascular neural regulation explored in the frequency domain. Circulation **84:** 482–492.

57. PAGANI, M., N. MONTANO, A. PORTA, *et al.* 1997. Relationship between spectral components of cardiovascular variabilities and direct measures of muscle sympathetic nerve activity in humans. Circulation **95:** 1441–1448.

58. FRATTOLA, A., G. PARATI, P. GAMBA, *et al.* 1997. Time and frequency domain estimates of spontaneous baroreflex sensitivity provide early detection of autonomic dysfunction in diabetes mellitus. Diabetologia **40:** 1470–1475.

59. PATTON, D.J., J.K. TRIEDMAN, M. PERROTT, *et al.* 1996. Baroreflex gain: characterization using autoregressive moving average analysis. Am. J. Physiol. **270**(Heart Circ. Physiol. **39**): H1240–H1249.

60. PARATI, G., J.P. SAUL, M. DI RIENZO & G. MANCIA. 1995. Spectral analysis of blood pressure and heart rate variability in evaluating cardiovascular regulation: a critical appraisal. Hypertension **25:** 1276–1286.

61. OMBONI, S., G. PARATI, M. DI RIENZO, *et al.* 1996. Spectral analysis of blood pressure and heart rate variability in autonomic disorders. Clin. Autonom. Res. **6:** 171–182.

62. MANCIA, G., F. PALEARI & G. PARATI. 1997. Early diagnosis of diabetic autonomic neuropathy: present and future approaches. Diabetologia **40:** 482–484.

63. CERUTTI, C., M. DUCHER, P. LANTELME, *et al.* 1995. Assessment of spontaneous baroreflex sensitivity in rats: a new method using the concept of statistical dependence. Am. J. Physiol. **268**(Regul. Integr. Comp. Physiol. **37**): R382–R388.

# Cardiorespiratory Interactions in Neural Circulatory Control in Humans

ABU S. M. SHAMSUZZAMAN AND VIREND K. SOMERS

*Divisions of Hypertension and Cardiovascular Diseases, Department of Internal Medicine, Mayo Clinic and Mayo Foundation, Rochester, Minnesota 55905, USA*

ABSTRACT: The reflex mechanisms and interactions described in this overview provide some explanation for the range of neural circulatory responses evident during changes in breathing. The effects described represent the integrated responses to activation of several reflex mechanisms, including peripheral and central chemoreflexes, arterial baroreflexes, pulmonary stretch receptors, and ventricular mechanoreceptors. These interactions occur on a dynamic basis and the transfer characteristics of any single interaction are, in all likelihood, also highly dynamic. Nevertheless, it is only by attempting to understand individual reflexes and their modulating influences that a more thorough understanding of the responses to complex phenomena such as hyperventilation, apnea, and obstructive sleep apnea can be better understood.

KEYWORDS: Chemoreflexes; Pulmonary afferents; Baroreflexes; Hypoxemia; Hyperventilation; Sleep apnea; Mueller maneuver

## INTRODUCTION

Neural control of the circulation represents the integrated response to diverse reflex, environmental, and homeostatic mechanisms. The interaction between cardiovascular and respiratory variables constitutes an important influence on neurally mediated changes in cardiac and vascular control. This brief review will seek to identify some of the key areas where interactions between the cardiovascular and respiratory systems result in distinct and functionally important changes in neural circulatory control. In particular, the specific effects of the chemoreflexes, pulmonary afferents, and baroreflexes will be examined, with an emphasis on the interactions between these. The implications of these interactions in conditions of hypoxemia, hyperventilation, and sleep apnea will also be addressed.

## CHEMOREFLEX RESPONSES TO HYPOXEMIA, HYPERCAPNIA, AND APNEA

The chemoreflexes exert profound influences not only on breathing, but also on cardiovascular function. Our current understanding of the stimuli, mechanisms, and

Address for correspondence: Virend K. Somers, M.D., Ph.D., Divisions of Hypertension and Cardiovascular Diseases, Department of Internal Medicine, Mayo Clinic and Mayo Foundation, 200 First Street SW, Rochester, MN 55905. Voice: 507-284-3591; fax: 507-284-1161.
somers.virend@mayo.edu

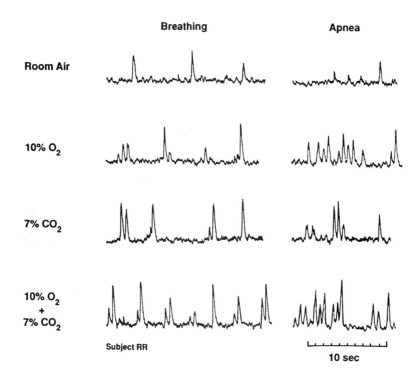

**FIGURE 1.** Direct intraneural recordings of sympathetic nerve activity measured during exposure to room air, isocapnic hypoxia (10% $O_2$/90% $N_2$ + titrated $CO_2$), hyperoxic hypercapnia (7% $CO_2$/93% $O_2$), and hypoxic hypercapnia (10% $O_2$/7% $CO_2$/83% $N_2$), during spontaneous breathing **(left)** and during end-expiratory apnea **(right)**. Sympathetic activity is a function of both burst frequency and burst amplitude. Three important points should be made: (1) sympathetic activity during breathing increased more with hypercapnia (7% $CO_2$) than with hypoxia (10% $O_2$); (2) apnea caused a markedly greater enhancement of sympathetic nerve activity during hypoxia (10% $O_2$) than during hypercapnia (7% $CO_2$); and (3) there was an additive effect of combined hypoxia and hypercapnia on sympathetic nerve activity. (Reproduced with permission from Somers *et al.*[4])

neural pathways involved in peripheral chemoreflex activation are summarized in an excellent recent review by Guyenet.[1] The central chemoreceptors are believed to be located on the ventral surface of the medulla and are less well understood. The influences of central chemoreceptors in cardiorespiratory control have also been covered in a recent and comprehensive review by Taylor *et al.*[2]

The peripheral chemoreflexes, located in the carotid bodies, respond primarily to hypoxemia and elicit hyperventilation, tachycardia, and increased sympathetic vaso-constrictor activity.[3,4] Hyperventilation in turn activates the pulmonary afferents, thereby inhibiting or buffering the sympathetic response to hypoxemia.[4] During apnea, when the inhibitory influence of the pulmonary afferents is eliminated, there is a striking potentiation of the sympathetic vasoconstrictor response to hypoxemia (FIGS. 1 and 2).[5]

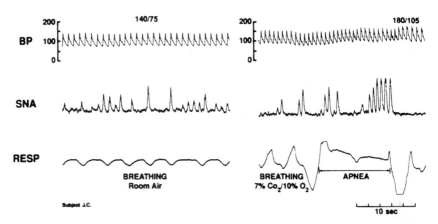

**FIGURE 2.** Intra-arterial blood pressure, sympathetic nerve activity, and respiration recorded in a subject while breathing room air **(left)** and during breathing and apnea when exposed to hypercapnic hypoxia (7% $CO_2$/10% $O_2$/83% $N_2$) **(right)**. Note the marked increase in blood pressure (from 140/75 mmHg during room air to a peak of 180/105 mmHg) and in sympathetic nerve activity with apnea during hypercapnic hypoxia (simulated sleep apnea). (Reproduced with permission from Somers *et al.*[5])

For purposes of understanding the cardiovascular components of peripheral chemoreceptor activation, it is important to recognize that cessation of breathing during apnea also elicits the primary cardiac response to peripheral chemoreflex activation, namely bradycardia (FIG. 3).[6,7] While slight cardiac slowing is evident in many normal subjects at the end of maximal voluntary apnea, the bradycardic response during apnea in FIGURE 3 represents an extreme of the distribution of cardiac responses to apnea in normal subjects. Note also that, in this subject, profound bradycardia during apnea was highly reproducible, even when tested over a year later. This response nevertheless serves to illustrate the simultaneous activation of vascular sympathetic and cardiac vagal drives. This combination of sympathetic vasoconstriction and vagal bradycardia constitutes part of what is generally understood as the diving reflex. This unique response incorporates simultaneous activation of *cardiac* vagal and *vascular* sympathetic responses. In effect, this diving reflex response redirects blood flow towards the heart and brain, two organs in which reflex sympathetic vasoconstriction during hypoxia and apnea does not occur.

Hypercapnia, acting primarily through the central chemoreceptors in the brain stem,[8] but also in part through the peripheral chemoreceptors, also triggers hyperventilation and increased sympathetic traffic to peripheral blood vessels (FIG. 1). Hypercapnia does not induce vagally mediated bradycardia as seen during hypoxia. Nevertheless, apnea during hypercapnia (with consequent elimination of hyperventilation) also results in potentiated sympathetic traffic, although this is less marked than is seen with hypoxemia. This differential interaction between ventilation and sympathetic activation, such that apnea during hypoxemia increases sympathetic drive more strikingly than does apnea during hypercapnia, may in part be the functional consequence of the anatomic proximity of the peripheral chemoreceptors and

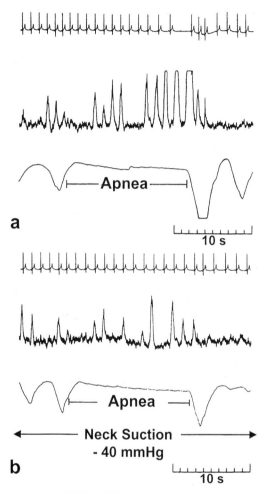

**FIGURE 3.** Recordings of SNA, ECG, and respiration showing **(a)** bradycardia and a-v block during apnea in a single patient (no. 1). Apnea during neck suction (baroreflex activation) **(b)**, however, results in an attenuated SNA response and less bradycardia, suggesting that baroreflex activation inhibits both sympathetic and parasympathetic responses to hypoxia. Neck suction alone induced slight cardiac slowing (data not shown). (Reproduced with permission from Somers *et al.*[5])

the pulmonary afferents, both synapsing in anatomically adjacent regions in the nucleus tractus solitarius.

When hypoxemia and hypercapnia are administered simultaneously in normal humans, there is a synergistic increase in minute ventilation.[9] Sympathetic activation is also greater than that induced by either of the individual stimuli alone. This enhanced response to the combined hypoxemic-hypercapnic stimulus is indicative of the potency of the chemoreflexes not only in increasing ventilation, but also in modulating neural circulatory control.

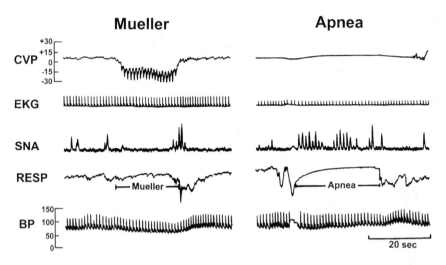

**FIGURE 4.** Recordings of central venous pressure (CVP), electrocardiogram (EKG), sympathetic nerve activity (SNA), respiration (RESP), and blood pressure (BP) during a Mueller maneuver as compared to end-expiratory apnea in the same subject. In contrast to apnea, the Mueller maneuver resulted in an initial profound suppression of sympathetic activity despite the fall in BP. SNA increased in the latter part of the Mueller maneuver. Release of both the Mueller maneuver and apnea resulted in increases in BP and sympathetic inhibition. CVP recordings for the period of apnea reflect the mean pressure levels. (Reproduced with permission from Somers *et al.*[5])

## THE MUELLER MANEUVER

Inspiration against a closed airway is also known as the Mueller maneuver. It is important that the reflex responses occurring during a Mueller maneuver be differentiated from those occurring during voluntary apnea. This is particularly true in understanding cardiorespiratory interactions during obstructed breathing, such as may occur during obstructive sleep apnea. In the setting of significant obstruction and potentiated respiratory drive, such as would occur during hypoxia and/or hypercapnia, inspiration against an obstructed airway can generate dramatic negative intrathoracic pressures resulting in distortion of cardiac configuration.[10,11] During 20 seconds of inspiration against a closed airway in normal subjects, the Mueller maneuver elicits substantial reductions in blood pressure with paradoxical decreases in sympathetic traffic and elimination of any increases in heart rate (Fig. 4). With maintenance of the Mueller maneuver over a full 20-second period, in the latter part of the Mueller maneuver, there is evidence for recovery of sympathetic traffic, heart rate, and blood pressure.

While it is not completely certain as to why sympathetic traffic, blood pressure, and heart rate are all reduced in the early phases of the Mueller maneuver, these responses would be consistent with activation of a depressor reflex. This reflex, possibly induced by increases in transmural cardiac pressure, distortion of the cardiac chambers, and activation of mechanical afferents in the infero-posterior wall of the

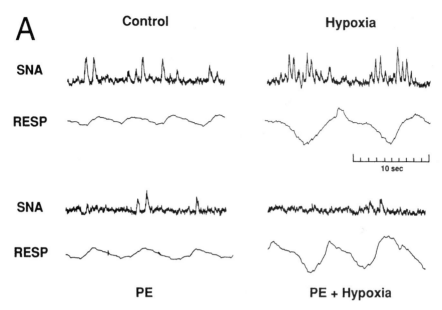

**FIGURE 5A.** Recordings of sympathetic nerve activity (SNA) and respiratory tracings (RESP) in a single subject at baseline (control) (**top left**) and during hypoxia (**top right**), PE infusion (**bottom left**), and the combination of hypoxia and PE infusion (**bottom right**). Note that hypoxia alone increased SNA, whereas PE suppressed SNA. Most importantly, hypoxia during PE resulted in a slight further suppression of SNA (compare to the response to the cold pressor test in FIG. 5C). (Reproduced with permission from Somers *et al.*[13])

left ventricle, will elicit vasodepressor and cardioinhibitory responses. Increases in transmural pressure causing stimulation of intrathoracic aortic arch receptors may also contribute to the depressor responses evident during the Mueller maneuver. The neural circulatory responses, particularly during the early part of the Mueller maneuver, illustrate the potential mechanotransduction effects of breathing and cardiac receptors on neural circulatory control.

## BAROREFLEX-CHEMOREFLEX INTERACTIONS

Animal studies have shown that activation of arterial baroreceptors inhibits both ventilatory and vasoconstrictor responses to peripheral chemoreflex stimulation.[12] Studies in humans have confirmed an interaction between the chemoreflex responses to hypoxemia and baroreflex activation (FIG. 5A).[13] Specifically, when the arterial baroreflexes are activated by raising blood pressure, there is complete elimination of the sympathetic response to peripheral chemoreflex activation. It is important that this interaction appears to differentially affect peripheral, as compared to central, chemoreflex responses. Indeed, arterial baroreflex activation has a much lesser inhibitory effect on the sympathetic responses either to hypercapnia (FIG. 5B) or to a nonspecific stimulus such as the cold pressor test (FIG. 5C). Again, this differential

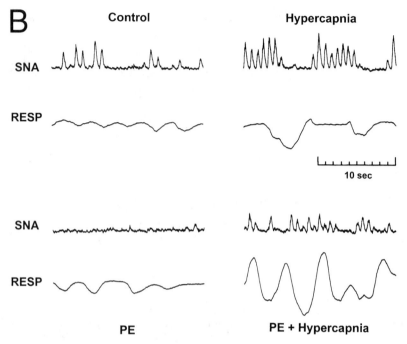

**FIGURE 5B.** Recordings of sympathetic nerve activity (SNA) and respiratory tracings (RESP) in a single subject at baseline (control) **(top left)** and during hypercapnia **(top right)**, PE infusion **(bottom left)**, and hypercapnia imposed during PE infusion. Note that hypercapnia alone increased SNA, and PE suppressed SNA. However, despite the suppression by PE, superimposed hypercapnia (unlike hypoxia) still elicited a substantial SNA response. (Reproduced with permission from Somers *et al.*[13])

interaction may be explained by the anatomical proximity of synapses of the arterial baroreceptor afferents and peripheral chemoreceptor afferents in the nucleus tractus solitarius.

The interaction between the baroreflex and the chemoreflex may also have implications for understanding the bradycardic responses to hypoxemia and apnea. Raising blood pressure and activating the arterial baroreflex results in bradycardia. Chemoreflex activation in the setting of apnea also elicits bradycardia. When chemoreflex activation and apnea occur in a setting of increased baroreflex activation, the bradycardic response is attenuated (FIG. 3). Thus, the arterial baroreflex inhibits not only the chemoreflex-mediated sympathetic vasoconstrictor response, but also the vagal bradycardic response.[14]

Baroreflex-chemoreflex interactions may have relevance to disease states in which baroreflex function is impaired,[14] including hypertension, heart failure, and perhaps premature birth. The normal buffering influence of the baroreflex and the chemoreflex may be diminished in these situations, resulting in excessive potentiation of chemoreflex sensitivity with consequent exaggerated sympathetic activation and/or bradyarrhythmias during hypoxemia and apnea.

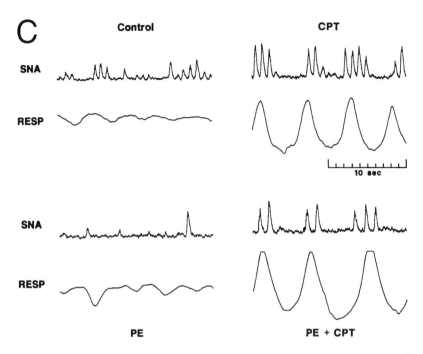

**FIGURE 5C.** Recordings of sympathetic nerve activity (SNA) and respiratory tracings (RESP) in a single subject at baseline (control) **(top left)** and during cold pressor test (CPT) **(top right)**, PE infusion **(bottom left)**, and the CPT imposed during the PE infusion. Baroreflex activation by PE did not abolish the SNA response to CPT (compare to the response to hypoxia in FIG. 5A). (Reproduced with permission from Somers *et al.*[13])

## HYPERVENTILATION AND THE BAROREFLEX

As described above, increases in blood pressure, acting via the baroreflex, inhibit the ventilatory responses to chemoreflex activation. Conversely, the phases of respiration have direct short-term effects on cardiovascular control. Inspiration impairs the cardioinhibitory baroreflex response.[15,16] Respiration also has distinct and contrasting effects on efferent sympathetic nerve traffic, which is inhibited during inspiration and enhanced during expiration as discussed earlier. Vagolytic effects of inspiration contribute to sinus arrhythmia, with relative tachycardia during inspiration and heart rate slowing during expiration.[7,16,17] The effects of more sustained ventilatory changes on baroreflex characteristics also have direct relevance to understanding cardiovascular control in physiologic situations such as hyperventilation induced by exercise[18] and in pathological situations such as hyperventilation induced by hypoxia or hypercapnia.

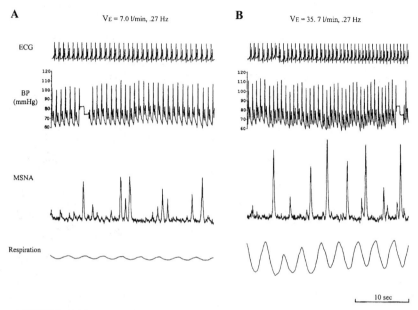

**FIGURE 6.** Electrocardiogram (ECG), finger blood pressure (BP), muscle sympathetic nerve activity (MSNA), and respiration in a single subject during quiet breathing (**A**) and isocapnic hyperventilation (**B**). Inspiration (upward deflection) is followed by suppression in MSNA during isocapnic hyperventilation. Inhibition of MSNA after inspiration is accompanied by facilitation after expiration. Hyperventilation induces an increase in BP, but also an increase in heart rate and MSNA, suggesting a blunting of baroreflex gain. (Reproduced with permission from van de Borne *et al.*[19])

These conditions result in simultaneous tachycardia, sympathetic activation, and blood pressure increases, all accompanied by hyperventilation. Recent data show that hyperventilation in the absence of hypocapnia or other disturbances in arterial blood gas tension is associated with an increase in blood pressure, tachycardia, and no change in sympathetic drive (FIG. 6).[19] The absence of reflex cardiac slowing and/or sympathetic inhibition in response to higher blood pressure during hyperventilation is suggestive of attenuation of baroreflex control of heart rate and sympathetic traffic during hyperventilation (FIG. 7). Changes in respiratory frequency alone, in the absence of hyperventilation, did not affect baroreflex gain. Therefore, the changes in baroreflex characteristics occurring during hyperventilation appear to be a function of the hyperventilation per se and not exclusively a consequence of the effects of central command on baroreflex gain. Thus, hyperventilation per se, in the absence of muscle exercise, joint movement, or direct baroreflex inhibitory effects of the chemoreflex, may contribute to simultaneous increases in blood pressure and heart rate during physiological and pathological conditions such as dynamic exercise or chemoreceptor stimulation. Baroreflex inhibition by hyperventilation may thus constitute a permissive mechanism allowing simultaneous increases in blood pressure, heart rate, and sympathetic traffic during exercise on chemoreflex activation.

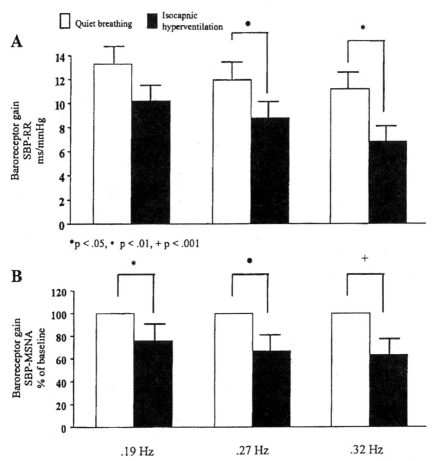

**FIGURE 7.** Baroreceptor gain of the sinus node (**A**) and sympathetic outflow (**B**) during quiet breathing (*open bars*) and isocapnic hyperventilation (*filled bars*) while respiration was paced at 0.19, 0.27, and 0.32 Hz. Attenuated baroreceptor gain during hyperventilation was evident at all respiratory frequencies (*$p < 0.05$; $^\bullet p < 0.01$; $^+ p < 0.001$; quiet breathing versus isocapnic hyperventilation). (Reproduced with permission from van de Borne *et al.*[19])

## SUMMARY

The reflex mechanisms and interactions described in this brief overview provide some explanation for the range of neural circulatory responses evident during changes in breathing. The effects described represent the integrated responses to activation of several reflex mechanisms, including peripheral and central chemoreflexes, arterial baroreflexes, pulmonary stretch receptors, and ventricular mechanoreceptors, among others. These interactions occur on a dynamic basis and the transfer characteristics of any single interaction are, in all likelihood, also highly dynamic. Nevertheless, it is only by attempting to understand individual reflexes and their modulating influences that a more thorough understanding of the responses to complex phenomena such as hyperventilation, apnea, and obstructive sleep apnea can be better understood.

## ACKNOWLEDGMENTS

We would like to express our gratitude to Sandra Hein for expert typing of this manuscript. A. S. M. Shamsuzzaman is a Fogarty Fellow of the National Institutes of Health and a recipient of the Perkins Memorial Award from the American Physiological Society. V. K. Somers is an Established Investigator of the American Heart Association and is supported by NIH Grant Nos. HL65176, HL61560, and RR00585. We express our appreciation to colleagues who have contributed to much of the work described in this brief review.

## REFERENCES

1. GUYENET, P.G. 2000. Neural structures that mediate sympathoexcitation during hypoxia. Respir. Physiol. **121:** 147–162.
2. TAYLOR, E.W., D. JORDAN & J.H. COOTE. 1999. Central control of the cardiovascular and respiratory systems and their interactions in vertebrates. Physiol. Rev. **79:** 855–916.
3. WADE, J.G., C.P. LARSON, JR., R.F. HICKEY et al. 1970. Effect of carotid endarterectomy on carotid chemoreceptor and baroreceptor function in man. N. Engl. J. Med. **282:** 823–829.
4. SOMERS, V.K., D.C. ZAVALA, A.L. MARK & F.M. ABBOUD. 1989. Influence of ventilation and hypocapnia on sympathetic nerve responses to hypoxia in normal humans. J. Appl. Physiol. **67:** 2095–2100.
5. SOMERS, V.K., A.L. MARK & F.M. ABBOUD. 1992. Circulatory regulation during hypoxia and hypercapnia. *In* Hypoxia, Metabolic Acidosis, and the Circulation, pp. 3–20. Oxford University Press. London/New York.
6. DE BURGH DALY, M. & M.J. SCOTT. 1962. An analysis of the primary cardiovascular reflex effects of stimulation of the carotid body chemoreceptors in the dog. Am. J. Physiol. **162:** 555–573.
7. DE BURGH DALY, M., J.E. ANGELL-JAMES & R. ELSNER. 1979. Role of carotid-body chemoreceptors and their reflex interactions in bradycardia and cardiac arrest. Lancet **1:** 764–767.
8. GELFAND, R. & C.J. LAMBERTSEN. 1973. Dynamic respiratory response to abrupt change of inspired $CO_2$ at normal and high $PO_2$. J. Appl. Physiol. **35:** 903–913.
9. SOMERS, V.K., D.C. ZAVALA, A.L. MARK & F.M. ABBOUD. 1989. Contrasting effects of hypoxia and hypercapnia on ventilation and sympathetic activity in humans. J. Appl. Physiol. **67:** 2101–2106.
10. CONDOS, W.R., R.D. LATHAM, S.D. HOADLEY & A. PASIPOULARIDIES. 1987. Hemodynamics of the Mueller maneuver in man: right and left heart micromanometry and Doppler echocardiography. Circulation **76:** 1020–1028.
11. SCHARF, S., R. BROWN, K. WARNER & S. KHURI. 1989. Intrathoracic pressures and left ventricular configuration with respiratory maneuvers. J. Appl. Physiol. **66:** 481–491.
12. HEISTAD, D.D., F.M. ABBOUD, A.L. MARK & P.G. SCHMID. 1974. Interaction of baroreceptor and chemoreceptor reflexes: modulation of the chemoreceptor reflex by changes in baroreceptor activity. J. Clin. Invest. **53:** 1226–1236.
13. SOMERS, V.K., A.L. MARK & F.M. ABBOUD. 1991. Interaction of baroreceptor and chemoreceptor reflex control of sympathetic nerve activity in normal humans. J. Clin. Invest. **87:** 1953–1957.

14. SOMERS, V.K., M.K. DYKEN, A.L. MARK & F.M. ABBOUD. 1992. Parasympathetic hyperresponsiveness and bradyarrhythmias during apnea in hypertension. Clin. Auton. Res. **2:** 171–176.
15. ECKBERG, D.L., Y.T. KIFLE & V.L. ROBERTS. 1980. Phase relationship between normal human respiration and baroreflex responsiveness. J. Physiol. **304:** 489–502.
16. MANCIA, G. & A.L. MARK. 1983. Arterial baroreflex in humans. *In* Handbook of Physiology: The Cardiovascular System, Peripheral Circulation, and Organ Blood Flow. Section 2, volume III, part 2, chapter 20, pp. 755–793. Am. Physiol. Soc. Bethesda, MD.
17. ANREP, G.V., W. PASCUAL & R. ROSSLER. 1936. Respiratory variations of heart rate. II. The central mechanism of the respiratory arrhythmia and the interrelations between the central and the reflex mechanisms. Proc. R. Soc. Lond. **B119:** 218–230.
18. RAVEN, P.B., J.T. POTTS & X. SHI. 1997. Baroreflex regulation of blood pressure during dynamic exercise. Exercise Sport Sci. Rev. **25:** 365–389.
19. VAN DE BORNE, P., S. MEZZETTI, N. MONTANO *et al.* 2000. Hyperventilation alters arterial baroreflex control of heart rate and muscle sympathetic nerve activity. Am. J. Physiol. (Heart Circ. Physiol.) **279:** H536–H541.

# Arterial Baroreceptor and Cardiopulmonary Reflex Control of Sympathetic Outflow in Human Heart Failure

JOHN S. FLORAS

*Mount Sinai Hospital and University Health Network Department of Medicine, University of Toronto, Toronto, Canada M5G 1X5*

ABSTRACT: Several observations indicate that the arterial baroreflex control of sympathetic nerve activity is preserved, even in advanced heart failure. These include: (1) augmentation of muscle sympathetic nerve activity burst amplitude and duration following a premature beat; (2) rapid recognition of changes in blood pressure induced by ventricular arrhythmias; (3) muscle sympathetic alternans and a steep inverse relationship between changes in diastolic pressure and the subsequent sympathetic burst amplitude during pulsus alternans; (4) similar inhibition of muscle sympathetic nerve activity in subjects with normal and impaired left ventricular systolic function by increases in intrathoracic aortic transmural pressure; (5) documentation, by cross-spectral analysis, of similar gain in the transfer function between blood pressure and muscle sympathetic nerve activity in these two groups; and (6) during sodium nitroprusside infusion, similar reflex increases in total body norepinephrine spillover in normal and heart-failure subjects. When nonhypotensive lower-body negative pressure was applied to test the hypothesis that selective reduction of atrial and pulmonary pressures would exert a cardiac sympathoinhibitory response in heart failure, there was no effect in control subjects, but cardiac norepinephrine spillover fell by 25% ($P < .05$) in those with systolic dysfunction. In summary, human heart failure is characterized by a rapidly responsive and sensitive arterial baroreflex, and by activation of a cardiac sympathoexcitatory reflex related to increased cardiopulmonary filling pressures.

KEYWORDS: Arterial baroreceptor reflex; Cardiopulmonary baroreceptor reflex; Heart failure; Humans; Microneurography; Sympathetic nervous system

## INTRODUCTION

Blunted arterial baroreflex control of heart rate is a characteristic feature of human heart failure. It has therefore been assumed that baroreflex inhibition of the sympathetic nervous system is also impaired. However, observations from our laboratories indicate that the arterial baroreflex control of sympathetic nerve activity is preserved, even in advanced heart failure.

Address for correspondence: Mount Sinai Hospital, Suite 1614, 600 University Avenue, Toronto, Ontario, Canada, M5G 1X5. Voice: 416-586-8704; fax: 416-586-8702.
john.floras@utoronto.ca

## EVIDENCE FOR SYMPATHETIC NERVOUS SYSTEM ACTIVATION
## IN HUMAN HEART FAILURE

Two means of exploring the contribution of arterial and cardiopulmonary reflexes to the regulation of sympathetic outflow in humans are microneurography, which permits the direct, beat-to-beat quantification of efferent sympathetic nerve discharge to vascular beds in skeletal muscle,[1] and the isotope dilution method developed by Esler.[2] With the latter, total body norepinephrine clearance and spillover into plasma can be determined from concentrations of cold and labeled neurotransmitter in plasma, drawn during steady-state infusion of tritiated norepinephrine in tracer concentrations. If the venous effluent from the heart, kidney, brain, or another vascular bed is collected simultaneously with an arterial sample, the difference in tritiated norepinephrine between vein and artery can be used to calculate its local extraction (Extr). Organ-specific norepinephrine spillover (NES) can be determined from the following equation: $NES = [(NE_v - NE_a) + (NE_a \times Extr)] \times PF$, where $NE_a$ and $NE_v$ represent the arterial and venous concentrations of unlabeled norepinephrine and PF plasma flow.[2]

Plasma norepinephrine concentrations are elevated in asymptomatic left-ventricular dysfunction and increase further with the progression to overt congestive heart failure.[3] At this more advanced stage, total body norepinephrine spillover is increased by a factor of 2, and norepinephrine clearance reduced by about a third.[4] In healthy subjects, approximately 25% of total body norepinephrine spillover arises from the kidney and about 2% from the heart.[2] In severe heart failure renal norepinephrine spillover increases 2- to 3-fold, and cardiac norepinephrine spillover 5- to 10-fold.[4] In patients with end-stage heart failure, under assessment for cardiac transplantation, cardiac norpinephrine spillover becomes a potent marker of premature mortality.[5]

The radio-tracer kinetic technique quantifies the rate at which neuronally released norepinephrine appears in plasma, rather than sympathetic nerve traffic or the rate of release of the neurotransmitter from sympathetic nerve endings. Therefore, spillover might be increased because of enhanced prejunctional modulation of norepinephrine release by $\beta_2$-adrenoceptor agonists (e.g., epinephrine[6,7]), or angiotensin II,[8] or by decreased uptake of norepinephrine from the neurovascular junction.[2] This ambiguity was resolved when direct microneurographic evidence for increased efferent muscle sympathetic burst frequency was obtained from older patients with advanced congestive heart failure.[9,10] We extended these findings to young subjects with dilated cardiomyopathy, and noted, as well, a positive relationship between sympathetic burst frequency and resistance in the calf, the vascular bed distal to the recording electrode.[11] More recently, Rundqvist et al. described a selective increase in cardiac adrenergic drive in patients with mild to moderate heart failure, prior to any detectable elevation in total body or renal norpinephrine spillover or in muscle sympathetic nerve activity.[12]

What mechanism or mechanisms might be responsible for these observations? Sympathetic activation in human heart failure has been ascribed to loss of inhibitory modulation by arterial or cardiopulmonary baroreceptor reflexes.[13] However, there is emerging evidence that excitatory reflexes also participate in this process. Since congestive heart failure can be defined as a syndrome in which filling pressures are elevated so as to maintain cardiac output sufficient for adequate tissue perfusion, engagement of ordinarily quiescent mechanosensitive cardiopulmonary afferents with sympathoexcitatory actions may be an important early stimulus to generalized or cardiac-specific adrenergic activation in this condition.

I will review current evidence related to these proposed mechanisms and develop the theme that sympathetic activation in human heart failure arises as a result of both loss of inhibitory modulation, and activation of excitatory systems.

## ARTERIAL BAROREFLEX REGULATION OF SYMPATHETIC NERVOUS SYSTEM ACTIVITY

Blunted arterial baroreflex control of heart rate in heart failure was first described by Eckberg et al.[13] These authors infused phenylephrine to raise systolic blood pressure, and noted that parasympathetically mediated bradycardia in response to this stimulus was attenuated in patients with ventricular dysfunction. Subsequent investigators infused phenylephrine and sodium nitroprusside to both raise and lower systolic blood pressure, and thereby induce reflex increases and decreases in pulse interval, respectively. Slopes for baroreflex sensitivity (expressed either as ms/mmHg or as bpm/mmHg) generated from these data were consistently steeper in healthy controls than in heart-failure patients.[14,15] Because baroreceptor afferent nerve discharge in experimental models of ventricular systolic dysfunction is less responsive to changes in local distending pressure,[16,17] it seemed reasonable to conclude that baroreflex restraint of central sympathetic outflow was also impaired in human heart failure.[13]

However, several difficulties with this interpretation emerged. First, it became apparent that mechanisms specific to the neural regulation of heart rate, and not sympathetic outflow, attenuate responses to pressor and depressor stimuli in heart failure. Impairment of vagal ganglionic transmission can account for much of the loss of reflex bradycardia,[18] whereas downregulation or desensitization of myocardial β-adrenergic receptors[19] will render the sinoatrial node less responsive to any increase in neurally released norepinephrine-evoked reflexively by a fall in blood pressure. Second, results of experiments involving muscle sympathetic nerve activity (MSNA) were inconsistent.[14,15,20] Ferguson et al. studied patients with marked depression of ejection fraction and elevated pulmonary diastolic pressure and reported a significant reduction in the sympathoneural response to nitroprusside, but not to phenylephrine.[14] This study had the historical advantage of studying patients free of vasoactive medication. However, the heart-failure patients, on average, were more than twice as old as the healthy young control subjects studied. In contrast, Grassi et al. described an impairment of both limbs of the reflex control of MSNA that worsened with the progression of heart failure.[15] Dibner-Dunlap et al. adopted a different protocol, in which phenylephrine was infused at the peak depressor response to nitroprusside. These authors observed similar gains in the arterial baroreflex control of MSNA in healthy and heart-failure subjects,[20] whereas reflex responses to stimuli that raised and lowered cardiac filling pressure without affecting systemic blood pressure were markedly attenuated. They concluded that impairment of the cardiopulmonary reflex was the principal defect in the regulation of sympathetic outflow in human heart failure.[20,21] Third, the principal representations of MSNA in these experiments were as bursts/min, or as the product of bursts/min and burst amplitude. However, these bursts are pulse synchronous, and in advanced stages of heart failure muscle sympathetic activity burst incidence (i.e., bursts/100 cardiac cycles) is often 90–100%. Because the heart-rate response to phenylephrine or nitroprusside is so attenuated, there is then little or no opportunity to modify sympathetic nerve activity if calculated as burst frequency (bursts/min). For example, in contrast to a healthy individual with a resting burst incidence of 25 or 30, in whom nitroprusside evokes a reflex increase in heart rate of 20 beats/min, in a heart failure patient with a resting burst incidence of 90 or 95 and a higher resting heart rate nitroprusside may evoke a reflex increase in heart rate of only 5 beats/min. As a result of this attenuated heart-rate response, pulse-synchronous neural discharge in the subject with heart failure might increase at most by 5 or 6 bursts/min. Consequently, if the observations of Ferguson et al.[14] are restated in terms of $\Delta$MSNA units·min$^{-1}$/$\Delta$beats·min$^{-1}$/$\Delta$mmHg diastolic blood pressure, then phenylephrine reduced mean values for MSNA by approximately 3.4 units in control subjects, and by 11.6 units in heart failure patients. Nitroprusside increased MSNA by 32 units·min$^{-1}$/beats·min$^{-1}$ in control subjects and by 40 units·min$^{-1}$/beats·min$^{-1}$ in heart-failure patients. Corresponding values for the sympathetic activation induced by nitroprusside for every mmHg reduction in diastolic blood pressure are approximately 4.6 units in control subjects, and 3.7 units in heart failure. When expressed, as by the authors, as changes for every mmHg reduction in mean arterial pressure, mean values in the two groups are virtually identical: 3.23 vs. 3.38 units. Interestingly, the reduction in the muscle sympathetic nerve response in heart failure in the experiments by Grassi et al.[15] was also proportional to the smaller heart-rate responses to both stimuli. In a subsequent experiment from this group, chronic treatment with angiotensin-converting enzyme-inhibition enhanced, in parallel, reflex heart rate and muscle sympathetic nerve responses to phenylephrine, but had no effect on either response to nitroprusside.[22]

## EVIDENCE FOR PRESERVED ARTERIAL BAROREFLEX CONTROL OF SYMPATHETIC NERVE ACTIVITY IN HUMAN HEART FAILURE

A number of observations from our laboratory have fundamentally altered our concepts of reflex regulation of sympathetic nerve activity in human heart failure.

### Pulse Synchronicity

Preservation of the characteristic pulse-synchronous nature of MSNA, even in end-stage heart failure, is perhaps the first clue that some arterial baroreflex regulation of central sympathetic outflow is maintained. By contrast, we had documented loss of pulse-synchronicity in a sarcoma patient with functional sinoaortic deafferentation and paroxysmal hypertension as a result of 4570 rads delivered to the entire cervical area, partial mastoid area, high axillae, and superior mediastinum, followed by bilateral aorto-internal carotid bypass with saphenous vein grafts.[23] Changes in blood pressure induced by nitroprusside or phenylephrine had no effect, whereas decreases in cardiac filling pressure with lower-body negative pressure produced a marked increase in muscle sympathetic burst frequency.

## Augmentation of Sympathetic Burst Amplitude and
## Duration following Premature Beats

It is important to distinguish between the reflex effects of baroreceptor afferent nerve firing during systole, and afferent nerve silence during diastole. Systolic stimulation of baroreceptor discharge will increase parasympathetic, and decrease afferent sympathetic outflow reflexively. Baroreceptor silence during diastole eliminates the tonic inhibition of efferent sympathetic outflow.[24] Thus the long pause and decay in diastolic blood pressure that follows a ventricular premature beat should result in increased sympathetic multifiber burst amplitude, duration, and area. Indeed, each of these increase as the coupling interval of the premature to the preceding beat decreases. In contrast, increases in diastolic blood pressure arising from postextrasystolic beats inhibit sympathetic discharge or cause neural silence.[25] This extrasystolic augmentation of sympathetic burst amplitude, duration and area, and postextrasystolic suppression in response to changes in diastolic pressure is replicated in heart failure (FIG. 1). Moreover, in end-stage heart failure closely coupled premature beats

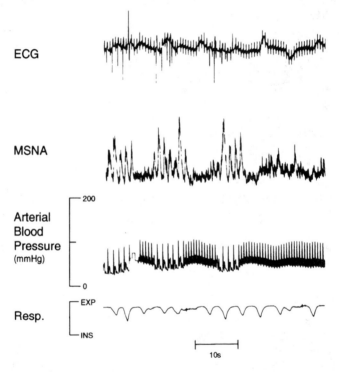

**FIGURE 1.** The electrocardiogram (ECG), mean voltage neurogram for MSNA, blood pressure, and respiratory excursions in a young man with end-stage heart failure due to dilated cardiomyopathy. Paroxysms of ventricular bigeminy result in a doubling of the blood pressure cycle length, a longer diastolic period, and lower diastolic blood pressure. These changes are registered immediately by the arterial baroreceptors and result in a corresponding increase in the duration of the sympathetic burst and a marked increase in burst amplitude. These are reversed with restoration of sinus rhythm.

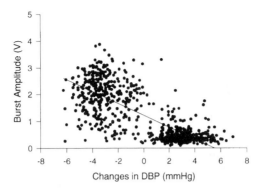

**FIGURE 2.** Inverse relation between MSNA, burst amplitude (V), and the change in DBP from the preceding cardiac cycle $(n - 2)$ to the DBP for the cardiac cycle immediately before this burst $(n - 1)$ over a 7-min sampling period $(n = 712; r = -0.767)$. Note the two clusters reflecting the presence of alternans. When DBP rises from one cardiac cycle to the next, MSNA burst amplitude is extremely low or suppressed; conversely, the highest sympathetic burst amplitudes are seen in response to a fall in DBP.

often fail to generate sufficient force to open the aortic valve. Under these circumstances, the arterial baroreceptors respond immediately to perceived changes in diastolic blood pressure and the duration of the blood-pressure cycle rather than to cardiac frequency (FIG. 1).

### Sympathetic Alternans

In 1997 we described alternation in the amplitude of MSNA in three patients with severe heart failure.[26] In the index patient with pulsus alternans, the amplitude of sympathetic bursts was inversely related to changes in the preceding diastolic (not systolic) pressure with a lag time of 1.2 to 1.3 s, indicating that these oscillations in burst amplitude were determined primarily by changes in this component of blood pressure. Spectral analysis of the blood pressure and microneurographic signals identified two spectral peaks, one at the cardiac frequency and a second peak, with greater spectral power, at the alternans frequency (i.e., at half the heart rate). The latter peak for both blood pressure and MSNA disappeared when alternans was abolished by nitroglycerin. We interpreted this "sympathetic alternans" in synchrony with pulsus alternans, and the rapid transduction of changes in the diastolic blood-pressure afferent signal to the amplitude of sympathetic outflow (FIG. 2), as indicating that the arterial baroreflex control of MSNA must be active and rapidly responsive in this condition. Although the "sensitivity" of this spontaneous relationship was not quantified, it is interesting to note that the doubling of sympathetic burst amplitude observed, in FIGURE 2, in response to a 2 mmHg drop in diastolic blood pressure is roughly comparable to the 5-fold increase in spontaneous MSNA burst incidence that normotensive healthy subjects experience in response to a 10-mmHg change in diastolic blood pressure.[27]

Comparison of sympathetic responses to blood-pressure perturbations in subjects with normal and impaired left-ventricular systolic function permits alternative calculations of arterial baroreflex gain, and provides further evidence in support of the preceding interpretation.

### Acute Inhibition of MSNA by the Mueller Maneuver

Somers *et al.* have described, in detail, the effects of the abrupt increase in negative intrathoracic pressure evoked by a Mueller maneuver on central venous pressure, blood pressure, heart rate, and MSNA in healthy volunteers.[28] Concordant decreases in central venous pressure, systolic blood pressure, and MSNA were observed over the first 10 s of this stimulus. To explain why these hemodynamic changes elicited a decrease rather than an increase in central sympathetic outflow, these authors proposed that abrupt increases in atrial and ventricular transmural pressure stimulated cardiac receptors with inhibitory reflex effects on noradrenergic tone.

This abrupt decrease in intrathoracic pressure will also increase transmural pressure in the intrathoracic aorta, and stimulate aortic arch baroreceptor discharge with inhibitory effects on sympathetic outflow.[29] In healthy humans, aortic baroreceptors play a greater role than carotid baroreceptors in the reflex modulation of MSNA.[30] Because the compromised myocardium is much more sensitive to changes in afterload than the normal left ventricle, patients with heart failure are unable to sustain resting blood pressure, stroke volume, and cardiac output in response to the generation of $-30$ cm $H_2O$ during a Mueller maneuve.[31] From the interaction between carotid and aortic baroreceptor reflexes, one might anticipate less reflex sympathoinhibition in response to the this stimulus in those with heart failure. However, when we related changes in MSNA in response to changes in intra-aortic diastolic transmural pressure at the onset of the Mueller maneuver, the gain of this measure of the aortic baroreceptor reflex was similar in those with marked left-ventricular systolic dysfunction ($-2.9 \pm 1.5$ bursts/100 heart beats/mmHg) and age-matched healthy controls ($-1.5 \pm 0.4$ bursts/100 heart beats/mmHg).[32]

### Cross-spectral Analysis of Gain in the Transfer Function between Blood Pressure and MSNA

Periodic oscillations in blood pressure and heart rate at frequencies between 0 and 0.5 Hz are mediated primarily by the autonomic nervous system. Because changes in blood pressure modulate sympathetic outflow via the arterial baroreflex, MSNA should exhibit similar periodicity. Indeed, the mean voltage neurogram displays fluctuations in muscle sympathetic nerve discharge synchronous with changes in blood pressure, heart rate, and respiration. We therefore submitted these signals to frequency-domain analysis, and to cross-spectral analysis, in order to characterize harmonic and nonharmonic components of variations in MSNA and to compare these in men with normal and impaired ventricular function. In the frequency domain, the strength of such relationships can be quantified in terms of transfer-function magnitude or gain (ratio of output/input power) and coherence (an index of the concordance between input and output signals at each frequency). The gain and coherence between MSNA, blood pressure, heart rate, and breathing frequency spectra were also calculated and compared.[33]

Muscle sympathetic burst frequency was 68% higher in the heart-failure subjects, whereas breathing frequency and heart rate were similar. There was no difference

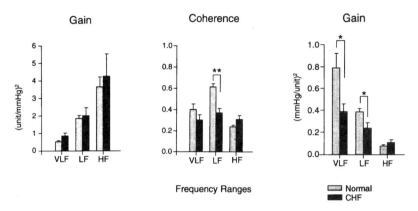

**FIGURE 3.** Mean values for gain of transfer function from BP to MSNA (representation of arterial baroreflex control of sympathetic nerve activity; **left graph**) and gain of transfer function from MSNA to BP (**right graph**) in normal subjects (*light bars*) and patients with heart failure (*dark bars*). **Middle graph**: Coherence between these two variables. VLF, 0–0.05 Hz; LF, 0.05–0.15 Hz; HF, 0.15–0.5 Hz.**$P < 0.01$. *$P < 0.05$. (From Ando *et al.*[33] Reprinted with permission from the American Physiological Society.)

with respect to total power, harmonic power, and nonharmonic power in the neural spectrum from 0 to 0.5 Hz, but low-frequency power was reduced in heart failure. There was less coherence between blood pressure and MSNA in the low-frequency range (0.05–0.15 Hz), but there was similar spectral power in both groups within the very low-frequency (0–0.05 Hz) and high-frequency (0.15–0.5 Hz) ranges.

Transfer-function analysis provided novel insight into mechanisms potentially responsible for these differing spectral patterns. The gain of the transfer function relating changes in blood pressure (stimulus) to changes in MSNA (response), which can be considered a representation of the arterial baroreflex control of MSNA, was similar across all frequency bands in the two groups. Similar gains would be anticipated if transduction of the blood pressure signal by an active arterial baroreflex was preserved in heart failure. This has been demonstrated in one experimental model of heart failure.[34] Moreover, and also consistent with the results of animal studies,[35] the arterial baroreflex acted as a high-pass filter, with transfer-function gain greatest within the high-frequency range (FIG. 3).

By contrast, there was a progressive loss of gain in the transfer of MSNA oscillations to blood pressure from the very low-, to low-, to high-frequency bands, in both heart failure and healthy subjects (FIG. 3), analogous to the neuroeffector junction acting as a low-pass filter.[36] This concept is consistent with the known frequency response characteristics of vascular resistance vessels to neurally released norepinephrine. This low-pass function therefore opens up the high-frequency component of this otherwise closed-loop circuit to study (FIG. 4). Transfer of MSNA oscillations into blood pressure in the very low-frequency and low-frequency ranges was significantly lower in heart failure (FIG. 3). This loss of modulation within the

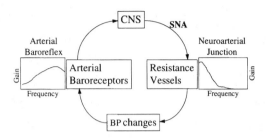

**FIGURE 4.** Representation of closed-circuit loop, with low-pass filtering of spectral power at neuroeffector junction, and augmented gain of arterial baroreceptor transduction of BP oscillations at high frequencies. This conceptual framework would explain the observations summarized in FIGURE 3. The reduction in LF spectral power in heart failure may arise at any point in this circuit, whereas HF spectral power in MSNA must be due primarily to arterial baroreceptor properties and signal transduction within central nerve system (CNS). (From Ando et al.[33] Reprinted with permission from the American Physiological Society.)

low-frequency range seems best explained by impaired neuroeffector transduction.[33]

Coherence between respiratory and neural oscillations was also similar in heart failure and healthy subjects. We therefore concluded that the higher sympathetic discharge rate in heart failure must be caused by factors other than the loss of regulation by inhibitory influences arising from arterial baroreceptors and pulmonary stretch receptors, and sought out alternate inhibitory or excitatory mechanisms for this phenomenon.

### Neurochemical Evidence

My colleagues Newton and Parker[37] have explored the effect of baroreceptor unloading on total body and cardiac norepinephrine spillover in patients with impaired and normal ventricular systolic function. Sodium nitroprusside was titrated to achieve similar hemodynamic responses in control and heart-failure subjects. Total body norepinephrine spillover increased, reflexively, to a similar extent in both groups, again indicating preservation of the arterial baroreflex control of sympathetic outflow in heart failure. By contrast, nitroprusside elicited a significant increase in cardiac norepinephrine spillover in those with normal ventricular function, but not in subjects with heart failure, suggesting reduced baroreflex control of cardiac sympathetic activity.

### Interpretation

The weight of evidence therefore obliges us to conclude that the arterial baroreflex control of sympathetic activity is intact and rapidly responsive in human heart failure. As a corollary, these observations would also indicate that the analysis of spontaneous changes in blood pressure and MSNA provides insight into arterial baroreflex function that is not available from the traditional vasoactive drug method. There may be five reasons as to why the pharmacological approach may have limited applicability to heart failure. First, responses calculated as burst frequency, which is a function of cardiac frequency, will be constrained secondarily to any primary disturbance in the baroreceptor–heart-rate reflex. Impairment of this reflex is significantly greater in heart failure than in hypertension, or with age. Second, as illustrated earlier, interpretation of arterial baroreflex gain is highly dependent upon the variables used to represent stimulus and response. For example, the attenuated sympathetic activation, in response to nitroprusside, reported by Ferguson et al.[14] was a function of their expressing changes in MSNA in terms of percentage rather than absolute increases. Because resting MSNA was 2- to 3-fold higher in their heart-failure population, expression of changes as a percentage will underestimate the true response of this group. There would appear to be no a priori rationale for expressing these data as relative increases. Indeed, in an earlier publication these authors expressed the MSNA response to a nonbaroreflex-mediated stimulus (the cold pressor test) in terms of Δunits/100 heart beats, and reported an identical increase in MSNA in heart-failure and control subjects, despite 3- to 4-fold higher baseline values for MSNA in the former group.[38] Third, atrial pressures are also affected by phenylephrine and nitroprusside.[15] Fourth, perturbations such as pulsus alternans cause smaller fluctuations in blood pressure that may lie more within the linear segment of the blood-pressure–MSNA relationship in heart failure. Fifth, blood-pressure changes caused by these interventions are slow in onset, whereas studies in anaesthetized rabbits[35] and conscious humans[39] indicate that baroreceptors are more responsive to high- than to low-frequency oscillations in blood pressure. For example, when static and sinusoidal neck pressure are applied to stimulate carotid baroreceptors, the greatest effect on MSNA is observed at the highest stimulus frequency. In contrast, there is little or no effect on muscle sympathetic outflow when negative pressure is applied as a ramp over 12 s, that is, analogous to the slower time course over which vasoactive drugs alter blood pressure.[39]

## EVIDENCE FOR ALTERED CARDIOPULMONARY REFLEX REGULATION OF SYMPATHETIC NERVOUS SYSTEM IN HEART FAILURE

There are two lines of evidence in humans that support the concept that the primary defect in the baroreceptor regulation of the sympathetic nervous system in human heart failure lies within reflexes arising from cardiac and pulmonary venous afferents.[20,21] In some patients, lower-body negative pressure elicits forearm vasodilation rather than vasoconstriction.[40] Activation of vagal afferents with inhibitory reflex effects on sympathetic outflow, in response to acute increases in ventricular contractile force, possibly due to release of pericardial constraint, has been offered as a potential mechanism for this paradoxical response.[40,41] Middlekauff et al.[42] unloaded cardiopulmonary baroreceptors by phlebotomy, and also observed a reduction in the reflex forearm vasoconstrictor response to this stimulus in heart-failure patients. Intriguingly, the renal cortical vasoconstrictor response, as assessed by positron emission tomography, was preserved. However, sympathetic outflow was not quantified in these experiments.[40–42] Dunlap et al. recorded MSNA and noted marked attenuation of reflex responses to stimuli that raised and lowered cardiac filling pressure without affecting systemic blood pressure.[20] Ferguson *et al.*[14] also reported attenuated muscle sympathetic nerve responses to changes in right atrial pressure in heart failure, but these occurred in the setting of concomitant hypertension and hypotension induced by phenylephrine and nitroprusside, respectively. In our laboratory, nonhypotensive lower-body negative pressure increased total body norepinephrine spillover significantly in subjects with normal ventricular systolic function, whereas there was only a trend, not significant, toward higher values for total body norepinephrine spillover in those with impaired ventricular systolic function.[43] In summary, there is substantial evidence for loss of cardiopulmonary reflex regulation of central sympathetic outflow to the periphery, and in particular, to skeletal muscle, in human heart failure.

The description of a significant positive relationship between pulmonary capillary wedge pressure and cardiac norepinephrine spillover[44] suggests a paradoxical excitation of sympathetic outflow at high left atrial pressure. Wang and Zucker documented sensitization of sympathetic afferents in the pacing- induced canine model of heart failure, and speculated that enhancement of this reflex might contribute to increased sympathetic nerve traffic in chronic heart failure.[45] Is there evidence in humans for activation, by increased filling pressure, of a cardiac-specific sympathoexcitatory reflex, arising from myelinated cardiac afferent nerves? If present, this could account for the selective increase in cardiac norepinephrine spillover in mild to moderate heart failure, prior to any detectable elevation in total body or renal norepinephrine spillover, or in muscle sympathetic nerve activity, as described by Rundqvist *et al.*[12] Consistent with this concept, Kaye *et al.*[46] infused sodium nitroprusside to lower both atrial and arterial pressure in patients with severe pulmonary hypertension secondary to heart failure and found a reduction in cardiac norepinephrine spillover. This observation stimulated us to construct a lower-body negative-pressure chamber that allowed for the simultaneous measurement of cardiac hemodynamics and neurochemistry. We hypothesized that a selective reduction in cardiac filling and pulmonary pressures in the absence of measurable changes in systemic arterial pressure would inhibit cardiac norepinephrine spillover in patients with congestive heart failure. Patients were submitted to nonhypotensive and hypotensive lower-body negative pressure. Nonhypotensive lower-body negative pressure reduced cardiac filling pressures in both groups. Stroke volume and cardiac output fell. This intervention resulted in a significant reduction in cardiac norepinephrine spillover in the heart-failure group, but no change in age-matched control subjects with normal left-ventricular systolic function. With hypotensive lower-body negative pressure there was a significant increase in cardiac norepinephrine spillover in the control group, but no significant elevation above baseline in subjects with heart failure. These findings suggest that a reduction in cardiopulmonary filling pressure leads to a reduction in efferent cardiac sympathetic tone. This withdrawal cannot be explained by activation of ventricular mechanoreceptors due to increases in systolic force,[40,41] since stroke volume and cardiac output fell. These changes occurred in the absence of any reduction in systemic blood pressure, implying that increases in cardiac filling pressures can activate mechanoreceptor afferents with specific cardiac sympathoexcitatory consequences. Since there is an inverse relationship between cardiac norepinephrine spillover and prognosis in advanced heart failure,[5] these findings suggest that therapies directed at normalizing cardiac filling pressures may have a beneficial effect on outcome.

## SUMMARY, CONCLUSIONS, AND FUTURE DIRECTIONS

From the available evidence in human heart failure, we conclude (1) the arterial baroreflex control of heart rate is impaired; (2) the arterial baroreflex control of efferent sympathetic nerve activity is rapidly responsive, with preserved sensitivity; (3) the cardiopulmonary reflex control of muscle sympathetic nerve activity is impaired; and (4) increased filling pressures appear to increase cardiac norepinephrine spillover by activating a cardiac-specific sympathoexcitatory reflex. However, in our view these several mechanisms are insufficient to account for the time course and magnitude of adrenergic activation in heart failure, nor the dynamic fluctuations in sympathetic nerve discharge that occur in the absence of any change in cardiac or peripheral hemodynamics, but in response to apnea, or other stimuli. Thus far we have elucidated four additional mechanisms that likely contribute to sympathetic activation in heart failure: adenosine, through a sympathoexcitatory reflex mediated via stimulation of the angiotensin $AT_1$ receptor,[47] increases in venous pressure in skeletal muscle,[48] a metaboreflex arising from skeletal muscle,[49] and sleep-related breathing disorders.[50] Intense activation of the sympathetic nervous system, and its entrainment by the pattern of breathing, is one of the most serious adverse consequences of obstructive and central apnea for the failing left ventricle. This magnitude of this burden is highlighted by our recent report on the largest series of patients with congestive heart failure studied with overnight polysomnography.[51] Of these 450 men and women, approximately one-third had obstructive sleep apnea, one-third central apnea due to Cheyne-Stokes respiration, and only one-third were free of sleep- related breathing disorders. A better understanding of the several mechanisms responsible for sympathetic activation in heart failure, and their interactions, should lead to novel therapeutic strategies for this debilitating condition.

### REFERENCES

1. WALLIN, B.G. & J. FAGIUS. 1988. Peripheral sympathetic neural activity in conscious humans. Ann. Rev. Physiol. **50:** 565–576.
2. ESLER, M. *et al.* 1988. Assessment of human sympathetic nervous system activity from measurements of norepinephrine turnover. Hypertension **11:** 3–20.
3. FRANCIS, G.S. *et al.* 1990. Comparison of neuroendocrine activation in patients with left ventricular dysfunction with and without congestive heart failure: a substudy of the Studies of Left Ventricular Dysfunction (SOLVD). Circulation **82:** 1724–1729.
4. HASKING, G.J. *et al.* 1986. Norepinephrine spillover to plasma in patients with congestive heart failure: evidence of increased overall and cardiorenal sympathetic nervous activity. Circulation **73:** 615–621.
5. KAYE, D.M. *et al.* 1995. Adverse consequences of high sympathetic nervous activity in the failing human heart. J. Am. Coll. Cardiol. **26:** 1257–1263.
6. FLORAS, J.S. *et al.* 1988. Epinephrine facilitates neurogenic vasoconstriction in humans. J. Clin. Invest. **81:** 1265–1274.
7. NEWTON, G.E. & J.D. PARKER. 1996. Acute effects of beta 1-selective and nonselective beta-adrenergic receptor blockade on cardiac sympathetic activity in congestive heart failure. Circulation **94:** 353–358.
8. ZIMMERMAN, B.G. 1978. Actions of angiotensin on adrenergic nerve endings. Fed. Proc. **37:** 199–202.
9. LEIMBACH, W.N. *et al.* 1986. Direct evidence from intraneural recordings for increased central sympathetic outflow in patients with heart failure. Circulation **73:** 913–919.

10. FERGUSON, D.W. *et al.* 1990. Clinical and hemodynamic correlates of sympathetic nerve activity in normal humans and patients with heart failure: evidence from direct microneurographic recordings. J. Am. Coll. Cardiol. **16:** 1125–1134.

11. HARA, K. & J.S. FLORAS. 1996. After-effects of exercise on haemodynamics and muscle sympathetic nerve activity in young patients with dilated cardiomyopathy. Heart **75:** 602–608.

12. RUNDQVIST, B. *et al.* 1997. Increased cardiac adrenergic drive precedes generalized sympathetic activation in human heart failure. Circulation **95:** 169–175.

13. FLORAS, J.S. 1993. Clinical aspects of sympathetic activation and parasympathetic withdrawal in heart failure. J. Am. Coll. Cardiol. **22:** 72A–84A.

14. FERGUSON, D.W. *et al.* 1992. Effects of heart failure on baroreflex control of sympathetic neural activity. Am. J. Cardiol. **69:** 523–531.

15. GRASSI, G. *et al.* 1995. Sympathetic activation and loss of reflex sympathetic control in mild congestive heart failure. Circulation **92:** 3206–3211.

16. DIBNER-DUNLAP, M.E. & M.D. THAMES. 1989. Baroreflex control of renal sympathetic nerve activity is preserved in heart failure despite reduced arterial baroreceptor sensitivity. Circ. Res. **65:** 1526–1535.

17. WANG, W. *et al.* 1990. Carotid sinus baroreceptor sensitivity in experimental heart failure. Circulation **81:** 1959–1966.

18. BIBEVSKI, S. & M.E. DUNLAP. 1999. Ganglionic mechanisms contribute to diminished vagal control in heart failure. Circulation **99:** 2958–2963.

19. BRISTOW, M.R. 1993. Changes in myocardial and vascular receptors in heart failure. J. Am. Coll. Cardiol. **22:** 61A–71A.

20. DIBNER-DUNLAP, M.E. *et al.* 1996. Enalaprilat augments arterial and cardiopulmonary baroreflex control of sympathetic nerve activity in patients with heart failure. J. Am. Coll. Cardiol. **27:** 358–364.

21. DIBNER-DUNLAP, M. 1992. Arterial or cardiopulmonary baroreflex control of sympathetic nerve activity in heart failure? (Lett.). Am. J. Cardiol. **70:** 1640–1642.

22. GRASSI, G. *et al.* 1997. Effects of chronic ACE inhibition on sympathetic nerve traffic and baroreflex control of circulation in heart failure. Circulation **96:** 1173–1179.

23. AKSAMIT, T.R. *et al.* 1987. Paroxysmal hypertension due to sinoaortic denervation in humans. Hypertension **9:** 309–314.

24. SANDERS, J.S. & D.W. FERGUSON. 1989. Diastolic pressure determines autonomic responses to pressure perturbation in humans. J. Appl. Physiol. **66:** 800–807.

25. WELCH, W.J. *et al.* 1989. Enhancement of sympathetic nerve activity by single premature ventricular beats in humans. J. Am. Coll. Cardiol. **13:** 69–75.

26. ANDO, S. *et al.* 1997. Sympathetic alternans. Evidence for arterial baroreflex control of muscle sympathetic nerve activity in congestive heart failure. Circulation **95:** 316–319.

27. WALLIN, B.G. & M.D. SUNDLOF. 1979. A quantitative study of muscle nerve sympathetic activity in resting normotensive and hypertensive subjects. Hypertension **1:** 67–77.

28. SOMERS, V.K. *et al.* 1993. Autonomic and hemodynamic responses and interactions during the Mueller maneuver in humans. J. Auton. Nerv. Syst. **44:** 253–259.

29. ANGELL JAMES, J.E. 1971. The effects of changes of extramural, 'intrathoracic', pressure on aortic arch baroreceptors. J. Physiol. (Lond.) **214:** 89–103.

30. SANDERS, J.S. *et al.* 1989. Importance of aortic baroreflex in regulation of sympathetic responses during hypotension. Evidence from direct sympathetic nerve recordings in humans. Circulation **79:** 83–92.

31. BRADLEY, T.D. *et al.* 2001. Hemodynamic effects of simulated obstructive apneas in subjects with and without heart failure. Submitted.

32. BRADLEY, T.D. *et al.* 2001. Effects of simulated obstructive apneas on sympathetic discharge to muscle in humans with normal and impaired cardiac function. Submitted.

33. ANDO, S. *et al.* 1997. Frequency domain characteristics of muscle sympathetic nerve activity in heart failure and healthy humans. Am. J. Physiol. **273** (Regul. Integrative Comp. Physiol. **42**): R205–R212.

34. MASAKI, H. *et al.* 1994. Dynamic arterial baroreflex in rabbits with heart failure induced by rapid pacing. Am. J. Physiol. **267** (Heart Circ. Physiol. **36**): H92–H99.

35. IMAIZUMI, T. *et al.* 1993. Contribution of wall mechanics to the dynamic properties of aortic baroreceptor. Am. J. Physiol. **264** (Heart Circ. Physiol. **33**): H872–H880.
36. ROSENBAUM, M. & D. RACE. 1968. Frequency-response characteristics of vascular resistance vessels. Am. J. Physiol. **215:** 1397–1402.
37. NEWTON, G.E. & J.D. PARKER. 1996. Cardiac sympathetic responses to acute vasodilation. Normal ventricular function versus congestive heart failure. Circulation **94:** 3161–3167.
38. OREN, R.M. *et al.* 1991. Sympathetic responses of patients with congestive heart failure to cold pressor stimulus. Am. J. Card. **67:** 993–1001
39. BÅTH, E. *et al.* 1981. Effects of dynamic and static neck suction on muscle nerve sympathetic activity, heart rate and blood pressure in man. J. Physiol. (Lond.) **311:** 551–564.
40. FERGUSON, D.W. *et al.* 1983. Effects of propranolol on reflex vascular responses to orthostatic stress in humans: role of ventricular baroreceptors. Circulation **67:** 802–807.
41. ATHERTON, J.J. *et al.* 1997. Diastolic ventricular interaction in chronic heart failure. Lancet **349:** 1720–1724.
42. MIDDLEKAUFF, H.R. *et al.* 1995. Evidence for preserved cardiopulmonary baroreflex control of renal cortical blood flow in humans with advanced heart failure. A positron emission tomography study. Circulation **92:** 395–401.
43. AZEVEDO, E.R. *et al.* 2000. Reducing cardiac filling pressure lowers norepinephrine spillover in patients with chronic heart failure. Circulation **101:** 2053–2059.
44. KAYE, D.M. *et al.* 1994. Neurochemical evidence of cardiac sympathetic activation and increased central nervous system norepinephrine turnover in severe congestive heart failure. J. Am. Coll. Cardiol. **23:** 570–578.
45. WANG, W. & I.H. ZUCKER. 1996. Cardiac sympathetic afferent reflex in dogs with congestive heart failure. Am. J. Physiol. **271** (Regul. Integrative Comp. Physiol. **42**): R751–R756.
46. KAYE. D.M. *et al.* 1998. Differential effect of acute baroreceptor unloading on cardiac and systemic sympathetic tone in congestive heart failure. J. Am. Coll. Cardiol. **31:** 583–587.
47. RONGEN, G.A. *et al.* 1998. Angiotensin $AT_1$ receptor blockade abolishes the reflex sympatho-excitatory response to adenosine. J. Clin. Invest. **101:** 769–776.
48. CHEN, X. *et al.* 1995. Effects of forearm venous occlusion on peroneal muscle sympathetic nerve activity in healthy subjects. Am. J. Cardiol. **76:** 212–214.
49. NOTARIUS, C.F. *et al.* 2001. Impact of heart failure and exercise capacity on sympathetic responses to handgrip exercise. Am. J. Physiol. **280** (Heart Circ. Physiol.) H969–H976.
50. BRADLEY, T.D. & J.S. FLORAS. 1996. Pathophysiologic and therapeutic implications of sleep apnea in congestive heart failure. J. Card. Failure. **2:** 223–240.
51. SIN, D.D. *et al.* 1999. Risk factors for central and obstructive sleep apnea in 450 men and women with congestive heart failure. Am. J. Resp. Crit. Care Med. **160:** 1101–1106.

# Cerebral Autoregulation in Orthostatic Intolerance

RONALD SCHONDORF, JULIE BENOIT, AND REUBEN STEIN

*Autonomic Reflex Laboratory, Department of Neurology, McGill University, Sir Mortimer B. Davis Jewish General Hospital, Montreal, Quebec, Canada H3T 1E2*

ABSTRACT: Many of the primary symptoms of orthostatic intolerance (fatigue, diminished concentration) as well as some of the premonitory symptoms of neurally mediated syncope (NMS) are thought to be due to cerebral hypoperfusion. Transcranial Doppler measurements of middle cerebral artery blood velocity (CBV) is at present the only technique for assessing rapid changes in cerebral blood flow, and hence for evaluating dynamic cerebral autoregulation. However, controversies exist regarding data interpretation. At syncope, during the collapse of blood pressure (BP), diastolic CBV diminishes, whereas systolic CBV is maintained. Some consider this increase in CBV pulsatility to be indicative of a paradoxical increase in cerebrovascular resistance (CVR) prior to syncope. Others note that mean CBV decreases much less than does mean BP, implying that cerebral autoregulatory mechanisms are intact and functioning at syncope. Similarly, there is no evidence of impaired dynamic cerebral autoregulation, as measured by standard linear transfer-function analysis, in patients with NMS. Some patients with exaggerated postural tachycardia (POTS) have been found to have an excessive decrease in CBV during head-up tilt. Controversy exists as to whether this decrease results from an excessive sympathetic outflow to the cerebral vasculature or from hyperventilation. However, many other equally symptomatic patients with a similar hemodynamic profile of exaggerated tachycardia during head-up tilt have normal CBV changes during this maneuver and have normal dynamic cerebral autoregulation as determined by transfer-function analysis. Whether these discrepancies reflect different pathologies in patients with POTS is currently unknown.

KEYWORDS: Neurally mediated syncope; Postural tachycardia; Fourier analysis

## ORTHOSTATIC INTOLERANCE: A BRIEF OVERVIEW

Assumption of an upright posture causes translocation of approximately 800 mL of blood from the intrathoracic venous compartment to veins of the buttocks, pelvis, and legs.[1] The normal compensatory cardiovascular response to this orthostatic stress is a neurogenically mediated increase in heart rate (HR) and in systemic vascular resistance. As these compensatory reflexes become overwhelmed, premonitory symptoms of restlessness, malaise, nausea, and diminished concentration develop

Address for correspondence: Ronald Schondorf, Ph.D., M.D., Department of Neurology, Sir Mortimer B. Davis Jewish General Hospital, 3755 chemin de la Côte St. Catherine, Montreal, Quebec, Canada H3T 1E2. Voice: 514-340-8222, ext. 4767 or 3525; fax: 514-340-7567.
ronald.schondorf@mcgill.ca

and ultimately syncope occurs if the orthostatic stress is not terminated. In some patients these symptoms may develop minutes before the abrupt cardiovascular collapse that is the hallmark of neurally mediated syncope (NMS).[2] Since most patients with intermittent NMS are otherwise healthy normal individuals who can pursue a normal range of activities of daily living, we regard NMS as being *an episodic* orthostatic intolerance. Several recent reviews summarizing our current state of knowledge concerning the pathophysiology of NMS have been recently published.[3–5]

There is also a significant patient cohort that chronically or frequently has symptoms to stressors of orthostatic tolerance that would have minimal or no effect on normal subjects. These patients predictably develop symptoms of disabling fatigue, dizziness, diminished concentration, tremulousness, palpitations, chest discomfort, and nausea while standing. Syncope occurs infrequently. Simple activities such as eating, showering, or low-intensity exercise may profoundly exacerbate these symptoms and may significantly impair even the most rudimentary activities of daily living.[6–9] This *chronic* orthostatic intolerance is a disorder that disproportionately (3–4 times more frequent) affects young women. The illness may develop subacutely and is often preceded by a viral-like illness.[10] The most common hemodynamic abnormality associated with chronic orthostatic intolerance is an exaggerated postural tachycardia (POTS) of greater than 30 beats/min within 5 min of standing that is associated with symptoms of orthostatic intolerance. In more florid POTS, the absolute HR is greater than 120 beats/min.[8,10,11] Orthostatic hypotension is not present in POTS.[12] Other hemodynamic abnormalities occasionally seen in chronic orthostatic intolerance include postural diastolic hypertension[13] and delayed orthostatic hypotension.[14] The pathophysiology of POTS is complex, and more than one etiology for this condition is likely. A restricted autonomic neuropathy, excessive venous pooling, diminished plasma volume or red cell mass, cardiac β-adrenergic hypersensitivity, brainstem dysfunction, diminished cardiovagal baroreflex sensitivity, and enhanced baseline sympathetic activity have all been found in select groups of patients with POTS.[7,8,11,15,16] Impairment of the norepinephrine transporter has been recently detected in one family.[17]

The true prevalence of orthostatic intolerance is unknown and even rudimentary estimates are hard to obtain. One recent estimate suggests that as many as 500,000 Americans may suffer from some form of orthostatic intolerance.[18] The difficulty in obtaining true prevalence estimates relates to the fact that these patients' complaints are often dismissed because of the nonspecific nature of the symptoms reported. Some are diagnosed incorrectly as having panic disorder or chronic anxiety.[19] Orthostatic intolerance may be a frequent yet unappreciated contributor to patient morbidity. For example, we have recently shown that 40% of young previously productive patients (predominantly women) who have been diagnosed by experts as having chronic fatigue syndrome have clinical and laboratory evidence of orthostatic intolerance.[6,19] The prevalence of chronic fatigue syndrome in the United States has been recently estimated at approximately 422 per 100,000 adults.

## CEREBRAL AUTOREGULATION IN ORTHOSTATIC INTOLERANCE

Whereas many of the associated symptoms of chronic orthostatic intolerance seem to be related to a hyperadrenergic state (palpitations, tremulousness, chest tightness), other symptoms such as lightheadedness and diminished concentration are thought to reflect cerebral hypoperfusion. Some of the premonitory symptoms of NMS appear similar to those of orthostatic intolerance and some have suggested that patients with NMS may also have a primary disorder of cerebral perfusion.[20] The cerebral vasculature has the intrinsic ability to maintain cerebral blood flow constant over a wide range of perfusion pressures.[21,22] This cerebral autoregulation is critical to the determination of cerebral perfusion not only under normal conditions but also under conditions of severe orthostatic stress. For example, many patients with autonomic failure who have profound orthostatic hypotension while standing have minimal symptoms of cerebral hypoperfusion, because the accompanying decrease in cerebral perfusion during upright posture is small.[23,24] The remainder of this review discusses evidence for the notion that cerebral perfusion and autoregulation are impaired in patients with NMS or POTS. Since most measures of cerebral perfusion in these patients have been made using transcranial Doppler, we will briefly review the principles and pitfalls of this methodology. The techniques of assessing cerebral autoregulation will then be discussed, and finally the evidence for disordered cerebral autoregulation in NMS and in POTS will be evaluated.

## TRANSCRANIAL DOPPLER

A 2-MHz range-gated ultrasound probe is used to insonate the intracranial vessels. The actual signal measured is a reflection from erythrocytes moving within the vessel of interest. The moving column of blood within the sample volume of interest contributes to a mixture of Doppler shifts. The various frequencies contained within these Doppler shifts are decomposed via spectral analysis, and a velocity profile is displayed.[25] By convention the maximal envelope of the velocity profile is used. The velocity actually measured is proportional to the cosine of the angle of insonation (the ideal signal would be measured at an angle of $0°$). Most studies have insonated the middle cerebral artery (MCA) via the transtemporal window because of the relative thinness of the squamous temporal bone,[26] and because the trajectory of this vessel is most parallel to the Doppler signal (lowest angle of insonation). The Doppler probe is firmly strapped in place with an adjustable headband to minimize probe shifts during upright posture.[27,28]

Transcranial Doppler measures cerebral blood velocity (CBV) rather than cerebral blood flow. This can represent a significant limitation in methodology, because MCA CBV can only be considered to be an index of cerebral blood flow if MCA lumen area does not change.[29] The following observations suggest that MCA CBV provides a reasonable approximation of cerebral blood flow during standardized laboratory conditions: carotid blood flow is closely correlated with MCA velocity;[30] MCA diameter does not change significantly during craniotomy;[31] a recent study using MRI did not find changes in MCA lumen diameter during orthostatic stress simulated by lower-body negative pressure or during hypo- or hypercapnia;[32] estimates of cerebral perfusion using transcranial Doppler correlate well with symptoms of orthostatic intolerance[23] and with estimates of cerebral oxygenation measured with near-infrared spectroscopy over a wide range of BP in patients with autonomic failure.[33] There are conditions, however, where MCA diameter does not remain constant. For example, increases in MCA diameter may occur during severe hypercapnia,[34] and MCA vasoconstriction may occur after nitric oxide synthase inhibition.[35] Under these and other similar conditions, CBV may not provide adequate estimates of cerebral blood flow.

## ESTIMATING CEREBRAL AUTOREGULATION

Many measurements of cerebral autoregulation have evaluated the change in mean cerebral blood flow as a function of change in mean cerebral perfusion pressure without considering the time course or the dynamics of autoregulation. In most instances, changes in mean perfusion pressure are induced pharmacologically or via reflexly mediated changes in mean BP.[22] The range and number of perfusion pressures sampled is often limited to two points. Measurements that essentially regard cerebral autoregulation as static are of use in providing information concerning the overall efficiency of the process.[22] However, it is now evident that cerebral autoregulation is to a large degree a dynamic process that rapidly compensates for naturally occurring or induced fluctuations in cerebral perfusion pressure.[22,36] Dynamic cerebral autoregulation has been studied following transient changes in BP induced by rapid deflation of large cuffs previously placed around the upper thigh,[37] following transient carotid artery compression,[38] or by performance of the Valsalva maneuver.[28,39] None of these techniques are amenable to the study of patients during orthostatic stress. Moreover, none of these methods defines the ability to counteract the BP fluctuations that normally occur during orthostasis.

Using standard linear transfer-function analysis, dynamic cerebral pressure autoregulation may also be modeled as a frequency-dependent phenomenon approximating a high-pass filter.[22,40,41] This analysis has been used extensively in the study of autoregulation of other vascular beds.[42,43] The signature of a dynamic autoregulating system is easily recognizable. At frequencies where autoregulation is operant, fluctuations in blood flow lead those in BP and normalized gain is <1, indicating the presence of an active mechanism that limits the transfer of BP fluctuations into flow. At higher frequencies, where autoregulation is no longer operant, normalized gain is >1, because vascular compliance amplifies BP fluctuations into flow. Fluctuations in MCA CBV also precede mechanically generated BP fluctuations, but only when cerebral autoregulation is intact.[44,45] Estimates of cerebral autoregulation obtained using linear transfer methods accord well with those obtained using the thigh-cuff deflation technique.[41] The limitations of linear transfer analysis techniques have been addressed extensively.[41,46,47] More recent models of dynamic cerebral autoregulation using nonlinear analysis have yielded slightly more accurate results under more limited conditions of measurement.[47]

## CEREBRAL AUTOREGULATION IN NMS

Although isolated cases of cerebral hypoperfusion without hypotension have been reported in patients with unexplained recurrent syncope,[48,49] in general there appears to be little evidence that static autoregulation is impaired during head-up tilt-induced syncope.[27] A typical example of head-up tilt-induced syncope is shown in

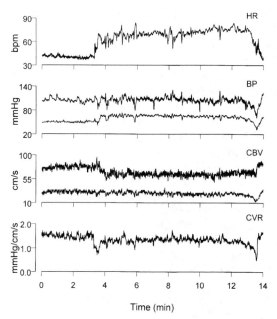

**FIGURE 1.** Typical beat-to-beat profiles of HR, systolic and diastolic BP, systolic and diastolic CBV, and calculated CVR from a patient with neurally mediated syncope during a supine baseline period and during 80° head-up tilt.

FIGURE 1. FIGURE 2 shows the averaged profile of the last 4 min preceding syncope constructed from data recorded from 49 subjects with NMS. From these two figures it is evident that CBV is maintained during the initial decline in BP and that only diastolic CBV decreases during syncope, whereas systolic CBV is maintained. Several investigators have obtained similar results.[20,27,50]

Two vastly different interpretations have been assigned to the data obtained during head-up tilt that depend on the index used to infer cerebrovascular resistance (CVR). Gosling's pulsatility index (systolic CBV-diastolic CBV)/mean CBV, can be used as an index of distal CVR if BP and HR are relatively stable.[51,52] The obvious increase in CBV pulsatility at syncope has prompted some to suggest the existence of a *paradoxical* vasoconstriction that must overwhelm dynamic cerebral autoregulation and contribute to the loss of consciousness at syncope.[20] In contrast, we have argued that the limited decrease in mean CBV in the face of large decreases in mean BP at syncope constitutes clear evidence of relatively preserved dynamic cerebral autoregulation.[27] Moreover, in many instances there is a clear divergence between pulsatility index and CVR.[28] In an experimental rabbit model of syncope, drug-induced hypotension or hypotensive hemorrhage provokes a significant decrease in CVR and a concomitant increase in pulsatility index.[52] Therefore, although under stable conditions a qualitative relationship does exist between pulsatility and CVR, it is doubtful that this index can serve as an adequate index of CVR during the rapid BP decrease at syncope. The etiology for the selective decline in diastolic CBV at syncope is still unclear. We have suggested that collapse of downstream vessels may

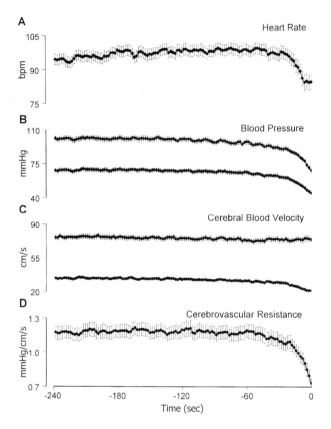

**FIGURE 2.** Profile of the last 2 min of beat-to-beat cardiovascular and cerebrovascular parameters back-averaged from the trough of the blood pressure at syncope ($n = 49$). Note that cerebral blood velocity is maintained during the initial gradual decline in blood pressure. As syncope developed, there was a precipitous decrease in heart rate, systolic, and diastolic blood pressure, diastolic cerebral blood velocity, and calculated cerebrovascular resistance. Systolic cerebral blood velocity does not change during syncope.

occur as diastolic BP decreases below the critical closing pressure of cerebral vessels.[27,36]

More recently, we have applied the linear transfer-analysis techniques discussed as an ancillary means of evaluating dynamic cerebral autoregulation prior to syncope.[53] FIGURE 3 is a representative sample analysis from the 3 min prior to the onset of syncope of the subject whose profile is shown in FIGURE 1. Forty-nine subjects with NMS and 15 control subjects have been analyzed. We have shown that (1) autoregulation is operant at frequencies lower than 0.14 Hz; (2) in the 3 min preceding syncope, dynamic cerebral autoregulation of subjects with NMS does not differ from that of controls; (3) dynamic cerebral autoregulation does not change over the course of head-up tilt in patients with NMS or in control subjects; and (4) dynamic cerebral autoregulation is unaffected by the degree of orthostatic intolerance, as inferred from

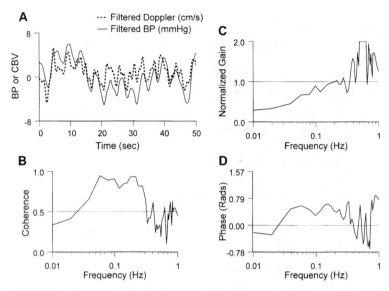

**FIGURE 3.** Linear transfer-function analysis yields a precise relationship between fluctuations in CBV and BP from the subject with syncope shown in FIGURE 1. Data are sampled from the last 3 min preceding syncope. Representative filtered data segment (**A**) shows that oscillations in BP and CBV are coherent. There is substantial coherence (**B**) in a frequency band from 0.03 to 0.3 Hz. Below 0.2 Hz transfer gain (**C**) is <1.0, indicating active cerebral autoregulation. Admittance phase (**D**) is positive, suggesting that flow leads pressure in the frequency band at which autoregulation is operating.

latency to onset of syncope. These observations complement the earlier conclusions of intact dynamic cerebral autoregulation in NMS.

Finally, other data obtained using techniques other than transcranial Doppler also suggest that cerebral autoregulation is preserved in NMS. EEG abnormalities (diffuse high-amplitude slow waves or disappearance of EEG activity) during head-up tilt-induced syncope are recorded only at clinically evident syncope and at a time when BP is no longer measurable by auscultation.[54] Multifocal myoclonus, visual, or auditory hallucinations may be associated with such profound cerebral hypoperfusion at syncope.[55] However, the EEG record is normal prior to syncope, indicating that at this point cerebral perfusion is still well preserved. Similar inferences can also be drawn from near-infrared spectroscopic measurements of cerebral oxygenation at syncope.[56]

## CEREBRAL AUTOREGULATION IN POTS

As noted earlier, the symptoms of lightheadedness and diminished concentration during orthostatic stress in POTS are often attributed to diminished cerebral perfusion.[28,57–59] To date, two groups of investigators have recorded significantly larger decreases in CBV, and hence very elevated CVRs during orthostatic stress from an

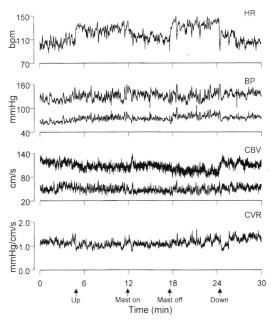

**FIGURE 4.** Typical beat-to-beat profiles of HR, systolic and diastolic BP, systolic and diastolic CBV, and calculated CVR from a patient with POTS during a supine baseline period, during 80° head-up tilt (*arrows*) and during a supine recovery period. During head-up tilt, MAST pants were inflated for approximately 5 min (*arrows*) in order to diminish venous pooling. During inflation, heart rate decreased. Symptoms of fatigue and lightheadedness were significantly improved without any significant change in cerebral perfusion.

approximate total of 45 patients with POTS.[28,57–59] In contrast, we have found no laboratory evidence of cerebral hypoperfusion in 24 patients with POTS.[60] These discrepancies highlight the fact that POTS remains a complex and multifactorial disorder that is incompletely understood. Nonetheless, in this section we will attempt to reconcile some of these discrepancies in order to focus on the gaps in our understanding of the symptoms of POTS.

FIGURE 4 is an example of a recording from a patient with POTS while supine and during head-up tilt. After approximately 7 min of head-up tilt, MAST pants were inflated in order to minimize venous pooling. This inflation was associated with a significant decrease in HR and with a definite relief in the symptoms of orthostatic intolerance (including lightheadedness) without any significant change in CBV. Deflation of MAST pants was associated with an increased HR and a return of symptoms again without any change in CBV. In none of our 24 patients was there an increase in CVR once a correction for the change in hydrostatic pressure during upright posture was applied. Moreover, the change in CVR did not differ from that of normal control subjects. These data suggest that in this subgroup of POTS static cerebral autoregulation is maintained.

Our patients were similar in age and gender to those described by others and had a similar hemodynamic profile. All patients described by the Vanderbilt group [57,59] appeared to conform to those with florid POTS, whereas many of the patients described by the Mayo group[58] did not fit this definition. Inclusion criteria for orthostatic intolerance required a 30-beats/min HR increment from baseline and an absolute HR of >100 beats/min for >60% of a 10-min tilt. Fourteen of our 24 patients had florid POTS, and all 24 conformed to the Mayo inclusion criteria. We found no difference in the CBV or CVR profiles between the two subgroups, although by definition the absolute HR attained during orthostatic stress were significantly different.

Many of the patients with POTS in the Mayo study exhibited an excessive decrease in end tidal $CO_2$ during orthostatic stress.[58] The symptoms of cerebral hypoperfusion and the decline in CBV were reversed by $CO_2$ rebreathing. Although neither tidal volume nor alveolar ventilation were measured, it was suggested that hyperventilation occurred as patients increased depth of respiration to increase venous return. We have not observed hyperventilation in our patient subset. If cerebral hypoperfusion is simply a maladaptive attempt to offset the increased venous pooling of POTS, then these patients may have normal cerebral autoregulation during head-up tilt. However, the Mayo group have also documented abnormally prolonged CBV recovery during phase IV of the Valsalva maneuver, an observation that might suggest that autoregulation is impaired in some of their patients with POTS.[28] We have applied linear transfer-analysis techniques to evaluate dynamic cerebral autoregulation in 24 patients with POTS. FIGURE 5 is a representative sample analysis from the 3 min prior to inflation of the MAST pants of the subject whose profile is

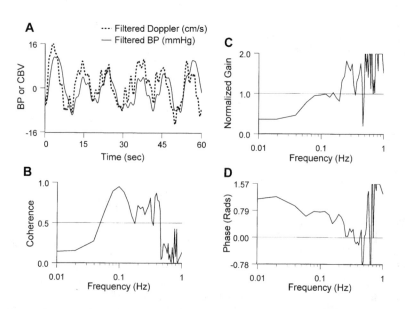

**FIGURE 5.** Representative filtered data segment (**A**) and transfer functions from the POTS patient shown in FIGURE 3. Data are sampled from the last 3 min preceding MAST pants inflation. There was substantial coherence (**B**) in a frequency band from 0.05 to 0.3 Hz. Below 0.08 Hz transfer gain (**C**) was <1.0, indicating active autoregulation. Admittance phase (**D**) was positive in this frequency band, suggesting that flow leads pressure.

shown in FIGURE 4. As for patients with NMS, we found no evidence of impaired dynamic cerebral autoregulation in POTS.

Infusion of the α-adrenergic receptor antagonist phentolamine or the α-receptor agonist phenylephrine each attenuated the decrease in CBV during head-up tilt in POTS.[57] End tidal $CO_2$ was not measured in these patients. These data prompted the suggestion that the increase in CVR in POTS is due to a primary sympathetically mediated increase in cerebral vasoconstriction. Although the role of the sympathetic nervous system in limiting autoregulatory breakthrough during hypertension has been well established,[61] there is little evidence at present that sympathetic activity contributes significantly to resting cerebrovascular tone at normocapnia[62] and during normotension.[63] Moreover reflexly mediated sympathetic cerebral vasoconstriction is evoked only by very large decreases in BP.[64]

Clearly, additional work is required. It remains unclear why some patients with POTS hyperventilate during orthostatic stress, while others with similar symptoms of *cerebral hypoperfusion* do not. We have not found evidence of impaired dynamic cerebral autoregulation during orthostatic stress in our patient subgroup, but this analysis has yet to be applied to other patients recorded in other laboratories. Is there a referral bias in the patients selected by some laboratories for detailed study, or are the patients studied typical of those with POTS encountered elsewhere? Lastly, if cerebral autoregulation and perfusion are maintained in many patients with POTS, then what is the pathophysiology of the symptoms of lightheadedness and diminished concentration that are ubiquitous in POTS? Clarification of these and other questions will permit more rational treatment and relief of symptoms of patients with orthostatic intolerance.

## ACKNOWLEDGMENTS

This work was supported by grants to Ronald Schondorf from The CFIDS Association of America and the Fondation des Maladies du Coeur du Québec.

## REFERENCES

1. BLOMQVIST, C.G. & H.L. STONE. 1983. Cardiovascular adjustments to gravitational stress. *In* Handbook of Physiology. The Cardiovascular System. Peripheral Circulation and Organ Blood Flow: 1025–1063. American Physiological Society. Bethesda, MD.
2. NOVAK, V., G. HONOS & R. SCHONDORF. 1996. Is the heart "empty" at syncope? J. Auton. Nerv. Syst. **60:** 83–92.
3. MOSQUEDA-GARCIA, R., R. FURLAN, J. TANK, *et al.* 2000. The elusive pathophysiology of neurally mediated syncope. Circulation. **102:** 2898–2906.
4. BENDITT, D.G. 1997. Neurally mediated syncopal syndromes: pathophysiological concepts and clinical evaluation. Pacing Clin. Electrophysiol. **20:** 572–584.
5. ROBERTSON, R.M., E. MEDINA, N. SHAH, *et al.* 1999. Neurally mediated syncope: pathophysiology and implications for treatment. Am. J. Med. Sci. **317:** 102–109.
6. SCHONDORF, R. & R. FREEMAN. 1999. The importance of orthostatic intolerance in the chronic fatigue syndrome. Am. J. Med. Sci. **317:** 117–123.
7. JACOB, G. & I. BIAGGIONI. 1999. Idiopathic orthostatic intolerance and postural tachycardia syndromes. Am. J. Med. Sci. **317:** 88–101.
8. LOW, P.A., T.L. OPFER-GEHRKING, S.C. TEXTOR, *et al.* 1995. Postural tachycardia syndrome (POTS). Neurology **45:** S19–S25.

9. STREETEN, D.H. 1999. Orthostatic intolerance: a historical introduction to the patho-physiological mechanisms. Am. J. Med. Sci. **317:** 78–87.
10. SCHONDORF, R. & P.A. LOW. 1993. Idiopathic postural orthostatic tachycardia syndrome: an attenuated form of acute pandysautonomia? Neurology **43:** 132–137.
11. LOW, P.A., R. SCHONDORF, V. NOVAK, et al.1997. Postural tachycardia syndrome (POTS). *In* Clinical Autonomic Disorders, P.A. Low, Ed.: 681–697. Lippincott-Raven. Philadelphia.
12. LOW, P.A., T.L. OPFER-GEHRKING, S.C. TEXTOR, et al. 1994. Comparison of the postural tachycardia syndrome (POTS) with orthostatic hypotension due to autonomic failure. J. Auton. Nerv. Syst. **50:** 181–188.
13. STREETEN, D.H., G.H. ANDERSON, JR., R. RICHARDSON, et al. 1988. Abnormal orthostatic changes in blood pressure and heart rate in subjects with intact sympathetic nervous function: evidence for excessive venous pooling. J. Lab. Clin. Med. **111:** 326–335.
14. STREETEN, D.H.P. & G.H. ANDERSEN. 1992. Delayed orthostatic intolerance. Arch. Intern. Med. **152:** 1066–1072.
15. JACOB, G., F. COSTA, J.R. SHANNON, et al. 2000. The neuropathic postural tachycardia syndrome. N. Engl. J. Med. **343:** 1008–1014.
16. FARQUHAR, W.B., J.A. TAYLOR, S.E. DARLING, et al. 2000. Abnormal baroreflex responses in patients with idiopathic orthostatic intolerance. Circulation **102:** 3086–3091.
17. SHANNON, J.R., N.L. FLATTEM, J. JORDAN, et al. 2000. Orthostatic intolerance and tachycardia associated with norepinephrine-transporter deficiency. N. Eng. J. Med. **342:** 541–549.
18. ROBERTSON, D. 1999. The epidemic of orthostatic tachycardia and orthostatic intolerance. Am. J. Med. Sci. **317:** 75–77.
19. SCHONDORF, R., J. BENOIT, T. WEIN, et al. 1999. Orthostatic intolerance in the chronic fatigue syndrome. J. Auton. Nerv. Syst. **75:** 192–201.
20. GRUBB, B.P., G. GERARD, K. ROUSH, et al. 1991. Cerebral vasoconstriction during head-upright tilt-induced vasovagal syncope. A paradoxic and unexpected response. Circulation **84:** 1157–1164.
21. PAULSON, O.B., S. STRANDGAARD & L. EDVINSSON. 1990. Cerebral autoregulation. Cerebrovasc. Brain Metab. Rev. **2:** 161–192.
22. PANERAI, R. 1998. Assessment of cerebral pressure autoregulation in humans-a review of measurement methods. Physiol. Meas. **19:** 305–338.
23. NOVAK, V., P. NOVAK, J.M. SPIES, et al. 1998. Autoregulation of cerebral blood flow in orthostatic hypotension. Stroke **29:** 104–111.
24. THOMAS, D.J. & R. BANNISTER. 1980. Preservation of autoregulation of cerebral blood flow in autonomic failure. J. Neurol. Sci. **44:** 205–212.
25. AASLID, R.1992. Development and principles of transcranial doppler. *In* Transcranial Doppler, D.W. Newell and R. Aaslid, Eds.: 1-8. Raven Press. New York.
26. FUJIOKA, K.A. & C.M. DOUVILLE.1992. Anatomy and freehand examination techniques. *In* Transcranial Doppler, D.W. Newell and R. Aaslid, Eds.: 9–31. Raven Press. New York.
27. SCHONDORF, R., J. BENOIT & T. WEIN. 1997. Cerebrovascular and cardiovascular measurements during neurally mediated syncope induced by head-up tilt. Stroke **28:** 1564–1568.
28. LOW, P.A., V. NOVAK, J.M. SPIES, et al. 1999. Cerebrovascular regulation in the postural orthostatic tachycardia syndrome (POTS). Am. J. Med. Sci. **317:** 124–133.
29. KONTOS, H. 1992. Assessment of cerebral autoregulation dynamics. Stroke **23:** 1031.
30. LINDEGAARD, K.F., T. LUNDAR, J. WIBERG, et al. 1987. Variations in middle cerebral artery blood flow investigated with noninvasive transcranial blood velocity measurements. Stroke **18:** 1025–1030.
31. GILLER, C.A., G. BOWMAN, H. DYER, et al. 1993. Cerebral arterial diameters during changes in blood pressure and carbon dioxide during craniotomy. Neurosurgery 1993 **32:** 737–741.
32. SERRADOR, J.M., P.A. PICOT, B.K. RUTT, et al. 2000. MRI measures of middle cerebral artery diameter in conscious humans during simulated orthostasis. Stroke **31:** 1672–1678.

33. HARMS, M.P.M., W. COLIER, W. WIELING, *et al.* 2000. Orthostatic tolerance, cerebral oxygenation, and blood velocity in humans with sympathetic failure. Stroke **31:** 1608–1614.
34. VALDUEZA, J.M., B. DRAGANSKI, O. HOFFMANN, *et al.* 1999. Analysis of $CO_2$ vasomotor reactivity and vessel diameter changes by simultaneous venous and arterial Doppler recordings. Stroke **30:** 81–86.
35. WHITE, R.P., C. DEANE, P. VALLANCE, *et al.* 1998. Nitric oxide synthase inhibition in humans reduces cerebral blood flow but not the hyperemic response to hypercapnia. Stroke **29:** 467–472.
36. AASLID, R.1992. Cerebral hemodynamics. *In* Transcranial Doppler, D.W. Newell and R. Aaslid, Eds.: 49–55. Raven Press. New York.
37. AASLID, R., K.F. LINDEGAARD, W. SORTEBERG, *et al.* 1989. Cerebral autoregulation dynamics in humans. Stroke **20:** 45–52.
38. SMIELEWSKI, P., M. CZOSNYKA, P. KIRKPATRICK, *et al.* 1996. Assessment of cerebral autoregulation using carotid artery compression. Stroke **27:** 2197–2203.
39. TIECKS, F., C. DOUVILLE, S. BYRD, *et al.* 1996. Evaluation of impaired cerebral autoregulation by the Valsalva maneuver. Stroke **27:** 1177–1182.
40. BLABER, A.P., R.L. BONDAR, F. STEIN, *et al.* 1997. Transfer function analysis of cerebral autoregulation dynamics in autonomic failure patients. Stroke **28:** 1686–1692.
41. ZHANG, R., J.H. ZUKERMAN, C.A. GILLER, *et al.,* 1998. Transfer function analysis of dynamic cerebral autoregulation in humans. Am. J. Physiol. **274:** H233–H241.
42. HOLSTEIN-RATHLOU, N. 1993. Oscillations and chaos in renal blood flow control. J. Am. Soc. Nephrol. **4:** 1275–1287.
43. ABU-AMARAH, I., D.O. AJIKOBI, H. BACHELARD, *et al.* 1998. Responses of mesenteric and renal blood flow dynamics to acute denervation in anesthetized rats. Am. J. Physiol. **275:** R1543–R1552.
44. DIEHL, R.R., D. LINDEN, D. LÜCKE, *et al.* 1995. Phase relationship between cerebral blood flow velocity and blood pressure—A clinical test of autoregulation. Stroke **26:** 1801–1804.
45. BIRCH, A.A., M.J. DIRNHUBER, R. HARTLEY-DAVIES, *et al.* 1995. Assessment of autoregulation by means of periodic changes in blood pressure. Stroke **26:** 834–837.
46. ZHANG, R., J.H. ZUCKERMAN & B.D. LEVINE. 2000. Spontaneous fluctuations in cerebral blood flow: insights from extended-duration recordings in humans. Am. J. Physiol. **278:** H1848–H1855.
47. PANERAI, R.B., S.L. DAWSON & J.F. POTTER. 1999. Linear and nonlinear analysis of human dynamic cerebral autoregulation. Am. J. Physiol. **277:** H1089–H1099.
48. FREDMAN, C.S., K.M. BIERMANN, V. PATEL, *et al.* 1995. Transcranial Doppler ultrasonography during head-upright tilt-table testing. Ann. Intern. Med. **123:** 848–849.
49. GRUBB, B.P., D. SAMOIL, D. KOSINSKI, *et al.* 1998. Cerebral syncope: loss of consciousness associated with cerebral vasoconstriction in the absence of systemic hypotension. Pacing Clin. Electrophysiol. **21:** 652–658.
50. DIEHL, R.R., D. LINDEN, A. CHALKIADAKI, *et al.* 1999. Cerebrovascular mechanisms in neurocardiogenic syncope with and without postural tachycardia syndrome. J. Auton. Nerv. Syst. **76:** 159–166.
51. BRAGONI, M. & E. FELDMANN.1996. Transcranial Doppler indices of intracranial hemodynamics. *In* Neurosonology, C.H. Tegeler, V.L. Babikian and C.R. Gomez, Eds. Mosby. St. Louis.
52. CZOSNYKA, M., H.K. RICHARDS, H.E. WHITEHOUSE, *et al.* 1996. Relationship between transcranial Doppler-determined pulsatility index and cerebrovascular resistance: an experimental study. J. Neurosurg. **84:** 79–84.
53. SCHONDORF, R., R. STEIN, R. ROBERTS, *et al.* 1999. Transfer function analysis of cerebral autoregulation in normal control subjects and in patients with neurally-mediated syncope. Clin. Auton. Res. **9:** 208.
54. AMMIRATI, F., F. COLIVICCHI, G. DI BATTISTA, *et al.* 1998. Electroencephalographic correlates of vasovagal syncope induced by head-up tilt testing. Stroke **29:** 2347–2351.
55. LEMPERT, T., M. BAUER & D. SCHMIDT. 1994. Syncope: a videometric analysis of 56 episodes of transient cerebral hypoxia. Ann. Neurol. **36:** 233–237.

56. MADSEN, P., F. POTT, S.B. OLSEN, *et al.* 1998. Near-infrared spectrophotometry determined brain oxygenation during fainting. Acta Physiol. Scand. **162:** 501–507.
57. JORDAN, J., J.R. SHANNON, B.K. BLACK, *et al.* 1998. Raised cerebrovascular resistance in idiopathic orthostatic intolerance—Evidence for sympathetic vasoconstriction. Hypertension **32:** 699–704.
58. NOVAK, V., J.M. SPIES, P. NOVAK, *et al.* 1998. Hypocapnia and cerebral hypoperfusion in orthostatic intolerance. Stroke **29:** 1876–1881.
59. JACOB, G., D. ATKINSON, J. JORDAN, *et al.* 1999. Effects of standing on cerebrovascular resistance in patients with idiopathic orthostatic intolerance. Am. J. Med. **106:** 59–64.
60. SCHONDORF, R., R. STEIN, J. BENOIT, *et al.* 2000. Transfer function analysis of cerebral autoregulation in patients with orthostatic intolerance (OI), postural tachycardia syndrome (POTS) and chronic fatigue syndrome (CFS). Clin. Auton. Res. **10:** 224.
61. HEISTAD, D. & H. KONTOS.1982. Cerebral circulation. *In* Handbook of Physiology—The Cardiovascular System III. 137–182. American Physiological Society. Bethesda, MD.
62. JORDAN, J., J.R. SHANNON, A. DIEDRICH, *et al.* 2000. Interaction of carbon dioxide and sympathetic nervous system activity in the regulation of cerebral perfusion in humans. Hypertension **36:** 383–388.
63. SANDOR, P. 1999. Nervous control of the cerebrovascular system: doubts and facts. Neurochem. Int. **35:** 237–259.
64. FITCH, W., E.T. MACKENZIE & A.M. HARPER. 1975. Effects of decreasing blood pressure on cerebral blood flow in the baboon. Circ. Res. **37:** 550–557.

# Familial Orthostatic Tachycardia Due to Norepinephrine Transporter Deficiency

DAVID ROBERTSON,[a] NANCY FLATTEM,[a] TAHIR TELLIOGLU,[a] ROBERT CARSON[a], EMILY GARLAND,[a] JOHN R. SHANNON,[a] JENS JORDAN,[b] GIRIS JACOB,[c] RANDY D. BLAKELY,[a] AND ITALO BIAGGIONI[a]

[a]Autonomic Dysfunction Center, Vanderbilt University, Nashville, Tennessee 37232-2195, USA

[b]Clinical Research Center, Franz Volhard Klinik, Berlin, Germany

[c]Recanati Autonomic Dysfunction Center, Rambam Medical Center, Haifa, Israel

ABSTRACT: Orthostatic intolerance (OI) or postural tachycardia syndrome (POTS) is a syndrome primarily affecting young females, and is characterized by lightheadedness, palpitations, fatigue, altered mentation, and syncope primarily occurring with upright posture and being relieved by lying down. There is typically tachycardia and raised plasma norepinephrine levels on upright posture, but little or no orthostatic hypotension. The pathophysiology of OI is believed to be very heterogeneous. Most studies of the syndrome have focused on abnormalities in norepinephrine release. Here the hypothesis that abnormal norepinephrine transporter (NET) function might contribute to the pathophysiology in some patients with OI was tested. In a proband with significant orthostatic symptoms and tachycardia, disproportionately elevated plasma norepinephrine with standing, impaired systemic, and local clearance of infused tritiated norepinephrine, impaired tyramine responsiveness, and a dissociataion between stimulated plasma norepinephrine and DHPG elevation were found. Studies of NET gene structure in the proband revealed a coding mutation that converts a highly conserved transmembrane domain Ala residue to Pro. Analysis of the protein produced by the mutant cDNA in transfected cells demonstrated greater than 98% reduction in activity relative to normal. NE, DHPG/NE, and heart rate correlated with the mutant allele in this family. Conclusion: These results represent the first identification of a specific genetic defect in OI and the first disease linked to a coding alteration in a $Na^+/Cl^-$-dependent neurotransmitter transporter. Identification of this mechanism may facilitate our understanding of genetic causes of OI and lead to the development of more effective therapeutic modalities.

KEYWORDS: Norepinephrine; Tachycardia; Orthostatic intolerance (OI); Norepinephrine transporter (NET); Mitral valve prolapse

Address for correspondence: David Robertson, M.D., Autonomic Dysfunction Center, AA3228 MCN, Vanderbilt University, Nashville, TN 37232-2195. Voice: 615-343-6499; fax: 615-343-8649.

david.robertson@mcmail.vanderbilt.edu

527

## INTRODUCTION

When homeostatic adjustments to the upright posture fail, disabling symptoms may occur.[1] These symptoms are often described as dizziness, visual changes, discomfort in the head or neck, poor concentration, or weakness. Palpitations, tremulousness, fatigue, and anxiety may be seen. In severe cases, there may be altered breathing pattern and syncope.

In 1925, Bradbury and Eggleston[2,3] reported such symptoms in profound orthostatic hypotension, and proposed that failure of the autonomic nervous system could cause them. Successful symptomatic pharmacotherapy with a sympathomimetic amine was reported in 1928.[4] Such patients, with intact central neurological function and no evidence of secondary autonomic neuropathy are now said to have pure autonomic failure.

## DIVERSITY OF AUTONOMIC DYSREGULATION

In the subsequent 70 years, there has been much improvement in our understanding of the heterogeneity of orthostatic disorders and autonomic failure (for review see Ref. 5). Although each etiology has its own characteristic clinical pattern and natural history, the conceptualization of autonomic failure reported by Bradbury and Eggleston has continued to dominate the literature and the textbooks. In English-speaking countries, until recently there has been a focus on severe orthostatic disorders that led to the neglect of more subtle presentations, such as orthostatic intolerance (OI). In Central Europe, there was a different intellectual tradition that drove a tenfold greater frequency of diagnosis of subtle orthostatic disorders than that seen in the United States and the United Kingdom.[6–8] The diversity of presentation of orthostatic disorders was noted in a careful study of "arterial orthostatic anemia" by Bjure and Laurell in 1927.[9] Much of the subsequent history of the concept of OI is discussed by Streeten.[10,11] Streeten proposed a classification of milder orthostatic disorders roughly calibrated with the severity of the impairment. This patient population is heterogeneous[12–21] and has been referred to by many names, as follow:

- Hyperadrenergic orthostatic hypotension[18]
- Orthostatic tachycardia syndrome[19,20]
- Postural orthostatic tachycardia syndrome[16]
- Postural tachycardia syndrome[16,52]
- Hyperadrenergic postural hypotension[29]
- Sympathotonic orthostatic hypotension[53]
- Hyperdynamic β-adrenergic state[17]
- Idiopathic hypovolemia[12]
- Orthostatic tachycardia plus[54]
- Sympathicotonic orthostatic hypotension[10]
- Mitral valve prolapse syndrome[55–57]
- Soldier's heart[58]
- Vasoregulatory asthenia[10]

- Neurocirculatory asthenia[10]
- Irritable heart[59]
- Orthostatic anemia[9]
- Chronic fatigue syndrome[60]

## ORTHOSTATIC INTOLERANCE

Patients with abnormal heart-rate response to upright posture have long been recognized, including individuals with sinoatrial,[22] atrial,[23] and ventricular[24] tachycardias provoked by standing. Among those with sinoatrial orthostatic tachycardia according to the criteria of Streeten[10] are many patients with posture-related symptoms of weakness, fatigue, chest discomfort, dizziness, anxiety, and occasionally presyncope or syncope (TABLE 1).[25,26] Some have mitral-valve prolapse by auscultatory or echocardiographic criteria. The raised heart rate on standing might be an important clue to understanding pathophysiology in these patients. This orthostatic tachycardia has caused investigators to consider several interesting possibilities to explain the disorder. If there were a circulating vasodilator,[27] or a reduced "effective" blood volume,[12,28] the orthostatic tachycardia might be an appropriate and healthy autonomic compensatory response mediated through the baroreflex to maintain adequate blood pressure and cardiac output.[29] However, the compensatory response is hemodynamically inadequate as can be seen in FIGURE 1, which shows a more rapid than normal decline in middle cerebral artery (MCA) blood velocity with tilt in orthostatic intolerance patients, even though blood pressure does not fall.[30,31]

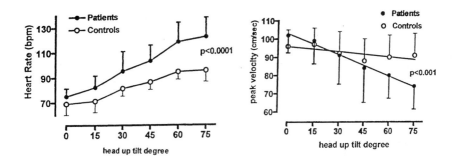

**FIGURE 1.** Transcranial Doppler of MCA patients with orthostatic intolerance and normal subjects during upright tilt. Note that as the angle of tilt is gradually decreased, MCA flow velocity fell more steeply in the patients than in the normal subjects, even though blood pressures were comparable. This suggests that relative vasoconstriction might be occurring in the cerebral vasculature during this upright stimulus.

TABLE 1. Contrasting features of pure autonomic failure and orthostatic intolerance

| PAF | OI |
| --- | --- |
| Hypotension | Tachycardia |
| Syncope early | Syncope late |
| Onset after 50 | Onset before 50 |
| Male = female | Female ≫ male |
| Low norepinephrine | High norepinephrine |

## COULD REDUCED NOREPINEPHRINE CLEARANCE UNDERLIE ORTHOSTATIC INTOLERANCE?

Virtually all explanations of the physiological and biochemical abnormalities in OI have focused on alterations in norepinephrine release (i.e., compensatory,[11] excessive,[32] or disordered[33]). An alternative explanation is an abnormality in synaptic norepinephrine clearance. Approximately 80–90% of norepinephrine released into many synapses is cleared by neuronal reuptake via the presynaptic norepinephrine transporter (NET), while the remaining 10–20% spills over into the circulation or extraneuronal tissue.[34] It is noteworthy that drugs inhibiting NET (e.g., cocaine, amphetamines, tricyclic antidepressants) may elicit findings typical of OI (i.e., tachycardia, orthostatic symptoms, and elevated plasma catecholamines). Furthermore, recent reports suggest a genetic component to OI, such as might be encountered in a disorder associated with impairment of a gene product underlying catecholamine metabolism.[35,36]

## THE NOREPINEPHRINE TRANSPORTER (SCL6A2) AS A CANDIDATE GENE

The norepinephrine (NE) transporter (NET) is the major mechanism of NE removal from the synaptic cleft. The expression and function of the NET is tightly controlled by mechanisms at both the transcriptional and second-messenger levels. A single gene encodes the NET at all noradrenergic synapses. It is therefore likely that polymorphisms in this gene product play a significant role in system physiology. We therefore hypothesized that abnormal NET function might underlie orthostatic intolerance.

## ASSESSMENT OF FUNCTION OF NET AT THE BEDSIDE

When we encountered twins (in a Swedish-American family of 10 siblings) with typical symptoms of OI, we undertook a systematic evaluation employing bedside physiological, biochemical, and pharmacological tests. The proband was a 33-year-old female with a 20-year history of exertional and orthostatic provocation of tachy-

**TABLE 2. Orthostatic blood pressure, heart rate, and plasma catecholamines**

Supine and upright blood pressure and heart rate

| | | | supine | upright |
|---|---|---|---|---|
| proband | sbp | | 120 | 110 |
| | dbp | (mmHg) | 74 | 72 |
| | h | (bpm) | 80 | 109 |
| twin | | | | |
| | sbp | (mmHg) | 132 | 156 |
| | dbp | (mmHg) | 74 | 95 |
| | h | (bpm) | 79 | 131 |
| controls | | | | |
| | sbp | (mmHg) | 108 ± 2 | 106 ± 3 |
| | dbp | (mmHg) | 63 ± 2 | 67 ± 3 |
| | h | (bpm) | 65 ± 2 | 83 ± 4 |

Supine and upright plasma catecholamines

| | | | supine | upright |
|---|---|---|---|---|
| proband | | | supine | upright |
| | NE | (pg/mL) | 269 | 923 |
| | Epi | (pg/mL) | 11 | 23 |
| | DHPG | (pg/mL) | 824 | 968 |
| | DHPG/NE | | 3.06 | 1.05 |
| twin | | | | |
| | NE | (pg/mL) | 199 | 911 |
| | Epi | (pg/mL) | 22 | 116 |
| | DHPG | (pg/mL) | 480 | 1068 |
| | DHPG/NE | | 2.41 | 1.17 |
| controls | | | | |
| | NE | (pg/mL) | 200 ± 20 | 485 ± 50 |
| | Epi | (pg/mL) | 25 ± 3 | 49 ± 4 |
| | DHPG | | 1104 ± 115 | 1379 ± 133 |
| | (pg/mL) | | | |
| | DHPG/NE | | 5.52 | 2.84 |

NOTE: Systolic blood pressure (sbp), diastolic blood pressure (dbp), and heart rate (hr) were determined on multiple occasions in the proband and twin and on one occasion in each of eight normal volunteers. Norepinephrine (NE), epinephrine (Epi), and dihydroxyphenylglycol (DHPG) were determined once each in the proband and twin and once in each of eight normal volunteers. Data are presented as mean ± SEM. To convert pg/mL to nmol/L, divide by 169 for norepinephine and 183 for epinephrine.

cardia, dyspnea, concentration difficulty, and syncope. She had volatile blood pressure and heart rate during or following anesthesia with each of her three Caesarean sections. Standard treatment for syncope (β-blockers, compression stockings, fludrocortisone) had been unsatisfactory. Implantation of a dual-chamber pacemaker seemed to decrease the frequency of syncope, but symptoms of orthostatic intoler-

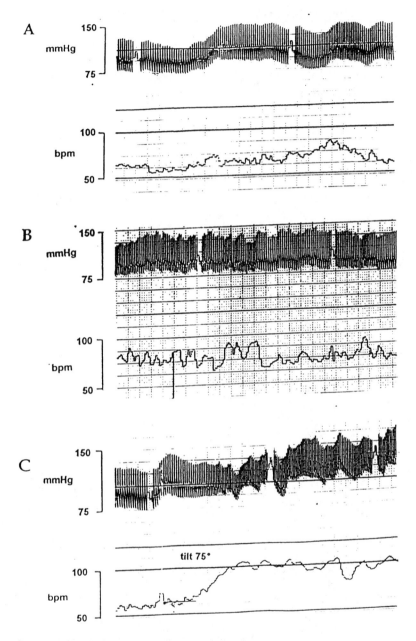

**FIGURE 2.** Beat-by-beat BP determinations by photoplethysmography (Finapres) and continuous HR recording illustrate spontaneous excursions of up to 50 mmHg and 25 bpm, respectively, in (**A**) the proband, and (**B**) her identical twin. (**C**) With tilt, BP, and HR volatility is intensified. In these tracings no external stimuli could be identified that were giving rise to the changes in BP and HR [other than the upright tile in (**C**)].

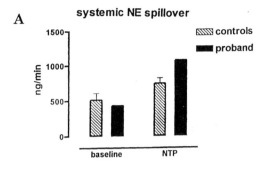

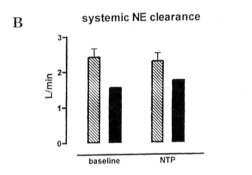

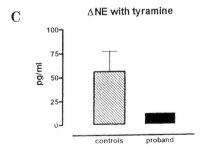

**FIGURE 3.** Systemic norepinephrine kinetics in the proband as compared to controls. It can be seen that after the stimulus of NTP, systemic norepinephrine spillover is enhanced in the proband as compared to controls in (**A**). In (**B**), it can be seen that in both the baseline state and after NTP, the proband has reduced systemic norepinephrine clearance. In (**C**), intravenous tyramine elicits less of an increase in plasma norepinephrine in the proband as compared to the controls, consistent with tyramine being unable to get access to its site of action in the neuronal terminal. Such access is by the norepinephrine transporter.

ance persisted. An echocardiogram revealed mild mitral regurgitation and possible mitral-valve prolapse. The proband's identical twin also had a history of mitral-valve prolapse and syncope as well as multiple symptoms worsened by stress and upright posture.

The proband and her twin were admitted to the General Clinical Research Center at Vanderbilt University Medical Center. They were placed on a caffeine-free, low monoamine diet containing 150 mEq $Na^+$ and 70 mEq $K^+$ per day for 3 days. All medications had been discontinued at least 2 weeks prior to admission. After fasting supine overnight, blood pressure, heart rate, and plasma catecholamines were measured supine and after standing. At least 2 h after breakfast, standard autonomic function testing was performed as previously described.[37] Urine was collected over a 24-h period for catecholamines and catecholamine metabolites. In the proband and a group of normal volunteers, systemic norepinephrine spillover and clearance and plasma norepinephrine concentrations were determined before and at the maximal blood pressure increase after an intravenous injection of 3 mg tyramine. Supine and upright blood pressure and heart rate, plasma catecholamines, norepinephrine spillover and clearance, and tyramine-mediated plasma catecholamine responses were compared to responses among subjects in a group of 10 normal volunteers (8 females, 2 males, $33 \pm 2$ years). In seven additional siblings and the proband's mother, blood pressure and heart rate were determined after 20 min supine and 5 min standing. Blood was obtained for determination of plasma catecholamines after 20 min supine and then after 30 min upright. In addition, blood was obtained from the proband, all nine of her siblings and her mother for DNA analysis.

## AUTONOMIC TESTING

Autonomic reflexes in both the proband and her twin were intact. The proband and twin had volatility of blood pressure and heart rate (FIG. 2). Supine and upright blood pressure, heart rate, and plasma catecholamines of the proband and her twin as compared to control subjects[38] are depicted in TABLE 2. The plasma levels of dihydroxyphenylglycol [DHPG, the intraneuronal monoamine oxidase (MAO) metabolite of norepinephrine][39] in the proband and her twin were low relative to the plasma level of norepinephrine. In normal controls, the supine DHPG/norepinephrine ratio was approximately 5:1, while in the proband and her twin the ratio was approximately 2:1. With standing, the ratios in normal controls averaged 3:1, while in the proband and twin they were 1:1. Urinary norepinephrine was elevated outside the normal range in both the proband and her twin.

## SYSTEMIC NOREPINEPHRINE SPILLOVER AND CLEARANCE

Arterial norepinephrine concentration at rest was slightly elevated in the proband compared to controls (280 pg/mL vs. $204 \pm 18$ pg/mL). This greater concentration was primarily due to decreased NE clearance since, despite a lower norepinephrine spillover rate in the proband (436 ng/min in the proband vs. $514 \pm 98$ ng/min in controls; FIG. 3A), norepinephrine clearance in the proband was less than half that of normal controls (1.56 vs. $2.42 \pm 0.25$ L/min; FIG. 3B). With nitroprusside (NTP) infusion, norepinephrine spillover increased to 1072 ng/min in the proband, but only 745 ± 75 ng/min in control subjects (FIG. 3A). Norepinephrine clearance did not change appreciably after NTP in either the proband (1.76 L/min) or the control group (2.31 ± 0.24 L/min) (FIG. 3B).

## IMPAIRED RESPONSE TO TYRAMINE

Tyramine is an indirectly acting amine that exerts its effect by releasing cytosolic norepinephrine. To cause norepinephrine release, tyramine must first be taken up into the neuron by NET.[40,41] Intravenous injection of 3 mg tyramine increased plasma norepinephrine by 56 ± 21 pg/mL in normal controls, but only 12 pg/mL in the proband (FIG. 3C).

## IDENTIFICATION OF A MISSENSE MUTATION (A457P) IN NET

The combination of low plasma DHPG/norepinephrine ratio, decreased plasma norepinephrine clearance, and blunted response to tyramine focused our attention on a potential defect in NET in the proband. The presence of a similar syndrome in her twin suggested a genetic origin. Direct sequence analysis of the human norepineph-rine transporter (hNET) gene (SLC6A2) in the proband revealed no divergence from previously published sequences in exons 1 through 8 and 10 through 15. In addition, all exonic boundaries preserved canonical gt/ag donor/acceptor sequences. Howev-er, two novel polymorphisms were identified within exon 9, one silent (c154a) and one missense (g237c) mutation. (The number in parenthesis refers to the location in the GenBank sequence for exon 9.) The proband was heterozygous for both the c154a and g237c polymorphisms. The g237c mutation resulted in a coding alteration of alanine to proline (A457P) within a highly conserved region of transmembrane

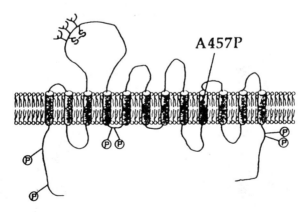

**FIGURE 4.** Location in NET of the A457P mutation. The structure of NET encompass-ing 12 membrane domains is shown. The arginine-to-proline mutation at amino acid 457 is shown in the 9th transmembrane domain.

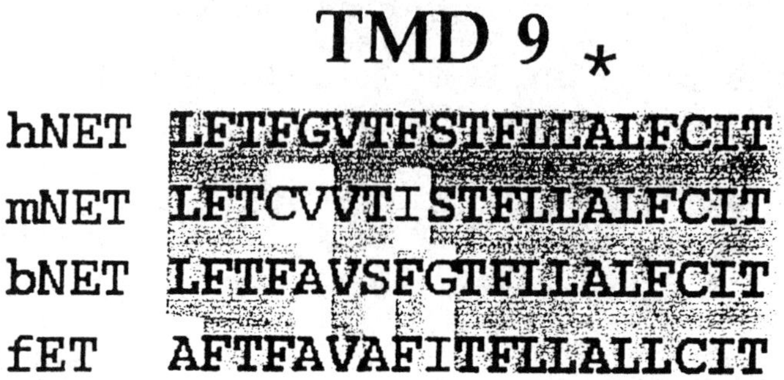

TMD 9
*
hNET LFTFGVTFSTFLLALFCIT
mNET LFTCVVTISTFLLALFCIT
bNET LFTFAVSFGTFLLALFCIT
fET AFTFAVAFITFLLALLCIT

**FIGURE 5.** The alanine at this site is highly conserved over several species. In TMD 9, an *asterisk* indicates the location of the alanine in the human (hNET), the mouse (mNET), the cow (bNet), and the frog (fNet).

domain (TMD) 9 (FIGS. 4 and 5). Alanine is present at this site in the transporter in other human subjects and in the cow, rat, mouse, and frog.

## THE A457P MUTATION RENDERS NET NONFUNCTIONAL

Heterologous expression of NET in parallel with NET A457P cDNAs revealed that [$^3$H]NE uptake is severely compromised by the A457P mutation. Chinese hamster ovary (CHO) cells transiently transfected with NET cDNA display a >10-fold elevation in norepinephrine transport activity over vector transfected cells. CHO cells transiently transfected with A457P NET cDNA possessed ≤2% of the uptake

NE uptake ($10^{-18}$ mol/ cell/ min)
0.30
0.25
0.20
0.15
0.10
0.05
0
wild type
A457P
control

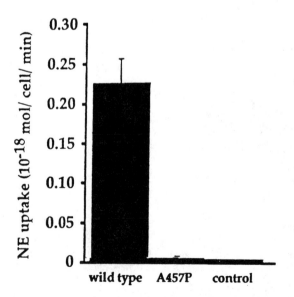

**FIGURE 6.** The A457P NET was essentially nonfunctional in CHO cells. These *in vitro* studies illustrate that norepinephrine is not taken up into cells with the mutated norepinephrine transporter, though it readily is taken up into cells with the wild-type transporter.

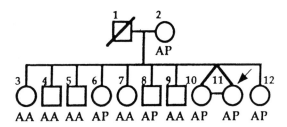

**FIGURE 7.** Among the siblings, 5 had the mutant A457P (P) allele and 5 were homologous for the wild type (A).

activity of the wild-type NET transfected cells (FIG. 6). Multiple clones were tested and all were found to be devoid of transport activity in a different cell host.

## SEGREGATION OF A457P MUTATION WITH PHENOTYPE

When genotyped by ASO, the proband's mother and 4 of her 8 siblings, including her twin (FIG. 7), were found to be heterozygous for the mutant allele (AP), whereas other family members were homozygous for the AA allele. Independently, we obtained heart rates and plasma catecholamines from the family. Supine heart rates displayed a trend toward elevation associated with the AP genotype ($p = ns$). However, upon standing, the heart rate was significantly greater in family members carrying the A457P mutation (AP) than in family members homozygous for the A457 genotype (AA) (FIG. 8). Similarly, supine plasma norepinephrine tended to be greater in AP than AA family members, whereas upright norepinephrine was significantly greater in AP individuals. Finally, the plasma DHPG/norepinephrine ratio was significantly greater in AA individuals than in AP individuals with both supine and upright postures (FIG. 8).

## SUMMARY OF CLINICAL EVIDENCE OF NET IMPAIRMENT

Bedside physiological, pharmacological, and biochemical tests in the proband indicated a defect in norepinephrine reuptake. Supine resting heart rate was within normal range, but about 10 bpm greater than age-matched controls,[42] and rose substantially with upright posture. This heart-rate change was paralleled by an increase in plasma norepinephrine, which rose almost fourfold with upright posture. Such changes could occur as a result of either an increase in release or a decrease in clearance of norepinephrine.[34,43] The proband's blunted plasma norepinephrine increase with tyramine, and her reduced systemic norepinephrine clearance compared to normal subjects were consistent with impaired norepinephrine reuptake as the primary deficit. The relationship of plasma DHPG and norepinephrine provided further evidence of impaired norepinephrine reuptake. Some NE taken up into the neuron by NET reaches the vesicles where it is stored for re-release, but much is converted

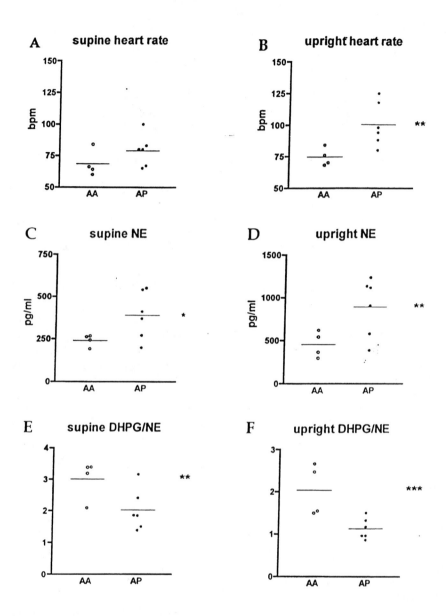

**FIGURE 8.** Orthostatic variables among family members with normal (AA) or mutant (AP) allele of NET. The heart rate changes were significantly higher in subjects with the A453 polymorphism (AP) vs. the wild type (AA) in the upright posture. Plasma norepinephrine was higher in family members with A453 as compared to the wild-type norepinephrine transporter. These catecholamine changes were particularly dramatic when the ratio of DHPG to norepinephrine was examined. DHPG is partially dependent upon norepinephrine uptake through the norepinephrine transporter, and lower than expected levels of DHPG were seen in family members with A457P.

to DHPG by MAO.[34] DHPG can then enter the circulation and serve as a marker of norepinephrine uptake and MAO activity.[39] The relatively low DHPG compared to norepinephrine in the plasma of the proband and her twin are consistent with impaired NET activity.

## CONTRIBUTION OF NET IMPAIRMENT TO OI CARDIOVASCULAR PATHOPHYSIOLOGY

NET deficiency could explain a number of clinical features in patients with OI. Elevated supine heart rate, elevated plasma norepinephrine associated with relatively decreased plasma DHPG, the reduced norepinephrine response to tyramine,[37] reduced systemic norepinephrine clearance,[37] and the disparity of the change in heart rate and plasma norepinephrine as compared to sympathetic nerve activity with upright posture[33] could all be attributed to impaired NET activity. In addition, we have observed that while many OI patients have a greater increase in diastolic blood pressure with upright posture than controls, their increase in heart rate is disproportionately greater.[37] This phenomenon may also be explained by NET deficiency. The noradrenergic synaptic clefts in the heart are approximately three times narrower than the synaptic clefts in the vasculature.[44] Therefore, removal of synaptic norepinephrine in the heart is far more dependent on NET than it is in vascular beds.[45] Thus, one would expect a disproportionate effect on heart rate and myocardial contractility as compared with blood pressure if NET were dysfunctional. That is precisely what is observed in patients with OI. It is also noteworthy that desmethylimipramine (DMI, desipramine), which blocks NET, elicits a similar hemodynamic profile when administered to patients in a comparable age group.[46] The drug raised supine blood pressure slightly, and increased supine and standing heart rate significantly. The upright blood pressure associated with this heart-rate increase was not different from placebo. These data were consistent with the concept that reduced NET function could elicit orthostatic tachycardia.

## COMPLEXITY INTRODUCED BY CNS EFFECTS OF NET IMPAIRMENT

The preceding features primarily represent manifestations of peripheral NET impairment. Central nervous system NET impairment is considerably more complicated. Noradrenergic and adrenergic neurons located at several sites in the central nervous system (e.g., the *nucleus tractus solitarii* [NTS] and the ventrolateral nuclei in the medulla) are involved in cardiovascular regulation. Increasing concentrations of norepinephrine, epinephrine, and their congeners in the NTS greatly reduce blood pressure and heart rate in the rat[47,48] by binding to $\alpha_2$-adrenoreceptors. In other areas, the opposite effect may by observed through activation of $\beta_2$-adrenoreceptors.[49] Agents that stimulate central $\alpha_2$-adrenoreceptors (e.g., clonidine and $\alpha$-methyldopa), and thus mimic increased central norepinephrine concentrations in sensitive areas, are widely used to reduce central sympathetic outflow. The prominent side effects of such agents include fatigue, a common complaint of patients with OI.[37] Acute pharmacological blockade by one DMI dosage regimen of NET caused a decrease in microneurographic sympathetic outflow,[50] presumably by increasing norepinephrine concentration in central synapses. Similarly, with central nervous system NET deficiency, one would expect a decrease in the indices of sympathetic tone. Yet, in the proband and in many patients with OI, central sympathetic tone does not appear to be suppressed under acute experimental conditions.[32,51] Thus chronic NET impairment, or perhaps compensatory (e.g., baroreflex) responses to it, may further complicate the phenotype. Peripheral and central impairment of NET could disrupt the fine control of autonomic balance. A limited capacity to clear synaptic norepinephrine might prolong the duration and increase the intensity of adrenoreceptor stimulation resulting from sympathetic nerve electrical activation. The supranormal and prolonged synaptic norepinephrine concentrations interacting with baroreflex-mediated withdrawal of sympathetic nerve traffic could coarsen blood-pressure and heart-rate patterns. This coarsening of sympathetic modulation could result in a spontaneous cycle of variability in heart rate and, to a lesser extent, vascular tone. Volatility of heart rate in patients with OI has been reported[57] and was evident in the proband.

## SUMMARY

The identification of NET deficiency[20] provides a pathophysiologic focus that potentially brings together the cardiac (mitral valve prolapse), autonomic, and central nervous system manifestations of OI that have heretofore eluded us. This discovery allows us to explore the systemic physiology of a mutation that may provide new insights into a range of disorders encompassing cardiovascular, psychiatric, and endocrinologic perturbations.

## ACKNOWLEDGMENT

This work was supported in part by NIH Grants M01 RR00095, 5P01 HL56693, 1U01NS33460, NASA Grant NAS 9-19483, and the Nathan Blaser Shy-Drager Research Program.

## REFERENCES

1. ROBERTSON, D. 1994. Genetics and molecular biology of hypotension. Curr. Opin. Neurol. **3:** 13–24.
2. BRADBURY, S. & C. EGGLESTON. 1924. Postural hypotension: a report of three cases. Am. Heart J. **1:** 73–86.
3. BRADBURY, S. & C. EGGLESTON. 1927. Postural hypotension: an autopsy upon a case. Am. Heart J. **3:** 105–106.
4. GHRIST, D.G. & G.E. BROWN. 1928. Postural hypotension with syncope: its successful treatment with ephedrine. Am. J. Med. Sci. **175:** 336–349.
5. ROBERTSON, D. Autonomic failure. 1995. *In* Handbook of the Autonomic Nervous System, A. Korczyn, Ed.: 129–148. Dekker. New York.
6. RIECKERT, H. 1982. Hypotone Dysregulation—eine deutsche Erkrankung? Münch Med. Wschr. **124:** 635–637.

7. KUNZE, M., B. GREDLER & K. STEINBACH. 1981. Hypotonie in Österreich: Ergebnisse einer Bevölkerungsbefragung. Wien. Med. Wschr. **131:** 253–256.
8. PEMBERTON, J. 1989 Does constitutional hypotension exist? Br. Med. J. **298:** 660–662.
9. BJURE, A. & H. LAURELL. 1927. Om abnorma statiska circulationsfenomen och därmed sammanhängande sjukliga symptom. Den arteriella orthostatiska anämin en försummad sjukdomsbild. Upsala Läkarförenings Förhandlingar **33:** 1–23.
10. STREETEN, D.H.P. 1987. Orthostatic Disorders of the Circulation: Mechanisms, Manifestations, and Treatment: 1–272. Plenum. New York.
11. STREETEN D.H.P. 1999. Orthostatic intolerance. A historical introduction to the pathophysiologic mechanisms. Am. J. Med. Sci. **317:** 78–87.
12. FOUAD, F.M., L. TADENA-THOME, *et al.* 1986. Idiopathic hypovolemia. Ann. Int. Med. **104:** 298–303.
13. ROBERTSON, D. 1999. The epidemic of orthostatic tachycardia and orthostatic intolerance. Am. J. Med. Sci. **7:** 75–77.
14. HOELDTKE, R.D. & K.M. DAVIS. 1991. The orthostatic tachycardia syndrome. J. Clin. Endocrinol. Metab. **73:** 132–139.
15. SCHONDORF, R. & P.A. LOW. 1993. Idiopathic postural tachycardia syndrome. Neurology **43:** 132–137.
16. ROSEN, S.G. & P. CRYER. 1982. Postural tachycardia syndrome: case report. Am. J. Med. **72:** 847–850.
17. FROHLICH, E.D., H.P. DUSTAN & I.P. PAGE. 1966. Hyperdynamic beta-adrenergic circulatory state. Arch. Intern. Med. **117:** 612–619.
18. JACOB, G. & I. BIAGGIONI. 1999. Idiopathic orthostatic intolerance and postural tachycardia syndromes. Am. J. Med. Sci. **317:** 88–101.
19. JACOB, G., F. COSTA, *et al.* 2000. The neuropathic postural tachycardia syndrome. N. Engl. J. Med. **343:** 1008–1014.
20. SHANNON, J.R., N.L. FLATTEM, *et al.* 2000. Orthostatic intolerance and tachycardia associated with norepinephrine-transporter deficiency. N. Engl. J. Med. **342:** 541–549.
21. SPRANGERS, R.L.H., K.H. WESSELING, *et al.* 1991. Initial blood pressure fall on standing up and exercise explained by changes in total peripheral resistance. Am. J. Physiol. **70:** 523–530.
22. MACLEAN, A.R., E.V. ALLEN & T.B. MAGATH. 1944. Orthostatic tachycardia and orthostatic hypotension: defects in the return of venous blood to the heart. Am. Heart J. **27:** 145–163.
23. FINE, M.J. & R. MILLER. 1940. Orthostatic paroxysmal auricular tachycardia with unusual response to change of posture. Am. Heart J. **20:** 366–373.
24. PETERS, M. & S.L. PENNER. 1946. Orthostatic paroxysmal ventricular tachycardia. Am. Heart J. **32:** 645–652.
25. KOSINSKI, D.J. & B.P. GRUBB. 1994. Neurally mediated syncope with an update on indications and usefullness of head-upright tilt table testing and pharmacologic therapy. Curr. Opin. Cardiol. **9:** 53–64.
26. KAUFMANN, H. 1995. Neurally-mediated syncope: pathogenesis diagnosis and treatment. Neurology **45:** 512–518.
27. STREETEN, D.H.P, L.P. KERR & C.B. KERR. 1972. Hyperbradykininism: a new orthostatic syndrome. Lancet **2:** 1048–1053.
28. EL-SAYED, H. & R. HAINSWORTH. 1995. Relationship between plasma volume, carotid baroreceptor sensitivity and orthostatic tolerance. Clin. Sci. **88:** 463–470.
29. CRYER, P.E., A.B. SILVERBERG, *et al.* 1978. Plasma catecholamines in diabetes. the syndromes of hypoadrenergic and hyperadrenergic postural hypotension. Am. J. Med. **64:** 407–416.
30. JORDAN, J., J.R. SHANNON, *et al.* 1998. Raised cerebrovascular resistance in idiopathic orthostatic intolerance: evidence for sympathetic vasoconstriction. Hypertension **32:** 699–704.

31. JACOB, G., D. ATKINSON, *et al.* 1999. Effects of standing on cerebrovascular resistance in patients with idiopathic orthostatic intolerance. Am. J. Med. **106:** 59–64.
32. NOVAK, V., J.M. SPIES, *et al.* 1998. Hypocapnia and cerebral hypoperfusion in orthostatic intolerance. Stroke **29:** 1876–1881.
33. FURLAN, R., G. JACOB, *et al.* 1998. Chronic orthostatic intolerance: a disorder with discordant cardiac and vascular sympathetic control. Circulation **98:** 2154–2159.
34. ESLER, M., G. JENNINGS, *et al.* 1990. Overflow of catecholamine neurotransmitters to the circulation: source, fate, and functions. Physiol. Rev. **70:** 963–985.
35. DESTEFANO, A.L., C.T. BALDWIN, *et al.* 1998. Autosomal dominant orthostatic hypotensive disorder maps to chromosome 18q. Am. J. Human Genet. **63:** 1425–1430
36. JORDAN, J., J.R. SHANNON, *et al.* 1999. Interaction of genetic predisposition and environmental factors in the pathogenesis of idiopathic orthostatic hypotension. Am. J. Med. Sci. **318:** 298–303.
37. MOSQUEDA-GARCIA, R. 1995. Evaluation of the autonomic nervous system. *In* Disorders of the Autonomic Nervous System, D. Robertson and I. Biaggioni, Eds.: 25–29. Harwood. London.
38. JACOB, G. & J.R. SHANNON. 1999. Abnormal norepinephrine clearance and adrenergic receptor sensitivity in idiopathic orthostatic intolerance. Circulation **99:** 1706–1712.
39. GOLDSTEIN, D.S., G. EISENHOFER, *et al.* 1988. Plasma dihydroxyphenylglycol and the intraneuronal disposition of norepinephrine in humans. J. Clin. Invest. **81:** 213–220.
40. BLAKELY, R.D., L.J. DE FELICE & H.C. HARTZELL. 1994. Molecular physiology of norepinephrine and serotonin transporters. J. Exp. Biol. **196:** 263–281.
41. DEMANET, J.C. 1976. Usefulness of noradrenaline and tyramine infusion tests in the diagnosis of orthostatic hypotension. Cardiology **61**(Suppl. 1): 213–224.
42. SHANNON, J.R., J. JORDAN, *et al.* 1998. Uncoupling of the baroreflex by $N_N$-cholingergic blockade in dissecting the components of cardiovascular regulation. Hypertension **32:** 101–107.
43. DAVIS, D., L.I. SINOWAY, *et al.* 1987. Norepinephrine kinetics during orthostatic stress in congestive heart failure. Circ. Res. **61:** I87–I90
44. NOVI, A.M. 1968. An electron microscopic study of the innervation of papillary muscles in the rat. Anat. Rec. **160:** 123–141.
45. GOLDSTEIN, D.S., J.E.J. BRUSH, *et al.* 1988. In vivo measurement of neuronal uptake of norepinephrine in the human heart. Circulation **78:** 41–48.
46. WALSH, B.T., C.M. HADIGAN & L.M. WONG. 1992. Increased pulse and blood pressure associated with desipramine treatment of bulimia nervosa. J. Clin. Psychopharmacol. **12:** 163–168.
47. GOLDBERG, M.R., C.S. TUNG, *et al.* 1982.. Evidence that alpha-methylepinephrine is an antihypertensive metabolite of alpha-methyldopa. Clin. Exp. Hypertens. Part A Theory Pract. **4:** 595–604.
48. TUNG, C.S., M.R. GOLDBERG, *et al.* 1983. Central and peripheral cardiovascular effects of alpha-methylepinephrine. J Pharm. Exp. Ther. **227:** 484–490.
49. ADLER-GRASCHINSKY, E. & S.Z. LANGER. 1975. Possible role of a beta-adrenoceptor in the regulation of noradrenaline release by nerve stimulation through a positive feedback mechanism. Br. J. Pharm. **53:** 43–50.
50. ESLER, M.D., G. WALLIN, *et al.* 1991. Effects of desipramine on sympathetic nerve firing and norepinephrine spillover to plasma in humans. Am. J. Physiol. **260:** R817–R823
51. SHANNON, J.R., J. JORDAN, *et al.* 1998. Sympathetic support of the circulation in idiopathic orthostatic intolerance (Abstr.). Circulation **98:** I-336.
52. LOW, P.A., T.L. OPFER-GEHRKING, *et al.* 1995. Postural tachycardia syndrome. Neurology **45:** 519–525.

53. POLINSKY, R.J., I.J. KOPIN, *et al.* 1981. Pharmacologic distinction of different orthostatic hypotension syndromes. Neurology **31:** 1–7.
54. KHURANA, R.K. 1995. Orthostatic intolerance and orthostatic tachycardia: a heterogeneous disorder. Clin. Auton. Res. **5:** 12–18.
55. BOUDOULAS, H., J.C. REYNOLDS, *et al.* 1980. Metabolic studies in mitral valve prolapse syndrome. Circulation **61:** 1200–1205.
56. GAFFNEY, F.A., E.S. KARLSSON, *et al.* 1979. Autonomic dysfunction in women with mitral valve prolapse syndrome. Circulation **59:** 894–901.
57. COGHLAN, H.C., P. PHARES, *et al.* 1979. Dysautonomia in mitral valve prolapse. Am. J. Med. **67:** 236–244.
58. FRASER, F. & R.M. WILSON. 1918. The sympathetic nervous system and the "irritable heart of soldiers." Br. Med. J. **2:** 27–32.
59. PEABODY, F., H. CLOUGH, *et al.* 1918. Effects of the injection of epinephrine in soldiers with "irritable heart." JAMA **71:** 1912–1919.
60. BOU-HOLAIGAH, I., P.C. ROWE, *et al.* 1995. The relationship between neurally mediated hypotension and the chronic fatigue syndrome. JAMA **274:** 961–967.

# Index of Contributors